Psychological Perspectives on Population

PSYCHOLOGICAL PERSPECTIVES ON POPULATION

EDITED BY

James T. Fawcett

BASIC BOOKS, INC.

PUBLISHERS

NEW YORK

© 1973 by Basic Books, Inc.
Library of Congress Catalog Card Number: 72–76920
SBN: 465–06673–9
Manufactured in the United States of America
DESIGNED BY VINCENT TORRE
73 74 75 76   10 9 8 7 6 5 4 3 2 1

FOREWORD

The joining of two scientific fields does not necessarily lead to better science. As Frank Lorimer has reminded us, "the marriage of demography and economics while both were immature—'Parson' Malthus officiating—resulted in a stormy and unfruitful union."[1] But such joinings, if they occur because the explanations of one discipline are experienced as inadequate and are therefore complemented by the explanations provided by a second discipline, may also constitute small-scale scientific revolutions.

The joining of psychology and demography is a case in point. Apart from rather unsatisfactory attempts (such as that of Malthus) to relate population growth to economic factors, the phenomena of births, deaths, and population increase were generally regarded as biological givens until the 1920s and 1930s. Then the sociological study of population phenomena began, and social structural variables came to be used extensively by demographers to explain both variations in fertility and trends in migration. The field sometimes called "social demography" thus arose alongside that of so-called "formal demography." It has only been since the 1960s, however, that more than a few psychologists have been interested and involved in population research. Now, in the early 1970s, the field of "psychology and population" seems to be quite firmly established.

As a result of this interest, a Task Force on Psychology, Family Planning, and Population Policy was established by the American Psychological Association in October 1969.[2] It has met frequently since then, and has stimulated both sessions at scientific meetings (the 1971 meetings of the APA had 12 sessions devoted to different aspects of the interrelation of psychology and population) and a number of research projects.

James T. Fawcett has been a member of the APA Task Force and is a major leader of this movement in psychology. His systematic review of the literature, *Psychology and Population*,[3] is the starting point for any serious

[1] Frank Lorimer, "General Survey," in *The University Teaching of Sciences: Demography*, ed. David V. Glass (Paris: UNESCO, 1957), p. 21. I am indebted to Dudley Kirk for calling this statement to my attention.

[2] APA Task Force on Psychology, Family Planning, and Population Policy, "Population and Family Planning: Growing Involvement of Psychologists," *American Psychologist*, 27, no. 1 (January 1972): pp. 27–30.

[3] James T. Fawcett, *Psychology & Population: Behavioral Research Issues in Fertility and Family Planning* (New York: The Population Council, 1970).

work in the field. By appreciating the need for the present volume, by planning its contents, by persuading so many highly-qualified psychologists to take the time to prepare these articles, and by his intelligent editing, Fawcett has contributed greatly to the field.

The contributions of psychology to population have many facets: witness the diverse contributions found between the covers of this book. In Chapter 2, for example, the Hoffmans present a new and important perspective on the value of children to parents, as one of the determinants of family size. In other chapters topics seldom dealt with systematically in the population literature are focused upon, such as the consequences of family size and population density (Chapters 7 and 8) and subjective reactions to particular methods of birth control (Chapters 9, 10, and 11). For many topics, the chapters of this book are as important for pointing out what is *not* known as for reviewing and synthesizing what can be learned from research.

This collaboration between psychology and population is part of a broader intellectual phenomenon: an awakening interest in population on the part of many other disciplines. Stimulated by the urgency of "the population problem," legal scholars, anthropologists, geographers, economists, and political scientists have joined sociologists and statisticians in the study of population. One finds articles dealing with population problems in other than sociological or demographic publications; conferences based on the theme of "population and _____" are a common occurrence; and applications to foundations and government agencies for fellowships and for research in population come from many directions.

From the point of view of psychology, *Psychological Perspectives on Population* is a major contribution toward an expansion of the traditional range of psychological interest and research. From the point of view of demography, Fawcett and his contributors have pointed in the direction of some solutions to old problems. And since a central problem of the social sciences is the relationship of the individual to society, since psychology and demography are the major disciplines that are more or less at the ends of the individual–society continuum, and since bearing children is a private act that is determined both in its timing and in its frequency by a host of social influences, the book may ultimately be judged not only as an instance of the application of psychology to an understanding of a social problem, but also as a contribution toward our understanding of social man.

David L. Sills

New York, N.Y.
1972

PREFACE

The articles collected in this book pertain to an area of study that has come to prominence so recently that it has yet to be adequately labeled, although the title "population psychology" seems to be gaining acceptance. That is perhaps as good a label as any for an area that actually represents the intersection between two traditional academic disciplines. The substantive topics for the area of population psychology come mainly from the field of demography or population studies, while the theoretical, conceptual, and methodological approaches to those topics come mainly from psychology. Publications such as this book should provide some markers around which a more specific definition of population psychology eventually will evolve.

Fertility and family planning provide the main themes for the book, since those are the topics to which psychologists have been most attracted. Attention is given to both determinants and consequences, at the psychological level, of fertility and family planning. What is meant by "the psychological level" is that the focus tends to be on the individual, or the individual within a small group, such as the family, rather than on a larger social aggregate, such as a group defined by economic or sociological characteristics. It is that orientation toward the behaviors and traits of individuals that distinguishes this book from most other writings in the population field. In some chapters, particularly those with a more theoretical orientation, an attempt is made to integrate the psychological with the socio-demographic levels of conceptualization and analysis.

In addition to the fertility and family-planning themes, some attention is given to urbanization, in terms of the consequences of population density. Migration is not treated at all, a regrettable lack that perhaps will be remedied by future work in population psychology.

Each chapter is intended to stand by itself as a comprehensive review of a topic or an approach to a topic. Not all chapters achieve that breadth of coverage, but such was the aim in the design of this book. The headings under which chapters are collected in Parts I–VII provide some coherence to the collection as a whole.

Since this is a "state of the art" report for a field still in its infancy, particular attention is given to questions about the kind of research that is needed in population psychology and how it can be done. The substantive conclusions that can be drawn from the material in the book are probably of lesser significance than the guidance that is offered for future work.

All of the chapters were specially prepared for this book under the sponsorship of The Population Council. I am grateful for that sponsorship and want to express special thanks to David Sills, Director of the Demographic Division of The Population Council, for his encouragement and good advice.

The preparation of this volume was facilitated by the activities of the American Psychological Association Task Force on Psychology, Family Planning, and Population Policy. It was through my connection with the Task Force that I came in contact with a number of the contributors to this book, and the efforts of the Task Force to heighten awareness of population issues among psychologists gave added impetus to the project.

The East-West Population Institute, with which I am currently affiliated, has provided important support in the later stages of preparation of this book.

I am, of course, especially grateful to the contributors, many of whom put aside other important work in order to prepare a chapter for this volume. The idea for this book sparked a great deal of enthusiasm, and I believe I can speak for the authors in expressing the hope that the contents will be of benefit both to psychologists who are interested in population issues and to population specialists who want to know about the perspectives offered by psychology.

JAMES T. FAWCETT

Honolulu, Hawaii
1972

THE AUTHORS

MARK APPELBAUM is Assistant Professor of Psychology and Associate Dean for Experimental and Special Studies at the University of North Carolina at Chapel Hill. Holding a B.S. in chemistry from Carnegie Institute of Technology and a Ph.D. in quantitative psychology from the University of Illinois, he was a post-doctoral fellow in the L. L. Thurstone Psychometric Laboratory at North Carolina prior to joining the faculty there. In 1970 he won the Standard Oil Foundation (Indiana) prize for distinguished undergraduate teaching.

KURT W. BACK is Professor of Sociology and Psychiatry at Duke University. He has previously served at the University of North Carolina, University of Puerto Rico, and the Bureau of Applied Social Research at Columbia, as well as at the Bureau of the Census and as part-time consultant with the Conservation Foundation. He received his Ph.D. in group psychology at the Research Center of Group Dynamics at M.I.T. He is author and co-author of numerous articles and several books, among them, *The Family and Population Control*, *The Control of Human Fertility in Jamaica*, *The Survey Under Unusual Conditions*, and *Slums, Projects and People*.

JUDITH M. BARDWICK is Associate Professor of Psychology at the University of Michigan. She earned a B.S. at Purdue University, an M.S. at Cornell University, and a Ph.D. at the University of Michigan. She has worked in the area of the psychology of women with particular research interest in relationships between psychological variables and reproductive physiology. She is a co-author of *Feminine Personality and Conflict*, author of *Psychology of Women*, and editor of *Readings in the Psychology of Women*.

MARC BORNSTEIN is a doctoral candidate in psychology at Yale University. He holds a B.A. in psychology from Columbia College. In 1970 he was awarded a Summer Internship for work at the Population Council. At Yale, he has done research in population studies, cognitive development, and visual psychophysics.

YVONNE BRACKBILL is Professor of Obstetrics and Gynecology and Pediatrics for Psychology, Georgetown University School of Medicine. She holds a B.A. from the University of California, an M.A. from the University of Colorado, and a Ph.D. from Stanford University. Her previous affiliations include San Jose State College, Johns Hopkins University, University of Denver, and University of Colorado. She is the author of numerous articles in professional journals, mainly in the area of child development, and she has co-authored or edited several books, including *Infancy and Early Childhood: A Handbook and Guide to Human Development*.

GEORGE P. CERNADA is the Resident Advisor for Taiwan for The Population Council. He holds a B.S. from Boston College and an M.P.H. from the School of Public Health of the University of California, where he was advanced to doctoral candidacy in 1971. He has worked closely with Asian family-planning programs since 1965. He recently edited and co-authored the volume, *Taiwan Family Planning Reader*, and has written numerous articles on family planning programs, particularly evaluation and communications aspects.

CATHERINE CHILMAN is Professor of Social Research and Director, Research Center, School of Social Welfare, University of Wisconsin, Milwaukee. She holds a B.A. from Oberlin College, an M.A. from the University of Chicago, and a Ph.D. in psychology from Syracuse University, where she also taught. A staff member of the U.S. Department of Health, Education, and Welfare for nine years, she directed a research and development unit concerned with social-welfare policy. Recently, she has been Curriculum Coordinator of a University of Michigan project for the training of social-work faculty from the developing countries in population and family planning. Author of many articles in professional journals and books and of *Growing Up Poor*, she has been a consultant to numerous federal agencies and has served on the boards of the *Journal of Marriage and the Family*, the National Council on Family Relations, the National Conference on Social Welfare, and SIECUS (Sex Information and Education Council of the United States).

JOHN A. CLAUSEN is Professor of Sociology and Research Sociologist at the Institute of Human Development, University of California, Berkeley. His B.A. and M.A. degrees were received from Cornell University and the Ph.D. from the University of Chicago. He has served as Chief of the Laboratory of Socioenvironmental Studies of the National Institute of Mental Health and as Director of the Institute of Human Development at Berkeley. His principal research and writing have been on the sociology of mental health and on the effects of social structure upon socialization through the course of life.

SUZANNE R. CLAUSEN has in recent years engaged in editorial work and translation as well as touring in both England and France. Her earlier research on the family entailed intensive participant observation as the mother of four sons. She received her B.A. from Cornell University and, more recently, an M.A. in French from the University of California at Berkeley.

THOMAS J. CRAWFORD is Assistant Professor of Psychology at the University of California at Berkeley. He holds a Ph.D. from Harvard University and taught at the University of Chicago before joining the Berkeley faculty. His research interests involve applications of models of attitude organization and change to social problems. His publications have dealt with topics in family planning, race relations, and experimental social psychology.

HENRY P. DAVID is Director of the AIR/Transnational Family Research Institute, Associate Professor in the Department of Psychiatry at the University of Maryland Medical School, and Research Adviser to Preterm Institute in Washington, D.C. He received his Ph.D. in clinical psychology from Columbia University, served for two years as Associate Director of the World Federation for Mental Health in Geneva, Switzerland, is the current Chairman of the American Psychological Association Task Force on Psychology and Family Planning, and is involved in the Cooperative Transnational Research Program in Fertility Behavior. His more than 100 publications include *Family Planning and Abortion in the Socialist Countries of Central and Eastern Europe* and *Child Mental Health in International Perspective*.

JAMES T. FAWCETT is Assistant Director of the East-West Population Institute and Associate Professor of Psychology at the University of Hawaii. He holds a B.S. from Pennsylvania State University, an M.S. from Yale University, and a Ph.D. from the University of California at Berkeley, all in psychology. He was associated with The Population Council for a number of years, including four years spent in Thailand, and has been a Visiting Scholar at the

University of Michigan. He is the author of *Psychology and Population: Behavioral Research Issues in Fertility and Family Planning.*

JONATHAN L. FREEDMAN is Professor of Psychology at Columbia University. He received his B.A. from Harvard University and M.S. and Ph.D. degrees from Yale University, then taught at Stanford before coming to Columbia. He is currently doing research on the effects of crowding on humans as well as on the determinants of compliance and mechanisms of long-term memory. His publications include *Deviancy* with Anthony Doob, a textbook, *Social Psychology* with Merrill Carlsmith and David Sears, and numerous articles. He is an associate editor of the *Journal of Experimental Social Psychology* and is on the boards of several other publications.

E. I. GEORGE is Dean, Faculty of Arts, and Professor and Chairman, Department of Psychology, University of Kerala, India. His Ph.D. is from London University and he is an Associate of the British Psychological Society. Currently he is President of the Indian Academy of Applied Psychology and is a member of the editorial board of the *Journal of Psychological Researches, Indian Journal of Experimental Psychology,* and *Journal of Applied Psychology.* His fields of special interest are clinical psychology, personality, social psychology, and population studies, and he has numerous publications in these areas. He is associated with several universities in India and is a member of the Expert Panel in Social Sciences of the University Grants Commission, New Delhi.

HARRISON G. GOUGH is Professor of Psychology and Chairman of the Department of Psychology at the University of California, Berkeley, and is also a research psychologist at the University's Institute of Personality Assessment and Research. His B.A., M.A., and Ph.D. degrees were taken at the University of Minnesota. In 1958–1959 he conducted cross-cultural studies in Italy on a Fulbright grant and extended this work in 1965–1966 in Rome under the Fulbright and Guggenheim awards. He has contributed extensively to the literature on personality testing and assessment and is the author of several well-known tests including the *Adjective Check List* and the *California Psychological Inventory.*

PAULA H. HASS is Assistant Professor of Sociology at Queens College of the City University of New York. She received her B.A. from Cornell University and her M.A. and Ph.D. degrees from Duke University. Dr. Hass previously served as Lecturer in Sociology at Duke University and Staff Researcher at the United Nations Population Division. Her empirical work has focused on female employment, fertility, and Latin-American demography.

LOIS WLADIS HOFFMAN is an Associate Professor at the University of Michigan with a joint appointment in the Department of Psychology and the Department of Population Planning. She holds a B.A. degree from the State University of New York at Buffalo, an M.S. from Purdue University, and a Ph.D. from the University of Michigan. She was a Research Associate at the Institute for Social Research, University of Michigan, for six years and has been on the faculty of the Psychology Department for five years. She has co-edited the *Review of Child Development Research,* Volumes I and II, co-authored *The Employed Mother in America,* and published articles on women's roles, the motivations for fertility, and the psychological development of the child.

MARTIN L. HOFFMAN is Professor of Psychology, University of Michigan, Ann Arbor. His B.S. degree is from Purdue University and his M.S. and Ph.D. are from the University of Michigan. He taught and did clinical work at Purdue University for four years and worked as Senior Research Associate at

the Merrill-Palmer Institute for twelve years before joining the University of
Michigan. He was chairman of the Doctoral Program in Developmental Psychology at Michigan for five years and co-editor of *Review of Child Development Research*, Volumes I and II. He now edits the *Merrill-Palmer Quarterly
of Behavior and Development*. He has written extensively on the effects of
childbearing practices on the child's social and moral development.

JOHN GRENVILLE HOLMES is Assistant Professor of Psychology at the University of
Waterloo. He was awarded his B.A. at Carleton University, Ottawa, and his
Ph.D. at the University of North Carolina at Chapel Hill. His previous appointment was at York University, Toronto, before joining the Waterloo
faculty. He is the past editor of *Representative Research in Social Psychology* and is engaged in research on group dynamics and the effects of
group membership on attitudes. His interests in population studies have
centered on group influence on family-size attitudes and husband-wife decision-making.

ANDIE L. KNUTSON is Professor of Behavioral Sciences in the School of Public
Health and Research Behavioral Scientist in the Institute of Human Development at the University of California, Berkeley. Professor Knutson is a
graduate of the University of Minnesota and received his M.A. and Ph.D. in
social psychology from Princeton University. Government appointments include chief of behavioral studies with the U.S. Public Health Service. He
holds Fellowships in the American Public Health Association, the American
Psychological Association, and the American Sociological Association. He is
the author of *The Individual, Society, and Health Behavior*.

SHIRLEY B. POFFENBERGER is a Research Associate in the Department of Population Planning, University of Michigan. She holds a B.A. in English from
the University of Colorado and an M.A. in Sociology from Michigan State
University. Her professional background includes a variety of teaching and
research experiences from nursery school to university level in the United
States and India. She and her husband, Thomas Poffenberger, first became
interested in the problems of pregnancy in 1948, when they both began to
publish research articles on that topic. Her other studies and publications
have related to child-rearing practices, social change, and communication.

THOMAS POFFENBERGER is Professor of Population Planning at the University of
Michigan. His B.A. in psychology, M.A. in sociology and Ed.D. in counseling
psychology were from Michigan State University. He was Associate Profes-
sor of Family Sociology at the University of California at Davis before spending seven years in India as Visiting Professor at Baroda University and as
consultant for the Ford Foundation with the Indian family-planning program.
He has also served as a consultant in Korea, Malaysia, Nepal, and Guatemala.
In 1968–1969 he was Senior Specialist at the Institute of Advanced Projects,
East-West Center, University of Hawaii. He has been Associate Editor of the
Journal of Marriage and Family Living and has published research articles
in the areas of developmental psychology, family sociology, and communication, motivation, and social change as they relate to fertility attitudes and
behavior.

EDWARD POHLMAN is Professor of Counseling Psychology at the University of the
Pacific. His Ph.D. is from Ohio State University. He was Visiting Professor at
the Central Family Planning Institute in Delhi in 1967–1969. Dr. Pohlman
has written or edited eight books and monographs, in print or in press,
including *The Psychology of Birth Planning*.

DAVID A. RODGERS is Head of the Section of Psychology and Research of the
Department of Psychiatry at the Cleveland Clinic Foundation. He holds a

B.S. degree in chemical engineering from the University of Oklahoma and a Ph.D. in psychology from the University of Chicago. Dr. Rodgers was on the faculty at the University of California at Berkeley for five years, studied at the Brain Research Institute of UCLA for a year, and was Head of the Medical Psychology Section of Scripps Clinic and Research Foundation in La Jolla, California, before coming to the Cleveland Clinic. He has published extensively on alcohol preference (primarily of mice), psycho-social effects of contraceptive procedures, and other matters that might be considered off-shoots of social role theory and clinical concerns.

NANCY F. RUSSO is Assistant Professor of Psychology at Richmond College of the City University of New York. Holding a Ph.D. in Social Psychology from Cornell University, she received her B.A. with highest honors from the University of California at Davis. She has taught at American University and held a position as Associate Research Scientist at The American Institutes for Research. Her major research interests are in the attitudes and behaviors of young people with respect to population, methods of birth limitation, and sex-role socialization.

M. BREWSTER SMITH is Professor of Psychology and Vice Chancellor for Social Sciences at the University of California, Santa Cruz. With a Stanford B.A. and M.A. and a Harvard Ph.D., he has taught at Harvard, Vassar, New York University, the University of California at Berkeley (where he was Director of the Institute of Human Development), and the University of Chicago (where he was chairman of the Psychology Department). He is author of *Social Psychology and Human Values* and co-author of *The American Soldier* and *Opinions and Personality*. He is a past president of the Society for the Psychological Study of Social Issues, and was Vice President of the Joint Commission on Mental Illness and Health.

VAIDA D. THOMPSON is Assistant Professor of Psychology at the University of North Carolina; she is also a Research Associate at the Carolina Population Center and is currently Acting Deputy Director of Academic Affairs at the Center. Professor Thompson's B.S. and M.A. degrees are from Florida State University; her Ph.D. is from the University of North Carolina. As a member of the American Psychological Association's Task Force on Psychology, Family Planning, and Population Policy, she has focused on the need for the training of psychologists in population. At her own institution, she has taught courses on psychology and population on all levels and is now chairman of a departmental committee which is establishing a graduate minor in population. Her work at Carolina Population Center has involved the development of interdisciplinary seminars on the graduate level and plans for undergraduate and graduate interdisciplinary programs which will include psychology. Her principal population research pertains to social psychological issues in population.

FREDERICK J. ZIEGLER is Director of the Mental Health Center of the Community Hospital of the Monterey Peninsula in Carmel, California. His M.D. is from Johns Hopkins University and his psychiatry residency was at the Johns Hopkins Hospital. He has been Psychiatrist-in-Charge of the Private Patient Clinic of the Johns Hopkins Hospital, Head of the Division of Psychiatry, Psychology and Neurology at the Scripps Clinic and Research Foundation in La Jolla, California, and Director of the Family Studies Program of the Cleveland Clinic Foundation. His publications have been primarily concerned with various aspects of hysterical conversion-reaction patients and psycho-social considerations involved in vasectomy and ovulation suppressor contraception.

CONTENTS

PART I

Psychological Perspectives on Fertility

PART II

The Social Context: Two Countries

PART III

Consequences of Family Size and Population Density

PART IV

Research on Methods of Birth Control

PART V

Some Measurement Issues in Fertility

PART VI

Research Related to Social Action Programs

PART VII

Training for Psychological Aspects of Population

PART I

Psychological Perspectives on Fertility

[1]

A SOCIAL-PSYCHOLOGICAL
VIEW OF FERTILITY

M. BREWSTER SMITH

In spite of the analytic fact that "the fertility of a population can be viewed as a resultant of many individual acts and decisions, made within a framework of biological and environmental constraints" (Smith, 1965, p. 70), it has not been very profitably so viewed heretofore. Fertility has remained almost unassailed a supra-individual *social* fact in the Durkheimian sense, a social rate with social correlates that graciously yields to demographic analysis but stands mute and enigmatic in the face of psychological scrutiny.

Demographic analysis of census data has become ever more sophisticated, as techniques have been developed to disentangle how particular age cohorts contribute to the fertility of populations and to describe and project the age structure of populations through time. With increased technical competence has come attendant conceptual sophistication about the potentialities of cohort analysis for the study of social change (Ryder, 1965). Structured interviews of well-defined population samples have served to supplement the census and to illuminate relationships that elude it, documenting the spread of contraceptive knowledge and use throughout American society, the narrowing of fertility differentials associated with socioeconomic status, and the persistence of religious and ethnic fertility differentials.

Typically such studies have found that when women of childbearing age are asked what they think is the ideal family size, their answers are adequately predictive of subsequent cohort fertility—but most inadequately predictive at the individual level, a severe handicap for psychological analysis. The most diligent attempt to discover psychological determinants of differential fertility—the so-called Princeton study (Westoff et al., 1961, 1963)—drew a blank, perhaps because ideal family size was used as the dependent variable and because the psychological instruments were admittedly weak. (Fawcett [1970] briefly reviews the major studies in this tradition; Hawthorn [1970] reviews the literature on fertility from a sociological perspective and also provides a good annotated bibliography.) A good deal can be said about the consequences for fertility of social status, social mobility, family structure, religious affiliation, and rural-urban residence, and about gross contrasts in fertility between the industrialized countries and the rest of the world. Since it is individual men and women, not cohorts or social strata, who have babies, these social facts should have their psychological counterparts, and a sound psychological perspective on fertility should be an essential component in developing social strategies to bring the growth of population under control. Unfortunately, little that is well established can be said from the psychological standpoint.

For psychologists this unsatisfactory state of affairs should pose an irresistible challenge, given substantial variance in fertility left unaccounted for by demographic methods and also given the plausible conjecture that at least substantial components of the variance that *is* accounted for demographically should be traceable in principle to mediating processes and dispositions at the individual level. Yet until very recently few psychologists have risen to the challenge; it is fervently hoped that many others will join in. The stakes are too high for us to accept the negative answer easily, especially when neither our theories nor our methods of measurement are in good enough order to make null results interesting or persuasive.

My part in the common endeavor is that of *amicus curiae*, not that of active investigator, so an even more modest stance befits me than the unsatisfactory research situation itself requires. In sketching some aspects of a social-psychological view of fertility, my aim will be to piece together scaffolding within which questions can be posed for research, rather than to present well-developed hypotheses ripe for empirical test. If the venture is worthwhile, it will be because the psychological variables that were previously lying to hand may not have been the right ones, and some of the more obvious questions from a psychological point of view remain to be pursued with proper diligence, or even to be asked. I will argue that much descriptive work at the psychological level needs to be done before fancier theorizing and hypothesis-testing are warranted.

My task is made more difficult by the disorder of contemporary social psychology, a border area claimed by both psychology and sociology in which a congeries of perspectives, concepts, and partial theories compete with one another without synthesis, and in which there is disagreement about methods and data. *The* social-psychological perspective cannot be represented consensually. In contrast with sociodemographic approaches, however, a social-psychological approach implies attention to individual behavior viewed as an interactive product of personal dispositions and situational properties, the former seen as the developmental resultant of previous interactions.

A focus at the individual level does not coincide with a psychological approach, of course; physiological and sociocultural factors affecting the events from conception to parturition can also be examined as they bear upon the individual. Two very generally relevant accounting schemes at the individual level provide a framework for the analysis of psychological and other factors affecting fertility: the reproductive causal sequence and the life cycle. It will be well to note them both at the outset.

As for the former, Davis and Blake (1956) point out that fertility change can be partitioned exhaustively among intercourse variables, conception variables, and gestation variables. Each step in the causal chain is the locus of nonpsychological influences; it is also at least potentially influenced by such psychological factors as motives, attitudes, habits, intentions, and decisions. Such an abstract analytical scheme does not tell us how the terms of fertility-relevant action are defined for the behaving individual: thus until the recent surprisingly radical shift in law and mores about abortion, gestation was a purely biological matter beyond the range of attitude and decision for many middle-class Americans. But the scheme reminds the psychologist to keep his search for the impact of psychological factors properly differentiated.

The relevance of the life cycle with its biologically and socially defined markers of puberty, adolescence, maturity, marriage, sequential childbearing, and middle age is as obvious to psychologists as it is to demographers. I note it here because it is well to be reminded that the psychological mediation of factors affecting fertility may differ systematically along the way as man and woman move through the cycle, and because the timing with which people move through the cycle (age of marriage, age of first child, for example) is one of the important determinants of fertility for which psychological mediation may be sought.

"The Tragedy of the Commons": Focal Problem for Policy and Research

In a now classic statement Garrett Hardin (1968) posed the problem of fertility control in a form that engages productively with social-psychological thinking. His parable of the commons dramatizes a structural feature that uncontrolled population growth shares with an interrelated parcel of contemporary social dilemmas, all of which hinge on the pressures that people are now bringing against an environment of limited resources as we reap the consequences of the passing of all mundane frontiers. Hardin writes:

The tragedy of the commons develops in this way. Picture a pasture open to all. It is to be expected that each herdsman will try to keep as many cattle as possible on the commons. Such an arrangement may work reasonably satisfactorily for centuries because tribal wars, poaching, and disease keep the numbers of both man and beast well below the "carrying capacity" of the land.

Finally, however, comes the day of reckoning, i.e., the day when the long-desired social stability becomes a reality. At this point, the inherent logic of the commons remorselessly generates tragedy.

As a rational being each herdsman seeks to maximize his gain. Explicitly or implicitly, more or less consciously, he asks: "What is the utility *to me* of adding one more animal to my herd?" This utility has two components:

1. A positive component, which is a function of the increment of one animal. Since the herdsman receives all the proceeds from the sale of the additional animal, the positive utility is nearly $+1$.
2. A negative component, which is a function of the additional overgrazing created by one more animal. But since the effects of overgrazing are shared by all the herdsmen, the negative utility for any particular decision-making herdsman is only a fraction of -1.

Adding together the component partial utilities, the rational herdsman concludes that the only sensible course for him to pursue is to add another animal to his herd. And another; and another. . . . But this is the conclusion reached by each and every rational herdsman sharing a commons. Therein is the tragedy. Each man is *locked in* to a system that compels him to increase his herd without limit—in a world that is limited. Ruin is the destination toward which all men rush, each pursuing his own best interest in a society that believes in the freedom of the commons. *Freedom in a commons brings ruin to all.* [P. 1244]

Just as the private utility to an individual of adding one additional car to the freeway exceeds his private share in the public disutility of ever more tangled traffic, just as the private gain from discharging pollution in the air or waters (also a commons) exceeds the private component of the shared cost of a deteriorating environment when this cost is treated as an "externality," so his share in the cost to all of a world clogged with people cannot balance the private gains to the behaving individual who wants more children (and people the world over presently want more children than are required for a stable population under existing conditions of health and mortality).

Hardin thus argues that the population crisis belongs to a class of problems for which there is no *technical* solution, in the sense of a solution that in principle is within the reach of science and technology. What is required, rather, is a political solution: "mutual coercion, mutually agreed upon," in Hardin's rendition of the Hobbesian social contract.

In a provocative and deeply pessimistic rejoinder the political scientist Crowe (1969) accepts Hardin's statement of the problem, but rejects as no longer feasible his conclusions for social policy. (He also chides Hardin for asserting what he says is a truism among social scientists: small matter, when so many social scientists still fail to see the structure of the problem as clearly.) In an increasingly "tribalized" world in which societies are fragmented into mutually alienated groups that diverge in ultimate values rather than in negotiable interests, how shall the social contract for political regulation be drawn? Matters are even more grim, says Crowe, because at the same time that the myth of value consensus has lost its force, the myth that the state holds a monopoly of coercive power has likewise been punctured by irreconcilable dissidents. If the population dilemma belongs to the class of problems that lack a technical solution, Crowe argues, these same problems now appear beyond the reach of political solution as well. Man's tragic predicament is deeper than Hardin supposed.

A temperamentally more sanguine and historically more sophisticated observer of the imperfections of modern government might take a less apocalyptic view than Crowe leaves us. But when ideological leaders of the black poor cry "genocide" at proposals for mild and voluntaristic programs of family planning, it should be easy to see what he is talking about. And one can hardly gainsay his complaint that little can be hoped for so long as scientists and technologists dump their insoluble problems on politics, while social scientists and politicians look to science and technology for magical solutions to the problems that *they* cannot solve—especially when precisely the same "insoluble" problems are at issue. We are in it together and had better cooperate.

Note, however, that when Hardin and Crowe write about problems that in principle lack a technical solution, they are talking about "hard" science and technology, and when Crowe writes about the lack of a political solution, he has in mind latter-day American politics. If we and our successors as American and world citizens are to grapple effectively with the potentially tragic problems—there is, of course, no guarantee that we will succeed— we cannot afford to accept either of these "givens."

The sense of impending catastrophe being promulgated by the apocalyptic writers and finding an appreciative audience in many of the younger generation may, after all, presage adaptive transformations in our political processes and institutions: faith in "business as usual" is waning. Facing the same ominous data, a more optimistic writer like Platt (1966) can envision the possibility that we stand on the threshold of "the step to Man"; human life may shift to a new and more desirable level if we can only manage to navigate these treacherous waters.

As for the first "given," the conception of science and technology surely must be broadened to include the social sciences, psychology among them. Hard science and politics-as-usual are not enough. And among the social sciences, the population problem is too important to be left to the demographers. As yet we have hardly begun the attempt to see if psychology and the social sciences can contribute to a solution that necessarily must have both technical and political ingredients.

If we follow Hardin, then the incentives governing individual decisions about procreation produce actions that now cumulate to the disadvantage of all—this is the motivational structure of the population problem. In the sphere of fertility the "Unseen Hand" that Adam Smith imagined as guiding individually self-interested economic actions so that they cumulate to the common good is clearly not working, any more than it works in the other spheres that govern man's ecological balance or in the economy as such. The pragmatic problem that we face is thus how to restructure the "dilemma of the commons" so that individual decisions can dependably cumulate to social advantage, so that net growth in population is brought to a halt. Insofar as decisional processes are involved, an engineering of incentives and constraints would seem to be called for, in which deliberate social policy replaces the mythical "Unseen Hand."

Of course, there are immense difficulties in the way of achieving an effective national population policy, let alone the effective international one that the facts require. These barriers also hinder the development of effective policy regarding any of the many matters that require comprehensive, long-term planning and implementation if the common good is to be advanced. Wildavsky (1964) is only one among many who have recently told us that the budgetary context of governmental decision-making enforces an incremental responsiveness to short-term pinches of the shoe that is the antithesis of comprehensive and effective policy. But these difficulties surely cannot excuse our giving up the attempt to design social policy on the basis of improved causal understanding before the attempt is fairly begun. The recent rapid shift in national attention to issues of population and ecology should give us heart.

The decision-making framework in which Hardin presents the dilemma of the commons fits very well with thoughtways now prevalent among social psychologists. Indeed, a number of psychologists have worked with formal models of decision-making; this approach has been reviewed by Taylor (1965) and by Becker and McClintock (1967). More broadly, "exchange theorists" such as Thibaut and Kelley (1959) have productively adapted the cost-benefit approach of economics for the analysis of a variety of social-psychological problems. But the analysis of behavioral alternatives in terms of their associated costs and gains, *as if* rational decision were involved, is much more widely shared. It rests on the insight of common-sense psychology that behavior is motivated and that motivation is governed by positive and negative incentives. The commons dilemma as Hardin poses it thus makes equal sense to the psychologist whose theoretical preferences turn him toward a cognitive theory of means and goals, to the stimulus-response behaviorist concerned with the shaping of behavior under the influence of the balance of "reinforcements" or rewards, and to the functional, personality-oriented psychologist who notes that people acquire and retain dispositions and behavior patterns that by and large work out for them adaptively in the balance of gratification. To insist that Hardin's phrasing of the dilemma should make sense to social psychologists of many stripes is not to minimize consequential differences that follow from these diverse preferences among strategies of theorizing. The point is rather that the practical dilemma is already shaped to present interesting theoretical problems for psychological research.

Decision-Making and Fertility: Some Research Questions

The remainder of this essay attempts to suggest at a more specific level some of the research problems that social psychologists might be concerned with if they take the commons dilemma seriously. For a starting point we may return to my statement, "*Insofar as decisional processes are involved* [italics added], an engineering of incentives and constraints would seem to be called for. . . ." A first empirical question thus has to do with the extent to which "decisions" *are* made in matters that affect fertility. A second concerns the terms in which decisions are made.

Whether or not having children is indeed a matter of decision surely varies with cultural group and with social stratum. At one extreme is the idealized case of the fatalistic traditionalist, for whom the appearance of offspring rests with the will of Allah; at the other, the voluntarism promulgated by the middle-class Planned Parenthood movement and fostered by the seemingly inevitable spread of a rational-technical orientation accompanying modern technology the world over. For the most part, as Rainwater (1960) has noted, the decision when it occurs is cast in negative terms—*not* to have (more) children, and failure to make a decision thus is likely to result in procreation. Even near the fatalistic pole, however, where the possibility of modern contraception does not exist in the range of choice, alternatives of delayed marriage, sexual abstinence, coitus interruptus, or abortion may have sufficient psychological reality to suggest the presence of ingredients of decision in childbearing. The involvement of decision would seem to be a matter of degree.

The second question is more complex, and points to a large area of *terra incognita* where careful descriptive social-psychological research is needed. What are the terms in which decisions are made? And how do nondecisional factors in the technological and social context influence these terms and thus affect fertility?

What are the units of decision, and how do they come to bear upon fertility-relevant behavior? *Do* marital partners decide upon a wanted family size? Or on an acceptable range? Or rather on the acceptability or desirability of a next pregnancy now? Are family decisions made in a short-run time perspective, like "incrementalist" government policy, or do some parents make their plans in a longer time perspective? Which parents? Who makes the decisions, with what degree of real or assumed consensus? What alternatives are weighed, and what considerations are seen as relevant? It is easy enough to ask questions about these matters in KAP surveys of knowledge, attitudes, and practices about birth control and family planning, but it is not so simple to determine whether the answers reflect real decisions that strategically affect fecundity or essentially epiphenomenal pseudo-decisions of little real consequence. Close phenomenological inquiry followed up longitudinally is needed to throw further light on these questions.

A careful mapping of what people take for granted as outside the range of decision or as setting the fixed terms of decision should be particularly fruitful in identifying limits on the present rationality of decision-making that suggest openings for substantial change in the outcome of decisions if the governing assumptions can be altered. A dramatic case in point is that of "pluralistic ignorance." The term was originated in a discussion of normatively regulated behavior by Katz and Schanck (1938), who wrote: "People will stay in line because their fellows do, yet, if they only knew that their comrades wanted to kick over the traces too, the institutional conformity of the group would quickly vanish . . ." (pp. 174–175). Such pluralistic ignorance was unearthed in the early Puerto Rican study by Hill, Stycos, and Back (1959), who found—contrary to the accepted tenet of cultural *machismo* that men are expected to want large families, especially of sons, as proof of their masculinity—that men were even more oriented toward small families than their wives. Since their wives were quite unaware of this fact, it was the false and vulnerable assumption that must have figured in their decision processes.

What people take for granted can undergo rapid change. For many devout Catholics the papal interdiction of "artificial" contraception must once have settled the matter, removing the possibility of efficient contraception from consideration as an alternative. After disagreement with this dictum had flared up among the priests and bishops of the post-Vatican II Church, however, the highly publicized controversy inevitably shifted the issues for decision on the part of the faithful. A dogma become moot no longer enjoys the privilege of automatically setting the terms of decision.

So with legally enforced norms that formerly excluded abortion in America or relegated it to a risky and expensive underworld.[1] The first crack in the armor of state law seems to have set in motion a process of

---

[1] Since this chapter was written, my attention has been called to the provocative paper by Namboodiri and Pope (1968), contrasting the implications of what they term the "economic" and the "normative" approaches to the explanatory analysis of human fertility. To the extent that economic considerations of utility apply, the values involved in decisions affecting family size fall into a hierarchy of preferences; to the extent that moral norms supervene, choices are made without consideration of utilities. The paper provides appropriate references developing each point of view and argues that "neither the economic nor the normative approach alone helps explain choice behavior in all situations"; determination of the extent to which either applies is an empirical matter.

The approach taken in the present essay is, of course, broadly "economic"; it underplays the role of moral norms, which, as Namboodiri and Pope suggest, may figure more prominently in regard to family size in nonindustrial societies than in industrially advanced ones. It should be noted, however, that norms vary in their consensuality and in their moral force; utilitarian considerations may often result in contranormative behavior. As a result, in the longer run the content of what is normative may shift under utilitarian pressures. Something of the sort may be happening in the United States in regard to the issue of abortion. These considerations argue against a sharp separation of the utilitarian and the normative.

rapid legal and normative change that has already made abortion figure in personal decisions on a scale that would have been unthinkable a few years ago. Was pluralistic ignorance involved in sustaining the former seemingly impregnable barriers? Or, as in the case of race relations, have we underestimated the responsiveness of the mores to legal initiative? In Chapter 9, Henry David examines the state of psychological research on abortion, research that may capture, it is to be hoped, some of the dynamics of the rapid change now in progress for the important light it could throw on the malleability of the terms of reproductive decisions.

The impact of developments in contraceptive and abortifacient technology will also depend on how they affect the terms of individual decision-making. There is the obvious factor of risk that enters into the cost-benefit balance: when the perceived risk entailed by a contraceptive technique can be reduced, its acceptability is enhanced. Akin are the effects to be anticipated from reducing the bother, mess, or unwelcome side effects of contraception. Elsewhere (Smith, 1965) I have stressed the psychological importance of differences between the various birth-control methods in how they package and structure the decision process. The existing methods can be ordered on a continuum from sterilization through the loop and the pill to the diaphragm and condom, according to the *scope* of consequences governed by a single decision. I argue that only those methods in which a single decision commits the person to effective birth prevention over many occasions of intercourse hold much promise in connection with population control; any method that requires a new decision to accompany each sexual act sets too stringent requirements for consistency of habit or internalization of controls to be effective in regulating behavior that is as impulsive and as private as sex. Moreover, the advantage should lie with methods that change the focus of decision from contraception to *conception*, so that pregnancy, not its prevention, requires active choice. Of presently available methods, only the imperfectly effective loop has this advantage for women for whom it is acceptable.

On these a priori psychological grounds, I would set considerably higher priority on improving the loop, or on developing an implanted long-term pill that can be neutralized at will by taking a complementary pill, than on further psychological research on many of the topics that I've been advocating! For persons continually at risk of conception, such technological measures should create a decision structure in which unwanted pregnancies could be reduced to a bedrock minimum. For persons only occasionally or unpredictably at risk—particularly the unmarried young—analogous considerations would give priority to the development of a safe, acceptable abortifacient for the morning after, a technological advance that would avoid the psychological and moral disadvantages of deliberately maintaining a constant state of readiness for sexual activity, as a regimen of the pill requires.

But convinced as I am of these armchair conclusions, research is clearly needed on just how proposed new techniques actually do get involved in the motivational and decision processes of their users. Clinical tests of new methods should always include systematic study of these matters.

The effects on fertility of differences or changes in the social structure and institutional context are also likely to be mediated by their influence on the terms of behavioral decisions that affect procreation. Davis (1967) counts on such mediation in his recent controversy with proponents of voluntaristic planned parenthood. In Davis's view support of family planning has misleadingly deflected potential support from more effective measures toward the control of population growth. He argues that only major social changes that entail the restructuring of incentives and the erosion of familistic values are adequate to change the fertility of a population. Planned parenthood, as he sees it, actually promotes rather than counteracts familistic values; moreover, it deals with trivial attitudes that cannot be expected to give leverage against the strong motives that underlie human fertility. One may differ with his verdict against the support of family planning (as I discuss the matter subsequently, I believe voluntaristic family planning and the programming of incentives are entirely compatible), yet accept his analysis of how social change can affect the motivational basis of fertility.

Plausible examples of these relationships are readily available. Thus the value of an additional child differs in an economy of farm or household industry versus one where prolonged education entails high costs and delays economic productivity until well after the capacity for independent adulthood has been reached. It likewise differs in a traditional society in which provision of sustenance to the aged and of ritual honor to the dead depends entirely on their progeny versus a secular society that provides for the social security of the aged. Corresponding differences in fertility rates follow. Yet it is difficult, indeed, to estimate in advance the net consequences for fertility of major social changes seen in process or contemplated as a matter of deliberate policy. There are no examples of success.

The structural changes now being fervently pressed by radical feminists would affect the terms of reproductive decisions as well as the values of parenthood. When few other options are socially available to women for creative self-realization, the values inherent in motherhood are likely to be seized upon and even magnified by default. If equal and adequate opportunities for women become available in what has previously been a man's world, however, motherhood—or at least compulsively repetitive motherhood—may less frequently be the most attractive alternative.

These conjectures need elaboration and testing in research. But I have carried the examples far enough to suggest that an adequate causal analysis, which is needed for the guidance of social policy, requires the joint application of sociological and psychological perspectives, which then become complementary rather than competitive. Controversies about which factors lend themselves most promisingly to strategic access are likely to be more illuminating, and less heated, than ones about the priority of social versus psychological causes, seen in the competitive terms of academic territoriality.

The loosely construed decision-making framework that I have found useful thus far must be still further qualified if it is not to become a Procrustean bed for the analysis of psychological factors in fertility. It is not always helpful to think of motivated human behavior in terms of decisions, even implicit ones. Behavior may be motivated and emitted without the weighing of alternatives. To try to compress the psychology of motivation into a decisional framework, with its implications of rationality, would surely be unwise. The quasi-rational component seems dependable enough, however, to make Hardin's analysis of the tragedy of the commons persuasive and to warrant the development of social strategies to shift the balance of incentives. In this connection it seems to me too bad that followers of B. F. Skinner's approach to the "experimental analysis of behavior" have not as yet turned their very considerable analytic and manipulative ingenuity to the population problem.[2]

In the broader realm of motivational processes relevant to fertility, the social psychologist is accustomed to focusing on beliefs, attitudes, and values as personal dispositions that, jointly with the person's appraisal of his situation of action, enter into the determination of what he does. The psychoanalytically oriented psychologist will be alert to deeper motivations that are less directly expressed. The burden of much of the foregoing, for the social psychologist, is to suggest that we do not yet have adequately clear ideas about *what* beliefs, attitudes, and values engage with reproductively relevant behavior. Naturalistically conceived research in depth along the lines of Rainwater's (1960, 1965) is needed if we are to discern the relevant units of psychological organization.

From Motives and Decisions to Planful Commitment: Internal versus External Control as a Promising Variable

People are not just bundles of beliefs, attitudes, and values that channel motives. These analytically distinguished structural components occur in the context of personality organization. Among the aspects of personality to which attention seems particularly promising in the present context is the way that people differ in the degree to which they are psychologically organized to carry out a planful course of action. As we ruefully know, there is many a slip between intention and realization, between expressions of attitude and consequential behavior. Progress toward the conceptualization and measurement of personality differences in this respect should be relevant to family planning.

[2] Lipe (1971) has partly filled this gap in a recent programmatic paper published after the completion of this chapter.

A recent social-psychological approach that gives considerable evidence of coming to grips with this problem deals with individual differences in the capacity for self-determination in terms of self-conceptions as being an "origin" or a "pawn" of social causation (De Charms, 1968) or in terms of generalized expectations as to whether the outcomes of one's actions are under internal or external control (Rotter, 1966; Lefcourt, 1966). As I have reinterpreted these convergent lines of research and theory elsewhere (Smith, 1972), what seems to be involved is a cluster of self-attitudes that tend to function as a self-fulfilling prophecy. People who are convinced that they are "origins," that their important outcomes are under their own control, behave so as to enhance the likelihood that their beliefs will be confirmed; so, unfortunately, do those who see themselves as "pawns" at the mercy of external forces. In his I-E scale (internal versus external control) Rotter has provided a convenient but rather crude and faulted measure of the variable, in terms of which there are validating indications that groups contrasting in actual social power differ as might be expected, and that the variable has behavioral consequences in line with our present interest in it.

More substantial clues are available that locus of control has a direct bearing on fertility-relevant behavior. In a study of undergraduates Mac-Donald (1970) reports that among the unmarried females who indicated that they had engaged in premarital coitus, substantially and significantly more of the respondents who were high in internal control than of those who were high in external control reported the use of some form of birth control. Essentially the same conceptual variable, differently approached, has been tapped by Williamson (1969) and others under the label "sense of efficacy." In the context of a major study of modernization, Williamson finds his measure to be related to favorable attitudes toward birth control. (See also Chapter 4 in this book.)

Still further supportive evidence has recently been reported by Keller, Sims, Henry, and Crawford (1970) in their suggestive intensive study of twenty lower-class Negro couples, half of whom were making effective use of contraceptives and half were not. (The subgroups were well matched; all were of childbearing age with at least two children; all were informed about contraception and had contraceptive services available.) Projective measures of feelings of efficacy, need for achievement (men only), and tendency to plan ahead were prominent among the measures that discriminated significantly between "users" and "nonusers," in a study presented as reestablishing the promise of a psychological approach to fertility.

In contrast with the measures of personality traits that have proved so disappointing in previous research on fertility, where the rationale for expecting any relationship has tended to be vague and intuitive at best, personal control or sensed efficacy is a variable that fills a well-defined theoretical gap. Voluntaristic programs of family planning, whether or not they are thought of as steps toward the control of population growth, crucially depend on the planfulness of their participants. If we can develop adequate measures of people's propensity to take command of their own fate, we will have brought into view an important ingredient in the success or failure of the voluntaristic strategy. We may also have discovered a "moderator variable" that helps to determine whether people act in terms of their expressed attitudes in matters of family planning.

The research priorities here seem clear enough. In the short run the Rotter scale or one or another of the several short scales of survey items that have been offered to tap the sense of efficacy should be applied in newly undertaken studies of attitudes and practices about birth control and family planning. But the indications are sufficiently strong that meaningful and substantial relations are to be found here to justify setting even higher priority on the development of a theoretically and psychometrically more adequate measure from the pool of items now available, taking into account the known deficiencies of the existing scales.

Concluding Considerations of Conceptualization and Strategy

The points I have chosen to emphasize are, I realize, a slim selection from the possible points of contact between social psychology and research on fertility and population. I have not dealt with the psychology of communication, persuasion, and attitude change, central topics of social psychology in which I have some personal investment, partly because these matters are treated elsewhere in this volume, but also partly because I am reluctantly convinced that these useful areas of social-psychological competence are unlikely to be the sites of major breakthroughs toward understanding what has eluded conventional demography. I have ignored the important area of small-group interaction as applied to communicative relationships in the family because it has been the preserve of social psychologists affiliated with sociology; I don't know enough about it.

In adopting a loose decision-making orientation as a point of departure for identifying research needs, I have risked presenting a rationalistic caricature of a realm of human behavior that is surely ridden with irrationality. In calling for research attention to limitations on rational decision, my preference for a cognitive theoretical approach has led me to stress factors in people's knowledge and beliefs, in their situations of action as they define them, that affect the terms of their decisions; I have slighted the barriers of habit and custom, less cognitively formulated, that also restrict people's options and need research attention.

Underlying my selection of topics is a set of appraisals and value judgments that govern what I would presently find most useful for learning about the social psychology of fertility, and the purposes of this book should be served best if I make them explicit. I am personally persuaded by

Hardin's analysis of the population problem as a "tragedy of the commons" and take seriously Crowe's elaboration of the difficulties that beset the search for a political solution. In these terms the problem is deadly serious: only the length of the period of grace that is left for us to find a solution seems to me open to debate. The world is limited; population will eventually cease to grow whatever we do. But unless deliberate policy intervenes, it will cease to grow because of the mortality of war, famine, disease, and environmental fouling and depletion—or because the quality of life has fallen to such a miserable level that in Hardin's equation the individual utilities for having children, plus and minus, finally balance out. The problem is so serious that even coercive measures have to be considered. According to Hardin's analysis, "jawboning" and educational approaches will not by themselves suffice.

But here my commitment to the value of human freedom insists on recognition. The values embedded in my view of human potentiality call for the expansion, not the contraction, of the range of human choice. Freedom and self-determination seem to me to make more difference to the quality of life than even clean air and green land. How to preserve the reality of choice, yet avoid the doom inherent in the commons tragedy?

To put the question thus seems to me to point unmistakably toward a deliberate social policy of incentives for family limitation—incentives provided directly to the potential parents, or produced indirectly via planned institutional changes that in turn modify the terms of reproductive decisions. A strategy of appropriately designed incentives would leave free choice to the individual—indeed, it would encourage planful choice—while it would steer the overall statistical outcome, as this outcome must be steered if we are to avoid catastrophe, by adjusting the nature or the value of the alternatives offered.

To speculate a bit further, I would see the strategy of direct incentives favored by Spengler (1969) as complementary to the reliance on major institutional change primarily stressed by Davis (1967). We are drastically inexperienced in the initiation and guidance of planned social change. Even if we can gird ourselves politically to bring it about, we will still lack the competence to steer it to produce just the effects on fertility that we want. At best the feedback features of the social system inherently involve time lags that preclude accurate guidance. To achieve a desired target of stable population replacement, then, the more sensitive control over decision structures that a program of direct incentives could provide seems an essential component of an effective social plan.

These are admittedly utopian speculations, but the seriousness of our predicament requires us to gain practice in utopian thinking. Closer to present realities is the discussion in Chapter 17 of some possible psychological contributions to the design of antinatalist incentives. I leave the further treatment of this topic to Pohlman, with the exception of declaring my conviction that any scheme of monetary incentives must rest upon a base of truly adequate income support. I would also note, with Chilman (1970), that other important human values besides stabilized population and freedom of choice are going to be deeply touched by any deliberate effort to limit population growth. Unanticipated and unwelcome side effects for the values presently realized in family life should be ferreted out imaginatively and monitored carefully.

To develop a policy of qualified voluntarism—voluntarism within a context of designed incentives—will require dependable and sophisticated knowledge about the terms in which people actually make the decisions that affect procreation and about the extent to which they make decisions at all. It is here that I have placed greatest emphasis in the present chapter. Developing such a policy also calls for knowledge of people's capacity for voluntary planning that is rational within a given incentive structure—the topic dealt with in the foregoing section.

In this bold—or rash?—endeavor, what help may we reasonably expect from social psychology? Here I have to return to my initial theme of modesty. In the face of discouraging prior efforts, I would hesitate to promise striking immediate gains from social-psychological research in the control of additional variance in fertility. But the sort of empirical mapping of relevant dispositions, situations, and decisional processes that I have called for might reasonably be expected to yield a clearer understanding of the causal nexus that underlies demographic correlations. This in turn should be relevant to the development of social policy.

From a strategic point of view technology and other components of people's situations of action are more likely to be accessible to change than are people themselves. Special attention might therefore be given to how people interpret and react to proposed innovations in social incentives and in contraceptive-abortifacient technology. Fortunately the evaluation of social programs is at last becoming a subject of potential interest to competent and imaginative social psychologists.

REFERENCES

Becker, G. M. and McClintock, C. G. 1967. Value: behavioral decision theory. *Annual Review of Psychology* 18:239–286.

Chilman, C. S. 1970. Probable social and psychological consequences of an American population policy aimed at the two-child family. *Annals of the New York Academy of Science* 175:868–879.

Crowe, B. L. 1969. The tragedy of the commons revisited. *Science* 166:1103–1107.

Davis, K. 1967. Population policy: will current programs succeed? *Science* 158:730–739.

Davis, K. and Blake, J. 1956. Social structure and fertility: an analytical framework. *Economic Development and Cultural Change* 4:211–235.

De Charms, R. 1968. *Personal causation. The internal affective determinants of behavior.* New York: Academic Press.

Fawcett, J. T. 1970. *Psychology and population.* New York: The Population Council.

Hardin, G. 1968. The tragedy of the commons. *Science* 162:1243–1248.

Hawthorne, G. 1970. *The sociology of fertility*. London: Collier-Macmillan.

Hill, R.; Stycos, J. M.; and Back, K. 1959. *The family and population control: a Puerto Rican experiment in social change*. Chapel Hill: University of North Carolina Press.

Katz, D. and Schanck, R. L. 1938. *Social psychology*. New York: Wiley.

Keller, A. B.; Sims, J. H.; Henry, W. E.; and Crawford, T. J. 1970. Psychological sources of "resistance" to family planning. *Merrill-Palmer Quarterly* 16:286–302.

Lefcourt, H. M. 1966. Internal versus external control of reinforcement. *Psychological Bulletin* 65:206–220.

Lipe, D. 1971. Incentives, fertility control, and research. *American Psychologist* 26:617–625.

MacDonald, Jr., A. P. 1970. Internal-external locus of control and the practice of birth control. *Psychological Reports* 21:206.

Namboodiri, N. K. and Pope, H. 1968. Social norms concerning family size. Paper presented at annual meeting of the Population Association of America, Boston, April 1968.

Platt, J. R. 1966. *The step to man*. New York: Wiley.

Rainwater, L. 1960. *And the poor get children*. Chicago: Quadrangle Books.

————. 1965. *Family design: marital sexuality, family size, and contraception*. Chicago: Aldine.

Rotter, J. B. 1966. Generalized expectancies for internal versus external control of reinforcement. *Psychological Monographs* 80, no. 1 (whole no. 609):1–28.

Ryder, N. B. 1965. The cohort as a concept in the study of social change. *American Sociological Review* 30:843–861.

Smith, M. B. 1965. Motivation, communications research, and family planning. In Mendel C. Sheps and Jeanne C. Ridley, eds., *Public health and population change: current research issues*. Pittsburgh: University of Pittsburgh Press. Pp. 70–89.

————. 1972. "Normality"—for an abnormal age. In D. Offer and D. X. Freedman, eds., *Modern psychiatry and clinical research: essays in honor of Roy R. Grinker*. New York: Basic Books. Pp. 102–119.

Spengler, J. 1969. Population problem: in search of a solution. *Science* 166:1234–1238.

Taylor, D. W. 1965. Decision making and problem solving. In J. G. March, ed., *Handbook of organizations*. Chicago: Rand McNally. Pp. 48–86.

Thibaut, J. W. and Kelley, H. H. 1959. *The social psychology of groups*. New York: Wiley.

Westoff, C. F.; Potter, R. G.; and Sagi, P. C. 1963. *The third child*. Princeton: Princeton University Press.

Westoff, C. F.; Potter, R. G.; Sagi, P. C.; and Mishler, E. G. 1961. *Family growth in metropolitan America*. Princeton: Princeton University Press.

Wildavsky, A. 1964. *The politics of the budgetary process*. Boston: Little, Brown.

Williamson, J. B. 1969. Subjective efficacy as an aspect of modernization in six developing nations. Unpublished Ph.D. diss., Harvard University. Cited in J. T. Fawcett, 1970, *Psychology and population*. New York: The Population Council.

[2]

THE VALUE OF CHILDREN
TO PARENTS

LOIS WLADIS HOFFMAN
AND MARTIN L. HOFFMAN

Introduction

What is the value of a child? The question has been answered endlessly in cave drawings, myths, religion, folk sayings, poetry, and popular songs. It has not been answered scientifically, however. We know that children are not only an inadvertent consequence of sex, for extensive use of birth control has neither eliminated them nor even brought their number down to a size commensurate with optimum population growth. We know they are not wanted for utilitarian reasons alone, for in the United States, where their cost far exceeds their practical worth, family size averaged 3.3 in 1960, and about 50 percent of American women considered four or more children ideal (Whelpton, Campbell, and Patterson, 1966; U.S. Department of Commerce, 1970). It is possible to list many nonutilitarian values that children might provide, but in most cases there is no evidence that these values are held by any sizable group. Data are virtually nonexistent on why certain values are important, why children seem to satisfy them, which of the values are salient at certain times, which actually motivate the parents to have a child. Indeed, the most impressive thing about the literature on the value of children and motivations for reproduction is that there are so few known facts.

In his recent book, Pohlman (1969) has taken an excellent first step by gathering together the motivations for childbearing that have appeared in the empirical and theoretical literature. The list he compiles is overwhelm-

NOTE: The authors are indebted to James T. Fawcett for suggesting that this chapter be written and for his help and encouragement through all phases of its preparation.

ing. It includes motives that operate at different levels of consciousness and with different degrees of primacy. It includes motives that appear to be contradictory, although clearly they may characterize different groups, or the same person at different times, or even the same person at the same time. But that is the nature of the problem. Motivations for children are complex, changing, and often ambivalent. The task is to document them, to sort them into meaningful conceptual schemes, and to study their interactions with other variables.

This chapter will not duplicate the complete coverage that is available in Pohlman's book and in Fawcett's monograph (1970). Instead a methodological critique will be presented in which issues of measurement and study design are discussed. This will take up the first section of the chapter. The research will be reviewed as it illustrates the methodological points. If much of this research is new and deals with unpublished manuscripts, this is partly a reflection of the recent upsurge of interest in the topic, and partly a deliberate attempt to complement rather than to overlap with the previous reviews. The second section of the chapter will be concerned with a conceptual scheme that attempts to organize the various materials on the value of children. A categorization of the values, drawn mainly from the relevant literature in a wide range of fields, will be presented, using available data illustratively. This will be followed by a theoretical model and a discussion of its use in organizing the values and guiding research. Throughout the chapter certain studies and topics are taken up in more detail than others because they are new, important, or necessary to illuminate particular points.

In this essay the *value of children* refers to the functions they serve or the needs they fulfill for parents. Our special interest is in the capacity of these values to affect the motivation to have children. *Motivation*, on the other hand, is closer to behavior; it refers to the predisposition to act. The motivation to have a child will depend to a considerable extent on the value of the child to the actor. The other factors that are involved, such as the "costs" of the child, will be discussed in the second section of this chapter. The motive for pregnancy per se is not a concern of this chapter.

Interest in the Value of Children

There are basically four reasons for studying the value of children to their parents. Three are directly relevant to the study of population and population planning: to affect motivations for fertility, to anticipate compensations that might be necessary should a smaller family size be achieved, and to predict fertility motivations and thus population trends. The fourth reason is only indirectly related to population: to consider the value of children as a possible influence on the parent-child relationship.

Interest in the value of children has been generated by concern about overpopulation and increasing appreciation of the fact that the desire for children is in excess of optimum population growth. Blake (1971) and others have argued persuasively that even if all couples had only those children they want and no others, a disastrous population explosion will occur. Improved means of birth prevention and the encouragement of their use is considered by these demographers to be an insufficient basis for an effective population policy. Accordingly a number of alternative approaches to decreasing family size have been advanced. One extreme suggestion (Hardin, 1970a, 1970b) advocates placing the decision about family size in the control of the state through involuntary sterilization at the birth of the nth child. Another suggestion is to increase the cost of having a child either directly through taxation or indirectly by giving parents a bonus for not having a child (Davis, 1967; Spengler, 1969; Kangas, 1970; see also Chapter 17). In a recent article Blake (1971) has pointed out, however, that a policy that penalizes fertility and leaves the desire for children untouched requires constant vigilance if it is to have any effect; it would also "create disaffection" (p. 219).

Examining the value of children then has two very practical purposes: (1) knowing these values may suggest means of satisfying them other than having children that may help reduce the very desire for children; and (2) if smaller family size should be achieved in some other way, the values may suggest appropriate forms of compensatory satisfactions that might be considered.

Studying the value of children should also facilitate prediction of population trends over time and across cultures. Fawcett (1970) notes that hypotheses about reproductive motives often involve the underlying theme that "social change brings about changes in the way children are valued, in relation to alternative sources of satisfaction" (p. 110). Failure to understand the increase in desired family size that began in the 1940s might thus be seen as a result of insufficient attention to the social changes that had altered the functions formerly served by children. Demographers had focused on the economic value of children, which was decreasing, but they ignored the social changes that were enhancing the noneconomic value of children.

The final reason for studying the value of children—because of the possible effects on the parent-child relationship—is related to population concerns because one of the arguments in support of birth planning and legalized abortion is that the unwanted child is rejected by his parents, with adverse consequences for his development.[1] This topic, however, is tangential to the major thrust of this chapter. Some of the studies will be considered in the section on measures, but there will be no attempt to deal with the conceptual issues.

[1] Indeed, many studies indicate that the rejected child suffers ill effects, but there are other reasons for rejection besides the possibility that the child was originally unwanted. Furthermore, a mistreated child may be highly valued; he may, for example, satisfy pathological parental needs. For the population argument studies are needed that examine the relationship between prenatal desire for the child and postnatal behavior toward the child.

Methodological Issues

This section of the chapter will be divided into three parts. The first will review and discuss attempts to measure the extent to which children are valued by parents. It will be our only effort to deal with the degree or quantity of this value. Measurement problems peculiar to the lower class will be singled out for special attention. The second part will deal with attempts to measure the particular values that children may satisfy, that is, the qualities for which they are valued. And the third will consider the kinds of studies that have been done and will focus on issues of research design.

How Much Are Children Valued?

Studies that deal with the extent to which children are valued generally seek data on the number of people who want some children, as opposed to none; the number of children that are wanted; and the amount of happiness that children provide.

Pohlman (1970) presents ample evidence for a "widespread desire for children" in the United States since World War II. Most American couples want more than two children. Having no children is viewed as a pitiable state, and having only one is viewed as undesirable for the child. Though the precise figures vary, only about 1 percent of the population want no children—whether asked before or after they become parents. A similar number want only one child.[2] The frequency starts piling up at two, and the average number of children wanted is between three and four. Today there appears to be less desire to remain childless in the United States than in European countries; this is a change from the Depression period when estimates placed the number favoring childlessness at somewhere between 6 and 11 percent (Thompson and Lewis, 1965).

Although the stated desire for having children and the report of how many one wants seems an easily accessible piece of data, even this operation has problems. A number of recent papers elaborate on these difficulties and suggest that the simple single questions currently in use should be replaced by multiple-item scales. Questions should deal with how strongly the respondent feels, under what conditions she would feel one way or another, and what influences other than her own attitude (e.g., her husband's view) would affect her fertility behavior. Fawcett (1971) notes that desired family size is not a good predictor of the respondent's subsequent fertility although the aggregate response is a good predictor of aggregate fertility. This sug-

[2] Blake (1971) reports data from a national sample of white Americans obtained in the summer of 1970: seven respondents out of 1,334 prefer a one-child family, and four respondents favor childlessness.

gests that the answers may "simply reflect what is usual and acceptable within the society" (p. 6). If this is so, desired family size would not even be a good predictor of aggregate fertility in periods of rapid social change. Such issues are discussed more fully in several unpublished papers (Mohanty, 1969; Mauldin, Watson, and Noe, 1971; Pohlman, 1970; and Fawcett, 1971) and elsewhere in this volume.

The assumption sometimes made that the desired number of children reflects how much they are valued is also questionable. Wanting a large family may be an indication of the *kind* of value children represent rather than the intensity of the desire for them. Rainwater (1965) found that when he asked his subjects why parents want a large family, the respondents who themselves wanted a small family said "love of children" (especially the men), but respondents who really wanted a large family answered in terms of specific gains such as a sense of accomplishment, the pleasure of watching them grow, and the happier atmosphere provided. On the other hand, data from the Princeton study do show a relationship between "liking children" and wanting a large family (Westoff, Potter, Sagi, and Mishler, 1961).

CHILDREN AS A SOURCE OF HAPPINESS

Data on the happiness children provide come mainly from outside the field of population research. In 1957 the Institute for Social Research at the University of Michigan conducted a national survey of mental health in which a representative sample of 2,460 adult Americans were interviewed about such matters as their feelings of happiness, unhappiness, worries, self-perceptions, and family relationships (Gurin, Veroff, and Feld, 1960). It is important to note for our purposes that when asked what their sources of happiness were, the two most frequently mentioned responses were economic-material and children. Each was mentioned by 29 percent of the sample. (The figures for children are even higher if responses referring to the family are included.) As sources of unhappiness, on the other hand, the economic category was again the highest, while children were mentioned by only 7 percent of the respondents. (Most of this latter group, as well as those who mentioned their marriage, were found to have more serious problems of adjustment, from which the authors conclude that the central life relationships are crucial for a sense of well-being.)

Another finding of interest was the greater ambivalence toward one's mate than toward one's children. This came through in a number of responses. The marriage was less frequently listed as a major source of happiness. Further, when parents described the "nicest things about marriage," they often mentioned external aspects such as a house, financial security, or the chance to have children. When they described the "nicest thing about having children" almost all of the responses dealt with the interpersonal relationship itself.

Children are a greater source of worries than of unhappiness. Fifteen percent of the sample named children as a source of worry while 18 percent named family health, which might include children. Economic worries led the list: they were mentioned by 41 percent.[3]

This predominantly positive portrait was undoubtedly heightened by the fact that some respondents were past the time of greatest involvement with their children. Older people recall fewer problems and are more positive in evaluating their parental experiences. Many worries of the parents of young children turn out to be unwarranted, and so from the wisdom of hindsight there were not many serious anxieties.

Another relevant question asked in this survey was "Thinking about a man's (woman's) life, how is a man's (woman's) life changed by having children?" The first answer given was coded as positive, neutral, or negative. The number of positive first responses rose from 40 percent for respondents in the twenty-one to thirty-four age group, to 42 percent for those between thirty-five and forty-four, to over half for those over forty-five. Women were more negative than men. Hoffman (1963a) asked this same question of 217 Detroit mothers of school-age children in intact families, and found that most of the responses were negative; four times as many were totally negative as totally positive and only half included anything that could be considered positive. The most common response was that the mother has less freedom (e.g., "They tie you down"). The preponderance of negative responses in this study might be expected because the respondents were all mothers of at least one grammar-school-age child whereas the national survey included fathers, older parents, and childless adults. Unfortunately, however, the two samples cannot really be compared because of differences in the coding unit: only the first response was coded in the national study, the total response in the Detroit study. Nonetheless, it is easy to imagine that a person's answers would be different at different stages in family life. Indeed, different responses might be expected if the mother of young children were asked that question at the bleak period of 5 P.M. when she and her children are hungry and irritable, the house is a mess, and supper must be prepared; and then asked it again several hours later when the children are asleep.[4]

THE PROBLEM OF CONCEPTUALIZING HOW MUCH CHILDREN ARE VALUED

How much a child is valued is obviously complicated and difficult to measure. The value indicated by one measure is often unrelated to that

---

[3] The first two sources named by the respondent were coded for the questions about happiness, unhappiness, and worries.

[4] It is interesting to contrast the results obtained in the Oakland Growth Study using an almost identical question: How is an adult's life changed by having children? The respondents were about forty-two years old and, unlike the two studies under discussion, the questionnaire was mailed rather than personally administered. Positive responses were given by 79 percent of the thirty-nine fathers and 89 percent of the forty-five mothers who returned the questionnaire. The authors wish to thank John Clausen for making these unpublished data available.

indicated by another—not because of inaccuracies in the measure but because of the multifaceted nature of the value of a child. Neither "nurturance needs" nor the "preference for babies over older children" were found by Westoff et al. (1961) to be related to the number of children desired, even though "liking children" did relate. Though a negative relationship might be expected between the satisfactions of parenthood and acknowledgment of problems and feelings of inadequacy as a parent, Gurin et al. (1960) found no relation—apparently because the question about "problems" evoked responses pertaining to external events, while the "inadequacy" item called forth intrinsic qualities of the respondent such as introspectiveness.

There is ambivalence toward all intense personal relationships. In some cases this ambivalence is so extreme as to be pathological. The "child beaters," for example, typically fight to retain custody of their "battered child." The work of Vogel and Bell (1960) illustrates the scapegoat role often played in the family by the disturbed child; the child's psychological maladjustment becomes an essential part of the family's integration. But even in normal situations there are many aspects to the child's value, and the concept will therefore need to be defined for the purposes of the particular study.

There are also differences in the value a parent places on each child. Sears, Maccoby, and Levin (1957), in a study of parent-child relations among suburban New England families with kindergarten children, found that mothers were more apt to recall delight over being pregnant when it was their first pregnancy, when a long time had elapsed since the previous one, or when existing children were all girls.

It seems clear that just as several measures are needed to obtain full information about the number of children desired, as mentioned earlier, the same is true with respect to any other aspect of the value of children. Furthermore, as we shall see later in the chapter, in many cases "How much are children valued?" may not be as useful a question as "For what purpose are they valued?"[5]

THE DESIRE FOR CHILDREN IN THE LOWER CLASS

The difficulty of estimating how much children are valued is highlighted in the studies of the lower class. In the United States, as elsewhere, the lower class has more children than the middle and upper classes. The question is do they really want more? To a considerable extent lower-class

_____

[5] One approach to the question of how valuable children are to parents might be to compare childlessness with parenthood. Some attention has been given to the adult's adjustment to the parent role (Rossi, 1968; Anthony and Benedek, 1970; Senn and Hartford, 1968; Lopata, 1971), but the data are scarce. Comparison between deliberately childless couples and parents has had even less attention. To compare the two groups with respect to indices of such variables as happiness, mental health, or self-actualization is difficult because of problems of self-selection; that is, would obtained differences reflect the effects of having or not having children, or factors that went into the original decision?

fertility appears to result from insufficient and ineffective use of contraception (Whelpton et al., 1966; Rainwater, 1960, 1965), but it is also true that the Protestant lower class reports a larger *desired* family size. An important question is if birth control were more acceptable, available, and trusted as effective, would the desired family size in the lower class decrease?[6]

Although the issue is beyond the scope of this chapter, there are many obstacles to contraception in the lower class. The techniques most frequently used—condom, withdrawal, and rhythm—are unpleasant, inconvenient, and ineffective. Furthermore, they are controlled by the man, whose interest in contraception is often less than that of the woman. Failure to use the diaphragm or coil seems in part the result of insufficient information. But Rainwater also interprets this hesitancy as reflecting the modesty of lower-class women and their embarrassment about discussing sexual matters with a doctor; indeed, Rainwater's lower-class informants often state this. Calling these women modest may seem inappropriate when they so openly discuss the intimacies of their sex life with the interviewer, but the interview and medical situations are different in several important respects. The interviewer was a woman, whereas few doctors are. Furthermore, a good interviewer, unlike a doctor, makes efforts to appear as close to the social class of her respondents as possible. Encounters with middle-class people and institutions are uncomfortable at best for the lower-class person, and the bureaucratic intimacy of a gynecological examination is not an attractive prospect. If a talk with a teacher produces anxiety in the lower class (Hess and Shipman, 1968) a gynecological examination must be extremely threatening. In addition the interviewer comes to the home, whereas the doctor's appointment must be planned in advance and requires going to an unfamiliar place. There are class differences in the willingness to plan and carry out an unpleasant action for the sake of a future reward and in the belief that a reward will be forthcoming. In this connection it should also be noted that most contraceptive techniques used by the lower class require constant diligence, and not having a baby requires far more sustained attention than having one. The effort and the impulse control needed do not appear to be characteristic of the American lower class (Schneider and Lysgaard, 1953).

Though lower-class resistance to effective contraception is a complex issue, it is important to distinguish the failure to use contraception from the desire for children. In considering "desired family size" demographers often neglect the parents' expectations. It is reasonable to assume that expectations are an influence on desired family size, however, and if they are, the widespread adoption of effective contraceptive techniques may not only reduce excess fertility, i.e., numbers of births in excess of desires, but also the number desired. Psychologists like Festinger would call it "dissonance reduction" and Aesop would call it "sweet lemons," but the number of children a couple tell themselves and others they want will be higher when their

[6] A similar question might be asked for Catholics. If the Catholic conscience allowed them to use birth control, would they continue to "want" large families?

expectations are higher. If birth control were practiced long enough for its effectiveness to be fully accepted, both actual and expected family size would drop. Desired family size would then also drop and become a more accurate reflection of the value of children.

Demographers know that having large families exerts a pull toward saying large families are desired because it is otherwise like wishing to do away with an existing child. There has been less sensitivity, however, to the manner in which desires are affected by expectations. Furthermore, the ambivalence about contraception that comes through clearly in Rainwater's rich data appears to be partly handled by the parents' selling themselves on large families. This is most obvious where the husband is resisting the wife's pressures to use the condom or withdrawal. His resistance may be based on passion, but it helps his conscience and his argument if he also likes children.

One other point should be made. These rationalizations operate on the individual level, but since similar processes are taking place with many persons who interact with one another, group norms may develop. It has been noted earlier that "desired family size" seems to reflect the pattern that is currently prevalent in one's group. But group norms, like individual attitudes, respond to environmental changes although usually more slowly. Thus as more congenial contraceptive techniques are developed and made more readily available to the lower class, and confidence in their effectiveness grows, it is reasonable to expect the desired family size to decrease, both as an individual goal and as a group norm.[7] It is consistent with this hypothesis that both the Indianapolis and Princeton studies found that among Protestant couples who successfully used birth control, family size was actually *smaller* in the lower than in the middle class (Westoff, Potter, and Sagi, 1963).

The social class differences in desired family size seem to have diminished in recent years according to Whelpton et al. (1966); in fact they found none. When the relationship is examined separately for religious groups, however, it is found that lower-class Protestants want more children than middle- and upper-class Protestants (Westoff et al., 1963; Blake, 1968; Rainwater, 1965). Part of this difference may be due to the rural background of many lower-class Protestants: thus as Westoff et al. (1963) note, "the negative association of fertility with socioeconomic status diminishes and tends to become positive among couples with several generations of urban living" (p. 239). Because of changes in contraceptive techniques and the increasing urbanization of the population, the negative relationship between social class and both desired and actual family size may be expected to diminish still further.[8]

[7] Berelson (1966) makes a very similar point—that the use of contraception leads to decreased births, which in turn leads to a decrease in desired family size as a personal goal and as a group norm.

[8] Other social changes might have a counterinfluence on the difference between classes,

It is very easy to offer psychological explanations of why the lower class wants more children than the middle class, and, indeed, we shall suggest some ourselves in the second section of this chapter. Until better measures are available, however, it is wise to view the basic premise with some skepticism.

For What Are Children Valued?

In the second section we will discuss more fully the qualities for which children are valued. Here we will review how these values have been measured. The most common method for studying the value of children to parents is to ask. This has varied from presenting respondents with attitudes with which they are to indicate degrees of agreement (Westoff et al., 1961; Stolka and Barnett, 1969), to sentence-completion items (Rabin, 1965; Rabin and Greene, 1968), open-ended questions (Gurin et al., 1960), interviews with mixed techniques, open-ended as well as objective items (Rainwater, 1965; Mueller, 1970; Mysore Population Study, 1961; Freedman, Whelpton, and Campbell, 1959), and focused or clinical-style interviews (Flapan, 1969). Meade (1971) and his colleagues have used story-completion items and also a technique of presenting respondents with descriptions of hypothetical families whose fertility decisions the respondents are asked to consider. Relevant data are also available from interviews used in studies of other topics (e.g., Coles, 1967; Komarovsky, 1967).

OBJECTIVE MEASURES

There has been so little attempt to study the value of children that generalizations about the usefulness of different measures are impossible to make. Thus the more objective measures have not proved useful despite their many practical advantages, but this may be due to the particular items used rather than to the general form of the items. For example, Stolka and Barnett developed four Likert-type scales—each with two or three items—to measure whether the value of children was to enhance a couple's prestige, fulfill the woman's major responsibility, carry out a religious duty, or achieve marital happiness. But most of the items were ill conceived. The three items making up the prestige scale, for example, all included the word prestige (e.g., "Having children should give a couple more prestige"). It seems unlikely that parents would think of prestige as a reason for having children and, even if it were a true reason, that they would care to admit it. Thus their finding that "woman's major responsibility" was the most widely accepted of the values studied may reflect only differences in the four measures.

Items used in the Indianapolis study reported by Swain and Kiser (1953)

---

however. For example, changes in women's roles may make alternatives to childbearing particularly attractive to middle-class educated women, and this could bring about a lower birth rate in that group.

have a similar problem. The questions suggest the answer. For example, one question was "Could anything give you as much satisfaction in life as having children of your own?" About 94 percent checked from the multiple-choice responses either "definitely no" or "probably no."

The measure used by Rabin consisted of incomplete sentences with multiple-choice endings designed to tap whether motivations for parenthood are altruistic (affection for children), fatalistic (fulfillment of expectations), narcissistic (the child will reflect glory upon the parent, prove adequacy), or instrumental. The items are so worded, however, that it is difficult to tell whether respondents are describing attitudes toward future children or toward their own parents. The measure has so far been used only with college students, few of whom are yet thinking of themselves as parents.

To measure the importance of reproduction for a woman's sense of femininity, Smith and Steinhoff (1971) have recently designed a set of questions (e.g., What kinds of things make you feel a woman?) with pre-coded responses that can be self-administered. The subjects are mothers who have just given birth or women about to receive a legal Hawaiian abortion, so the responses will be specific to this situation. This specificity is appropriate for the particular study, but the obtained data should not be generalized to other settings. The measure, on the other hand, might have more general use.

Researchers at Western Washington State College have been constructing several relevant measures (Meade, 1971; Cvetkovich, 1971). In one, the respondent is given a description of a hypothetical family and asked about family plans. This measure may reveal what aspects of the situation are salient for the respondent (e.g., economic or health factors), but it elicits few responses about the value of children. It is mentioned here, nevertheless, because the general idea of presenting subjects with a hypothetical family and asking specific questions is a promising one. Cvetkovich and Brislin (Cvetkovich, 1971) have developed a questionnaire consisting of four sub-scales, two of which deal specifically with the value of children and include such items as "There's a lot of truth in the saying 'a girl becomes a woman when she becomes a mother'" and "There has been more than one marriage saved by having children." These researchers have also used Dean's (1961) measure of alienation. As mentioned later in this chapter, one value of children may be to counteract feelings of alienation.[9] This research is in the preliminary stage and the measures have only been used with college students; thus their general utility remains to be seen.

Meade (1971) has also described a measure used so far only with college students, in which the respondent is presented with an opening sentence from which he is to write a composition. The opening sentences are: "They sat by the brook talking about the family they would have"; "He (She)

[9] Cvetkovich (1971) points out that extreme alienation can also lead to the wish to avoid having children, even though less extreme levels can underly a motive to have children in order to obtain a primary group.

looked at his (her) children with pride"; and "He (She) decided this was the last child." In general boys talked about money and costs, loss of personal freedom, and personal fulfillment or achievement satisfactions; girls talked more about love and happiness. In interpreting these sex differences it is important to stress that they are the same as those found in many areas of life (Hoffman, 1972).

The Princeton study (Westoff et al., 1961) developed measures of personality factors bearing on the motivation for having children—including among others manifest anxiety, nurturance needs, and achievement needs. These appear to be relevant to the value of children since their relationship to childbearing motivations and behavior is an indication of the value children serve. As personality measures, however, they are the major focus of another chapter. The Princeton study also developed some more direct measures of the value of children. The index of "liking for children," for example, consists of five Likert scale items. Though simple, the final items were selected with considerable care on the basis of pretests and factor analysis. If the results of the study have been disappointing the problem may lie in the hypotheses and the study design, as discussed elsewhere in this chapter, rather than in the measures, which in our view may have borne more than their share of blame. Further exploration of the Princeton data using the follow-up materials and more sophisticated variable analysis might prove worthwhile. And in developing new indexes of the value of children an investigator would be well advised to consider the approach to item selection used in the Princeton studies. This approach would be easier today because of the computers that were unavailable in the 1950s.

FOCUSED INTERVIEW

The focused interview used by Flapan yields rich data, but whether it will be useful remains to be seen. The aim of Flapan's study, a longitudinal one, is to identify configurations of childbearing motivations and relevant socioemotional conflicts; and then to relate these to behavioral and somatic reactions during the various stages of the woman's reproductive behavior (e.g., somatic responses during pregnancy) and also to her mothering behavior. The first published report gives a list of motives with illustrative excerpts from the data, but the motives listed do not add to those already in the literature, nor is the attempt made to specify the conditions under which one or another of them will be salient. Nevertheless, this is a pioneer attempt to obtain systematically depth materials about fertility motivation, and despite the limitation of the sample, the study, when completed, may make a significant contribution.

OPEN-ENDED QUESTIONS

Perhaps the most useful responses to date are those given by the subjects in Rainwater's two studies (1960, 1965). The method was a conversational depth interview—not quite so clinically oriented as Flapan's, but more probing and flexible than most interviews used in research. Rich data are quoted liberally and usefully arranged throughout both reports. They are not exploited quantitatively and hypothesis testing is minimal, but these are excellent exploratory studies nonetheless.

It is interesting how often some of the most revealing insights come not from answers to direct questions about fertility motivations, but from other questions in the same interview. For example, Rainwater found that the lower-class fathers who effectively practiced birth control, when asked to describe themselves, frequently reveal the importance of their children as a source of self-esteem. In general when the prevalence of a given value is to be ascertained, the coding procedures should take into account the fact that the response to a question may come through somewhere else in the interview.

In a study of economic values affecting family size in Taiwan, Mueller (1970) found that while only 12 percent of the respondents listed as a value of children the fact that they would support them in their old age, 73 percent actually expected such support (and 54 percent named children as their *only* means of old-age support). Accordingly she developed a scale of the perceived utility of children (and one of sensitivity to the cost of raising children) that was based on the responses to many different items in the interview. Mentions of the economic benefits of raising children in several different contexts were assigned weights and combined into an overall score. The measures thus obtained were effectively related to other variables. Having children is so culturally expected and overlaid with clichés that the answer to a more direct question or the first answer to a question may not be as true a reflection of the respondent's view as the responses he gives after he has had more of a chance to think about the topic. In coding interviews researchers should therefore consider the coding unit with care.

There are a number of studies that include specific items either designed for or capable of producing data on the value of children. Some of these have already been mentioned, like the questions about how children change one's life, the best thing about having children, the worst thing, and so forth. In addition a number of the KAP surveys[10] have included questions about why people would want a small or large family. The answers—when they are reported—seem shallow and ambiguous. A few studies pursued this line of inquiry further. For example, the Mysore Population Study (1961) followed the more open-ended question with specific probes such as "Do you think that with more children you will be better taken care of in your old age?" This study also attempted to ascertain which values were the more salient as motives for fertility.

[10] The KAP survey provides "basic factual data on existing levels of family planning knowledge, attitudes, and practice for the population surveyed at a particular point in time; it will usually also measure past practices of family planning, and fertility" (p. 5). At least 400 KAP surveys have been undertaken in seventy-two countries over the past thirty years (Mauldin et al., 1971).

The KAP surveys in general are criticized elsewhere (e.g., Mauldin et al., 1971). Some of the difficulties, however, may result from the cross-cultural nature of the project. Consider, for example, the problem of finding interviewers in relatively nonliterate areas sufficiently like the respondents to inspire rapport, yet capable of training in the techniques of uniform and objective interviewing. These difficulties were overcome to a considerable extent in the study by the Poffenbergers (1969). Since their study of an Indian village is reported in Chapter 5 of this volume, it will not be detailed here, but it may be cited as an example of the results that can be obtained with painstaking and time-consuming effort. In many cases the actual questions asked were very similar to those used in other studies, e.g., questions about the advantages and disadvantages of large and small families. There were important differences in the interviewer-interviewee rapport, however, owing largely to the fact that the interviewers were well trained and had long-established and trusted relationships with the respondents. The technique of interviewing may have been an additional contributing factor. Interviewers memorized the items and only wrote the responses down afterward. There was also a great deal of standardized probing. For example, the stated desired number of children was only part of the answer. Respondents were also asked about how many they would have if these were all girls. The coding of these responses, as in the Mysore study (1961) and in Mueller's study, did not look only to a single item but considered the entire interview.

NONVERBAL MEASURES

Thus far only verbally communicated measures have been discussed. The fact that children are valued for a particular quality can sometimes be demonstrated behaviorally. For example, if pregnancy were often found to occur when a wife's achievement in work or school seemed to challenge her husband's superiority in these areas, we might infer that one possible value of children (or pregnancy) is to reassert the wife's femininity or the husband's masculinity. Identifying situations in which births often occur may reveal motivations that are prevalent though unconscious and thus not amenable to verbal report. Research of this sort is needed, but such patterns are rarely useful as measures. In fact it is difficult to imagine a behavioral index of the value of children, with the possible exception of some work by ethologists. In these studies pictures were presented to men and women subjects, and pupil enlargement, previously established as an indication of excitation, was observed. As will be discussed later, women showed more pupil enlargement than men in response to pictures of infants. For most research purposes, however, measuring the value of children to individuals will usually require asking—whether directly or indirectly.

Social groups, on the other hand, might be differentiated on the basis of existing information. It is unlikely, for example, that children are valued for the financial support they can offer in old age in a country like Sweden where the government provides adequately for its aged. By considering how much care is provided for the aged, different countries might be ranked as to the degree to which children are valued for this reason. A country's rank might in turn be related to other variables, such as desired family size, sex preference, certain childrearing patterns, or response to family-planning programs. These cross-national comparisons, however, require considerable attention to the extraneous variables that must be controlled, and because of these variables the researcher would do well to consider explanations other than his original hypothesis that might explain the empirical relationships obtained.

SOME GENERAL MEASUREMENT ISSUES

From the foregoing it should be apparent that new measures need to be developed. To a great extent these will have to be designed for each study, but the development of acceptable measures that have general utility would be an especially valuable contribution.

In developing new measures, as in planning the research design, it is important to avoid an overly simplistic view. The value of children is an elusive and complex phenomenon. Both the content and the intensity of the value of children will vary at different times—at different stages in the life cycle and, as suggested earlier, even at different times of the day. The value of a baby is different from that of a child, and although not independent, both are different from the value of being a parent. The researcher might be interested in the value of a single child, of an additional child, of a small number, or of a large family. He might be interested in the value of children already on the scene, of a particular child, or the value of children as yet unborn.

Furthermore, these values operate at different levels of the personality and with different degrees of intensity. Often the respondent has difficulty reporting his feelings not because they are repressed but simply because he has never thought about anything so patent as parenthood. The most important motive may be the most deeply repressed. It may also be so obvious that the respondent does not think to name it. Yet some researchers code only the first response.

It is also true that the child can represent conflicting values—even to the same person—and the same value can evoke conflicting motives. There is a double-sided nature to the value of children; they may simultaneously gratify two seemingly contradictory needs. For example, Hoffman and Wyatt (1960) have pointed out that they may gratify needs for independence and dependence—in the same person and at the same time. Similarly children may provide a buffer against incorporation by the extended family and also a sense of belonging in an impersonal world. If they "tie you down" as many respondents say, this is not necessarily a negative value. These complexities are important to understand if the questionnaire or interview method is to be fruitfully used in the research on the values and motives involved in reproduction.

The researcher has a dilemma. The interview, or some such form of verbal communication, is probably necessary but it is fraught with problems. We will reiterate just a few that are implicit in the preceding discussion:

1. The answers evoked by a question vary greatly as a function of the wording. The several questions asked by Gurin et al. (1960) clearly indicate this. If a researcher plans to use data to make general statements about the population, to state which values are more dominant, for example, it is important that the values of the respondents and not the questionnaire wording determine the results. The data reported by Stolka and Barnett (1969) are questionable because of this problem.

2. If the research involves comparison between subjects it is important that each subject respond to the same question. While researchers can use uniform wording, how can they guarantee uniform interpretation? Clearly for this topic the lack of ambiguity in questions is particularly important. Pretesting procedures should focus on uniformity of question interpretation, and it should be recognized that a single question is rarely an adequate measure. A series of questions and more creative coding procedures, such as those used by Mueller (1970), would be helpful.

3. Sometimes differences between subjects reflect differences in response styles. It is important in reporting group differences not to be misled by these styles. For example, many of the differences reported between men and women in their valuation of children are not specific to this topic. Women in general tend to complain more, admit weakness more, seem more introspective, and be more concerned with affiliative relationships.

4. The use of indirect measures, such as the "hypothetical family" technique being developed at Western Washington State College, the Rabin measure, and some of the KAP and the Gallup questions, presents a problem. Is the respondent expressing his view about himself or about others? At the simplest level, when an American states that the "ideal family size in America" is four children, he may personally prefer two, but his answer may reflect his judgment that his own smaller preference is atypical. For example, Rainwater (1965) compared responses about ideal family size in America to responses about personal desires. Catholics gave smaller figures for the ideal American size than for themselves, and Protestants tended slightly to give larger figures. Clearly the answers to the questions about the ideal American size were in part a cognitive judgment. Similarly Rainwater asked his respondents why couples have large families and why they have small ones. The answers provide interesting data, but they are perceptions of others. Whether they also reflect the value of children to the respondents is problematic. Because of this ambiguity indirect measures should not substitute for direct ones unless there is a clear advantage to be gained, and the results should be interpreted cautiously.

5. While there is a need for practical measures with general utility that can be used in different cultures, the concept to be measured is multifaceted, complex, and frequently changing—even within the individual. A major objective of the present chapter is to conceptualize the value of children, since this is a step that must precede operationalization.

The Study Design

Most of the data on the value of children are descriptive materials including clinical studies, research of an anthropological or exploratory nature, and isolated findings or even single responses in studies that were primarily concerned with a different topic. These studies often present interesting and rich insights, but they do not yield information about the prevalence of any of the values or motives, nor do they relate these in any systematic way to other factors. Still even the response of a single informant can sometimes provide new insights. Clinical cases have often proved useful in this way, and much of the value of Rainwater's work is in his liberal use of quotations throughout the two books. Insightful respondents are particularly valuable when they speak for a group whose views are less readily available. Coles (1967), for example, quotes from one of his interviewees:

To me, having a baby inside me is the only time I'm really alive. I know I can make something, do something, no matter what color my skin is, and what names people call me. When the baby gets born I see him, and he's full of life; or she is; and I think to myself that it doesn't make any difference what happens later, at least now we've got a chance, or the baby does. You can see the little one grow and get larger and start doing things, and you feel there must be some hope, some chance that things will get better; because there it is, right before you, a real, live growing baby. The children and their father feel it, too, just like I do. They feel the baby is a good sign, or at least he's *some* sign. If we didn't have that, what would be the difference from death? Even without children my life would still be bad—they're not going to give us what *they* have, the birth control people. [P. 368]

While these kinds of data contribute ideas to include in a list of the values of children, they raise questions of how general such feelings are. Does the patient in psychiatric treatment speak for those who haven't made it to the couch? Does the introspective, lucid, lower-class woman speak for her more taciturn sisters? Does the anthropologist's informant typify his group? It is not enough to say that it seems likely that they do. The social scientist should know how representative these feelings are. He should also know when one or another value will predominate. Since there are many values involved the question becomes what is the hierarchy in any situational context? The new child may afford hope in the face of personal helplessness, but when does the future seem bright enough to make a new baby not a lottery ticket bought with one's last dime but an investment that warrants careful planning? Or when is hope so dim that even the lottery-ticket value is lost?

NORMATIVE DATA

The closest approximation to normative data yet available on the value of children in the United States is that provided by Rainwater: for example, the tables with precise and specific categories reporting responses to why people have large and small families by sex, race, and social class (1965, pp. 143–148). Yet because of the limitations of the sample (and the data analysis),[11] the major contribution of these studies remains the rich insights they afford.

Two demographic surveys in the United States (Freedman et al., 1959; Whelpton et al., 1966) included relevant questions, but the answers reported are not illuminating. In the earlier study only a brief summary of some responses is supplied. Results are reported more fully in the later study, but only the first response was used, the coded responses were not all at the same level, and over a quarter of the responses could not be coded at all.

Other studies on the topic are limited either by the measurement problems pointed out earlier or by the highly specific nature of the samples. The data obtained by Gurin et al. (1960) may include pertinent information on a well-selected national sample, but they have not been analyzed for this purpose. There is more normative information for developing countries like Taiwan, Ghana, and India than for the United States, since, as already mentioned, some of the KAP studies in those countries included questions about the reasons for preferring large and small families. Most of the reasons reported are utilitarian; children, especially males, are seen as economic assets and particularly as sources of support in old age.

STUDIES RELATING THE VALUE OF CHILDREN TO OTHER VARIABLES

Several studies of the relationship between the value of children and other variables have been done in the developing countries. Caldwell (1967), for example, studied differences in the value of children in three economically contrasting regions of Ghana, and the Mysore Population Study examined rural-urban differences in India. Mueller (1970) used the scales previously described to measure the economic utility of children in Taiwan, as perceived by the parents, and the extent to which the parents were concerned with the economic costs of children (i.e., the negative economic value). The economic values and costs were each studied in relation to possible independent variables such as education, income, desire for consumer goods, and urbanization of residence as well as two fertility-relevant dependent variables: desired family size and use of contraceptives.

The research by Day and Day (1969, 1970) used a very different methodology to test the hypothesis that the satisfactions a society provides may function as alternatives to fertility. Their approach is called "macro-sociological" and their hypotheses about the value of children are tested by

[11] For example, there is very little systematic hypothesis-testing in the study.

comparing different countries. Basically their theory is that natality will be low in countries offering abundant alternative personal satisfactions or where available instrumentalities are so scarce that natality is seen as risky. Countries are classified according to a prepared list of satisfactions and instrumentalities, and the hypothesis is tested by comparing their birth rates. This technique of comparing countries that contrast in certain relevant ways may be useful as an antidote to pat theories or as a source of hypotheses. The problem with using total countries as the unit of analysis, however, is that too many variables are operating simultaneously. For example, if it were found that in countries having ample opportunities for women to obtain professional training, birth rates were low, what would this tell us about the relationship between professional training and the birth rate? A culture has many interrelated parts and the presumed independent and dependent variables are part of this complex. They can therefore be expected to covary not necessarily because one leads to the other, but because they are two aspects of the same broad theme. Furthermore, one cannot use refined subsample analyses in order to zero in on the crucial variables and the precise way in which they influence one another because the N's are necessarily small. The Days thus far have presented data for only six countries, but even with the twenty they eventually hope to include the obstacles to creative statistical analysis will be great.

The only other study of note that reports relationships between the value of children and fertility variables is again Rainwater's. One outcome of this study was that women who wanted small families, in contrast to those who wanted large ones, tended to describe themselves in terms of their interests outside the family or their companionship with their husband—a "microsociological" finding supportive of the above view that alternative satisfactions may lessen the desire for fertility.

THE PRINCETON STUDY

The Princeton study has already been mentioned as being only indirectly relevant to our topic, but it will now be examined in some detail by way of illustrating certain further issues of research design. As noted above, this study has been heavily criticized for its measurement of psychological variables and its sample, but in our view the theory and research design may be more at fault. That is, the weak relationships found between the psychological variables and fertility may reflect (1) poorly selected dependent variables, (2) oversimplified psychological concepts, and (3) failure to consider the social setting in which the relationships operate and to examine them within different subgroups.

Dependent Variables. The families studied all had only two children at the time the research was originally undertaken. This homogeneous sample was well chosen for a number of research purposes. However, one of the dependent variables was "fertility-planning success." Although it was cleverly measured, it seems unlikely that in a sample of subjects having no more than two children this would be a sensitive variable. This may be why the expected correlation between "ability to defer gratification" and fertility-planning success was not obtained. It is interesting to note in this connection that Kar (1971) found a positive relation between a variable similar to deferment of gratification (called "future orientation") and contraceptive use, in a lower-class sample of California families with one or more children.

The hypothesis that the woman's nurturance needs would relate to desired family size was also not confirmed, and this, too, may be because of an ill-chosen dependent variable. It seems likely that nurturance needs should have a bearing on fertility, but why on the desire for a large family? If one imagines oneself as a mother of a small and then a large family, the latter does not conjure up scenes of nurturing so much as it does accomplishment or pride—often with others looking on in admiration. Indeed, this aspect of the large family is expressed by the respondents in Rainwater's study who wanted a large family, as previously noted. It would be useful to obtain data on the appeal of the large family as a prior goal, as opposed to ending up with a large family because one frequently wanted another child. Very possibly nurturance needs, as well as the preference for younger children (which also failed to relate to "desired family size"), would do better in relation to large families, planned but only one child at a time.

Oversimplification of Psychological Concepts. The independent variables were oversimplified in several respects. First, they were treated as though they were linear or dichotomous when in fact they more typically show a curvilinear relationship to the dependent variables. Anxiety is a case in point since a number of psychological studies show that it relates to performance in a curvilinear manner.[12] To treat it as a continuous variable diminishes its power. In addition (this point will be discussed more fully in Chapter 12) psychological variables are often more effective when considered in combinations as typologies. In the Princeton study all psychological traits were considered singly.

The "need for achievement" in women was expected to relate to the desire for small families. However, there are indications that women's achievement needs may be quite diffuse, and McClelland (1964) has noted the many areas, domestic as well as professional, in which the women scholars at the Radcliffe Institute for Independent Study express their achievement strivings. Furthermore, the Princeton hypothesis does not consider possible obstacles to the expression of achievement needs outside the home. While their hypothesis might have merit for the woman with high achievement needs who has the opportunity to pursue career goals, what about the woman who is blocked from such pursuits but encouraged in her domestic activities? The latter might express her frustrated achievement goals by

12 This point and several other related issues are discussed by Russo (1971).

wanting a very large family. Empirically the two types would cancel each other out yielding the kind of zero-order correlation actually found. This leads to the third point: the expression of a psychological state depends on the situation, and thus it is necessary to examine the relationship between independent and dependent variables separately for the different situations.

The Social Setting and Subgroup Analysis. It is rare in the social sciences to find a statistically significant and theoretically important relationship between two isolated variables. There are some sure-fire independent variables like social class or education, religion, sex, and rural-urban background. These relate to many different social behaviors such as fertility, childrearing practices, maternal employment rates, and juvenile delinquency, but they are too far removed in the chain of causality to explain them. What needs to be examined is the process by which the two variables are connected. What aspect of social class is important in determining the relationship? What changes can be predicted? What is the action program implied? To understand empirical relationships of this sort one often needs to examine the psychological factors that are involved.

On the other hand, to understand the relationship between a psychological trait and a fertility behavior and even to demonstrate it empirically, the researcher must consider the social context within which it occurs. Such relationships do not operate in a vacuum. The authors of the Princeton study indicate some awareness of this, but they do not incorporate it into their analysis. Although they often discuss the possibility of a relationship going one way or the other depending on surrounding circumstances, they do not examine it separately for the different circumstances. They do so for certain standard-control variables like religion, but not for theoretically derived ones that might more effectively differentiate the situation in ways that affect the relationship. To return to the previous example, whether or not the desire for children will express a particular need such as achievement depends on the alternative satisfactions available. The relationship between this need and the desire for children may be heavily influenced by the various opportunities present in the woman's life for achievement expression. As another example, the Princeton study, as well as several others, considered anxious-dependency as a variable affecting fertility desires, but this relationship, too, depends on what alternative acceptable roles exist. Under some conditions mothering a large brood may be the most protected and undemanding role available; under others it might be the most challenging. The task for the researcher is to specify the conditions under which one or another effect will occur and to demonstrate this empirically.

The basic point here is that the relation between a psychological variable and a fertility-relevant variable should be examined separately within relatively homogeneous subsamples,[13] the makeup of the subsamples to be

[13] An alternative approach that is more appropriate in some cases is to combine several independent variables and then to consider all of the logically possible types more or less

determined by the particular theory and relationship under study. It might, for example, be based on differences in opportunity structures; in husband-wife relationships; in attitudes of the community, the husband, or the wife. Subsample analysis often reveals different empirical relationships for each subgroup that are obscured when only the total sample is examined. And in some cases it may expose the relationship obtained in a large sample as the spurious result of group differences rather than the reflection of a psychological process. The importance of subsample analysis and the skills it requires have been discussed by Lazarsfeld (1955), Anastasi (1958), and Hoffman (1963b) in connection with other topics. Research on the psychological aspects of fertility would also benefit from its use.

Of particular interest in this connection is the failure of the Princeton study to take account of the social structure within which relationships between psychological factors and fertility occur. Just as the demographer's variables require psychological data to understand the process by which they affect behavior, the psychologist's variables must take account of the social structure if the theory is to be a dynamic one capable of predicting change.

The longitudinal study of married couples under the direction of E. Lowell Kelly found that women who were "anxious-dependent" had smaller families. The authors of the Princeton study, therefore, made a similar prediction. The data did not support it. But why should one expect the same relationship to prevail when Kelly's subjects were having their babies in the 1930s and those in the Princeton study were having theirs in the 1950s? During the intervening twenty years woman's role had undergone many changes. Technological advances had greatly improved the efficiency of household operations with modern appliances, commercial food-processing procedures, and no-iron fabrics. A number of childhood diseases had been conquered with inoculations and penicillin, thus alleviating a great deal of maternal anxiety. The standard of living was up, jobs for women were more available, and maternal employment rates had increased to the point where going to work was a possibility to consider once the youngest child entered the first grade. In the 1930s mothering one or two children was a respected full-time job; by the 1950s this was not as true. Under these conditions one might expect a change in the relationship between anxious-dependency (keeping in mind that this was half of a continuum and not a pathological state) and fertility.

The Princeton study has data on the woman's employment history, and the cities involved differ with respect to female employment rates. It would be interesting to see if the association between dependency and small-family desire is reduced when there are many employment opportunities,

---

equally. In the subgroup analysis the attention is focused on a particular relationship and the context is varied.

and heightened when there are few such opportunities—for example, when the woman has had little work experience or lives in a community where the norm is for mothers not to work. A study design that uses such operations will now be discussed.[14]

COMPARISON OF SOCIAL SETTINGS

The theoretical paper by Hoffman and Wyatt (1960) was originally part of a proposed research project that did not materialize, but the design has implications for our present concerns. The theory, in brief, follows. The increased desire for three or more children reflects in part a change in motivation in response to several social trends. One pertains to technologically induced changes in the role of women, for example, the housewife role, which has ceased to be a satisfying or even legitimate full-time pursuit. Another is the rise in maternal employment, to the point where it is likely to occur as a conscious possibility to a woman whose youngest child enters school. These trends, together with the prevalence in America of the Protestant Ethic, result in a pressure on the woman to choose between the housewife and employment roles. For those who dislike both alternatives having another baby can postpone the choice. It gives the woman the chance to avoid work as well as unacceptable leisure, to have a role that is socially approved, creative, and demands her very special attention, and finally to remain dependent and continue in a traditionally feminine, circumscribed pattern. Other relevant trends are the cultural emphasis on child-rearing and the prevalent belief in environmentalism and the importance of the mother for the child, which added creativity and significance to motherhood just as these qualities were disappearing from the housewife role. Finally there are the themes of loneliness and alienation. The new baby or a large family may signify companionship to the mother, a fusion of self and child, a tie to immortality, as well as a meaningful status in society.

This theory has four levels: (1) social conditions (e.g., simplification of the housewife role and the fact of extensive maternal employment); (2) individual personality factors (e.g., dependency), which are partly a response to the social conditions and partly independent of them; (3) the value to the mother of a new child or a large family, which is partly a function of

[14] The problems in the Princeton study pointed up here largely reflect the absence of a well-developed overall theory. In the study eight personality variables were considered. Anxious-dependency (manifest anxiety), need to nurture, need for achievement, and ability to defer gratification are discussed above. Another, "cooperation," was expected to relate to desired family size and success in family planning, but the basis for the prediction is unclear. The mother's "self-awareness" was expected to relate to successful family planning because it did in the pretest. Neither "cooperation" nor "self-awareness" related as predicted. The remaining variables, "compulsivity" and "ambiguity tolerance," appear to be two sides of the same coin and are highly correlated with each other ($r=.41$). The expectation that they would relate to a large desired family size seems reasonable, and the relationships obtained are small but statistically significant.

the interaction between (1) and (2); and (4) fertility plans, which are obviously affected by (3). For example, the pressures toward employment may interact with strong dependency needs to make the prospect of having a new baby attractive. An assumption of this model is that the value of a child is too multidimensional to carry a one-to-one relationship with any single personality trait. The analysis is depicted schematically in Figure 2–1.[15]

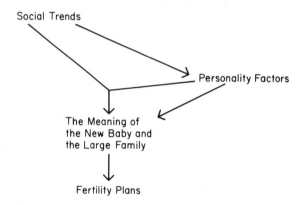

Figure 2–1. Relationships between the
Four Levels of the Theory.

Social Trends

Personality Factors

The Meaning of
the New Baby and
the Large Family

Fertility Plans

The theory requires a research design that taps all four of its levels. Limited space prevents a full treatment of the various types of measures that might be used, but we will discuss how the level of social conditions might be handled since this is perhaps the most difficult and challenging. In the particular study the aim was to handle the social conditions by operationalizing them in terms of contrasting situations within the same larger society and to keep the extraneous variables as similar as possible. Even within a society the social trends will affect some groups more than others. There are subgroup variations in the amount of time and effort required by the housewife role and its potential for creative satisfaction; the extent to which employment is a viable alternative; the nature and importance of childrearing beliefs; and the conditions that lead to alienation. The social situation of the respondent can be established through a variety of techniques, including interview questions about the respondent's friends and neighbors (e.g., whether they work, how they spend leisure time); her ties to the community and length of residence there; social and spatial distance from members of her extended family; belief in the Protestant Ethic. Though obtained through individual responses, such data can be the basis for

[15] The connection between the meaning of the new baby and fertility plans would actually be more complicated than it appears in Figure 2–1, because in this discussion the husband's views, practical matters, and competing factors are ignored.

operationally defining social conditions. (Most of the personality traits, and the value of a new baby and a large family, were to be tapped by focused and other types of depth interviews, projective tests designed specifically for the study, as well as more structured interview questions. Data on a fifth level, actual fertility behavior, were to be obtained in later follow-up interviews.)

Summary of Methodological Issues

The interest in research on the value of children is very new. It is inspired largely by concern with overpopulation and the belief that at least part of the solution will require curbing the desire for children. Because so little adequate data are available and because many studies on the topic will undoubtedly be launched in the next few years, it was decided to concentrate in this chapter on methodological issues, problems of conceptualization, and theory construction.

We discussed above the measurement and conceptualization of two questions: how much children are valued and for what qualities are they valued. The complex and multifaceted nature of the value of children was stressed. New though untried measures were reported to give the researcher interested in this area information about some of the possibilities, but a very basic need for instrumentation emerges from this review. When social problems are pressing there is a great temptation to cut short the laborious tasks of developing adequate measures, but it is in the end a disservice to report data that are not grounded in adequate research procedures.

Besides the complexities of conceptualizing and measuring the value of children, selected problems of interviewing procedures, the coding of data, and the interpretation of results were discussed. In dealing with issues of research design we stressed the need for normative data on the prevalence and salience of the value of children and for studies relating these values to independent variables, such as technological change, and to dependent variables, especially fertility motivation and behavior. The question of which fertility behavior (e.g., desired family size, wanting another child) is relevant for which value came up in discussing the Princeton study, as it will again in another context in the next section. In addition, attention was given to the unit of analysis (groups or countries versus individuals).

Particular stress was put on the need for more complex research designs. For a dynamic analysis relationships should be examined within specified social contexts. Predictions based on the interaction of variables will be far more worthwhile than the simple correlations between two variables that have characterized past research.

A Theoretical Approach

Clearly there is a need for a theoretical model useful for the study of variations in fertility behavior and more specifically of cultural differences and historical trends in the motivation to have children. One of the important dynamic elements in such a model is the way in which children are valued. In this section of the chapter we will present a scheme for conceptualizing the value of children so that this variable can be used in a wide variety of theories—sociological as well as psychological. We will also discuss in somewhat less detail the other elements to be considered in the theoretical model. Finally we will present our notions as to how these variables interact, respond to social change, and affect the motivation to have children.

A review of the literature reveals that the existing theories do not deal with the variety of values that might be served by children. Thus there are theories about the economic value of children, but their ability to make accurate predictions about fertility is limited by the fact that although non-economic values are acknowledged, they are not incorporated into the theories in any meaningful way. On the other hand, there are the "listers" who through empirical work or thoughtful analysis present long lists of the values (or of the motivations) with no effort even to organize them into useful homogeneous categories. The combinations are so helter-skelter that it is impossible to compare the empirical findings of one study with those of another or to relate the noneconomic values reported by parents to other variables measured in the study. The empirical groupings are generally based on classifying the respondents' answers to such questions as "What are the advantages of large families?" The resulting categories have been too broadly inclusive (e.g., advantages for the parent versus advantages for existing children in the family) or too vague (e.g., the respondent's "liking for children"), in either case lacking enough specificity to be useful; or they have been lacking in psychological unity (e.g., one study grouped the prestige that comes from having children with the assurance of the continuity of the family).

It seems then that a necessary first step is to provide a conceptual framework consisting of values that are anchored in particular psychological needs, tied to the social structure and influenceable by it, and subject to cultural variation. The values should be capable of being satisfied by some aspect of parenthood, although alternative satisfactions might be possible. They should be grouped on the basis of their psychological unity; that is, the values in a group would be based on relatively homogeneous needs. Another important aim is that the conceptual scheme be all-inclusive—capable of incorporating the many values that children provide in various cultures.

Toward these ends a set of values was constructed from a comprehensive examination of the research and theoretical literature. There has as yet been no real empirical search for a comprehensive list of values, however; and, indeed, as mentioned earlier, there is a paucity of useful normative data on those that are known. The list presented on pages 46–47 is best seen as a tentative and open code, subject to modification on the basis of future work.

There is one important value that is excluded—the biological value of children. This was deliberately omitted because it did not seem to fit the criteria of being tied to the social structure and being subject to cultural variation. The biological theories that deal with motives for pregnancy or maternal behaviors that occur as a result of pregnancy need not be a concern, for they do not deal directly with the motives for parenthood or the value of children. On the other hand, the recent work of the ethologists, although it does not fit into the value scheme, is quite relevant to the general topic, and it will be considered before discussing more fully the scheme and the theoretical model.

THE BIOLOGICAL VALUE OF CHILDREN—AN ETHOLOGICAL POSITION

The basic ethological point of view about maternal behavior, given by Lorenz (1965) and summarized by Hess (1970), is that:

. . . there is a releaser that is very widespread in the animal kingdom. This releaser is the quality we call "babyishness." If the young and adults of several species are compared for differences in bodily and facial features it will be seen readily that the nature of the differences is apparently the same almost through-out the phylogenetic scale. Limbs are shorter and much heavier in proportion to the torso in babies than in adults. Also, the head is proportionately much larger in relation to the body than is the case with adults. On the face itself the fore-head is more prominent and bulbous; the eyes large and perhaps located as far down as below the middle of the face, because of the large forehead. In addition, the cheeks may be round and protruding. In many species there is also a greater degree of overall fatness in contrast to normal adult bodies. [P. 20]

These physical attributes are further enhanced by behavioral ones such as clumsiness. When an object possesses some of these characteristics it releases in most people some typical affects and behavior patterns—mainly a desire for physical contact, holding, hugging, and cuddling. Bowlby (1958) stresses the baby's inborn reactions of crying, smiling, clasping, and follow-ing, which he claims serve to release appropriate caretaker affect and behavior. This is the basis for the strong bond between parent and child, which Bowlby calls the "primary tie."

Hess summarizes the findings of several relevant experimental studies. One study by Hess and Polt (1960) found that "women's eye pupils en-larged considerably when they looked at pictures of babies, whereas men's pupils showed very little change in size." In a later study by Hess (1967) people were shown drawings of human and animal faces that were progres-sively stylized "toward greater and greater babyishness in the appearance of the faces, culminating in the Walt Disney type portrayal of infant and animal babies." A positive correlation was found between the degree of babyishness in the drawings and the degree to which the viewers' pupils increased in size. Hess concludes that these findings support the ethological notion that the quality of babyishness definitely has positive appeal. He also suggests (Hess, 1970) that these findings show:

> . . . that in man as in other animals, social prescriptions and customs are not the sole or even primary factors that guarantee the rearing and protection of babies. This seems to indicate that the biologically rooted releaser of "babyishness" may have promoted infant care in primitive man before societies were ever formed, just as it appears to do in many animal species. Thus this releaser may have a high survival value for the species of man. [P. 21]

Thus the possibility that children have a biologically based value is not at all disproved, and there is a respected body of experimental findings that support it. Naturally this does not mean that all persons are equal in this regard, it does not mean that having children is a biological necessity, and it does not mean that the biological value is more compelling than the social ones. It does mean, however, that it may be one of the many factors that affect the motivation to have children, and as such precise prediction and control requires that biological factors be considered.[16] The biological hypothesis, however, is not useful for explaining cultural variations and historical trends. It has therefore been omitted from the value scheme and the discussion that follows.

The Value Scheme

The value scheme consists of nine categories or basic values; these are listed below. In the discussion of each value empirical data will be brought in only illustratively since, with the exception of some of the findings on the economic-utilitarian value, the data have the deficiencies pointed out in the first section of this chapter. Because of prevalent shortcomings and the lack of standardization in the measuring instruments, sampling and data-collection procedures, and coding categories, statistics would be misleading.

THE VALUE OF CHILDREN

1. Adult status and social identity
2. Expansion of the self, tie to a larger entity, "immortality"
3. Morality: religion; altruism; good of the group; norms regarding sexuality, impulsivity, virtue

---

[16] The idea of vulnerability to pregnancy because of a deeply felt but short-lived impulse to have a child comes up occasionally in the data reported by Rainwater (1965, p. 163). For example, a wife who has resolved to have no more children picks up a friend's baby and says to her husband, "You'd better get me out of here," and the husband reports "I feel the same way myself when I see a cute baby on TV or in a magazine." Whether based on biology or learning theory, such stimulus-based impulse motivation is particularly interesting since whether pregnancy is the outcome will depend on a number of conditions that are subject to social control. Consider, for

4. Primary group ties, affiliation
5. Stimulation, novelty, fun
6. Creativity, accomplishment, competence
7. Power, influence, effectance
8. Social comparison, competition
9. Economic utility

ADULT STATUS AND SOCIAL IDENTITY

More than finishing school, going to work, or even getting married, parenthood establishes a person as a truly mature, stable, and acceptable member of the community and provides him access to other institutions of adult society. This is especially true for women, for whom motherhood is also defined as their major role in life. It is not only that the mass media present all "adjusted" adult women as mothers, or that popular opinion stresses this view, but also that in the United States as elsewhere not many acceptable alternative roles are available especially for lower-class, uneducated women. Furthermore, females are typically socialized with the expectation that they will become mothers, and this is the major status that the child growing up in the nuclear family sees the mother enacting. The occupational pursuits of both parents are unreal to the child because they are enacted away from the home, but the mother's role at home is visible and, particularly when the children are young, more heavily stressed than any paid employment she might also have. The childhood fantasies of girls include being a mother; from an early age they view motherhood as the essence of being a woman, and they often find the concept of being an adult woman without children difficult to comprehend ("Is she a girl or a mommy?").

Motherhood is thus the normal culmination of the socialization process for girls. It signifies to all concerned that she is on the right track as a developing woman. This is perhaps why when asked "How does having children change a woman's life?" women will often give such responses as "children provide a goal in life," "they are a fulfillment," "you really grow up," and "having children is what women are made for"—although, as discussed earlier, negative responses to this question are also given.

Stolka and Barnett (1969), in one of the studies criticized earlier, report that women tend to view "women's role" as a more important reason for having children than prestige, religion, and marital happiness. The value of giving adult status and identity to women would appear to be most influential with respect to the first child. Subsequent births, however, may provide needed reconfirmation especially at certain points in the life cycle, for example, when the youngest child is old enough to go to school (Hoffman and Wyatt, 1960).

---

example, a birth-control technique that required a period of time—several weeks perhaps or at least a trip to the doctor—to restore fertility as compared to one that required a minor lapse in diligence against pregnancy.

EXPANSION OF THE SELF

Perhaps in response to the evanescent quality of life, many people feel the need to anchor themselves beyond their own lifetime. Having children may satisfy this need because it is a way of reproducing oneself, having one's characteristics reflected in another who will live longer, and thus attaining a kind of immortality. Swain and Kiser (1953) report that 75 percent of the respondents in the Indianapolis study, husbands and wives, gave affirmative answers when asked "Is one of your greatest satisfactions in being a parent knowing that after you are gone some part of you will live on in your children?" Seventy-three percent also gave affirmative answers to "Do you get a big 'kick' out of seeing your children do things they have seen you do?" Both questions, however, have the shortcoming indicated in the first section—they seem to invite acquiescence rather than introspective responses.

The "carrying on of the family name" or "continuation of the family" is a reason for wanting children that comes up often in American studies, such as Rainwater's, and also in studies in India (Mysore Population Study, 1961; Poffenberger, 1969), Ghana (Caldwell, 1967, 1968) and the Philippines (Guthrie, 1968). Men tend to express this view more often than women (Rainwater, 1965; Clare and Kiser, 1952; Mysore Population Study, 1961), although a slight reversal of this trend was found in one study (Caldwell, 1968). The potential salience of this value is indicated in the Poffenberger study, where Indian men were asked to state the benefits of having a wife. Though the question did not mention children, a frequently cited benefit was the continuation of the family lineage, e.g., "so our descent will continue" and "to continue the generation." This response was more common than sex, helping with problems, or caring for the children and second only to performing services for the husband and looking after his needs.

Children also help expand the parent's self-conception in two other ways. The first is by providing larger entities—the parent-child dyad, the family. The feeling that one has ties to the larger society, that one is an organic part of the community and its basic life processes, must inevitably be enhanced by the experience of having and rearing children. The second is by evoking new, and for most parents previously untapped, dimensions of personality, such as the feeling of being essential and the desire to protect another human being, which stimulate further development and expansion of the self.

Children are a tie to the past also, in that the parent passes on much that he received from his own parents—values, folklore, songs—to his own children. And in general children may help provide continuity and thus unify a person's emerging identity as a parent, with both (1) his childhood expectations of becoming a parent, which may also be the ultimate fulfillment of the motive to identify with his own parent, and (2) his future expectations, which revolve to a great extent around the growth and development of his child.

MORALITY

Childbearing is often viewed as a moral act—one that involves giving up one's own interest for the sake of another person, community welfare, religious tradition, or norms supporting impulse inhibition, hard work, and so forth.

Religion. Religion often contributes to the definition of parenthood as moral. As Pohlman (1969, p. 45) notes, in the Judeo-Christian tradition "children were often viewed as blessings from heaven and barrenness as a curse, sometimes as a punishment for some particular misdeed." Some religions teach that "children must be born in order to reach heaven, or to free souls from bondage, or to permit souls to go on their way in a cycle of transmigration" (p. 75). Rainwater (1965) points out that the fundamentalist religious orientation of some Negro lower-class mothers emphasizes the moral virtue inherent in motherhood. Some lower-class parents regard birth as a "token of heaven's favor." ("We've done everything we can to have one . . . I think we will have children when God feels we are worthy of them." "When we wanted a child we prayed. I really don't think I would have become pregnant except for prayer.") And according to some religions children are needed to perform one's death rituals. Sons are needed among Orthodox Jews, for example, to say prayers for their dead parents and among certain groups in India to "carry the dead bodies of their parents and burn them with care . . ." (Poffenberger, 1969). The view that having children is "God's will," "a sign of God's blessing," or "will fulfill God's commands" has been found in India (Poffenberger, 1969), Kenya (Dow, 1967; Heisel, 1968; Martin, 1970), East Java (Gille and Pardoko, 1966), and the Philippines (Guthrie, 1968).

The influence of Catholic ideology underlies one of the best documented findings in the fertility literature: that Catholics have a greater desire for large families than non-Catholics. Some specific findings of interest, reported by Rainwater (1965), are that in all classes but the lower-lower, Catholics want more children than Protestants; nearly 60 percent of middle-class Catholics say they want five or more children; and nine out of ten middle-class Catholic men who want large families include their religion as one of the reasons. On the other hand, Westoff et al. (1963) found that only a minority of Catholic women believed their religion favored large families although they knew it discouraged birth control.

Altruism. Having children provides the opportunity to be altruistic because of the sacrifices the parent must make. Not wanting a child may therefore make one appear irresponsible and selfish. Evidence for this and for the idea that a large family makes people feel virtuous was obtained by Rainwater (1965). In addition to the general perception of the deliberately childless woman as "totally self-involved," he also found that men who want large families see those who want small families as "simply catering to their own convenience and as selfishly concerned to have more goods and time" (p. 178). Over half the men who wanted large families characterized those who wanted small families as "selfish." Rainwater's interpretation is that part of these men's desire for large families stems from a wish to avoid a selfish identity and to be regarded by themselves and others as men who are willing to give of themselves. These findings were not obtained for women who, though they wanted large families, seemed to understand that wanting a small family might signify a concern for providing for the children rather than selfishness. Rainwater also reports that a subsample of middle-class mothers who criticized themselves for being too egocentric or selfish more often expressed a preference for large families than middle-class women who criticized themselves for other reasons. Rainwater's interpretation is that the women who want large families are "reaching out to embrace an identity in which they are loving and creative persons and to deny or overcome tendencies to seek purely self-centered gratifications" (p. 195).

Good of the Group. Having children may also provide the opportunity for a totally different kind of altruism: doing something to help perpetuate one's group. The desire to have large families for the "national good" has been found in Ghana (Caldwell, 1967, 1968) and Kenya (Dow, 1967; Martin, 1970). The Poffenbergers (1969) report that none of their Indian respondents mentioned national or community welfare as a reason for having large families, but a small number mentioned the importance of sons for maintaining the fame and status of their caste.

The current view in this country is that family size should be reduced—here and elsewhere. Barnett (1970) reports that although national public opinion polls in 1965 and 1967 found 54 percent considered population growth a serious problem, his own data indicate that "concern with population growth is distinct from an attitude emphasizing responsibility on the part of the individual married couple to limit its fertility because of overpopulation" (p. 60). Poffenberger, Bachman, and Weiss (1970) report that nearly two-thirds of a national sample of post-high school age boys recognized population growth as a potential problem for this country (although less important than Vietnam, race relations, pollution, and inflation). These were mostly white subjects. On the other hand, Buckhout and his colleagues (1971) found that black and Chicano college students supported the idea of having *more* children as a way of helping their group against the oppressive white majority. According to the authors "the consensus . . . was that the population explosion was not as bad as the 'white establishment' sees it." To the question, "Why do you consider it so important to have children?" a Chicano respondent said: "Because it is a natural role of humanity, and also because it is a hope that our *raza* has. We should double the actual number of Chicanos as soon as possible." The authors also state that the unfortunate semantic loading of the term "population control" produced a predictable reaction from the politically conscious black students; for example, "Black people need more power and you can't have power without people; birth control for blacks is legalized genocide. . . ." The equating of fertility with political power is also discussed by Newman (1970, p. 835), who describes newspaper accounts of the greater success of birth-control programs among Indian residents of Fiji than among Fijian residents. These accounts point up the political advantage—more voters—that will eventually accrue to the Fijians if the trend continues. (Newman makes the general point that when "one has been convinced that voter registration is important, it is not a long step to the idea that the more voters to register, the better," and she goes on further to suggest that the largest structural obstacle to acceptance of family planning is "distrust of policies carried out for subordinate groups by dominant groups, no matter how eloquently they are couched in terms of the subordinate group's self-interest.")

Norms Regarding Sexuality, Impulsivity, Virtue. In the United States motherhood has tended to be viewed as an end to sexuality. In the mass media being a mother (or loving one's mother) means virtue. The advertisements for hair dyes, for example, showing lovely ladies with babies and referring to their motherhood, clearly seem designed to take the wickedness out of dyeing one's hair. Rainwater (1960) reports that the lower-class men he interviewed frequently express concern about their wives "going bad." They tend to view "mother" and "good woman" as synonymous, and one way of being certain that a wife will stay a good woman is to have a houseful of children. Being a father is also an enormous source of self-respect for the lower-class man and may compensate for his moral and other shortcomings.

It seems likely in such a social context that pregnancy and motherhood will help a woman feel virtuous and give her a sense of worth where there are not many alternatives. She may also welcome the fact that motherhood gives stability and structure to her life and thus provides an escape from impulsivity and too much freedom—an anchor that keeps her from the wanton life that may sometimes beckon. Such feelings are apt to be unconscious, certainly not readily articulated in response to direct questions about children. A person easily thinks of the fact that children "tie you down" and may realize that he wants his spouse to be tied down, but he will not often be aware of his own desire to be tied down.[17]

[17] There are related moral factors concerning the use of contraceptives, but these are not taken up here because they do not bear directly on the value of children. For example, the lower-middle and lower classes, especially Catholics, often associate the use of contraceptive devices—condoms, in particular—with premarital sex and venereal disease (Rainwater, 1965). This association militates against their use within marriage where sex is supposed to be "respectable." A practical implication of this point is that where marital and extramarital sex are sharply differentiated with respect to morality, the use of contraceptives in marriage would be more acceptable if devices specifically for use in marriage were readily available.

As a final comment on social norms, it may be noted that bearing and rearing a large family also may be viewed as useful, difficult, and at times unpleasant work that does not permit idleness and therefore meets the requirements of the Protestant Ethic. One may feel virtuous for this reason. The special significance of the Protestant Ethic for the value of children comes up at several points in this chapter.

PRIMARY GROUP TIES, AFFILIATION

The affiliative value of children is particularly important and has been reported in a wide variety of cultures. The significance of the nuclear family as a bulwark against the impersonalization of modern society has been noted by Durkheim (1951), described by Cooley (1920), and reasserted in sociological and psychological writings through the years. Nothing in the intervening years has occurred to diminish the importance of the family as the major primary group. On the contrary, the increase in geographical mobility, the increased size and bureaucratization of various community institutions like schools, churches, and places of employment, all tend to increase the very special role of the nuclear family as the one important primary group that has permanence. Evidence for the "avoidance of loneliness" and companionship as reasons for having large families has been obtained among Americans and also among parents in other cultures (Whelpton et al., 1966; Rainwater, 1965; Caldwell, 1967; Heisel, 1968; Martin, 1970).

The possibility that children provide more affiliative value than a husband or wife comes up in a number of studies. In the national survey by Gurin et al. (1960), respondents, as noted earlier, felt more positive toward their children than toward their mates and stressed the interpersonal satisfactions of their parenthood but the extrinsic satisfactions of their marriage. In two studies the majority of respondents said they believed children were necessary for a happy marriage (Centers and Blumberg, 1954; Christopherson and Walters, 1958). In another study, lower-class wives indicated that children created a common interest with their husbands where little existed before (Lopata, 1971).

The affiliative value of children is apt to be especially important for the wife. Both Rainwater (1960) and Komarovsky (1967) stressed the desire on the part of the lower-class wife for more affection from her husband than she received. For these women children became a major source of affection. Rainwater (1965) in fact sees the effect of social class as largely taking place through the conjugal role organization of the family. The more segregated role relationship that characterizes the lower class contributes to marital dissatisfaction and thus is a primary contributor to large family size. In describing lower-class mothers, Rainwater (1960, p. 87) states: "Children come to represent an avenue of compensation for their husbands' lack of affection." He also suggests further:

Even when the sense of distance in the marital relation is not so great, these women often find it easier to relate to their children in affectionate ways than to their husbands. The children (at least when young) seem easier to manage and arouse fewer conflicts than does the difficult task of relating to grown men whom they do not understand too well and of whom they are often a little afraid. [P. 87]

In the middle class the husband's career sometimes prevents him from satisfying his wife's affective needs (Bailyn, 1970). And for the wife in both social classes the affection of her children may endure even though the marriage ends in divorce or widowhood. Although this chapter has focused on the married, it is possible that children are sometimes valued as a source of affection to unmarried women as well.

The focus here has been on the woman, and there are empirical data that suggest that women's needs for affection are greater than men's and that the socialization of men tends to inhibit their ability to supply affection to their wives (Hoffman, 1972). In describing the parent-child relationship women more often than men refer to love, affection, and companionship (Gurin et al., 1960; Meade, 1971). It is possible, however, that children provide for men one of the few relationships where they can express warmth and tenderness.

STIMULATION, NOVELTY, FUN

People want change and new experiences, especially when life is reasonably secure but dull and routine. To anticipate having children is to anticipate introducing a major change in one's life. Children add an element of unpredictability and excitement to the home. Observing them grow, develop, and change is a unique opportunity for the long-range and continuous experience of novelty and variety. Rainwater (1965) describes one of the mothers in his sample as feeling "more alive because of the variegated emotional exchange, both giving and getting, which her five-person household allows her." Several respondents stress that each additional child is a new experience. To quote two of Rainwater's respondents talking about the effects of children on the home atmosphere, "something new is always happening"; "there's never a dull moment around here."

Aside from stimulation and novelty, children can add an element of sheer pleasure, fun, and excitement. In playing with their children parents can legitimately experience the joy of reliving their own youth, both directly and vicariously, through the child. If upset about aging they can take up once again the role of a younger adult by having another child. Several studies in the United States and elsewhere attest to the widespread feeling that children are fun, a "pleasure to be with," and a "source of happiness" to their parents (Poffenberger, 1969; Komarovsky, 1967; Caldwell, 1967, 1968; Mysore Population Study, 1961; Heisel, 1968). This appears to be true for men as well as women, though there is some evidence that it is more true of women (Mysore Population Study, 1961; Poffenberger, 1969). In the Meade study using the projective story-telling technique already described, women college students stressed the joys and happiness that children bring to a greater extent than men (Meade, 1971).

By virtue of the spontaneity and lack of awareness of the parent's problems, children may often help the parent take his mind off his problems. The routine that children impose and their insensitivity to what, from the adult point of view, is a great concern or misfortune may help the parents maintain an equilibrium. Children conduct business as usual, and by their activity and play they may help the parents to feel that their worries are not so important, to put them in perspective, or to keep excesses of grief within socially required bounds. The fact that a child's play resembles his own when he was a child may also contribute to the parent's security since it communicates some stability in a world of change. The role of the child in distracting the parent from his worries has not been studied, but a respondent in the Mysore Population Study made a relevant comment: "No other thing in the world makes me forget my worries except children."

CREATIVITY, ACCOMPLISHMENT, COMPETENCE

When society advances beyond the subsistence level and large numbers of people have the necessities of life, needs for creativity, achievement, and accomplishment may emerge (Maslow, 1955), and rearing children may provide an outlet for such needs. Indeed, a central theme of the Hoffman-Wyatt formulation (1960) discussed earlier is that housework is no longer an avenue for creative expression, while the rearing of children, on the other hand, has gained recognition as a significant and challenging role even though it is also anxiety producing.

Parents may thus gain a sense of creativity, accomplishment, and achievement, not only from physically producing a child, but also from meeting the challenges and crises that inevitably occur as part of the rearing process and from observing the child's responses to their efforts. The view that parents gain such feelings from children has been found in upper-, middle-, and lower-class Americans, black as well as white (Centers and Blumberg, 1954; Rainwater, 1965). This view is generally expressed more often by men than women (Gurin et al., 1960; Meade, 1971).[18]

POWER, INFLUENCE, EFFECTANCE

In some cultures parenthood dramatically changes the power of the parent, particularly the mother. For example, in the Indian village studied by the Poffenbergers (Poffenberger, 1968; Poffenberger, 1969) the new bride moves into the village of her husband's family and lives in a subservient role to her mother-in-law. The emphasis in marriage is on her reproductive capacity and her major function is to bear sons, at least one of whom must live. If

---

[18] We have noted earlier that the affiliative value of children is more important to women than to men. The importance of achievement to males and affiliation to females is a sex difference found as early as the preschool ages (Hoffman, 1972). Rainwater (1965) reports a possibly contradictory finding in the upper-middle and upper-lower classes: women are more likely than men to give "accomplishment" and "sense of fulfillment" as reasons for having large families. Data are not presented, however, that would enable us to tell how much of the difference is in "achievement" alone.

she succeeds she gains some control over her own life and over her childless sisters-in-law. Eventually when her son marries and brings home a bride she comes into her own. "The shy young girl of 14 to 16 years who came to her in-law's family could become the powerful and dominating mother-in-law at a later stage in the family life cycle but she could gain this status in only one way—through having one or more living sons" (1969, p. 114).

Even in America there is evidence that for those wives who have very little power, motherhood provides them with the courage to make demands, and these demands are more respected than they would have been previously. The daughter-in-law with children seems to have more influence with her husband's family, and she can exert more influence on her husband as well, partly "for the sake of the children." Perhaps because motherhood gives the woman her official status as described earlier, her claim seems more legitimate in her own eyes, her husband's, and her in-laws'. Even with her own parents her motherhood serves a similar function. Not statistics, but descriptive materials support this hypothesis (Rainwater, 1965; Komarovsky, 1967). On the other hand, statistically, the *more* children she has, the less power the wife exerts even with social class and religion controlled (Hoffman, 1958, 1963d; Blood and Wolfe, 1960; Heer, 1963). An adequate analysis of the actual relationship between the mother's power and the number of children would have to consider the possibility of a curvilinear relationship. Furthermore, power in the family is a complex variable, and different aspects may operate quite differently. For example, more control over household routines may be accompanied by less control over major family decisions (Hoffman and Lippitt, 1960; Blood, 1963).

Children also afford both parents unique opportunities for another form of power—the chance to guide, teach, control, and generally exert enormous influence over another human being. The parents control the material and emotional supplies needed by the child, and for a considerable period they are physically stronger and allowed by law to use physical coercion to impose their will. Indeed, the power of a parent over a child is almost without parallel. The lower-class man and woman have few, if any, other opportunities to exercise power over others, and many of their interactions with others, on their jobs and in relations with various social agencies, place them in the position of the one over whom power is exercised. There is some evidence for the idea of a pecking order. For example, the more power assertive the lower-class man is toward his wife, the more power assertive the wife is toward the child. There are also data that the lower-class father is more power assertive toward his child than the middle-class father (M. Hoffman, 1963). However, there are no studies of the relation between class and the husband's direct assertion of power over his wife, although middle-class fathers do have a larger say in major family decisions (Blood and Wolfe, 1960).

Perhaps more important than any of the aspects of power discussed thus far is the "effectance" that having children represents. Having a child is one way to have an effect—an impact—on one's own life and on that of others. The significance of the new baby for change and stimulation has already been discussed. What is important here is that this effect is in the parent's control. Many of the values of children are expressed by the lower-class black woman in Cole's study quoted earlier, but an important theme in her response is this idea: the ability to have an effect lies rather exclusively in having children. For the lower classes of both sexes, for the very young, and for women of all classes, a new baby can be a major influence on their lives and those of others. There are few other such opportunities.

A few studies have examined relationships between the feeling of powerlessness and fertility behavior. Kar (1971) found that people who felt powerless were less likely to use contraceptives, and Groat and Neal (1967) found a similar variable positively related to family size, though only among Catholics. The authors of these studies offer different explanations for their findings, but it is possible that one value of children is that producing and molding a human being gives one a sense of "effectance," particularly when in general one feels powerless.

SOCIAL COMPARISON, COMPETITION

Children can give their parents prestige and competitive advantage in a variety of ways. The most obvious example is when the competition occurs with respect to number. This frequently occurs in nonindustrialized cultures (Newton, 1967) and sometimes in the United States. Where birth control is not practiced, the number of children is a public demonstration of the parents' sexuality, and Catholic couples, for example, often take pride in their fertility as a manifestation of potency, fecundity, and marital love. Particularly where finances are not severely strained, there may be considerable prestige in having a large, healthy, happy family. Whether the current concern with overpopulation is cutting into the prestigeful aspects of the large family is unknown. It does not seem to have had a remarkable effect on ideal family size (Blake, 1971).

Hoffman and Wyatt (1960) suggest several social comparison advantages of the large family. For example, the parent's expertise among his peers increases with increasing number. They also suggest that the other achievements of the woman, in community activities, career, or in physical attractiveness, are enhanced if she is also the mother of a large brood.

The competitive value of children can be expressed in other ways, however. For example, while competition with one's parents can lead to trying to outdo them in number of children produced, it can also lead to the opposite behavior. Having fewer children than one's parents can be an indication of planning, emancipation, and social mobility. Furthermore, competition with parents, siblings, friends, and enemies can lead to a concentration on quality rather than quantity. There are no relevant data, but it seems likely that children in the United States are valued, at least among some groups, more for their vicarious achievement possibilities than for their number. The batting average in the Little League and the financial or professional status eventually achieved by the child may be important sources of prestige to the parents.

ECONOMIC UTILITY

By far the most frequently studied value of children is their economic utility. In fact it is one of the few that has been directly linked to desired family size and even to contraceptive use. In Mueller's (1970) study in Taiwan the parents' perception of children as economically useful was found to be related positively to the desire for a large family. The sensitivity to the expenses involved in rearing children, "cost sensitivity," on the other hand, was also measured and found to be associated with the desire for a small family. Parents who saw little utility in having large families and those who indicated cost sensitivity were also more likely to practice contraception. Further, the perceived utility of children was negatively related to the parents' education and income; and the perceived costs were positively related to education and the desire for consumer goods.

That children in the developing countries, and particularly in areas where a rural economy predominates, are valued for economic reasons is well documented. The most common answers obtained in these areas to questions about why people want large families, why the respondent wants more children, and what is good about having children pertain to the economic value of children. The answers are usually phrased either in terms of the economically valuable work children perform when they are young or the old-age security they provide for the parents. In addition children may be economically valued for the "bridewealth" they bring in and also for their utility in assisting with household chores and the care of other children (Heisel, 1968; Dow, 1967; Martin, 1970; Guthrie, 1968; Mysore Population Study, 1961; Poffenberger, 1968; Caldwell, 1967, 1968; Newton, 1967).

The percentage of respondents who value children for economic reasons may be even higher than some of the figures indicate because other answers that are not coded as economic may nonetheless represent economic motives. For example, having many children to be sure one son will survive is often treated separately, although it may derive from the need for the son to care for the parents in their old age.[19] It is also interesting that in Mueller's research in Taiwan (1970), as mentioned earlier, only 12 percent of the respondents, when asked directly to list the advantage of a large family, included the financial help they would expect to receive from the children later in life. When asked about economic expectations in old age, however, fully 73 percent indicated that their children were to be their major source of support.

---

[19] This category may also include the noneconomic value of having a son to perform religious rituals after the parent's death or to carry on the family name. Unfortunately, as pointed out earlier, the quality of the responses and the coding of the data are typically too ambiguous to make such distinctions.

The importance of the economic value of children declines with increased industrialization and urbanization, the rise of cash in place of subsistence farming, increased pressures to send children to school, and an increase in the educational level of the parents. This pattern has been found within developing countries and in comparisons between countries (Caldwell, 1967; Siddiqui, 1967; Mueller, 1970). It should also be noted that the same parents who stress the economic value of children are not unaware of their economic cost. For a number of reasons, however, the positive economic values may come out ahead. In some cases, as often occurs in an agricultural economy, an economic need may exist for which there is no alternative but children. The nature of farming is such that there is a seasonal demand for labor rather than a steady demand. But finding workers who can be hired and fired depending on the seasons is difficult, especially when all the other industries are farms operating on the same schedule. The poor farmer cannot afford to pay for labor that is not needed, and the laborer cannot live in an area where there is no income for long periods. One's own children, on the other hand, can help with farm work even when very young. Despite their cost, therefore, having children may be viewed as a necessity.

Another example of the preeminence of the economic value of children occurs when the economy is so close to subsistence that saving for one's old age or disability is impossible; if there is no government or private charitable institution to provide adequate care under these circumstances, then where else can one turn except to one's children? Parents and relatives of one's own age will be in the same difficult position and cannot provide help. Furthermore, in some cases, as in many parts of India, it is possible only for sons to help, since the married daughter serves her husband and his family, not her own. It is interesting to note that a statistical computation by Heer and May (1968) indicated that in a country with a life expectancy of fifty years, five children would be necessary for the couple to be 95 percent certain that one son would survive until the father's sixty-fifth birthday. Poffenberger (1968) notes that this figure seems to be the very one the Indian villagers have arrived at also, undoubtedly using more empirical than statistical procedures. Clearly from their answers the villagers are aware that to be assured of a son for old-age care, a couple must bear more children than they can comfortably afford, and they usually arrive at a number between four and six.[20] It should also be noted in passing that whereas the "ability to defer gratification" is often treated by social scientists as though it were a special quality of the wealthier classes in industrialized nations, the poor Indian villagers in Poffenberger's study are willing to undergo considerable hardship in the early years of parenthood in order to obtain that support in old age. When asked why parents would want a *small* family, the usual response is in terms of the economic costs of children, yet these costs are tolerated for the expected benefits later in life.

[20] This is higher than the number they report as ideal (Poffenberger, 1968).

The negative value or cost of children is seen as economic in the developing countries particularly as the areas become more industrialized. At the same time that the economic assets of the child are declining, the economic liabilities are increasing. The child's ability to contribute financially to the wage-earning household is limited by his skills and the child labor laws. Furthermore, the child's help is less essential; that is, the farmer's own income may depend on his children, whereas the wage earner's income, however small, is independent of the family's efforts. Pressures to send children to school often accompany modernization trends, and thus the child's help is less available even though the school schedule in rural areas is sometimes adapted to the harvest needs. Schooling also involves added costs to the parents.

Various estimates have been made of the financial expenses involved in childrearing under different economic conditions, from subsistence farming through the various economic strata in America (Dublin and Lotka, 1946; Blood, 1962; Pohlman, 1969; Robinson and Horlacher, 1971). Complications and inconsistencies in these estimates arise because, apart from the actual cost of food, clothing, shelter, medical care, and education, there are different standards about what level of provision is adequate. Thus as economic well-being increases, the cost of each child increases because the standards become higher. In addition the parent's desire for competing consumer goods increases, and so also do the opportunities for the wife's employment, which become more difficult to take advantage of with additional children. Decreased-mortality effects, on the other hand, have not been considered and these would decrease financial costs; that is, in high-mortality areas parents may have to bear and care for several children for various periods in order to end up with one twelve year old. All of the estimates report that the cost of childrearing in absolute terms increases with an increased standard of living. It is also suggested, however, that as the income increases, the proportion of the total income that is spent on the child decreases. Robinson and Horlacher (1971) review various attempts to develop an economic theory of fertility. These use the economic theory model, but recognize the need to consider the nonmonetary value of children. The nonmonetary value of children, however, is, as stressed throughout this chapter, a complicated as well as crucial consideration. Furthermore, the whole issue of alternatives to children is not handled by the approaches to date, although it is clearly essential in predicting fertility. Where alternative sources of satisfaction are less, the desire for children might be greater.

Two different ways of looking at the social setting are implicit in the preceding discussion: rural versus urban and rich versus poor. The effects of urbanization are much clearer than the effects of wealth. In the rural setting as compared to the urban one the positive economic value of the child is high, the cost is low. With respect to wealth it can be said that in the absence of public provision the economic value of the child will be greater where the parents are too poor to save for old age and incapacities;

and furthermore, there may be differences in the kind of economic value a child may provide (e.g., ADC money versus help in the family business). But by and large there is no overwhelming effect of wealth on the child's economic contribution. On the other hand, wealth does affect the cost of the child as stated above: the absolute cost is greater among the wealthy, but the proportion of the income is less.[21]

The Economic-Utility Value of Children in the United States. The economic-utility value of children in the United States is very low. Although 75 percent of Rainwater's respondents mentioned economic costs as considerations concerning family size, no one mentioned children as economic assets. Only a few respondents mentioned the household help children give as a motivation for larger families. The Rainwater sample was an urban one, but in a national survey Whelpton et al. (1966) also found economic reasons the major ones given for a small family though never mentioned as a reason for a large one.[22] In short there is no evidence in the United States that children are raised for profit.

It is very likely true in the United States as elsewhere that the economic value of the farm child is greater than the city child and that his contribution starts at an earlier age, but there are no adequate data indicating that the value of the American farm child is seen by parents in economic terms nor that this is in itself a motive for fertility. With greater diversification of the economy and geographical mobility, it is easier to obtain hired hands when needed who do not need to be supported during the slack times; the laborers move to another area to seek jobs after the harvest. Thus children may be less essential to the farmer in America than in the developing countries. In any case there are better data on the value of children among farmers for India, Ghana, and Taiwan than for the United States.

The utility of children as household helpers may be lower in the United States than elsewhere because of the prevailing childrearing philosophies here. Although children do help with household tasks (Hoffman, 1958; Roy, 1963), parents are often concerned that children should not be overly burdened. In a study of third-through-sixth grade children Hoffman (1963c) found that less household assistance was given by children of employed mothers who liked their work than children of a matched sample of nonem-

---

[21] The nature of the competing economic goods may change with increased income to more durable goods, goods that require a long-term financial commitment, and goods that make more dramatic changes in one's life style. In fact the item being considered as an alternative to the child by the wealthier parent might be geared toward the very values that lead to the desire for the child, e.g., a summer home, travel. Such alternative goods would be more attractive and relevant and would also involve a commitment that postponed the additional child for many years.

[22] The figures are not comparable because Rainwater gives the percentage of respondents who gave any economic reasons; Whelpton et al. give the percentage who gave an economic reason as their first answer (54 percent). The questions were different also. In the latter study the questions actually followed a statement of desired or expected number and pertained to the reasons for not wanting a smaller family and for not expecting a larger one.

ployed mothers. In context the findings suggested that the employed mothers deliberately avoided imposing tasks on their children.

The Economic Setting and Noneconomic Values. The economic setting—whether the social class or the rural-urban dimension—may affect fertility behavior not just through its effect on the child's economic value but also because the life style associated with it may affect the noneconomic value of the child. Thus lower-class Americans may desire more children, as already noted, because they have fewer alternative sources of the non-economic values children provide. Children may be the lower-class man's only opportunities to feel effective, to have a sense of personal worth, to have power over another. The lower-class wife may find an affectionate response in her children that is lacking in her husband.

There is much in rural life to enhance the value of children aside from their economic contribution. Farm children are incorporated into the economic and social life of their parents to a degree that is rare in the city. An obvious example is the 4-H Club, but there are many other social gatherings that include the whole family and often have economic relevance. As a result, parents and children may be expected to have more in common, and any generation gap should be less severe than in urban families. The father can more readily envision himself as working and playing with a son who is identified with him and shares his interests—a replication of himself. Even though he has no children yet or only very young ones, this is what he sees around him and what he experienced with his own father. There is a continuity in the life style and frequently in the passing on of the farm ownership. All of this contributes to an extended sense of self in the father. Furthermore, the child has adult responsibilities at a very young age, such as driving a tractor at ten, and this also makes him more of a companion to the father. Finally, in the agricultural setting fertility per se is a meaningful value. Who wants a chicken that does not lay, or a bull that cannot effectively impregnate and produce good offspring? The cow that calves and gives milk is a proud possession. The whole concept of parenthood thus takes on a positive light, and this orientation may last even after the person so socialized has moved to the city.[23]

A Theoretical Model for Predicting Fertility Motivation

In the preceding discussion of the nine values that make up the scheme, some points have been made that should be highlighted:

Group Differences. Different values will be salient in different social structures and in different subgroups within a structure. In an agricultural setting, for example, the economic value of children will be high and so may certain noneconomic values such as "expansion of the self." For lower-class

[23] This last group of values is really derived from the economic value. That is, fertility is viewed so positively in the agricultural setting because of its past association with the economic value.

Americans the moral, competence, and power values are important; for lower-class women the affectional values are also probably high. There are differences between men and women, whites and blacks, and people in bureaucratic and entrepreneurial settings. Furthermore, these differences will change as other aspects of the social structure change, and as the relationship of the groups to the structure changes. Analysis of the societal factors involved is therefore important in predicting changes in fertility behavior.

Alternatives. To a considerable extent the differences between groups are a function of the alternatives to children that are available as sources of the values. Children may be particularly important to the lower class because they have fewer alternative sources of these values. To the extent that the role of housewife loses its potential for making a woman feel creative and competent, as well as moral in terms of the Protestant Ethic, the value of children may increase. As a final example, if India had an alternative to sons for economic security in old age, the value of children might diminish.

Values and the Number of Children Desired. Although all the values discussed are relevant to fertility, certain of them will affect the desire to have some children rather than none, others to have a new baby, and still others will be tied to a desire for many children. Which response is called forth by the value will be affected by the surrounding circumstances. To use examples that have already been cited, the economic value of children in India as old-age insurance requires a large family, as long as mortality rates are believed to be high and the sex of the child depends on chance. A change in either or both of these conditions would make it possible to obtain the same value with fewer children. Where social mobility is low and there is little possibility for the child to achieve, the achievement value may require having many children—the achievement being the sheer number of them. On the other hand, "my son, the doctor" represents the child as an achievement with the emphasis on quality.

For some values each successive child may be somewhat less important. That is, the first child transforms a girl into someone with status as adult and mother. The second may add substance to her role, but the impact is apt to be less. After she has a certain number of children, that value is fully satiated. The extent to which each successive child satisfies a value and the number needed for satiation will be different for the various values.

THE UNITS OF THE MODEL

The theoretical model consists of five classes of variables: (1) the value of children; (2) alternative sources of the value; (3) costs; (4) barriers; and (5) facilitators. *Values* have already been defined. *Alternatives* pertain to other avenues, besides children, for fulfilling a value. *Costs* refer to what must be lost or sacrificed to obtain a value in any particular way. The cost of children is usually expressed in economic terms or as the loss of freedom. The preponderance of economic reasons for having a small family has already been noted.[24] It has also been pointed out that "loss of freedom" was the modal answer given by mothers of elementary-school children in Detroit to the question "How does having children change a woman's life?" In the Detroit study another question asked was "What is the worst thing about having children?" Anxieties about the child's physical health and psychological and moral development were frequently mentioned (Hoffman, 1963a). These are also costs.

Barriers and *facilitators* refer to the factors that make it more difficult or easier to realize the particular value by having children. Among the barriers would be included economic depression or individual poverty, a shortage of space or housing, the mother's ill health, other demands on the mother's time, a belief that reproduction was wrong in view of the population explosion. Among the facilitators are economic prosperity, adequate space and housing, help with competing work and time demands, as well as pronatalist views either culturally prevalent or held by one's primary group.[25]

At its simplest the basic idea of the model is that fertility motivation can be analyzed in terms of these five concepts. They can be used to predict a given person's desire for children or the desires of a particular group. Changes elsewhere in the social structure might change any of the five and thus affect fertility motivation. Furthermore, if public welfare required a change in fertility motivation, a program could be launched by directing an attack toward these five points. The current suggestions for decreasing the desire for children can be so conceptualized. Both the suggestion to levy a tax on children and the proposal to offer financial rewards for nonfertility (Spengler, 1969; Kangas, 1970) attempt to cut down fertility motivation by increasing the cost. Attempts to convince the population of the need to keep family size down can be seen as efforts to erect barriers. These approaches, however, leave the hunger for children unsatisfied. They would thus meet with a great deal of resistance, and, indeed, evidence already mentioned indicates that concern with the population explosion, for example, does not have an overwhelming effect in curtailing family plans (Barnett, 1970). Moreover, if the restriction on family size were achieved through erecting costs and barriers without providing alternative satisfactions, fertility rates would rise again as soon as there was any weakening in these obstacles. In addition social discontent and other unintended consequences might result in the interim.

On the other hand, attention only to the value and alternatives is also inadequate because providing alternative satisfactions to one or more of the values might leave others still to be satisfied by having children. Further-

---

[24] The economic costs of children are reviewed in Pohlman (1969) and Robinson and Horlacher (1971).

[25] Just as there are costs, barriers, and facilitators that will affect motivations for children, there are costs, barriers, and facilitators that will affect motivations for the various alternative sources of the values.

more, the change involved in providing these alternatives might also have unanticipated effects on the costs, facilitators, or barriers. For example, if having children defines the American woman's major role, it would seem possible that an occupation could do this instead. Several recent writers have suggested this very approach, and some, as part of an antinatalist policy, have also advocated child-care centers and greater equalization between the sexes with respect to household and child-care activities in order to encourage women to seek employment. However, it is possible that the working women still want children for their other values, i.e., to satisfy other needs that are not met by their occupational pursuits. In this case child-care centers and role equalization *as a population policy* might back-fire since these changes would remove barriers to fertility and provide facilitators. The example of female employment as an alternative will be considered in detail since it is an application of the theoretical model that shows both its use and its complexities.

FEMALE EMPLOYMENT AS AN ALTERNATIVE TO MOTHERHOOD

Many articles in recent years have indicated a compatibility between the desire to curtail population growth and an increase in the occupational sphere of the woman's life. In some cases the authors suggest that female employment be encouraged in order to bring about a decrease in family size, and in some cases increased occupational opportunities have been seen as necessary compensation (e.g., Collver and Langlois, 1962; Hoffman, 1963a; Blake, 1965, 1969; Davis, 1967; Day and Day, 1969, 1970; Gill, 1970; Chilman, 1970; Farley, 1970).

It is well documented that working mothers in the United States have fewer children than comparable nonworking mothers and that among both children and adults, females who plan to work plan also to have smaller families (Ridley, 1959; Nye and Hoffman, 1963; Blake, 1965; Whelpton et al., 1966; Farley, 1970; Gustavus and Nam, 1970; U.S. Department of Labor, 1970). While the causal direction of these relationships has not been established, it is more than likely a mutually reinforcing pattern. Working is eased by curtailing family size, and willingness to curtail family size makes working more feasible and attractive. Furthermore, voluntary maternal employment may coexist with small family size because they are both manifestations of a similar orientation or role definition.

Before dealing with the employment-fertility relationship in terms of our model, a practical problem should be pointed out. Where will all the jobs come from? Won't a drop in the birth rate decrease the number of jobs available since a great many jobs, and particularly those now filled by women, involve providing services for children? As the percentage of children in the population is decreased, so, too, is the need for teachers, nurses, pediatricians, manufacturers and sellers of children's clothes and toys, and so forth, thus creating fewer jobs as we increase the number of job seekers (Rossi, 1965). This need not be an insurmountable problem, but it may require anticipatory planning and may entail considerable social and economic change.

Now let us look at the extent to which employment is an alternative to motherhood. There are two sets of relevant data. First, there is some evidence to suggest that employment is not an alternative in the United States, or at least not a very effective one, under present circumstances. The desire for large families may be lessened for employed women but not eliminated. Farley, for example, presents data that indicate over half of her respondents—all female graduate students at Cornell in May 1969—wanted three or more children.[26] Levine's data (1968) for graduate women at Yale are consistent with this, the majority wanting three or more children, and fully 82 percent of the women in law and medical schools wanting at least three. If highly educated women have such family plans, what about lower-class women who, as Chilman (1970) has pointed out, have less attractive jobs available and a life style that has centered around reproductive and childrearing functions?

Second, data from other cultures do not consistently support the idea of a negative relationship between employment and family size (Mysore Population Study, 1961; Safilios-Rothschild, 1969a; Gendell, 1965; Stycos and Weller, 1967). It has been pointed out by Stycos and Weller, Safilios-Rothschild, and Newman (1970) that where employment and mother roles are compatible, as where the extended family makes many surrogate mothers available, employment can be an adjunct to reproduction rather than an alternative, and the employment-fertility relationship may be depressed or nonexistent. Indeed, Stycos and Weller, in their study of fertility in Turkey, conceptualize female employment as though it were only a barrier to fertility. If they are correct, then the point made earlier might apply; that is, the policy of encouraging female employment by providing child-care facilities might have the adverse effect of enabling working women to have the larger families that the strain of the two roles heretofore has prevented. In terms of our model, if employment operates only as a barrier, help with child care will increase fertility, not decrease it.

In actuality female employment probably operates both as an alternative and as a barrier; for some groups it may be more of an alternative and for others, more of a barrier. Highly educated women are more likely to find intrinsically gratifying jobs that satisfy a number of the values now satisfied by children. Since child care and help with household tasks have been more available to this group, employment is not as major a barrier to having more children. The fact that employed women in this group have smaller families therefore suggests that employment may be a true alternative for them. The

---

[26] These figures are calculated from Farley's tables (1970) and are not reported in her analysis.

smaller family size of the less educated woman, on the other hand, may more often reflect employment as a barrier. Let us now examine the difference between classes in more detail.

There is considerable evidence that American women fear their own academic and career success and see it as a threat to their femininity. Komarovsky (1950) pointed up many years ago the pattern among college girls of holding back their intellectual ability because it was seen as jeopardizing their popularity. This has been discussed more recently by Maccoby (1963), Rossi (1965), Bardwick (1971), Hoffman (1972), and many others. Horner (1968) has shown that a story about a girl in medical school who is "at the head of her class" evokes anxiety responses in many college girls. The data suggest that career-oriented women may be concerned about their femininity. In America motherhood may be an antidote to these concerns. If careers for women became more acceptable and if opportunities for women were opened up, then the career might operate as a more attractive and less conflict-producing alternative to motherhood for those women whose education enabled them to obtain more interesting jobs. Looking at the list of values that children satisfy, the career might be more than an alternative *role* for this group of women. Depending on the particular career, almost any of the other values we have described might be obtained in this way—even the economic, which children in America rarely can provide. Childhood socialization practices, adult role prescriptions, and sex discrimination have all worked against this possibility (Hoffman, 1972), but new trends might make careers for women sufficiently acceptable that motherhood would not be necessary to prove one's femininity. Under these conditions the zero- and one-child family might become more prevalent for this group. Never modal, such small families have been more common among urban educated women in Western Europe than in the United States, and it would be interesting to study some of the differences between these two groups of women with respect to self-concepts, childrearing aims, conjugal relationships, and social roles (Safilios-Rothschild, 1969b).

For the less educated woman the picture is quite different. Elsewhere we have analyzed some of the alternative gratifications that even unskilled employment can offer women, including stimulation, a sense of competence, and money (Hoffman, 1963a). However, these satisfactions were analyzed primarily as supplements to motherhood and alternatives to housework. Can the kind of jobs available to the uneducated woman adequately fulfill the values now provided by children? It seems likely that they cannot, that the uneducated employed mothers want more children than they have, and that their smaller family size results from not having adequate supplementary help with child care and household tasks. Thus if such help were provided, as it should be for reasons irrelevant to fertility effects, this would reduce the barriers to having children, and these women could then have the benefit of both roles. Even the cost of having a new child would be reduced since the mother might not have to give up her job. Under these conditions we might well expect the fertility rates of the uneducated working mothers to rise.[27]

Another group of interest is those women who do not want to work. How would they respond to increased opportunities for women to work and to the emergence of cultural supports such as child-care facilities? One obvious result is that there would be fewer such women. It is also possible, though, following the Hoffman-Wyatt hypothesis, that they would experience the need to have *still more* children in order to compensate for their comparative indolence.

Complicated as this discussion has been, we did not mention the man on the scene, and yet a change in the value of children for women might be accompanied by a very different change for men. It has not been empirically established that the woman is the major one to study in predicting fertility, and in Rainwater's study of the lower class the men seem to have a greater role in determining family size than the women. There is a definite need to study husband-wife interactions and how fertility "decisions" are made. And, in fact, employment seems to affect husband-wife decision-making in general (Hoffman, 1963d; Blood, 1963; Safilios-Rothschild, 1970).

Conclusions

Clearly the model we have presented is not a magic helper. Furthermore, though it came out of a review of the literature, solid data on this topic are —with the exception of some of the studies on the economic-utility value— close to nonexistent. That is, there is very little evidence for the prevalence and salience of the values, whether they actually affect fertility behavior, and how they vary in response to social factors. This is a theoretical model to guide research, not a generalization from research. It is consistent with what is known, but what is known is grossly inadequate.

Though it is a working model subject to change, it can nevertheless serve as a useful framework for pointing out the relevant variables that should be considered before empirical studies on this topic are undertaken, and especially before any large-scale social effort is launched. Theory development and empirical work can concentrate on one particular aspect of the model, but the accumulation of knowledge might move more efficiently if the different projects kept the overall framework more or less in view. It is to be hoped that the framework might serve as a guide from which more specific theories are developed and around which these different theories might be integrated. Toward this goal we have tried to keep the model very

---

[27] One implication of this analysis is that education for women may have particularly important antinatalist implications. Not only would it help provide more women with opportunities for jobs that are alternatives to motherhood, but it would also have payoff in future generations, for the education of the mother predicts the career-orientation of the daughter (Levine, 1968).

general and versatile. In the final section of this chapter we present some research projects that would carry through on this plan.

For social planning, on the other hand, the entire model must always be kept in mind. This means that the social event or program in question must be examined for its probable effects on all nine values. Furthermore, to reduce the likelihood of unanticipated consequences, the larger social context should be examined. If the outcome depends on the interaction of values, alternatives, costs, barriers, and facilitators, and if these are part of a social system wherein change in one effects change in the others, then a social program that focuses exclusively on only one part might have unexpected—and unwanted—outcomes. We have discussed the idea of employment for women as a policy for reducing fertility—not to refute it but to highlight the kinds of issues that must be examined if a truly effective program is to be undertaken. Here we mention some additional possible alternatives to children that might be similarly analyzed and studied.

ADDITIONAL ALTERNATIVES

If change in fertility behavior requires attention to the values that children now provide and alternative satisfactions, there are a number of possible alternatives that might be considered.

1. The use of leisure time has been a recent concern in the United States, but it has not been considered in relation to fertility. The Hoffman-Wyatt hypothesis suggests that one reason for the larger family is to fill the time released from household tasks with a productive contribution to the family and with meaningful work, in accordance with the dictates of the Protestant Ethic.[28] Examination of the list of values (pp. 46–47) reveals that several might be satisfied through leisure-time activities, e.g., those numbered 1, 3, 5, and 6.

2. Recent years have seen the emergence of new family forms among young people, some of which might be considered for their possible value in curtailing fertility. The style of life in the commune obviously might satisfy some of the values currently satisfied by children. Furthermore, if there are values that can be satisfied only by rearing children the commune life might allow many adults to share in the experience of rearing a small number of children. Although typically commune families appear to be unstable, in part this may be the result of the commune's being in an early experimental stage, the emotional instability of many of its early devotees, and the frequent hostility of the surrounding community. If the population explosion is drastic enough to require involuntary sterilization as some have suggested (Hardin, 1970a, 1970b), then it seems reasonable to give serious

---

[28] It is possible that the Protestant Ethic has received its first major setback in the current youth culture. The questionable ordering of national priorities, highlighted by the country's persistence in an unpopular war, has led to a distrust of many established social values, among them the attitude toward work.

consideration to communal and perhaps other forms of family organizations that at first may seem outrageous. The fact of their spontaneous voluntary emergence makes it especially important that we learn more about them.

3. If many of the high-fertility groups are low in power and have less access to alternatives to children as sources of the values—all of which seems to be true—it follows that a more equal distribution of power and other resources might be a way of lowering the fertility rate.

The point here is that as long as children satisfy an important value for which there is no alternative, people will climb over a great many barriers and put up with a great many costs before they will diminish fertility. As long as children satisfy important values, even very trivial reasons for another child will seem valid.

Suggestions for Future Research. Interest in the value of children is so recent that the research needs include everything from measurement construction and validation to the more dynamic studies that test hypotheses about how these values are affected by social structure and respond to changes and how they in turn operate to affect childbearing motivations and behavior. The thrust of the entire chapter has been to highlight the need for conceptualization, theories, and sound empirical studies. The list that follows is only a small sample of the research that should be undertaken on this important topic.

1. Measures must be developed to assess the value of children and the salience of the different values. While some measures are needed for specific research purposes, there is also a need for instruments that will have general utility and can be used cross-culturally.

2. Data are needed on the hierarchy and potency of the values for different societies, subgroups within societies, and different ages and stages in the life cycle.

3. The relationship between the hierarchy of values held and the motivations for childbearing should be established. The units studied and compared could be groups or individuals. The balance among the values, alternatives, costs, barriers, and facilitators should be considered in these studies.

4. A given value or combination of values may be more closely tied to one kind of fertility motivation than another. What is the most relevant fertility variable: family-size plans, having another child, having a child of a particular sex, having a child at a particular time—such as soon or at a very young age—careless use of contraceptives and "accidental" pregnancies, an intense need to have at least one child rather than none?

5. The effects of specific events on the balance of values, alternatives, costs, barriers, and facilitators should be examined. These events could be sociocultural changes such as increased industrialization, urbanization, or redefinitions of cultural roles, or more microscopic events such as the youngest child starting kindergarten or a geographical move. There is a need here

for the thoughtful analysis of the probable impacts of these changes and for the development of dynamic theories that are then tested empirically.

Specific hypotheses of this sort have been suggested throughout the chapter—several, for example, dealing with changes in the woman's role, in orientations toward work and leisure, and in the distribution of power. All of these changes, as well as many others, actually are occurring—even within the United States. Since social change occurs at different rates for different segments of the population, it is possible to study the effects of these events on (a) the value of children, (b) the value-alternative-cost-facilitator-barrier pattern, and (c) the relationship between either (a) or (b) and motivations for childbearing.

6. At present there is interest in "social indicators" studies. These are national surveys repeated at regular intervals that tap certain important attitudes. With such studies it would be possible to know, rather than to guess, whether or not certain changes have occurred. This technique would be extremely valuable for measuring at intervals the value of children and the attractiveness of the alternatives to children for satisfying these values. For example, a study reported in 1958 by Weiss and Samuelson dealt with the meaning of various aspects of women's roles—volunteer work, marriage, maternity, employment, and leisure—and included a measure of the Protestant Ethic. A replication of this study or of key questions in it would be a useful index of social change.

7. The concept of alternatives to childbearing should be more fully explored. Certain alternatives might be considered and then examined for their effects on fertility motivation and behavior. Studies could investigate which of the nine values are supplied by the various possible alternatives and how fully. Attention might also be given to the effects of these alternatives on the other aspects of childbearing motivation—costs, facilitators, and barriers. Most of the relevant questions raised in this chapter with respect to maternal employment could be studied empirically. A similar analysis and empirical examination could be made of variant family forms such as the kibbutzim and the new American communes.

8. There are an endless number of specific studies that might be undertaken. For example, why is the educated urban woman in Western Europe more willing than her American counterpart to have fewer than two children? Is her husband more demanding, her Protestant Ethic less demanding, her household less mechanized? Is her femininity more secure or at least less tied to motherhood? Is the American passion for popularity a factor, so that the socialization aims of the American mother require that the child have a sibling to develop peer interaction skills? Is loneliness a particularly American concern that parents want to spare their children? Is it the greater availability of space in America?[29]

[29] Constantina Safilios-Rothschild (personal communication) has suggested that in Greece the extended family provides close ties among cousins, thus making sibling interaction less important.

9. What effect does the change in the self-concept of blacks and their access to power and social mobility have on the value of children among this group? It should be feasible to operationalize this social change in contemporary America because progress has taken place at different rates in different cities.

10. Differences in the value of children to men and to women should be assessed. The connection between these values and other aspects of each of their roles is important, for a change in the role of women will also involve a change for men, and thus predicted effects on the values for women might have a counteractive influence in men. Studies should also consider the interaction between the man and woman in childbearing "decisions." Control over childbearing shifts from one to the other with different birth-control techniques, and consideration of available and acceptable techniques should be part of such a study.

11. Studies should be undertaken to determine the effect of each child on the value to the parent of those not yet born. Rossi (1968) has written about the problems of adjusting to the parent role and the discontinuities involved. What effect does this experience of adjusting to parenthood have on the value of additional children? Many of Rainwater's subjects, for example, indicate that their desired family size decreased after the first.

12. Do special periods of vulnerability to childbearing occur? For example, as the child matures, the values he formerly fulfilled may diminish. Does the first recognition by the mother of this shift bring about a desire for another child that may lessen in intensity after a while?

13. It would be worthwhile to study differences in the value to parents of boys and girls, not just which is the more valued, but which values are more closely tied to each sex. Differences in sex preferences between groups and especially in response to social change should also be studied. As the certainty of filial support in old age declines, does the value of daughters increase? In several cultures daughters are considered closer or more loyal. Such studies are relevant to fertility, of course, because a strong sex preference will increase family size.

14. Developmental studies of the value of children might be undertaken that deal not only with childhood socialization experiences but with changes through the life cycle. Does early socialization have an effect, or is the value of children more dependent on events that occur later in life? At what point does parenthood, rather than some alternative, get attached to the person's developing needs? For example, is parenthood seen as a position in which to exercise power because a major aspect of early childhood involves being in the reciprocal relationship to a high-powered parent? (My parent has power over me; I will become a parent and have power.) Or are childhood experiences important primarily because of a general feeling toward childhood and family life as a happy or unhappy experience?

REFERENCES

Anastasi, A. 1958. Heredity, environment, and the question, "how?" *Psychological Review* 65:197–208.
Anthony, E. J. and Benedek, T., eds. 1970. *Parenthood: psychology and psychopathology.* Boston: Little, Brown.
Bailyn, L. 1970. Career and family orientations of husbands and wives in relation to marital happiness. *Human Relations* 23:97–113.
Bardwick, J. M. 1971. *The psychology of women: a study of biosocial conflict.* New York: Harper & Row.
Barnett, L. D. 1970. U.S. population growth as an abstractly perceived problem. *Demography* 7:53–60.
Berelson, B. 1966. KAP studies on fertility. In B. Berelson et al., eds., *Family planning and population programs.* Chicago: University of Chicago Press. Pp. 655–668.
Blake, J. 1965. Demographic science and the redirection of population policy. In M. C. Sheps and J. C. Ridley, eds. *Public health and population change.* Pittsburgh: University of Pittsburgh Press. Pp. 41–69.
———. 1968. Are babies consumer durables? A critique of the economic theory of reproductive motivation. *Population Studies* 22:5–25.
———. 1969. Population policy for Americans: is the government being misled? *Science* 164:522–529.
———. 1971. Reproductive motivation and population policy. *Bio Science* 21:215–220.
Blood, R. O. 1962. *Marriage.* New York: Free Press.
———. 1963. The husband-wife relationship. In F. I. Nye and L. W. Hoffman, eds., *The employed mother in America.* Chicago: Rand McNally. Pp. 282–305.
Blood, R. O. and Wolfe, D. M. 1960. *Husbands and wives: the dynamics of married living.* New York: Free Press.
Bowlby, J. A. 1958. The nature of the child's tie to his mother. *International Journal of Psychoanalysis* 39:350–373.
Buckhout, R. et al. 1971. The war on people: a scenario for population control? Unpublished manuscript, California State College, Hayward.
Caldwell, J. C. 1967. Fertility attitudes in three economically contrasting rural regions of Ghana. *Economic Development and Cultural Change* 15:217–238.
———. 1968. *Population growth and family change in Africa: the new urban elite in Ghana.* Canberra: Australian National University Press.
Centers, R. and Blumberg, G. H. 1954. Social and psychological factors in human procreation: a survey approach. *Journal of Social Psychology* 40:245–257.
Chilman, C. S. 1970. Probable social and psychological consequences of an American population policy aimed at the two-child family. In E. Milner, ed., *The impact of fertility limitation on women's life, career and personality.* New York: Annals of the New York Academy of Sciences. 175:868–879.
Christopherson, V. A. and Walters, J. 1958. Responses of Protestants, Catholics and Jews concerning marriage and family life. *Sociology and Social Research* 43:16–22.
Clare, J. E. and Kiser, C. V. 1952. Preference for children of given sex in relation to fertility. In P. K. Whelpton and C. V. Kiser, eds., *Social and psychological factors affecting fertility,* Vol. 3. New York: Milbank Memorial Fund. Pp. 621–673.
Coles, R. 1967. *Children of crisis: a study of courage and fear.* Boston: Little, Brown.
Collver, A. and Langlois, E. 1962. The female labor force in metropolitan areas: an international comparison. *Economic Development and Cultural Change* 10:367–385.
Cooley, C. H. 1920. *Social organization.* New York: Scribner's.
Cvetkovich, G. 1971. Assessing child planning policies. Paper presented at the Western Psychological Association, San Francisco, May 1971.
Davis, K. 1967. Population policy: will current programs succeed? *Science* 158:730–739.
Day, L. H. and Day, A. T. 1969. Family size in industrialized countries: an inquiry into

the social-cultural determinants of levels of childbearing. *Journal of Marriage and the Family* 31:242–251.

————. 1970. The social setting of low natality in industrialized countries. Paper presented at the International Sociological Association, Varna, Bulgaria, September 1970.

Dean, D. G. 1961. Alienation: its meaning and measurement. *American Sociological Review* 26:753–754.

Dow, T. E. 1967. Family size and family planning in Nairobi. *Demography* 4:780–797.

Dublin, L. I. and Lotka, A. J. 1946. *The money value of man.* New York: Ronald.

Durkheim, E. 1951. *Suicide.* Glencoe, Ill.: Free Press.

Farley, J. 1970. Graduate women: career aspirations and desired family size. *American Psychologist* 25:1099–1100.

Fawcett, J. T. 1970. *Psychology and population: behavioral research issues in fertility and family planning.* New York: The Population Council.

————. 1971. Attitude measures in KAP studies: an overview and critique. Paper presented at the Conference on Psychological Measurement in Family Planning and Population Policy, University of California, Berkeley, Calif., February 1971.

Flapan, M. 1969. A paradigm for the analysis of childbearing motivations of married women prior to the birth of the first child. *American Journal of Orthopsychiatry* 39: 402–417.

Freedman, R.; Whelpton, R. K.; and Campbell, A. A. 1959. *Family planning, sterility, and population growth.* New York: McGraw-Hill.

Gendell, M. 1965. *The influence of family building activity on woman's rate of economic activity.* Paper presented at the United Nations World Population Conference, Belgrade, Yugoslavia (mimeo).

Gill, D. G. 1970. Looking ahead: some social and individual consequences of mass acceptance of the two-child family in Britain. In E. Milner, ed., *The impact of fertility limitation on women's life-career and personality.* New York: Annals of the New York Academy of Sciences 175:847–863.

Gille, H. and Pardoko, R. H. 1966. A family life study in East Java: preliminary findings. In B. Berelson et al., eds. *Family planning and population programs.* Chicago: University of Chicago Press.

Groat, H. T. and Neal, A. G. 1967. Social psychological correlates of urban fertility. *American Sociological Review* 32:945–959.

Gurin, G.; Veroff, J.; and Feld, S. 1960. *Americans view their mental health.* New York: Basic Books.

Gustavus, S. O. and Nam, C. B. 1970. The formation and stability of ideal family size among young people. *Demography* 7:43–51.

Guthrie, G. M. 1968. Psychological factors and preferred family size. *Saint Louis Quarterly* 6:391–398.

Hardin, G. 1970a. Parenthood: right or privilege. *Science* 169:427.

————. 1970b. Letters. *Science* 170:259–262.

Heer, D. M. 1963. Dominance and the working wife. In F. I. Nye and L. W. Hoffman, eds., *The employed mother in America.* Chicago: Rand McNally. Pp. 251–262.

Heer, D. M. and May, D. A. 1968. Son survivorship motivation and family size in India: a computer simulation. *Population Studies* 22:199–210.

Heisel, D. F. 1968. Attitudes and practices of contraception in Kenya. *Demography* 5: 632–641.

Hess, E. H. 1967. Ethology. In A. M. Freedman and H. I. Kaplan, eds., *Comprehensive textbook of psychiatry.* Baltimore: Williams & Wilkins. Pp. 180–189.

————. 1970. Ethology and developmental psychology. In P. H. Mussen, ed., *Carmichael's manual of child psychology* Vol. 1. New York: Wiley. Pp. 1–38.

Hess, E. H. and Polt, J. M. 1960. Pupil size as related to interest value of visual stimuli. *Science* 132:349–350.

Hess, R. D. and Shipman, V. C. 1968. Maternal attitudes toward the school and the role of the pupil: some social class comparisons. In A. H. Passow, ed., *Developing programs for the educationally disadvantaged.* New York: Teachers College.

Hoffman, L. W. 1958. *Effects of the employment of mothers on parental power relations and the division of household tasks.* Ph.D. diss., University of Michigan. Ann Arbor: University Microfilms.

————. 1963a. The decision to work. In F. I. Nye and L. W. Hoffman, eds., *The employed mother in America.* Chicago: Rand McNally. Pp. 18–39.

————. 1963b. Effects on children: summary and discussion. In F. I. Nye and L. W. Hoffman, eds., *The employed mother in America.* Chicago: Rand McNally. Pp. 190–212.

————. 1963c. Mother's enjoyment of work and effects on the child. In F. I. Nye and L. W. Hoffman, eds., *The employed mother in America.* Chicago: Rand McNally. Pp. 95–105.

————. 1963d. Parental power relations and the division of household tasks. In F. I. Nye and L. W. Hoffman, eds., *The employed mother in America.* Chicago: Rand McNally. Pp. 215–230.

————. 1972. Early childhood experiences and women's achievement motives. *Journal of Social Issues* 28:129–155.

Hoffman, L. W. and Lippitt, R. 1960. The measurement of family life variables. In P. H. Mussen, ed., *Handbook of research methods in child development.* New York: Wiley. Pp. 945–1013.

Hoffman, L. W. and Wyatt, F. 1960. Social change and motivations for having larger families: some theoretical considerations. *Merrill-Palmer Quarterly* 6:235–244.

Hoffman, M. L. 1963. Personality, family structure, and social class as antecedents of parental power assertion. *Child Development* 34:869–884.

Horner, M. S. 1968. *Sex differences in achievement motivation and performance in competitive and non-competitive situations.* Ph.D. diss., University of Michigan. Ann Arbor: University Microfilms.

Kangas, L. W. 1970. Integrated incentives for fertility control. *Science* 169:1278–1283.

Kar, S. B. 1971. Individual aspirations as related to early and late acceptance of contraception. *The Journal of Social Psychology* 83:235–245.

Komarovsky, M. 1950. Functional analysis of sex roles. *American Sociological Review* 15:508–516.

————. 1967. *Blue-collar marriage.* New York: Vintage.

Lazarsfeld, P. F. 1955. Interpretation of statistical relations as a research operation. In P. F. Lazarsfeld and M. Rosenberg, eds., *The language of social research.* Glencoe, Ill.: Free Press. Pp. 115–125.

Levine, A. G. 1968. Marital and occupational plans of women in professional schools: law, medicine, nursing, teaching. Unpublished Ph.D. diss., Yale University.

Lopata, M. Z. 1971. *Occupation housewife.* New York: Oxford University Press.

Lorenz, K. Z. 1965. *Evolution and modification of behavior.* Chicago: University of Chicago Press.

McClelland, D. C. 1964. Wanted: a new self-image for women. In R. J. Lifton, ed., *The woman in America.* Cambridge, Mass.: American Academy of Arts and Sciences.

Maccoby, E. E. 1963. Woman's intellect. In S. M. Farber and R. H. L. Wilson, eds., *The potential of woman.* New York: McGraw-Hill.

Martin, W. T. 1970. Family planning attitudes and knowledge: a study of African families in Nairobi. Unpublished manuscript.

Maslow, A. H. 1955. Deficiency motivation and growth motivation. In M. R. Jones, ed., *Nebraska symposium on motivation.* Lincoln: University of Nebraska Press. Pp. 1–30.

Mauldin, W. P.; Watson, W. B.; and Noe, L. F. 1971. KAP surveys and evaluation of family planning programs. New York: The Population Council, January 1971 (mimeo).

Meade, R. 1971. Assessment of personal motivations for childbearing. Paper presented at the Conference on Psychological Measurement in Family Planning and Population Policy, University of California, Berkeley, Calif., February 1971.

Mohanty, S. P. 1969. Attempts at measuring family planning attitudes in India: an assessment of traditional and emerging techniques. Paper presented at the All-India Seminar on Models in Demographic Analysis, Demographic Training and Research Centre, Bombay, February 1969.

Mueller, E. 1970. Attitudes toward the economics of family size and their relation to fertility. Unpublished manuscript, University of Michigan.

Newman, L. F. 1970. Cultural factors in family planning. In E. Milner, ed., *The impact of fertility limitation on women's life-career and personality.* New York: Annals of the New York Academy of Sciences 175:833–840.

Newton, N. 1967. Pregnancy, childbirth, and outcome: a review of patterns of culture and future research needs. In S. A. Richardson and A. F. Guttmacher, *Childbearing— its social and psychological aspects*. Baltimore: Williams & Wilkins. Pp. 147–228.

Nye, F. I. and Hoffman, L. W. 1963. The socio-cultural setting. In F. I. Nye and L. W. Hoffman, eds., *The employed mother in America*. Chicago: Rand McNally.

Poffenberger, T. 1968. Motivational aspects of resistance to family planning in an Indian village. *Demography* 5:757–766.

———. 1969. Husband-wife communication and motivational aspects of population control in an Indian village. Central Family Planning Institute Monograph Series No. 10, December 1969.

Poffenberger, T.; Bachman, J. G.; and Weiss, E. 1970. Survey of population knowledge and attitudes of post high school age boys in the United States. Paper presented at the meeting on Student Knowledge of and Attitudes toward Population Matters, The Population Council, New York, December 1970.

Pohlman, E. H. 1969. *Psychology of birth planning*. Cambridge, Mass.: Schenkman.

———. 1970. Influencing people to *want* fewer children. Paper presented at the American Psychological Association Convention, Miami, Florida, September 1970.

Rabin, A. I. Motivation for parenthood. 1965. *Journal of Projective Techniques and Personality Assessment* 29:405–411.

Rabin, A. I. and Greene, R. J. 1968. Assessing motivation for parenthood. *Journal of Psychology* 69:39–46.

Rainwater, L. 1960. *And the poor get children*. Chicago: Quadrangle Books.

———. 1965. *Family design: marital sexuality, family size, and contraception*. Chicago: Aldine.

Ridley, J. C. 1959. Number of children expected in relation to non-familial activities of the wife. *Milbank Memorial Fund Quarterly* 37:277–296.

Robinson, W. C. and Horlacher, D. E. 1971. Population growth and economic welfare. *Reports on Population/Family Planning* No. 6:1–39.

Rossi, A. S. 1965. Barriers to the career choice of engineering, medicine, or science among American women. In J. A. Mattfeld and E. G. Van Aken, eds., *Women and the scientific professions*. Cambridge, Mass.: MIT Press. Pp. 51–127.

———. 1968. Transition to parenthood. *Journal of Marriage and the Family* 30:26–39.

Roy, P. 1963. Adolescent roles: rural-urban differentials. In F. I. Nye and L. W. Hoffman, eds., *The employed mother in America*. Chicago: Rand McNally.

Russo, N. F. 1971. Some observations on the role of personality variables in past and current fertility research. Paper presented at the Conference on Psychological Measurement in Family Planning and Population Policy, University of California, Berkeley, Calif., February 1971.

Safilios-Rothschild, C. J. 1969a. Sociopsychological factors affecting fertility in urban Greece: a preliminary report. *Marriage and Family Living* 31:595–606.

———. 1969b. Some aspects of social modernization in the United States and Greece. *Sociologie et Sociétés* 1:1. (Translation from the French original on mimeo.)

———. 1970. The influence of the wife's degree of work commitment upon some aspects of family organization and dynamics. *Journal of Marriage and the Family* 32:681–691.

Schneider, L. and Lysgaard, S. 1953. The deferred gratification pattern: a preliminary study. *American Sociological Review* 18:142–149.

Sears, R. R.; Maccoby, E. E.; and Levin, H. 1957. *Patterns of child rearing*. Evanston, Ill.: Row, Peterson, & Co.

Senn, M. J. E. and Hartford, C. 1968. *The first born: experiences of eight American families*. Cambridge, Mass.: Harvard University Press.

Siddiqui, H. R. 1967. Family, social engineering, and population programs: a study of physicians, government officials, lawyers, and professors in Pakistan. Unpublished Ph.D. diss., Cornell University.

Smith, R. and Steinhoff, P. 1971. The Hawaii pregnancy, birth control and abortion study. Paper presented at the Conference on Psychological Measurement in Family Planning and Population Policy, University of California, Berkeley, Calif., February 1971.

Spengler, J. J. 1969. Population problem: in search of a solution. *Science* 166:1234–1238.

Stolka, S. M. and Barnett, L. D. 1969. Education and religion as factors in women's attitudes motivating childbearing. *Journal of Marriage and the Family* 31:740–750.

Stycos, J. M. and Weller, R. H. 1967. Female working roles and fertility. *Demography* 4:210–217.

Swain, M. D. and Kiser, C. V. 1953. Social and psychological factors affecting fertility. *Milbank Memorial Fund Quarterly* 31:51–84.

Thompson, W. S. and Lewis, D. T. 1965. *Population problems.* New York: McGraw-Hill.

United Nations. 1961. *Mysore population study* (ST/SOA/Ser. A/34). New York: Department of Economics and Social Affairs.

U.S. Department of Commerce, Census Bureau. 1970. Statistical Abstracts of the United States. 91st edition. Washington, D.C.: U.S. Government Printing Office.

U.S. Department of Labor, Women's Bureau. 1970. *Who are the working mothers?* Leaflet 37, October 1970.

Vogel, E. F. and Bell, N. W. 1960. The emotionally disturbed child as the family scapegoat. In N. W. Bell and E. F. Vogel, eds., *A modern introduction to the family.* Glencoe, Ill.: Free Press. Pp. 382–397.

Weiss, R. S. and Samelson, N. M. 1958. Social roles of American women: their contribution to a sense of usefulness and importance. *Marriage and Family Living* 20:358–366.

Westoff, C. F.; Potter, R. G.; and Sagi, P. C. 1963. *The third child.* Princeton: Princeton University Press.

Westoff, C. F.; Potter, P. C.; Sagi, P. C.; and Mishler, E. G. 1961. *Family growth in metropolitan America.* Princeton: Princeton University Press.

Whelpton, P. K.; Campbell, A. A.; and Patterson, J. E. 1966. *Fertility and family planning in the United States,* Princeton: Princeton University Press.

[3]

FAMILY STRUCTURE AND
FERTILITY CONTROL

KURT W. BACK AND
PAULA H. HASS

Strangely the discussion of fertility rates and of changes in fertility under different conditions has omitted the human aspect. Only recently have demographers included sexual behavior and contraceptive practice in their research efforts (Stycos, introduction to Rainwater, 1960), and even here the approach has been curiously detached. Sexual behavior, birth, and their relationship occur within a highly affective context, and emotions such as love, tenderness, responsibility, and even craving for immortality give meaning to terms such as fertility rate. Theories of family structure and the relationship of family structure to fertility deal primarily with indicators of the affective relations between couples and with the relationship of couples to the rest of society. This link between personal affection and social integration becomes the interest of the psychologist and an avenue for his contribution to the problems of population control.

From a psychological as well as social point of view the family is the primary context of fertility and reproduction. Biologically conception and birth may óccur before and outside marriage; socially the family—the parents—speak for the child until he is responsible himself; and psychologically procreation and rearing of children occur within an affective relationship that is either the biological family or a family surrogate. It is therefore natural that scientists, scholars, and philosophers have looked to the family to explain fertility patterns and to fertility patterns to explain family relations.

For instance Bertrand Russell in *Marriage and Morals* (1929) has surmised that organized family life began when man first realized the existence of a relationship between conception and birth. Prior to this time sexual exclusiveness was unnecessary or misunderstood. Afterward, however, man was unwilling to support another man's children, and the exclusive sexual union was born. This kind of speculation, similar to Freud's theory of the primal horde, must remain an unproven theory; however, ingenious hypotheses of this kind have been proposed with the most important implicit assumption being the relationships between family, fertility, and economic as well as emotional concerns.

Thus Russell posits the origin of the family on strong emotions, jealousy and possessiveness, while acknowledging some rational base on responsibility for upkeep of the children. Correspondingly he predicted rational change in family relations when the relationship between intercourse and procreation became attenuated through the widespread use of efficient contraception. This capacity for control has been reached now. The sexual act and conception are again separated. Where conception is under human control the need for a stable family may diminish, and other new forms of family life may develop. Again, this is merely speculative.

However, we do have an array of data on the relation between family conditions and fertility. These data have been collected from many sources, and their purport is not always clear. We can begin to disentangle the relationship, however, noting the direction of the influence and thereby providing some measure of understanding and control of the future, as well as understanding of past and present conditions.

In available data one can discern a general trend of two concurrent changes. The family structure has changed from an extended kinship structure with a variety of functions in society to a nuclear family with little kinship relation and functions concentrating on affective interpersonal gratifications. Concomitant with the change in family structure was a reduction in fertility, mainly through the use and acceptance of various contraceptive methods—the so-called demographic transition from high fertility and high mortality to low fertility and low mortality.

It would be plausible to assume a logical connection between the two: namely, that the social and economic value of a large number of children declines with the loss of the family's function as an economic unit and with its comparative independence of the larger kinship structure and that under these conditions families plan to have fewer children; conversely the possibility of controlling fertility has made it possible to have small, socially mobile family units. This kind of reasoning assumes a rational planning of the total number of children and a certain automatic adjustment of fertility to material conditions.

Examined closely, the relationship between family structure and fertility is not as simple as some logical theories may have predicted. Children are frequently not planned rationally, and the long period between conception and birth may render the cause-and-effect relationship psychologically unmeaningful, even though intellectually the relationship is well understood. Thus in current fertility research the subtle variables of intrafamilial relationships and emotional attachments, and even the more stable social conditions of family formation, have proven themselves to be less predictive than fecundity and more general conditions in the society, such as education and religion (cf. Westoff, Potter, Sagi, and Mishler, 1961).

Thus on a global level we find relationships between fertility and level of education, urbanization, economic development, and religion; we also know that in the last analysis fertility depends on conception and death, that is, on the workings of intimate personal relations generally within a family context. The norms of family formation, structure, and relationships within a society are necessarily important in these fertility analyses, but the true meaning of the family variables has mainly eluded researchers. It may be the task of psychologists to investigate the change in family structure and fertility patterns through the mediation of the affective relations between the partners. We shall review the relevant evidence that has been collected; first, the relation between social structure factors and fertility and then between the functions of the family and fertility. After this we can hazard guesses and interpretations of the nature of the interrelations, suggest avenues of future research and make a few predictions of future developments.

Societal Family Structures and Fertility

Let us begin by delineating two different and extreme types of possible kinship structures. When priority is given to marital ties within the family structure, the kinship system is called a conjugal system. The independent nuclear family might be characterized as a conjugal kinship system. However, when blood ties between parents and children or between siblings are stressed, we have a consanguineous system. Thus, for example, in extended families the wife or husband may be viewed as an outsider whose needs must be subordinated to the wider kin group. At the simplest level of economic subsistence (hunting and gathering societies) there is a nuclear family system, emphasizing the conjugal ties; at the intermediate level (sedentary agriculture and herding) there is the extended family or consanguineous system; and with the industrial type of economy there is again a nuclear family system, emphasizing the conjugal kinship (Nimkoff and Middleton, 1968).

In societies in which the consanguineous relationships are more important there is evidence of a younger age at marriage, higher proportions of the population entering marriage, and greater incidence of plural marriage (polygamy). Marriages are arranged for social and economic reasons (kinship or economic factors, such as maintenance of property) and involve some type of exchange; residence is not neolocal, but matri- or patrilocal. Within marriage itself blood relatives take precedence over marital solidarity, sibling ties are strong, and large numbers of children are emphasized. Fertility is considered to be the natural concomitant of the union, ensuring the perpetuation of the kinship line, as well as providing children needed as economic assets and meeting the expectations of the couple, who view procreation as an inevitable outcome of marriage.

With regard to the nuclear family unit and conjugal kinship system, we shall focus our attention exclusively on the nuclear family operating within an industrial context and ignore the nuclear family operating in hunting and gathering societies, such as the Eskimo society. The nuclear family within the *industrial* society is characterized by a later age at marriage, greater incidence of celibacy, monogamy, individual choice of mate from a delimited field of eligibles, and neolocal residence. Within marriage the conjugal bond takes priority over kinship ties, and marriage is contracted on the basis of personal attraction as well as on ascriptive considerations, such as social class, religion, or ethnic category. Under these conditions the family's function of providing emotional gratification to its members assumes greater importance, and the function of reproduction becomes less salient.

These differences are not absolute; in fact recent work has demonstrated that even in highly industrialized societies kinship and the extended family remain important institutions (Litwak, 1960; Sussman, 1954, 1959). The real difference may be more subtle: members of industrialized societies as well as members of underdeveloped societies recognize the existence of a kin group and its distinction from the nuclear family. What is different is the emotional investment between the two, on the one side a diffuse loyalty to the whole kin group and on the other a distinct affective relationship within the nuclear family. Slater (1963) has shown that some discharge of affect outside the nuclear family is necessary for a society to survive. Therefore, a person can expend all his affect on his kinship group, and a kin group may be an exclusive unit to a degree that the nuclear family cannot be. These emotional correlates of different family structures may become significant in sexual behavior and fertility. Thus even though the actual distinction between societies with extended kinship patterns and with nuclear families is not as large as is sometimes depicted, the fact that different norms exist may have important effects on family relations.

A cursory glance at social trends in the last century or so will show the congruence of functional and emotional conditions in the two family types and the transition from one type to another. Moreover, it has been widely assumed that the extended family structure is an important *cause* of high fertility. However, there is an increasing amount of theoretical argument against such a proposition as well as some negative empirical evidence.

The basic argument in favor of the proposition is the theoretical viewpoint that both corporate kinship groups (clans and organized lineages) and extended families (both the residential and kin network variety) motivate and support early and near universal marriage and high marital fertility. On the other hand, societies that emphasize the independent nuclear or stem family and economic independence will tend to have low societal fertility. Where contraception is not widely practiced, later age at marriage and greater incidence of celibacy may function to produce lower fertility.

It is not assumed that the family system is the only or most important causal factor influencing fertility. In some situations economic, religious, ecological, or other nonfamilial factors may take precedence. Moreover, it is also realized that the family system may exert influence only in interaction with other factors, such as religious or cultural ideals regarding continuation of lineage, which are subsumed as part of an individual's motivation for marriage and reproduction (Lorimer, 1954; Davis, 1955; Davis and Blake, 1956, as cited in Burch and Gendell, 1970). In other words the lineage is used to achieve economic and emotional values important in the culture.

In response to these propositions the various theoretical counterarguments are presented by Burch and Gendell (1970) in their review of the literature on extended family structure and fertility. Stycos (1958) argues that in nonindustrial societies extended residential families or joint households are probably much less prevalent than cultural ideals suggest. Therefore, such residential arrangements can hardly explain high levels of societal fertility. Second, although the ideal may be prevalent its influence on actual fertility should be less than the influence of the actual family structure. Furthermore, Goode (1963a, 1963b) and others (Davis and Blake, 1956) argue that there is no inherent connection between the independent nuclear family system and low fertility. Rather Goode states that the fertility level will be decided in the interests of the couple alone, and not in terms of the interests of a wider kinship group. Thus it could be high (as on the American frontier) or low (as in an industrial city), depending on circumstances.

Goode's observations, as well as Stycos's statement on the relative prevalence of the extended family, are suggestive of a new approach. Let us return to the Nimkoff and Middleton (1968) work on economic and family systems. On the basis of secondary analysis of 549 of the 565 cultures in Murdock's World Ethnographic Sample, the authors have isolated five factors that appear to influence type of familial system (nuclear or extended) through their association with type of subsistence: (1) abundance and stability of the food supply; (2) degree of demand for the family as a unit of labor; (3) the amount of geographic mobility involved in subsistence activities; (4) the amount and nature of property; and (5) the degree of stratification in complex societies. The first of these factors is considered the most important. In short, relatively ample and regular food supply, high use of the family as a labor unit, low necessity for geographic mobility with respect to subsistence, and strongly developed concepts of property (especially land) as owned collectively rather than individually were associated with the maximum probability of extended familism. Moreover, in societies complex enough to have stratification (which presupposes a stable food supply and a concept of property) this factor was positively correlated with extended familism. The reverse conditions were associated with familism of the independent nuclear family type. It is possible that it is these factors, rather than the type of family system itself, that are related to fertility. Reference to these factors can perhaps clarify why fertility of the nuclear independent family on the American frontier was characterized as high, whereas for industrial cities it is low. On the frontier there was high demand for the family as a unit of labor, low geographic mobility involved in subsistence activities, property in the form of land, and high fertility.

Aside from theoretical arguments actual empirical evidence on the relationship between type of family system and fertility is quite limited. (See Burch and Gendell, 1970, for a more complete review of the literature.) With regard to preliterate societies Namboodiri (1967), interpreting ethnographic data for forty societies, finds that societies having extended residential families have higher fertility than those stressing independent nuclear family organization only if they also have kinship systems organized in terms of lineages.

Field studies in contemporary nonindustrial or industrializing nations are also available, but their findings are contradictory and inconclusive. Data that support the acceptance of the relationship between extended family structure and fertility are presented by Freedman, Takeshita, and Sun (1964) and by Liu (1967). Freedman and his associates, reporting on survey data for Taichung (1962–1963), find that for all women, with the exception of those thirty-five to thirty-nine years of age, living in a nuclear family (rather than in a stem or joint family) is linked to lower cumulative fertility, smaller desired family size, and use of fertility control, including abortion and sterilization. Recent studies in Taiwan also indicate that there is a tendency for ever married women aged fifteen to forty-nine in nuclear families to have lower age-standardized cumulative fertility than those in joint families. This is true for the total island, cities, urban townships, and rural townships. However, differences, while consistent, are not large (Liu, 1967).

Inconsistent and contrary evidence on the relationship between extended family and fertility is presented by Nag (1967) and Pakrasi and Malaker (1967). Nag (1967) presents evidence on 3,725 ever married women living in seven rural villages of West Bengal, representing different Hindu and Muslim castes. He finds substantial numbers of women living in joint families, but some tendency for these women to have fewer children ever born. However, when age-standardized rates are computed from the Nag data by Pakrasi and Malaker (1967), the differentials are reduced and in one group they are reversed.

A similar study done by Pakrasi and Malaker (1967) involving 1,018 married couples in Calcutta is also available. Pakrasi and Malaker find substantial numbers of women living in joint families, particularly women who have been married for shorter periods of time. Controlling for marital duration and social class, they conclude that in general women in joint families have lower cumulative fertility than those in simple families. The only exception to these findings is in the lowest class comprised of unskilled and skilled manual laborers. Here the differential is reversed in two of four marital duration categories. Both Nag and Pakrasi and Malaker cite previous studies in India that yield approximately the same results.

Despite the evidence of these few studies regarding the relationship between residence in an extended family and fertility, the evidence must still be considered inconclusive.

Burch and Gendell (1970) list the following methodological problems yet to be dealt with adequately in these studies. With regard to the time reference of the theory, Burch and Gendell state that many relevant empirical cases only occur in the past, and recent appropriate data are unavailable. Moreover, as Freedman (1963) cautions, studies of contemporary societies, such as those summarized above, may be largely irrelevant. If modernization has occurred in Latin America, Taiwan, and other developing nations, these societies would already have undergone substantial mortality declines. Mortality in turn affects fertility and would largely modify the traditional family structures; it may destroy the relationship that might have existed previously between family structure and fertility. Second, with the exception of Namboodiri's work (1967) the studies described above use the individual woman as the unit of analysis. Without the use of aggregate data these data cannot indicate if *societies* in which extended families predominate have higher levels of fertility than do societies in which nuclear families prevail. Third, there are differences in the definition of key variables. As Burch and Gendell (1970) indicate, theories linking the extended family with high fertility differ in meaning according to the concepts and definitions of extended family and fertility that are used. Thus, for example, Nag (1967), Pakrasi and Malaker (1967), and Liu (1967) each use a different definition for the joint family. Moreover, all three fail to distinguish between collateral and generational extension and the actual size of the extended family. There are also various measures of fertility employed, and cumulative fertility is often compared to current residence; this lack of conceptual clarity may help explain the differences in study findings. Finally other authors indicate the difficulties involved with contrary causal forces. Stycos (1958) and others have suggested that the extended family in some circumstances may want its members to have fewer children and may try to motivate them in this direction. This may be especially true in contemporary India for couples who are not the head of the household in which they are living (Rele, 1963). Thus one would want to control for the variable, relationship to family head. Second, Driver (1963) and Nag (1967) have suggested that women in joint households have inter-course less frequently because of lack of privacy and the pressure of kin to obey cultural taboos. It is suggested that future field studies should take a more dynamic view of household structure and should be alert to the possibility that causation may run from fertility to family structure as well as from family structure to fertility.

The field studies complement the evidence of the comparative studies, but some additional cautions must be made. In principle this caution is based on the problem of ecological correlation. Societies may differ in fertility according to their norms of family formation, but within any particular society the families that live as nuclear families may not differ in the same way from those that live in extended families. Thus within a society a family type may be related to a particular social class position or educa-tional status, and without proper controls one might measure the effect of these social status variables but not of family structure. A particular diffi-culty here is that family structure may vary over the life cycle, giving a misleading correlation between cumulative fertility and residential family type. This factor is especially important given the continual investigation of the joint family in India. As Nag (1967) and Pakrasi and Malaker (1967) indicate, there are substantial numbers of women living in joint family systems, particularly at shorter marital durations. The Indian joint family is characteristic of just one stage in the life cycle, and people typically pass through several stages during their lifetime. The process begins as the sons marry and remain in the parental home with their wives, thus re-sembling extended families. Upon the death of the father the true joint family comes into existence. The sons remain in the parental home, and the joint family remains intact until the younger siblings have completed their education and have married. At that time the joint family breaks up into smaller nuclear residential units, each son and his wife and children, if any, setting up a separate residence and dividing the family property (Gore, 1965). Therefore, it is most likely that many of the women, especially those in middle marital durations, who are currently categorized as living in independent nuclear families have *previously* resided in joint family systems. Women with longer marital durations, especially those in the ever married samples (including widows), may have recently reentered a joint family system, as their older sons have married and brought their wives into the family of procreation.

In addition, Palmore, Klein, and bin Morzul (1970) have pointed out the importance of "availability." Even in an extended family system, mortality and migration may result in fact in absence of relatives beyond the nuclear family. Thus, the actual distribution of nuclear and extended families can be determined as much by availability as by social norms. Conversely Las-lett (1965, pp. 90–92) has pointed out that, because of increased life ex-pectancy, extended families are more frequent now than they were in preindustrial times.

It is not clear from the available data whether the family-size ideals and the norms of a society influence fertility or whether actual participation in a nuclear or extended family leads to differential fertility. To gain some insight into these questions we must turn to the available evidence on family interaction and its effects and discuss questions that are closer to the field of social psychology.

Familial Interaction and Fertility

There is a body of empirical evidence concerned with the relationships between family members within the nuclear family in industrialized societies and the effects of these relationships on contraceptive behavior and fertility. One central characteristic of families that differentiates them from each other and has important consequences for their contraceptive and fertility behavior lies in the nature of the role relationship between husband and wife in the nuclear family. Indeed, Stycos (1962) concludes that one of the facilitating conditions for effective fertility control is the extent to which family structure facilitates sharing of goals and knowledge: effects of segregation of sexes, dominance patterns, ease of communication, stability of conjugal bonds, and articulation of family with other social institutions.

On a societal basis it is theorized that male-dominant family systems are causally related to high fertility. The authority of the husband, the importance of demonstrating virility in terms of numbers of male offspring, as well as the assumed economic value of male children, the separation of the husband from involvement with childrearing routines, the low status of the woman, and her limited opportunities for experience in nondomestic roles are elements of the patriarchal system that are thought to be causal social antecedents of high fertility. The absence of fertility planning and the rigidity of marital roles are also characteristic of such societies. This hypothesis has been applied across cultures (Lorimer, 1954) and within cultures (Westoff et al., 1961; Westoff, Potter, and Sagi, 1963; Hill, Stycos, and Back, 1959).

Sociologists contend that modern urban family systems tend toward egalitarianism (Goldberg, 1959). Ramifications of this trend are to be found in the increased employment of women outside the house, the greater involvement of husbands in matters concerning fertility, the greater use of birth control, and lower fertility (Westoff et al., 1961).

A few studies have investigated elements of the patriarchal system and their relationship to the absence of fertility planning. Thus Hill and his associates (1959), in their study of lower-class Puerto Rican couples, investigated the phenomenon of machismo and sexual mores, such as intense sexual jealousy and suspicion of marital fidelity of the wife. Various other studies have also focused on male dominance in decision-making and other attributes of the marital relationship.

Machismo

Machismo is a complex of male sex-role expectations, incorporating attitudes toward sex (early and extensive premarital and extramarital sex relations for men, manifestations of fertility through rapid production of children, especially sons, and negative views toward male contraceptive techniques within the marital relationship); attitudes toward women (domination); attitudes toward work (a disregard and devaluation of any type of domestic responsibilities, especially the practicalities of daily home life); and attitudes toward authority (physical strength as a means of settling disagreements and roughness as a way to relate to the weak or subordinate). These attitudes are acquired and reinforced by the male peer group (DeHoyos and DeHoyos, 1966; Stycos, 1968).

With respect to machismo Hill et al. (1959) conclude that it has little effect on fertility. The authors find no linear relationship between machismo (as measured by an index of male anxiety) and communication with the wife, extent of activities prohibited to her, and the amount of birth control practiced. However, the highest scoring men on the machismo scale did exhibit the machismo pattern: prohibiting more activities to their wives, talking less to them, and experiencing less success with birth control, although there was no difference in the extent of birth control being practiced. Upon further examination it was found that these men are young (not yet having proven their virility) or very old (past the period of accepted maximum virility), and thus their real influence on fertility is minimal. Moreover, as a group they desire fewer children.

In conclusion one cannot accept the sequence of childhood training, adult machismo, and a desire for many offspring as an explanation for high fertility, at least within the lower class (Hill et al., 1959). Unfortunately the narrow sampling base of the Puerto Rican study does not permit rigorous testing of the relative influence of machismo within the society. Nor can it assess the effect of machismo as a cultural belief. Although there is little evidence that individuals who have the traits of machismo want more children, the *belief* among men and women that this complex of values exists may lead them to higher fertility than members of societies in which these beliefs do not exist.

Female Matrimonial Fidelity and Modesty

With respect to sexual mores there is evidence that the complex of matrimonial fidelity for women affects fertility control. Briefly stated, the complex requires that a woman avoid any act that might be regarded by a jealous husband as a threat to his sexual monopoly of her. With regard to the marital relationship the husband is to be treated in terms of respect and formality; the wife is supposed to demonstrate modesty and avoid discussion of intimate topics (Cruz, 1967).

There is some empirical evidence that this sexual custom affects fertility control. Stycos (1968) states that some lower-class Puerto Rican males raise serious objections to birth control on the grounds that it undermines male authority and promotes infidelity. Likewise Rainwater (1960) observes that lower-class men in his U.S. sample desire larger families because children keep mothers at home and thereby help keep them good as well as submissive. Moreover, men want to believe that their wives are innocent and too modest to discuss such matters as sex and birth control (Hill et al., 1959).

Wives also possess attitudes that inhibit the use of contraception. First, they are too reluctant to initiate the subject of birth control, having been taught that reticence on sexual matters is an attribute of a good woman, and by definition the wife is always a good woman. A woman is very reluctant to suggest to her husband that she use contraceptive methods for fear he suspect her of wanting to engage in extramarital sexual activity without being detected (Hill et al., 1959; Stycos, 1968). Moreover, wives are reluctant to attend birth-control clinics because of the latter's public nature and the frequent necessity for a medical examination (Stycos, 1968; Hill et al., 1959). The influence of these attitudes on fertility behavior is indicated by the findings of a negative relationship between the modesty score and discussion of birth control and a relationship between the modesty score and attendance at birth-control clinics (Hill et al., 1959). Rao (1959) cites similar patterns of male dominance, poor communication, and modesty as detrimental to family planning in India. And Kazen and Browning (1967) reach similar conclusions in their study of Mexican-Americans.

Husband-Wife Dominance and Conjugal Role Relationships

With respect to dominance in the marital relationship or conjugal role relationship, Rainwater (1965) has suggested three types. Joint conjugal role relationships are those in which the predominant pattern of marital life involves shared or interchangeable activities. Specifically these couples plan events together, share task performance to a greater extent, and share leisure-time interaction. Not only do they see the functional efficacy of this sharing, but they stress the interpersonal value of it. Segregated role relationships refer to relationships that emphasize a formal division of labor within the family.

> . . . couples in the more segregated relationships tend to have less communication with each other, to go their own ways more, to have more serious financial and interpersonal problems, and to be generally less family-centered in their conceptions of themselves. . . . Husbands in segregated relations were more often seen as disloyal to the family; they spent more time away from home in male-centered activities that made their wives uneasy about the stability of the relationship and about financial security. [Rainwater, 1965, p. 232]

Finally intermediate role relationships are not sharply polarized in either the jointly organized or highly segregated direction.

Many studies have noted the association between socioeconomic status and type of conjugal role relationship both in developed countries, such as the United States and England, and in developing countries, especially those of Latin America. Numerous other studies have investigated the relationship between dominance or type of conjugal role relationship and desired family size, fertility, and contraceptive effectiveness.

With regard to the relationship between husband-wife dominance or type of conjugal role relationship and desired family size, findings are contradictory. It can be argued that the more egalitarian the household (or the less segregated the conjugal role relationship), the fewer the number of children desired by the wife since interests other than fertility may be pursued. Hoffman and Wyatt (1960) propose that women who see themselves as oriented to their husbands or to outside interests should not want as large a family as those women who think of themselves mainly in terms of interests in children and homemaking. Rainwater's data on 409 respondents from three U.S. cities (1965) support the conclusion that preference for a small or medium-sized family is associated with joint conjugal role relationships, orientation primarily to husbands or to outside interests, and anxiety on the part of the wife about coping with homemaking tasks. Larger family preferences are associated with relationships of intermediate segregation, orientation toward children and home, and concern about excessive egocentrism. It is possible that wives who feel they are not free to participate extensively in the lives of their husbands have a tendency to want more children in order to fill a gap that would not otherwise exist. Blood and Wolfe (1960) make a similar interpretation of comparable findings on a middle-class Detroit sample of households.

On the other hand, Rainwater's data (1965) indicate that for the husband the relationship is in the same direction, but it is not statistically significant. Moreover, the findings do not hold in the lower-lower class of the Rainwater sample. Data from the longitudinal Study of Family Growth in Metropolitan America (Westoff et al., 1961; Westoff et al., 1963) provide no clear support for the hypothesis that women who have better "adjustment to the mother role" want and therefore have more children. Women who wanted more children were as liable as others to want out-of-home activities. With regard to dominance patterns and desired number of children, the authors also found a slight negative correlation between dominance patterns in social life and nonsocial areas and the number of children desired by the wife (—.06 and —.09). Where dominance patterns between husband and wife approach the egalitarian and wife-dominant pattern, the correlations slightly favor a larger number of additional children desired. Likewise analysis of currently mated Latin-American women mated at least five years and living in seven metropolitan areas indicates that the wife's report of egalitarianism in decision-making with regard to important financial decisions and childrearing is not associated with family-size preference in Buenos Aires, Río de Janeiro, Bogotá, Mexico City, Panamá City, or Caracas. In the seventh city, San José, Costa Rica, there is a positive association, indicating larger family-size preferences among those women who report egalitarian decision-making in the home (Hass, 1971).

With regard to conjugal role relationship and fertility, measured as the number of children ever born, findings are also contradictory. Some studies have demonstrated that the less segregated the conjugal role relationship, the lower the fertility, whereas other studies have not.

In developed countries studies have failed to demonstrate this relationship. The Indianapolis Study proved quite inconclusive (Kiser and Whelpton, 1953). Herbst (1957) reports no relationship found between dominance patterns and fertility in an Australian sample. And analysis of 731 Detroit households (Blood and Wolfe, 1960) indicates a lack of association between patterns of dominance in decision-making per se and fertility. Finally Westoff et al. (1963) found that patterns of dominance in running the home, determining the social life, and determining nonsocial areas, and extent of help available to the wife were not associated with the number of pregnancies since the birth of the second child. With regard to these findings one should keep in mind the problems of different aspects of decision-making involved, limited samples, limited range of fertility variation, and incomplete fertility levels.

Research in developing countries has indicated the existence of this relationship, although the research designs often fail to incorporate controls on relevant variables such as age at union or marital duration. Hill et al. (1959), in their study of lower-class Puerto Rican couples, conclude that familism (as measured in high authority of the husband, subordination and restriction of the wife's behavior in working outside the home and in other types of participation) appears closely related to fertility in that the more restrictive family types have higher fertility rates. Stycos (1968) reports that within the lower class both men and women who feel that having a large number of children ties down their spouses and helps to keep them faithful, indeed, have higher fertility. Similarly DeHoyos and DeHoyos (1966), in a study of 101 married women in Ciudad Juarez, Mexico, conclude that 22 percent of the husbands with small families and 44 percent of those with large families are involved in the Mexican amigo system, implying a lack of sharing in recreation. Contradictory evidence is obtained from fertility surveys conducted in seven Latin-American metropolitan areas by the United Nations Demographic Center for Latin America (CELADE). Analyzing subsamples of currently mated women, mated at least five years, Hass (1971) concludes that the wife's report of greater sharing in decision-making with regard to important financial decisions and childrearing is associated with lower fertility in only one city sample of currently mated women, i.e., Río de Janeiro. On the other hand, with respect to another familial variable, sharing of leisure, it is indicated that greater leisure-time interaction is associated with lower fertility in only two city samples: Mexico City and Panamá City. Significant differences in fertility are especially evident among the well educated and among those women mated at a later age. Findings remain the same when controls for women's educational attainment, age at union, and marital duration are instituted (Hass, 1971). Another survey of fertility in metropolitan Latin America (Weller, 1968) also concludes that the pattern of dominance with respect to having an additional child bears little relation to cumulative fertility in a San Juan, Puerto Rico, housing sample.

With respect to contraception contradictory findings also exist. However, the majority of studies seem to indicate that for certain subgroups of the population the less segregated the role relationship, the greater the use of an effective birth-control method and the earlier the inception of its use. One possible explanation for the relationship is that couples in more joint conjugal role relationships are less inhibited about sex and therefore able to practice contraception with less embarrassment. Another possibility is that these couples communicate more effectively and are able to cooperate in all areas, including contraception.

Utilizing the concept of conjugal role relationship to explain differences in the effectiveness of contraceptive practice met with little success in Rainwater's (1965) study of middle-class couples. Rainwater concludes that within the middle class differentiating factors in effectiveness of contraception are difficult to distinguish. Both before and after the birth of the last wanted child over 90 percent of the middle-class Protestant couples are effective practitioners. Second, the concept was not useful in differentiating lower-class contraceptive usage prior to the birth of the last wanted child. After this point, however, when serious attempts at contraception are begun in the lower class, marked differences are found. Rainwater notes: ". . . after the birth of the last wanted child the relationship is stronger—only 26 percent of those in highly segregated relationships are effective practitioners compared to 67 percent of those in less segregated relationships" (1965, pp. 231–232). The relationship holds when controls for religion and race are also instituted. Lower-class couples in less segregated role relationships have greater and more effective use of contraceptive methods and use methods that are technically more effective, particularly feminine methods, such as the diaphragm, pill, cream, or jelly alone.

Little research has been conducted in developing countries concerning the degree of segregation in the conjugal role relationship and the use and timing of contraception. Hill et al. (1959), in their study of lower-class Puerto Ricans, conclude that the more restrictive the family organization, the lower the proportion using contraceptive methods, the more irregular and shorter the use, and the later the initiation of contraception (beyond the point of desired children). These habits result in a much lower effectiveness in family planning and the highest number of unwanted pregnancies.

Contradictory evidence is again obtained from analysis of the seven fertility surveys conducted in Latin America. Controlling for women's educational attainment, age at union, and marital duration, it appears that greater sharing in decision-making, as reported by the wife, is associated with more extensive usage of contraception in the Buenos Aires sample alone; and there is a significant relationship between greater sharing of decision-making and earlier use of contraception only in the Bogotá sample. Differences are especially evident among the less-educated women in these samples.

With respect to sharing of leisure-time interaction Hass (1971) also reports that greater leisure-time interaction is associated with greater contraceptive usage in only two city samples: Buenos Aires and Caracas. There is no significant relationship between sharing of leisure-time interaction and parity at first contraception in any of the seven city samples.

Another study of fertility in metropolitan Latin America (Weller, 1968) also indicates that dominance patterns with respect to who makes the final decision on whether or not to have another child appear to be unrelated to the extent of contraceptive usage in a San Juan, Puerto Rico, housing sample. With respect to parity at which contraception is begun, Weller (1968) reports that timing of contraceptive use is latest among the husband-dominant couples and earliest among the egalitarian and wife-dominant couples.

Aside from the studies indicating the existence of a relationship within the lower class (Rainwater, 1965; Hill et al., 1959), other studies do not reach similar conclusions. Westoff et al. (1961) conclude that where dominance patterns in social and nonsocial areas between husbands and wives approach the egalitarian and wife-dominant patterns, the correlations only slightly favor fertility-planning success (.06 and .08). Similar correlations are found with regard to birth-spacing intervals. In a later reinterview of the sample (Westoff et al., 1963) the authors conclude that patterns of dominance and extent of help available to the wife are poor indicators of fertility performance. Although no tabulations of the correlations are presented, the authors assert that the ability to control fertility showed no association with any of these dominance and household aid variables.

How can these disparate findings be evaluated and explained? Westoff et al. (1961) doubt the relevance of the findings on dominance and fertility control in Puerto Rico. They suggest that the small correlations (.10 to .25) between male dominance and fertility control in the Puerto Rican data (Hill et al., 1959) are "nearly random" and constitute "weak if not questionable evidence" (Westoff et al., 1961, pp. 299, 306). Third, they state that weak correlations—significant or not—aid little in explaining and predicting births. Fourth, the authors suggest that researchers may have been mistaken in treating husband-wife dominance as a fixed entity. They suggest that several events, including both female employment and having another child, may enlarge the wife's sphere of activity, her power and authority. Thus the degree of male dominance may be a result as well as a cause of birth-planning variables.

With regard to the dispute on relative size of correlations Pohlman (1969) notes that the Westoff et al. correlations in the first survey (1961, p. 301, table 94; pp. 312–313, tables 103, 104) are consistently in the predicted direction even within religious and social class subgroupings. Although the correlations are small superficiality and insensitivity of measurement in large-scale sample surveys may explain this. Pohlman (1969) therefore posits that

if the etiology of fertility is indeed very complex, the presence of even small correlations may be worthy of some note. . . . In short, it would seem premature to conclude that patterns of husband-wife dominance in some areas may not be influential on either contraception or family-size desires. [P. 349]

We can also offer two other explanations, based on the samples and timing of the studies. It is quite possible that the special nature of the Family Growth in Metropolitan America samples accounts for a slight association in the first survey and a lack of association in the second. All women in the first interview had just had their second child prior to the interview. Thus in both studies we are dealing with women who may still be bearing wanted children. As indicated from the Rainwater study (1965), "Before the birth of the last wanted child, conjugal role organization seems but weakly related to effective or ineffective practice" within the lower class (pp. 231–232). Within the middle class factors differentiating effectiveness of contraception were difficult to distinguish both before and after the birth of the last wanted child. It is therefore probable that the samples of lower-class respondents in the United States (Rainwater, 1965), Puerto Rico (Hill et al., 1959), Buenos Aires, Bogotá, and Caracas samples (Hass, 1971) contain greater numbers of couples who have already borne their last wanted child, and, therefore, dominance and type of conjugal role relationship may have increased predictive power. Unfortunately this still leaves unanswered the absence of any relationship between type of conjugal role relationship and contraceptive usage in the Río de Janeiro, San José, Mexico City, and Panamá City samples (Hass, 1971) and the San Juan sample (Weller, 1968).

Finally it is also important to realize that the Puerto Rican fertility studies and the CELADE studies were conducted prior to the advent or widespread use of coitus-independent methods of contraception (the pill and IUD). As Fawcett (1970) indicates, these new methods depend less on cooperation than traditional contraceptive methods and presumably require different motivation than the motivation required for use of traditional methods, sterilization, or abortion. Thus women in the Family Growth in Metropolitan America studies and the Rainwater study have greater access to coitus-independent methods, and their capability of achieving contraceptive effectiveness would depend less on husband-wife dominance within the marital relationship.

The somewhat contradictory results of the relation between conjugal role relationship and fertility lead us to reexamine the basis of the assumed relationship between the two. The argument really rests on two separate steps. First, it is assumed that couples in segregated relationships want a larger family than those in joint conjugal role relations; second, it is assumed that families with joint role relationships can limit their family more effectively. The first argument harks back to the structural relationship, the segregated family being closer to the kinship structure and the joint family closer to the conjugal family. Thus the change in fertility patterns may have little to do with the role structure of the family, but may be a correlate of a global change, namely, modernization. We could easily imagine that some conjugal joint role families, concentrating mainly on their homes and their relationships, may want a large family sharing the responsibility for the bringing up of the children. Thus the consequence is not so much a question of the role relationships themselves but of their intended use. The second problem is somewhat different but may also be more psychological than structural. All types of role relationships may result in effective action: organizations with segregated roles are frequently created for higher efficiency in reaching specified goals. On the other hand, some goals are reached easier by a joint role relationship. It is not the nature of the structures but whether they function properly that makes them successful or not. Experiments in social psychology (Thibaut et al., 1960; Shaw, 1964) have shown that attunement of the communication process and activities to the tasks to be accomplished is of primary importance. Thus we shall turn now to the intermediate variables leading to fertility in the family context—marital communication, sexual gratifications and marital adjustment.

Marital Communication

Rainwater theorizes that the amount and quality of marital communication is an important factor of conjugal role relationships and contributes to greater contraceptive effectiveness among jointly organized couples. Studies in developed countries (Rainwater, 1965) and developing countries such as Puerto Rico (Hill et al., 1959) and Mexico (DeHoyos and DeHoyos, 1966) indicate that controlling for social class, there is a relationship between degree of segregation of conjugal role relationship and general communication. We may then ask what are the consequences of communication on fertility and contraceptive usage?

First, marital communication is necessary if discussions on desired family size and discussions on contraceptive usage are to exist. In certain cases casual discussion may indicate the expectation of a large family, and couples may not think it necessary to discuss family planning until fairly late in the childbearing history, as in the case of Catholics in the United States (Rainwater, 1965). In most cases, however, casual or late discussion may reflect weak motivations for a small family or lack of knowledge on specific methods of contraception, as in the case of Jamaica. In Jamaica Stycos and Back (1964) found that only a minority (38 percent) of their lower-class Jamaican respondents had ever discussed family size with their husbands. Moreover, those who wanted no more children were no more likely to have discussed the matter than those who did want more. Another reason for casual or late discussion may be the wife's attempt to avoid suspicions of marital infidelity.

In the absence of effective communication each of the mates makes assumptions about the other according to cultural stereotypes. In static cultures these assumptions may be satisfactory, but in societies undergoing rapid social change the stereotypes may not be realistic. Thus, for example, the Puerto Rican study found that husbands attribute more modesty (a cultural ideal) to their wives than their wives actually possess, and wives assume greater virility drives and desires for children (another cultural ideal) than their hsubands actually possess (Hill et al., 1959; see also Stycos, 1968).

A second consequence is that knowledge about contraception is not pooled. In Puerto Rico it was found that comparing the responses of over 300 couples, in only a fifth of these instances did the husband and wife know the same number of methods. Thus much of the knowledge possessed individually failed to affect behavior because it was not exchanged. Moreover, it was found that in every age and educational category those who discussed family-size ideals knew more birth-control methods (Hill et al., 1959; Stycos, 1968).

Third, couples with effective communication are more likely to use birth control, as noted in studies in Israel (Bachi and Matras, 1964); in Peru, (Stycos, 1968); in Jamaica (Stycos and Back, 1964), where communication with the spouse seems to be of outstanding importance in the continued use of contraception; and in Puerto Rico (Hill et al. 1959), where communication was best correlated with use of birth-control clinics, number of birth-control methods known and the number used, whether birth control had ever been used, length of use, regularity of use, and success of use.

Sexual Gratification

The degree of sexual gratification varies quite markedly by social class, and within the lower class also by type of conjugal role relationship (Rainwater, 1965; Kinsey et al., 1953). In turn sexual gratification appears to be related to contraceptive effectiveness in U.S. samples. In short, American women expressing greater sexual gratification seem able to accept and discuss contraception more easily. Rainwater (1965) comments:

> A highly segregated conjugal role relationship makes it difficult for couples to function in the close cooperation required for both mutually gratifying sexual relations and effective contraceptive practice. In this context, contraception tends to become a bone of contention in relation to the wife's wish to avoid anything connected with sex, and her anxiety about becoming pregnant coupled with the difficulties she experiences in doing anything to prevent it. [P. 280]

Thus among lower-class white and black Protestants a positive relationship exists between effectiveness at contraception and the extent to which the wife indicates that she finds sexual relations with her husband gratifying. The relationship does not hold for Catholics—as long as their families are not larger than they wanted, their religious views are not tested by excess fertility.

Within the middle class sexual gratification is also related to effective practice before the birth of the last wanted child for both Catholics and Protestants (Rainwater, 1965). Among couples who express mutual enjoyment of the sexual relationship, almost 90 percent were also effective contraceptive users. Among those couples in which one partner enjoyed sexual relations more than his or her spouse, only about half of the couples were effective planners. Rainwater offers two possible explanations. First, as previously stated, couples with unequal enjoyment of sexual relations may find it difficult to cooperate in using contraception regularly and therefore effectively, or the lack of regular or effective contraception may reinforce unequal enjoyment of sex because of fear of pregnancy. On the other hand, Rainwater suggests that couples who do find anxiety in their sexual relationship may tend to delay effective contraception in the unconscious hope that additional children will improve the relationship. In such relationships there would be little emphasis on family planning and spacing of children (Rainwater, 1965; Sloman, 1948).

Landis et al. (1950) and others (Rutherford, Banks, and Coburn, 1962) also find a significant tendency for wives who feared another labor and childbirth to have a less satisfactory sexual adjustment or "postpartum frigidity." Likewise wives (but not husbands) who mistrust the contraceptive method they use report a less satisfactory sexual relationship. Terman

(1938) reports a similar finding. Finally Babchuk and LaCognata (1960) also provide evidence agreeing with Rainwater that couples with more sexual and marital relationship problems are less successful in using the same contraceptive methods.

Cross-cultural data, however, have failed to replicate Rainwater's and Babchuk's and LaCognata's findings. Hill et al. (1959) report that self-ratings of sexual satisfaction seem to be associated with male dominance in the marital relationship and the holding of traditional values, i.e., the segregated conjugal role relationship. The authors report that lower-class Puerto Rican wives who are least satisfied with the sex relationship are the most likely to have practiced birth control over a long period, if they have practiced it at all. There is a nonsignificant indication that sexually dissatisfied wives also practice birth control more successfully. Dissatisfaction appears more frequently in dominant wives, working wives, and wives who are striving-oriented in their values.

Rainwater (1960) also found examples of this particular kind of woman in his sample of lower-class Americans. The woman who rejects sexuality, but nonetheless is effective at contraception, merely separates the two phenomena. Since she considers contraception very much in her own interest she is better able to accept feminine methods of contraception than are other kinds of rejecting or ambivalent women.

Marital Adjustment

As a final factor let us review the literature on the relationship between marital adjustment and fertility and contraceptive effectiveness. Many studies have tried to correlate marital adjustment and family size (Blood and Wolfe, 1960; Burgess and Cottrell, 1939; Christensen and Philbrick, 1952; Farber and Blackman, 1956; Westoff et al., 1961; Westoff et al., 1963; Landis and Landis, 1963; Reed, 1946; and Terman, 1938). As Pohlman (1969) indicates in his excellent review of the topic, the cause-and-effect relationship is difficult to identify in cross-sectional studies and even in the one major longitudinal study (Westoff et al., 1963). Second, some studies fail to control for relevant variables such as marital duration or socioeconomic status. After reviewing the findings Pohlman (1969) concludes:

> It seems clear that there is no single correlation between children and marriage happiness. A happier marriage may lead some people to be more willing to have children; a marriage threatening breakup may lead others to want and have children. Children may promote marital happiness in some cases; and children, especially unwanted children, may hurt marital happiness in others [P. 98].

With regard to contraceptive effectiveness Kiser and Whelpton (1953) report that among Indianapolis couples marital adjustment (a happy marriage, little disagreement over family matters, and little desire to improve spouse) is directly related to successful family planning, both with respect to preventing unwanted pregnancies and to success in having as many children as desired among the "number and space planned" couples. There is other evidence also that *unwanted* children seem to lead to poorer marital adjustment (Burgess and Cottrell, 1939; Reed, 1946), although even here the cause-and-effect relationship is difficult to determine.

Research in Puerto Rico (Hill et al., 1959) concludes likewise. Marital happiness (willingness to remarry the same person and self-rating of satisfaction in marriage) is positively related (.23) to general communication between spouses; and agreement on marital issues appears to be significantly related to success in fertility control, although the correlation is small (.10).

Summary

The survey of the evidence shows mainly contradictory evidence for many of the hypotheses linking family structure and fertility. The difficulty seems to rest in the destinction between comparative studies and field research, between comparing families in different societies and families within the same society. The hypotheses are mainly derived from the comparative studies and evidence indicating that changes in family values, role relationships, and interaction patterns differ in societies that have reduced their fertility. These hypotheses are then tested on different family styles within a society. The conditions for adhering to a certain family pattern within a society may be more idiosyncratic, e.g., relating to the life cycle or the specific personality and status relations of the two partners, rather than to the differences in macrosocial factors.

In this light we may review the evidence that we have assembled. We find that many of the supposed factors affecting desire for offspring are in fact not operative. In this regard we discussed in detail the findings about machismo. Desire for a large number of offspring may be a cultural norm distinguishing societies, but it cannot be easily related to the simple personality traits that have been mentioned. We have concluded that there are some factors that influence cooperation between partners and, therefore, achievement of childbearing goals. These factors include distrust of marital fidelity, sexual modesty, and the resulting lack of communication between spouses who see each other as strangers and even potential enemies in the sexual sphere. Within the lower class degree of role segregation seems to be the best indicator of the kind of social change that makes effective action possible, while in upper and middle classes this change has already been achieved, and degree of role segregation is no longer an indicator. Finally the data on sexual gratification should be interpreted in this light. Under conditions in which egalitarian, freely communicating relationships lead to better marriages, these measures do relate to success in contraception; but in many societies other types of marriage patterns, in which success is not dependent on deep emotional relationships, are accepted, and here the expected correlations do not hold and are even reversed. It would be the psychologist's task to focus on affect as the important variable and determine its dependence on cultural norms as well as its effect on fertility goals and success in achieving them under different social standards.

Concentrating on affect as the central variable may also shift the focus in another way. There is almost always an implicit assumption in fertility studies that the number of children is a definite goal that may be shifted. It is not clear, however, to what degree family size is a real goal for many people. Looking at affect as the primary variable, we are led to a process orientation, namely, that even with planning, children are planned one by one, depending on the situation of the family, the marital relationship, and the satisfaction of the wife among other factors. We may look at the marital relationship and fertility as a continuing process, where the particular economic and affective situation lead to the conception of a child, and the birth and maturation of the child change the family situation. Excess fertility may be best understood by considering the situation under which the high parity are born and not by focusing on a decision of a couple to have many children. In this regard Fortney (1971) has related the incidence of "accidental" pregnancies among U.S. middle-class women to lack of satisfaction with available and alternative nonfamilial roles.

Changes and reassessment occur more extensively through changes in marital status. The simplified model of global decision-making on family size is also reflected in the decision of many studies to include only couples where both members are married only once. Although this makes for a neater study design, it is becoming more and more unrealistic in present-day society. Not only are broken marriages and remarriages more and more frequent, but new forms of marriage or lasting relations without marriage are emerging and being recognized. Changes in family life of this kind cannot fail to have a profound effect on the distribution of affect as well as on fertility patterns. We can conclude this chapter by discussing current available evidence on how these possible changes in family structure may affect fertility.

Prospects for the Future

The sexual revolution has focused interest on possible alternative forms of the family for future generations. Thus Margaret Mead (1970) has suggested the possibility of marriage in two steps. The first step, individual marriage, would be "a licensed union in which two individuals would be committed to each other as individuals for as long as they wished to remain together, but not as future parents" (pp. 80–81). As the first step in marriage this arrangement would not include children. In contrast the second type of marriage, parental marriage, would always follow an individual marriage. It would have its own license, ceremony, and responsibilities and would be explicitly directed toward the formation of a family (Mead, 1970). This proposal reiterates Russell's (1929) earlier suggestion of limited trial marriage, especially for students.

Albert Ellis has examined group marriage as a possible alternative. In its strictest form group marriage consists of a relatively small number of adults living together, having sexual access to one another, sharing labor, goods, and service, and rearing children together. In its looser form group marriage consists of communal or tribal marriage where a larger group of adults live in a cooperative community and have theoretical sexual access to all members, although in fact their sexual access may be limited to only a few members of the group. Small-scale group marriage has apparently been reasonably common throughout history, and there have been isolated incidences of more large-scale group marriage, such as the Oneida Community in upstate New York. More recent experiments have involved the Kerista movement and various other reports of group marriage in the literature of sexually liberal organizations. From these reports Ellis (1970) concludes, ". . . it can be seen that group marriage unquestionably exists today in the United States and in other parts of the world. But it leads a somewhat checkered career, never seems to become exceptionally well established, and is largely practiced by unstable groups which have a hard time getting started and an even more difficult time remaining in existence" (pp. 91–92). Ellis believes that it is highly unlikely that group marriage will ever fully replace monogamic mating, or even that the majority of Westerners will voluntarily choose it instead of our present system of monogamy. However, he concludes that it is highly probable that a sizable minority of individuals will participate in some type of simultaneous sex relationship, including nonmonogamic unions or a form of group marriage, on an intermittent or temporary basis rather than on a permanent basis.

One is tempted to ask what would be the consequences of such marital arrangements on fertility and contraceptive usage? Insight into this problem can be obtained if we examine some of the current literature relating type of union to fertility. Much of our knowledge is based on investigations in the Caribbean where nonlegal types of unions are important.

In the English-speaking Caribbean three categories of unions have been identified and investigated: the visiting relationship (a nonlegal arrangement involving noncohabitation); the common-law union or consensual union (a nonlegal arrangement involving cohabitation); and the legal union (legal cohabitation). Roberts (1955, 1957, 1969) presents data on fertility differentials in the English Caribbean by type of union and concludes that in terms of period rates highest fertility at all ages is recorded for married women; the second highest fertility is experienced by women in common-law unions; and at a considerably lower level are the fertility rates for women in visiting unions. Several measures of completed fertility give essentially the same pattern. Fairly similar results are found in data for Martinique (Leridon et al., 1970), thus disputing the widely held view that illegitimacy of union increases fertility.

On the other hand, evidence from other parts of Latin America and the Caribbean is frequently at variance or even contradictory to these previous findings. Thus, for example, common-law marriages in Puerto Rico are far more fertile than those in Jamaica, and consequently fertility differentials are almost nonexistent (Jaffe, 1959) or even reversed (Stycos, 1968). Urban fertility surveys further complicate the findings. Fertility is higher for the consensually married than for the legally married in the cities of Caracas, Mexico City, and Panamá City (where consensual unions are more prevalent). However, fertility of the consensually married is lower in Bogotá, Buenos Aires, and San José (Miró, 1966). Mortara (1961) concludes that differences in the proportions of couples consensually married among Latin-American countries have little explanatory value for intercountry fertility differentials and concludes that no important overall fertility differences exist between the two types of union.

The disparities in these research findings indicate that other important variables related to type of union and fertility must be examined and their influence estimated. In an excellent review of the topic Mertens (1970) concludes that one must take into account differential characteristics of unions: age at onset, frequency of sexual relations, first age of childbearing, and spacing patterns. For example, Roberts (1955, 1957, 1969) states that on the average women in visiting unions and consensual unions are first exposed to pregnancy at a younger age than are women in legal marriages; however, the intervals between unions and therefore periods of nonexposure to pregnancy are greater for women in visiting unions than for those in the other two types.

With regard to frequency of sexual intercourse within unions Stycos (1968) states that frequency of sexual relations differs in different unions. Moreover, within every type of union frequency of sexual relations is affected by the rank order of the union. Thus, for example, women in visiting unions have more infrequent sexual relations than women in the other two types of unions. However, the average monthly frequency of intercourse shows a substantial increase after the first visiting union. Other differential characteristics indicated by Mertens (1970) are stability, incidence of induced abortion, and mortality of the partners, all of which are related to exposure to pregnancy. Moreover, we would also want information on educational attainment and contraceptive usage of the partners. Finally Mertens urges that marital status be conceptualized as a dynamic process, involving not only a change in partners throughout time but a change in type of union over time. He remarks that stability is an especially important variable. Instability of reproductive unions may affect fertility in contradictory ways. For instance, unstable unions may serve to reduce fertility if they create interunion periods during which a woman is not exposed to the possibility of pregnancy and periods at the end of the union during which frequency of sexual relations decreases. On the other hand, instability may increase the motivation for childbearing by encouraging additional offspring with each new partner (Blake, 1954). Moreover, Mertens cautions that change in itself should not necessarily be viewed as instability, since it may indicate a process to strengthen bonds by transition to a more stable type of union (1970). The desire to shift is caused by the prestige of the legal union and a concern for the legitimation of the children. Thus the shift could be selective of those who have offspring and could thus inflate fertility of legal unions. Finally in keeping with the dynamic view Mertens suggests making classifications on fertility according to the initial and terminal types of union.

With regard to two-stage marriage and group marriage we must take into consideration these same variables. Thus two-stage marriage might serve to raise the age of first childbearing and therefore lower fertility if couples are encouraged to enter individual marriage prior to parental marriage. On the other hand, the legalization of two-stage marriage might serve to maintain the same age at union if people simply enter individual marriage at younger ages and are therefore ready for parental marriage at approximately the same age in which they otherwise enter monogamous unions. In hypothesizing possible effects one would be concerned also with the relative stability of individual marriage as well as with the interunion period between individual marriages.

With regard to the familial interaction variables, individual marriage presupposes widespread discussion and usage of effective contraception since it precludes the presence of children. Moreover, one would suspect that the decision to enter parental marriage would follow the attainment of marital adjustment and sexual adjustment (and therefore contraceptive effectiveness) and would be followed by discussion on family-size ideals.

With regard to group marriage we would want to know the frequency of sexual intercourse within unions and the stability of unions, not only with regard to number of partners and interunion periods of nonexposure, but also with regard to change in type of union over time from group marriage to monogamous marriage. If frequency of sexual relations is higher or additional offspring with each partner is desired in group marital arrangements, one might hypothesize higher fertility. On the other hand, if interunion periods are relatively long, or economic considerations are taken into account and pressure is placed on members to maintain the size of the group because of problems of self-support, one could hypothesize reduced fertility. Finally, as Ellis notes, in larger communal living arrangements unions may approach a simple monogamous arrangement between two commune members, and one would not necessarily expect fertility from such a union to differ from the fertility of a legal monogamous union.

Again, with regard to the familial interaction variables one would suspect the attainment of marital adjustment and sexual adjustment (and therefore contraceptive effectiveness) among *stable*, long-term partners. One would also suspect that the demands of childrearing—the restriction of freedom, as well as the necessity for child care and child support—might act as a deterrent against childbearing, especially among members in recently established communal marriages, who are probably oriented to outside activities and marital partners rather than to home and children.

From the evidence that we have been able to assemble it is not possible to conclude what demographic consequences the dissolution of the conjugal family may have, if the family is dissolving at all. This reminds us of our earlier conclusion that the change from corporate kinship groups to the conjugal family was less the cause of fertility reduction than a concomitant part of the same social change. Both these conclusions remind us that these changes do not occur in a vacuum, but within a larger cultural context. In this perspective we have to evaluate the fertility effects of possible future family patterns.

The growth of communes and new types of voluntary transient relationships may be a sign of diffuse and shallow affect, lack of individual commitment, and assumption of responsibility by a larger group or the whole society for the offspring. In this case we can expect increased fertility as a result of attempts to give meaning to each union by producing a child; casual attitudes toward individual relationships and toward responsibility to one's own children; and relative ease of parenthood with the provision of communal child-care centers. However, the same individuals who look for these new forms may also have values concordant with preservation of the environment, the "ecological panic," and the ideology of Spaceship Earth. Imbued with a culture of this kind, they may adopt a rigorous population-planning policy, restricting the growth of each group and exerting individual control, even through radical birth-control measures. Both alternatives would have important effects upon personality and affective relations of parents and offspring; they would lead to impressive changes until a new relatively stable society could be reached.

Our excursion into possible futures has shown again that family structure by itself cannot be taken as a main determinant of fertility patterns. The fertility goals are dependent on the larger values of the society; the effectiveness of the family in achieving them is dependent on subtle affective interactions. Family structure is a mechanism through which the social values are transferred into the planning of a couple; it is also the framework within which the interpersonal relations are acted out.

REFERENCES

Babchuk, N. and LaCognata, A. 1960. Crises and the effective utilization of contraception. *Marriage and Family Living* 22:254–258.

Bachi, R. and Matras, J. 1964. Family size preferences of Jewish maternity cases in Israel. *Milbank Memorial Fund Quarterly* 2, part 1:38–56.

Blake, J. 1954. Family instability and reproductive behavior in Jamaica. In *Milbank Memorial Fund annual conference*. New York: Milbank Memorial Fund. Pp. 24–41.

Blood, R. O. and Wolfe, D. M. 1960. *Husbands and wives: the dynamics of married living*. New York: Free Press.

Burch, T. K. and Gendell, M. 1970. Extended family structure and fertility: some conceptual and methodological issues. *Journal of Marriage and the Family* 32:227–236.

Burgess, E. W. and Cottrell, L. S. 1939. *Predicting success or failure in marriage*. Englewood Cliffs, N.J.: Prentice-Hall.

Christensen, H. T. and Philbrick, R. E. 1952. Family size as a factor in marital adjustment of college couples. *American Sociological Review* 17:306–312.

Cruz, L. 1967. Brazil. In R. Patai, ed., *Women in the modern world*. New York: Free Press. Pp. 209–225.

Davis, K. 1955. Institutional factors favoring high fertility in underdeveloped areas. *Eugenics Quarterly* 2:33–39.

Davis, K. and Blake, J. 1956. Social structure and fertility: an analytical framework. *Economic Development and Cultural Change* 4:211–235.

DeHoyos, A. and DeHoyos, G. 1966. The amigo system and alienation of the wife in the conjugal Mexican family. In B. Farber, ed., *Kinship and family organization*. New York: Wiley. Pp. 102–115.

Driver, E. D. 1963. *Differential fertility in central India*. Princeton: Princeton University Press.

Ellis, A. 1970. Group marriage: a possible alternative? In H. A. Otto, ed., *The Family in search of a future: alternative models for moderns*. New York: Appleton-Century-Crofts. Pp. 85–97.

Farber, B. and Blackman, L. S. 1956. Marital role tensions and number and sex of children. *American Sociological Review* 21:596–601.

Fawcett, J. T. 1970. *Psychology and population: behavioral research issues in fertility and family planning*. New York: The Population Council.

Fortney, J. A. 1971. "Role preference and fertility: an exploration of motivation for childbearing." Unpublished Ph.D. diss., Duke University.

Freedman, R. 1963. The sociology of human fertility: a trend report and bibliography. *Current Sociology* Vol. 10–11. (Republished: Oxford, Basil Blackwell.)

Freedman, R.; Takeshita, J. Y.; and Sun, T. H. 1964. Fertility and family planning in Taiwan: a case study of the demographic transition. *American Journal of Sociology* 70:16–27.

Goldberg, D. 1959. The fertility of two-generation urbanites. *Population Studies* 12:214–222.

Goode, W. J. 1963a. Industrialization and family change. In B. F. Hoselitz and W. E. Moore, eds., *Industrialization and society*. Paris: UNESCO. Pp. 240–250.

———. 1963b. *World revolution and family patterns*. New York: Free Press.

Gore, M. S. 1965. The traditional Indian family. In M. F. Nimkoff, ed., *Comparative family systems*. Boston: Houghton Mifflin. Pp. 209–231.

Hass, P. H. 1971. Maternal employment, fertility, and contraceptive usage in metropolitan Latin America. Unpublished Ph.D. diss., Duke University.

Herbst, P. G. 1957. Family living—patterns of interaction. In O. A. Oeser and S. B. Hammond, eds., *Social structure and personality in a city*. New York: Macmillan. Pp. 164–179.

Hill, R.; Stycos, J. M.; and Back, K. 1959. *The family and population control: a Puerto Rican experiment in social change*. Chapel Hill: University of North Carolina Press.

Hoffman, L. W. and Wyatt, F. 1960. Social change and motivations for having larger families: some theoretical considerations. *Merrill-Palmer Quarterly* 6:235–244.

Jaffe, A. J. 1959. *People, jobs, and economic development.* Glencoe, Ill.: Free Press.

Kazen, P. M. and Browning, H. L. 1967. Sociological aspects of the high fertility of the U.S. Mexican-descent population: an exploratory study. Unpublished manuscript, Population Research Center, University of Texas.

Kinsey, C.; Pomeroy, W. B.; Martin, C. R.; and Gebhard, P. H. 1953. *Sexual behavior in the human female.* Philadelphia: W. B. Saunders.

Kiser, C. V. and Whelpton, P. K. 1953. Resume of the Indianapolis study of social and psychological factors affecting fertility. *Population Studies* 7:95–110.

Landis, J. T. and Landis, M. G. 1963. *Building a successful marriage.* Englewood Cliffs, N.J.: Prentice-Hall.

Landis, J. T.; Poffenberger, T.; and Poffenberger, S. 1950. The effects of first pregnancy upon the sexual adjustment of 212 couples. *American Sociological Review* 15:766–772.

Laslett, P. 1965. *The world we have lost.* New York: Scribner.

Leridon, H.; Zucker, E.; and Cazenove, M. 1970. *Fécondité et famille en Martinique: Faits, attitudes et opinions.* Paris: INED-PUF.

Litwak, E. 1960. Occupational mobility and extended family cohesion. *American Sociological Review* 25:9–21.

Liu, P. K. C. 1967. Differential fertility in Taiwan. In contributed papers, *International Union for the Scientific Study of Population, Sydney conference, 1967.* Sydney, Australia. Pp. 363–370.

Lorimer, F. 1954. *Culture and human fertility: a study of the relation of cultural conditions to fertility in non-industrial and transitional societies.* Paris: UNESCO.

Mead, M. 1970. Marriage in two steps. In H. A. Otto, ed., *The family in search of a future: alternative models for moderns.* New York: Appleton-Century-Crofts. Pp. 75–84.

Mertens, W. 1970. Fertility and family planning research in Latin America: an overview of recent developments. Paper presented at the Conferencia Regional Latinoamericana de Población, Mexico City.

Miró, C. A. 1966. Some misconceptions disproved: a program of comparative fertility surveys in Latin America. In B. Berelson et al., eds., *Family planning and population problems: a review of world developments.* Chicago: University of Chicago Press. Pp. 615–634.

Mortara, G. 1961. *Le unioni coniugali libere nell'America Latina.* Rome: Facolta di Scienze Statistiche Demografiche ed Attuariali. Pp. 116–120.

Nag, M. 1967. Family type and fertility. In *Proceedings, world population conference, 1965.* New York: United Nations 2:160–163.

Namboodiri, N. K. 1967. Fertility differentials in non-industrial societies. Unpublished mimeographed paper.

Nimkoff, M. F. and Middleton, R. 1968. Types of family and types of economy. In R. F. Winch and L. W. Goodman, eds., *Selected studies in marriage and the family.* New York: Holt, Rinehart & Winston. Pp. 35–42.

Pakrasi, K. and Malaker, C. 1967. The relationship between family type and fertility. *Milbank Memorial Fund Quarterly* 45:451–460.

Palmore, J. A.; Klein, R. E.; bin Morzul Ariffin. 1970. Class and family in a modernizing society. *American Journal of Sociology* 76 (November): 375–398.

Pohlman, E. 1969. *The psychology of birth planning.* Cambridge, Mass.: Schenkman.

Rainwater, L. 1960. *And the poor get children.* Chicago: Quadrangle Books.

———. 1965. *Family design: marital sexuality, family size, and family planning.* Chicago: Aldine.

Rao, M. K. 1959. Progress in family planning in Bagalore. *Journal of Family Welfare* (Bombay) 6:16–23.

Reed, R. B. 1946. Interrelationship of marital adjustment, fertility control, and size of family. In P. K. Whelpton and C. V. Kiser, eds., *Social and psychological factors affecting fertility.* New York: Milbank Memorial Fund 1:259–301.

Rele, J. R. 1963. Fertility differentials in India: evidence from a rural background. *Milbank Memorial Fund Quarterly* 41:183–199.

Roberts, G. W. 1955. Some aspects of mating and fertility in the West Indies. *Population Studies* 8:212–217.

————. 1957. *The population of Jamaica.* London: Cambridge University Press.

————. 1969. Fertility in some Caribbean countries. Paper presented at the London Population Conference, London.

Russell, B. 1929. *Marriage and morals.* New York: Horace Liveright, Inc.

Rutherford, R. N.; Banks, A. L.; and Coburn, W. A. 1962. Frigidity in the female partner with special reference to postpartum frigidity: some clinical observations and study programs. In W. S. Kroger, ed., *Psychosomatic obstetrics, gynecology, and endocrinology.* Springfield, Ill.: Thomas. Pp. 400–414.

Shaw, M. E. 1964. Communication networks. In L. Berkowitz, ed., *Advances in experimental social psychology.* New York: Academic Press. Vol. 1.

Slater, P. E. 1963. On social regression. *American Sociological Review* 28:339–364.

Sloman, S. S. 1948. Emotional problems in "planned for" children. *American Journal of Orthopsychiatry* 18:523–528.

Stycos, J. M. 1958. Some directions for research on fertility control. *Milbank Memorial Fund Quarterly* 36:126–148.

————. 1962. Experiments in social change: the Caribbean fertility studies. In C. V. Kiser, ed., *Research in family planning.* Princeton: Princeton University Press. Pp. 305–333.

————. 1968. *Human fertility in Latin America: sociological perspectives.* Ithaca, N.Y.: Cornell University Press.

Stycos, J. M. and Back, K. W. 1964. *The control of human fertility in Jamaica.* Ithaca, N.Y.: Cornell University Press.

Sussman, M. B. 1954. Family continuity: selective factors which affect relationships between families at generational levels. *Marriage and Family Living* 16:112–120.

————. 1959. The isolated nuclear family: fact or fiction. *Social Problems* 6:333–340.

Terman, L. 1938. *Psychological factors in marital happiness.* New York: McGraw-Hill.

Thibaut, J. W.; Strickland, L. H.; Mundy, D.; and Goding, E. F. 1960. Communication, task demands, and group effectiveness. *Journal of Personality* 28:156–166.

Weller, R. H. 1968. The employment of wives, dominance, and fertility. *Journal of Marriage and the Family* 30:437–442.

Westoff, C. F.; Potter, R. G.; and Sagi, P. C. 1963. *The third child.* Princeton: Princeton University Press.

Westoff, C. F.; Potter, R. G.; Sagi, P. C.; and Mishler, E. G. 1961. *Family growth in metropolitan America.* Princeton: Princeton University Press.

[4]

MODERNIZATION, INDIVIDUAL
MODERNITY, AND FERTILITY

JAMES T. FAWCETT
AND MARC H. BORNSTEIN

In this chapter we will be concerned with three different but related sets of data pertaining to *modernization,* a societal-level process; *individual modernity,* a person-level pattern of traits; and *fertility,* which may be measured at the aggregate level as fertility rates or at the individual level as the number of children born to a woman or to a couple. We will first elaborate upon the distinction between modernization and individual modernity, then discuss the reasons for attempting to relate research on these topics to fertility.

Modernization is the term usually used to describe the movement of socioeconomic systems toward higher levels of development, as revealed by cross-national comparisons and by changes in socioeconomic indices over time. As noted by Lerner (1968), the level of such indices in the industrialized, urbanized, technologically oriented nations has produced an image of what is modern, providing a goal for the aspirations of less developed nations and stimulating among social scientists "efforts to conceptualize modernization as the contemporary mode of social change that is both general in validity and global in scope" (p. 387). In social-science terms modernization is viewed necessarily as a multivariate phenomenon, but there is not a consensus as to which variables should appropriately be included or emphasized. The scales or dimensions used to define modernization include diverse kinds of variables, and their components are often labeled differently depending upon the professional interests or theoretical orientation of the investigator. The study of modernization is thus to a large degree ad hoc, and relevant work can be discerned within the traditions of various disciplines: the folk-urban dichotomy from anthropology and sociology, the underdeveloped-developed and agrarian-industrial contrasts from economics, the traditional-modern comparisons of societies and people from several of the social sciences, including psychology.

Studies specifically labeled as pertaining to modernization have dealt mainly with societal-level variables, such as levels of literacy or education, average per-capita income, proportion of population living in urban areas or engaged in industrial occupations, number of radios or newspaper circulation per capita, indices of power consumption, and so on. Recently, however, attention has focused upon the measurement of individual modernity or modernism. Operationally this approach requires the collection of response data from individuals through sample surveys, personality tests, attitude scales, and the like, within a research design that attempts to distinguish between modern and traditional individuals. The basic research hypothesis is that people who would be sociologically classified as more modern, such as urban factory workers, will be similar to each other with respect to certain measurable psychological characteristics; moreover, that a modern group (factory workers) will differ from a traditional group (farmers) on these same characteristics. A general model underlying many studies of individual modernity is that exposure to uniformities in the immediate social and physical environment, such as the work situation, will result in cross-cultural uniformities in certain behaviors and psychological traits. (The differences among several analytic and causal models of modernization are discussed by Weiner [1966] in the introduction to his useful collection of articles on this topic.)

Individual modernity then is a pattern of psychological characteristics related to societal modernization. Research on individual modernity has been both descriptive and explanatory, with causal relationships viewed as operating in two directions: social change affects the modal characteristics of individuals, and the characteristics of individuals can hamper or facilitate social change. The interaction between societal modernity and individual modernity is apparent in Lerner's (1968) description of five major components of modernization: self-sustaining growth in the economy; public participation in the polity; diffusion of secular-rational norms in the culture; mobility in the society; and "a corresponding transformation in the modal personality that equips individuals to function effectively in a social order that operates according to the foregoing characteristics" (p. 387).

In the present context we are interested in traits associated with individual modernity because of the relationship between modernization and fertility. In general people in modern societies have fewer children. An examination of the psychological characteristics that distinguish modern and traditional individuals may provide some insight into the complex personal processes that intervene between social change and fertility change.

The practical significance of this topic is highlighted by recent discussions in the population literature concerning "reproductive motivation" and population policies (cf. Berelson, 1969; Blake, 1965, 1968, 1969; Chilman, 1970; Davis, 1967; Spengler, 1969). A central controversy in the population field revolves around the necessity, desirability, and effectiveness of several alternative approaches to population limitation: the provision of programs and facilities to eliminate unwanted childbearing; the alteration of fertility patterns through direct means such as persuasion, incentives, or penalties; and the changing of institutional conditions that are assumed to affect reproductive motivations, such as the availability of nonfamilial roles for women. We cannot discuss here the details of this controversy, but would point out that the research reviewed in this chapter is relevant to an understanding of the relationship between social conditions and reproductive motivations. Existing knowledge about that relationship stems mainly from macroanalytic studies that bypass the individual level of analysis. By including the individual level (e.g., by showing that education affects fertility through changes in certain personal traits) research on individual modernity can contribute to the knowledge required as a basis for population policy recommendations. If fundamental reproductive motives are in fact derived from social and economic conditions, then better knowledge about the components of that relationship and the intervening processes should inevitably suggest points at which accelerated change is most feasible, culturally acceptable, and likely to be effective.

Having expressed such an ambitious goal, we must note forthwith that it will not readily be achieved. By tracing the relationships among modernization, individual modernity, and fertility some insight may be gained as to the ways in which certain social conditions affect fertility outcomes via changes in individuals, but the picture is fragmentary at best and much of the evidence is indirect. A stance of modesty is therefore appropriate, but we present the following review in the hope that it will be viewed as a provocative and potentially productive research area, which should complement other approaches to the study of fertility.

We will begin by reviewing some of the findings and hypotheses from traditional fertility research that are pertinent to social modernization. Following that we will summarize recent research on individual modernity, emphasizing the variables relating modernity to fertility. Finally we will discuss the implications of these research results.

Modernization and Fertility Change

Demographic analyses have shown consistent relationships between modernization and fertility in a number of ways: fertility changes associated with societal changes over time (the demographic transition); fertility comparisons among groups within a society (urban-rural, educated-uneducated); and fertility comparisons among societies (industrialized nations and developing nations). In general a more advanced level of modernization has been shown to be negatively correlated with fertility. Few social phenomena are as well documented as the inverse relationship between modernization and fertility (see Adelman and Morris, 1966; Ryder, 1959; United Nations, 1953).

This broad generalization must immediately be followed, however, by certain qualifications and exceptions. While it is true that there is consistent evidence for a long-term inverse relationship between modernization and fertility, a direct, positive relationship has been shown for shorter time periods and for subgroups within a society (see Gendell, 1967; Heer, 1966). When more refined measurements are applied, pertaining both to ways of classifying populations and to indices of fertility, it is found that the general trend admits of many variations, irregularities, and even reversals. For this reason and because sociodemographic analyses do not in any event account for much of the variation in fertility, hypotheses have been developed that attempt to specify the variables and processes that intervene between socioeconomic stratification indices and fertility. Some of these hypotheses are essentially psychological or sociopsychological in nature. That is, they deal with ways in which individuals may differentially perceive, interpret, or react to their immediate social setting, with special reference to the consequences for family-size preferences, contraceptive performance, and actual fertility. It is beyond the scope of this chapter to review systematically such hypotheses, but we will attempt to summarize major themes. More comprehensive discussions may be found in Fawcett (1970), Freedman (1963), and Hawthorn (1970).

Before describing some of the social-psychological themes related to fertility change, we would note that these can be incorporated only loosely within a theoretical framework. There does not exist a systematic and comprehensive theory of fertility, although some useful attempts have been made to develop conceptual schemes that incorporate diverse kinds of variables (Freedman, 1967; Hill, Stycos, and Back, 1959; Mishler and Westoff, 1955). Also Davis and Blake (1956) have provided an exhaustive classification of "intermediate" variables through which fertility change must be effected, grouped under the three general categories of intercourse variables, conception variables, and gestation variables. Yaukey (1969) has suggested that separate attention should be given to social and psychological factors affecting Davis's and Blake's intermediate variables and to the relationships between the intermediate variables and fertility. This research strategy is proposed as a substitute for the traditional macroanalytic approach of correlating social stratification variables directly with fertility. The study of modernization and fertility change is, of course, an example of that traditional approach, while the studies of individual modernity tend more toward Yaukey's proposed focus on social and psychological factors related to the intermediate variables.

Also congruent with Yaukey's proposal are the analyses based on survey data that relate modernization indices to family-size preferences and practice of contraception. Such analyses are available for a number of developing countries where fertility surveys have been conducted, often using indices that combine attitudinal responses and information pertaining to socio-economic status, ownership of modern goods, and so on (see Freedman and Takeshita, 1969; Goldberg and Litton, 1969; Hawley and Prachuabmoh, 1966; Lapham, 1971). A comparative analysis of survey data from seventeen countries has been provided by Berelson (1966). In general the findings are supportive of the macrolevel relationship between modernization and fertility: those respondents classified as more modern in surveys are more likely to want fewer children and to practice contraception.

It should also be noted that because of differing analytic perspectives of investigators, the same data have been classified in different ways in studies of modernization, individual modernity, and fertility. For example, fertility rates have been taken as contributing to the pace of modernization, as resulting from the modernization process, or as being an essential part of the definition of modernization. A concept such as "values" has been used in some studies as a social stratification index, focusing on commonalities among religious or cultural groups, while in other studies attention has been directed to differences in specific value orientations within social categories (cf. Clifford, 1971; Kahl, 1968; Spengler, 1966). There has also been con-siderable overlap between the categories used to define social class and modernity; that is, in comparative perspective the higher social classes have been viewed as more modern.

Such disparities of views are reflected in the review of research that follows. Our own conceptual preference should, however, be made clear. We consider that data pertaining to traits of individuals (attitudes, values, personality characteristics) are essential to an understanding of how social and environmental factors have an effect on fertility outcomes and that these personal variables should in general be studied *in relation to* social stratification variables. We would want to know, for instance, how education affects a person's life aspirations and what part children play in that pattern of aspirations for people at different levels of education. The research design required for this kind of understanding is, of course, complex, and few examples are available, as noted by Rosen and Simmons (1971):

> The paucity of social psychological studies of fertility across several com-munities and social classes, along a continuum from rural village through tradi-tional city to modern industrial metropolis, has made it difficult to identify the linkages between macro-structural and psychological levels of analysis. What specifically are the intervening mechanisms which connect a macro-structural phenomenon such as industrialization to individual action, as expressed in fertility decline? [P. 51]

A sociopsychological perspective of this kind has not been entirely absent from the population literature, of course, and it is to a review of such considerations in the context of modernization that we now turn.

Cultural and Religious Values

Prominent among the themes that relate modernization processes to fertility change are the effects of changes in cultural and religious values. In broad terms modernism is characterized as an outlook that is incompatible with certain traditional values that in themselves tend to be pronatalist in nature. The modern individual is not only less firmly bound to such traditional values, but also is likely to hold new values that may have antinatalist implications. The kinds of values most frequently discussed in relation to fertility are those pertaining to family relationships and to religious systems.

In Chapter 3 of this volume Back and Hass review thoroughly the studies of family and fertility in the context of modernization, so we need not repeat their observations. We will note only that people who would usually be classified as more modern, by virtue of their socioeconomic status, urban residence, industrial occupation, and so forth, are more likely to value a conjugal relationship that is more flexible, verbal, and egalitarian, all of which seem to be conducive to low fertility. Individuals in such unions are also apt to be located at a considerable psychological distance from the authority of the previous generation (see Kahl, 1968; Rainwater, 1965; Yaukey, 1961). In addition the modern family is subject to different perceptions of environmental constraints (a topic that will be discussed below), particularly if the family is located in an urban setting.

The strength of commitment to religion, referred to as religiosity or religiousness, has been found to vary inversely with numerous modern traits. We are not concerned here with the effects of different religious systems on the fertility of adherents, although those effects have been shown to be powerful, but with the degree of adherence of individuals within specific religions and the relationship of that variable to fertility. This, too, is important, as illustrated by studies of several religions in different countries (Stycos, 1968a; Westoff, Potter, and Sagi, 1963; Yaukey, 1961). Pronatalist injunctions for the faithful are characteristic of many religions, most notably Islam and Catholicism. To the extent that these value prescriptions have behavioral outcomes, and it would be wrong to assume that they have none, the strength of commitment to a religion will have an effect on fertility. Moreover, some religious value systems contain elements not bearing directly on fertility but likely to have an effect, e.g., an emphasis on family solidarity or on the authority of men over women (see Kirk, 1966).

While religiosity tends to be related inversely to the variables used to define modernity (which, as noted above, are also in large part social class indicators), the relationship is by no means a consistent one; variations can be noted for specific religions, and there are interaction effects among religiosity, economic resources, and fertility (see Hawthorn, 1970). Modernity seems to have less of an effect on religiosity among Muslims, for instance, and American Catholics at higher educational and economic levels tend to show stronger religious commitment and higher fertility (Miro and Rath, 1965; Yaukey, 1961). Nonetheless, the erosion of traditional religious and familial values is surely a significant part of the connection between modernization and fertility change.

Social Structure Effects

A social system that encourages social mobility and, by extension, individual social aspirations has been logically regarded as having antinatalist implications. The underlying assumption here is that large families are in most cases a hindrance to upward mobility, so individuals with high aspirations are likely to restrict their fertility. This plausible hypothesis has not received clear research confirmation (Duncan, 1966; Westoff et al., 1963); however, it deserves mention in the present context because extent of mobility is one of the defining characteristics of a modern social system. Indeed, one social scientist has proposed that the number of life options available within a society be used as *the* definition of modernity (Safilios-Rothschild, 1970).

An element of social structure assumed to be of critical importance toward understanding fertility is the type of roles available to women and specifically the availability of nonfamilial roles, especially work roles. Considerable evidence is available showing an inverse relationship between labor-force participation of women and fertility, although the causal connection is not always clear—for example, women may work because they are subfecund, or women may voluntarily limit their fertility because they want to work. Moreover, the relationship is not always strong, especially in agrarian societies. Stycos and Weller (1967) have proposed that relationships with fertility would be clearer if women's occupations were classified according to whether they are incompatible with the demands of childbearing. The social status associated with the job is also an important consideration, as shown by Rosen and Simmons (1971). Potentially important, though not yet well understood, are the effects of availability of children's day-care facilities on the relationship between female work roles and fertility.

Perceptions of Environment and Resources

A topic that cuts across many others is the way in which people perceive their environment and the resources available to them, and how they relate these perceptions to size of the family. An obvious and perhaps critically important example is parents' perceptions of infant and child mortality. Given a certain desired family size, how many pregnancies are needed to achieve it? The significance of this issue in India is stressed in Chapter 5 by the Poffenbergers. A decline in infant and child mortality is a major characteristic of modernization and, of course, of the first phase of the demographic transition. Factors that are not well understood are the lag in

individual perceptions of the decline in mortality and the connection between such perceptions and reproductive behavior. Available data suggest,
however, that perceptions about mortality and fertility do not mirror current
reality, and substantial differences exist between generations and among
strata within a society (see Stycos, 1968b).

With regard to resources available to the family the following question
may be asked: are children viewed by parents as competitive with other
sources of satisfaction? In the case of extreme poverty the issue may, of
course, be survival rather than satisfaction. However, given sufficient resources so that some substitutions permit the maintenance of a large or a
small family, questions may be raised about the bases on which such tradeoff
decisions are made. This approach brings in the economists' framework for
efficient decision-making, using cost, income, and preference variables.
Robinson and Horlacher (1971, pp. 19–27) have reviewed applications of
economic decision theory to fertility, with attention to presumed differences
among societies at different stages of development. It is important to note
that this approach incorporates psychological as well as economic variables
since the satisfactions and costs of children are importantly emotional in
content, and it does not presuppose a conscious, rational weighing of alternatives. What it does do is focus attention on children as serving certain
functions, some of which might be served by alternatives to children, and
it provides an analytic framework within which diverse kinds of variables
can be incorporated.

An important theme in the population literature, especially in connection
with the demographic transition, is the differing economic functions of
children in agrarian and industrial societies. Coale (1967) for instance
notes that:

> In an urban industrial society children are less of an economic asset and more
> of an economic burden than in a rural society. The economic disadvantage of
> children is increased by laws restricting child labor and making education
> mandatory. [P. 168]

Freedman (1962), discussing the contraction of fertility differentials
among subgroups in the United States, speculates that ". . . the functions of
children and of the family are becoming more similar in different major
social strata" (p. 221). In one of the few studies focusing explicitly on
parental perceptions of the economic costs and benefits of children, Mueller
(1970) finds that perceptions differ among social strata in Taiwan and that
these variables have an independent effect, when compared with social
classification variables, in explaining family-size preferences and contraceptive use.

The functional approach has also been found useful for explaining the
interaction of variables found to have a powerful effect on fertility, such as
education and family structure. Noting the pervasive inverse relationship
between levels of literacy and fertility, Freedman (1963b) says:

I suggest that with increased education and literacy the population becomes involved with the ideas and institutions of a larger modern culture. If the individual is, or believes he is, part of a larger nonfamilial system, he begins to find rewards in social relationships for which large numbers of children may be irrelevant. [P. 232]

Heer (1969) has examined in detail the possible relationships between increased education and fertility, pointing out that a rise in income that accompanies education may enhance fertility, but that other effects of education, such as awareness of new goals and activities, tend to reduce the relative preference for children or to raise their relative cost. In this analysis also fertility is seen as being basically related to perceptions of available resources.

Finally, on what appears to be a more sophisticated level, modern man is coming to recognize his place in an ecological balance with nature and to regard overpopulation as disruptive. Possibly this perception will in the long run be linked to personal childbearing decisions and have an effect on societal fertility.

Personal Traits

The sociopsychological themes related to fertility just discussed—cultural and religious values, social structure, perceptions of environment and resources—tend to be viewed mainly as affecting family-size preferences. That is, they are aspects of the person's life space that may determine whether he desires a large or a small family ("large" and "small" being defined relatively within a given cultural setting). By contrast personal traits tend to be discussed in relation to the degree of efficacy in limiting the family to a desired size, or, as in the case of fatalistic attitudes, as indicating whether "desired" family size has any meaning at all for the individual.

Personal traits seen as related to both modernization and fertility are frequently viewed (explicitly or implicitly) as being derived from the demands of the sociocultural environment, i.e., as functionally related to a given setting. Such traits could be developed either through adaptive socialization practices or through standardization of behavior patterns at any stage of development.

For instance orientation toward the future and planfulness are cognitive and behavioral aspects of personality organization sometimes thought to be less prominent among individuals who are less modern. This differentiation is ascribed in part to the observation that such qualities are not demanded by agrarian settings or low-status occupations (see Hill et al., 1959). The relevance of future-orientation and planfulness to fertility is obvious, as exemplified in the phrase "family planning."

The population literature pertaining to personal traits consists more of discussion than of data, and the few attempts made by population researchers to measure personality characteristics have not been notably successful (see Chapter 12 in this volume). Moreover, population studies have seldom been designed to *compare* personal traits in modern and traditional populations. For that perspective we turn now to the topic of individual modernity.

The Measurement of Individual Modernity

We will begin the review of research on individual modernity by focusing on two recent studies that have in common two pertinent characteristics: (1) they attempt to derive operationally a multivariate definition of individual modernity or modernism; and (2) they include as part of this definition measurement of fertility or related variables. We will discuss general aspects of the two studies, then raise some methodological issues connected with the comparative study of modernity. After that we will describe several dimensions of individual modernity—subjective efficacy, orientation to time, and openness to change—that seem especially relevant to fertility. To substantiate the connection between these sets of traits and fertility, we will draw upon evidence both from the studies that have attempted to measure individual modernity and from other, more specialized, comparative psychological studies.

Two Studies of Individual Modernity

The two studies that we will describe in some detail are the Harvard Project on Social and Cultural Aspects of Development, referred to hereafter as the Harvard Project, which was carried out in six developing countries (Inkeles, 1966, 1969a, 1969b; Inkeles and Smith, 1970; Schuman, Inkeles, and Smith, 1967; Smith and Inkeles, 1966; Williamson, 1970); and the comparative study of modernism in Brazil and Mexico by Kahl (1968).

As noted above, these studies are distinctive in that they include both multivariate measurement of modernity and analyses of fertility-related variables. Other studies that have made important contributions to the measurement of modernity, but without particular attention to fertility, include the work of Lerner (1958) in the Middle East, the research carried out in Africa by Doob (1960, 1969), the attitude scales applied in Africa, Australia, and Hong Kong by Dawson (Dawson, 1967, 1969; Dawson, Law, Leung, and Whitney, 1971), and the research on urbanization and modernism in Turkey by Schnaiberg (1970a, 1970b). These studies will not be described here, but we will refer to pertinent findings from them in the discussion that follows.

The Harvard Project was based upon extensive structured interviews with more than 6,000 young men in Argentina, Chile, India, Israel, Nigeria, and

East Pakistan. The respondents in each country were selected to represent groups presumed to have different degrees of exposure to modernizing influences: farmers living in traditional rural communities; recent migrants to the city; urban dwellers engaged in traditional occupations; urban dwellers with experience in more modern industrial occupations; and students in secondary schools and universities. The rationale for the project was stated by Smith and Inkeles (1966) as follows:

Basically, we assumed that modernity would emerge as a complex but coherent set of psychic dispositions manifested in general qualities such as a sense of efficacy, readiness for new experience, and interest in planning, linked, in turn, to certain dispositions to act in institutional relations—as in being an active citizen, valuing science, maintaining one's autonomy in kinship matters, and accepting birth control. . . . We assumed these personal qualities would be the end product of certain early and late socialization experiences such as education, urban experience, and work in modern organizations such as the factory. [P. 355]

The interview instrument was derived from a large set of items designed to tap more than thirty themes thought relevant to modernity. Those themes are listed in Table 4–1 (from Smith and Inkeles, 1966). In another report

TABLE 4-1

Themes Used by Smith and Inkeles (1966) to Define Psychosocial Modernity

Political activism	Growth of opinion valuation
Role of aged	Political identification
Educational aspirations	Extended kinship obligations
Occupational aspirations	Kinship obligation to parental authority
Calculability of people's dependability	Mass media valuation
Calculability of people's honesty	Openness to new experience—places
Change perception and valuation	Openness to new experience—people
Citizens political reference groups	Particularism—universalism
Consumption aspirations	Planning valuation
Consumer values	Religious causality
Dignity valuation	Religious-secular orientation
General efficacy	Social class attitudes
Efficacy and opportunity in life chances	Time (punctuality) valuation
Efficacy of science and medicine	Technical skill valuation
Family size—attitudes	Women's rights
Family size—birth control	Coed work and school
Growth of opinion awareness	

Inkeles (1966, pp. 141–144) describes nine themes pertaining to attitudes and values that he considers as central to the definition of modern man, on the basis of initial analysis of the data. These may be summarized as follows:

1. Readiness for new experience and openness to innovation and change
2. The disposition to hold opinions about a large number of issues that arise not only in the immediate environment but also outside of it; awareness of the

diversity of opinions held by others; opinions of others not automatically accepted or rejected on the basis of their status or power

3. Time orientation toward the present or the future, rather than the past; acceptance of fixed hours and schedules, punctuality

4. Orientation toward, and belief in, planning and organizing as a way of handling life

5. Efficacy; a belief that man can learn to dominate his environment to achieve his goals

6. Calculability; confidence that other people and institutions can be relied on to fulfill their obligations; belief in a reasonably lawful world under human control

7. Awareness of the dignity of others and a disposition to show respect for them, as revealed particularly in attitudes toward women and children

8. Faith in science and technology

9. Belief in distributive justice, that rewards should be given according to the person's contribution, not because of special properties or status of the person

A major finding of the Harvard Project is the coherence of a modernity syndrome across cultures, suggesting that ". . . men everywhere have the same structural mechanisms underlying their socio-psychic functioning, despite the enormous variability of the culture content which they embody" (Smith and Inkeles, 1966, p. 377). Similar evidence seems to be emerging from other studies, although there is some dispute about the propriety of the measuring techniques, as used in the cross-cultural context, and the interpretations derived from them (Schnaiberg, 1970b; Stephenson, 1968; Strauss, 1969).

Williamson (1970) has dealt specifically with the fertility-related data from the Harvard Project, and his findings show both similarities and differences across cultures. Using the data from factory workers in five countries, Williamson analyzed the relationships among ideal family size, subjective efficacy (an index derived from responses to fourteen questions), and favorability toward birth control. Ideal family size and subjective efficacy were analyzed both as independent variables and as intervening variables in relation to a variety of social indicators, such as education, skill level, information level, income, and so on. The results show that: (1) the "psychological" variables, ideal family size and subjective efficacy, have slightly stronger predictive power than the social indicators with respect to attitudes toward birth control; (2) ideal family size and subjective efficacy function more as independent determinants of favorability toward birth control than as intervening variables between the social variables and favorability toward acceptance of birth control; (3) there is considerable variability across samples in the level of the relationships for both independent and intervening effects. In sum the Williamson study provides a thorough analysis of the relationships among some aspects of modernity that are relevant to fertility. The concept of subjective efficacy will be discussed in greater detail below.

The research by Kahl (1968) is in many respects similar to the Harvard

Project, although more limited in scope. Kahl's interviews were conducted with 627 men in Brazil and 740 men in Mexico, representing three residential characteristics (provincials, migrants, metropolitans) and several occupational levels (ranging from unskilled manual through high-status white-collar workers). All respondents were salaried workers in businesses or factories.

The Kahl Project was designed as ". . . a study of those value orientations that are the principles used by men to organize their occupational careers. It seeks to delineate and to measure a set of values that represents a 'modern' view of work and life" (p. 4). To that end Kahl, like Inkeles and his co-workers, developed a questionnaire with sets of items designed to tap certain themes relevant to modernity (or "modernism," the term used by Kahl). Beginning with fourteen value scales, Kahl identified through subsequent analyses seven regarded as the "core" of modernism in both Brazil and Mexico: activism; low integration with relatives; preference for urban life; individualism; low community stratification; mass media participation; and low stratification of life chances. These rather uninformative labels are fleshed out by the following summary portrait:

A modern man is an activist; he believes in making plans in advance for important parts of his life, and he has a sense of security that he can usually bring those plans to fruition. Unlike the fatalistic peasant who follows the routines of life and shrugs his shoulders to indicate that much of what happens will be beyond his control, the industrial man attempts to organize the future to serve his own purposes.

To carry out these plans, the modern man is willing to move away from his relatives and to depend upon his own initiative. For him, nepotism is more a burdensome responsibility than a mechanism of security. Similarly, he is an individualist who avoids extreme identification with people in his own work group. Therefore he says that he would prefer to express his own ideas and make his own decisions even if his peers disagree.

The context in which the modern man prefers to carry out his plans is the open scene of the big city. He finds that the stimulation of urban life and its opportunities is strong, and he develops sufficient skill with urban modes to feel at ease in making new friends in the city.

He perceives the city as a place which is not rigidly stratified—that is, he sees it as open to influence by ordinary citizens like himself. Similarly, he sees life chances or career opportunities as open rather than closed; a man of humble background has a chance to fulfill his dreams and rise within the system. He participates in urban life by actively availing himself of the mass media. He reads newspapers, listens to the radio, discusses civic affairs. [P. 133]

Congruent with the findings from the Harvard Project, Kahl reports that "the general value syndrome of modernism . . . was supported by the field data in both Brazil and Mexico" (p. 21). He found also that social status predicted modernism scores better than geographical residence (large cities versus small towns), concluding, "It seems that position in the social structure determines the degree of modernism, and nationality differences are not important" (p. 21). Socioeconomic status actually accounted for only about a third of the variance in modernism, although this relationship might have been stronger if the sample had included the peasant farming class. As Kahl points out elsewhere, socioeconomic status is a catchall classification, and it is precisely for this reason that the study of values is important: to capture some of the subjective differences and variations in personal experience that are known to exist within status categories.

In a separate analysis Kahl assessed the role of personal values as determinants of ideal family size. An interesting cross-national difference emerged. In both Brazil and Mexico it was found that modern values were helpful in predicting ideal family size (with socioeconomic status and residence held constant), but the correlation between values and ideal family size was higher in Mexico. In fact modern values were the best predictor of ideal family size among the three independent variables in Mexico, where ideal family size is high. In Brazil, however, where ideal family size is smaller, location of residence was the best predictor, and the degree of association was stronger. Kahl speculates that this difference is due to a pattern of traits in Brazilian culture that facilitates transition to the small-family norm once urbanization begins.

Some Methodological and Substantive Issues

The Harvard Project and the research by Kahl are important beginnings in the search for a syndrome of individual modernity and in the effort to link modernity to fertility change. In the next section we will discuss some specific aspects of individual modernity that seem significant for fertility. Before doing that, however, we must note some important limitations and criticisms pertaining to the studies just described.

From the rather special perspective taken here, namely, our interest in fertility, it is regrettable that these investigations have dealt only with male respondents. That focus is understandable since both projects were designed especially to assess the effects of occupational experience as a modernizing influence and because men in developing countries are more likely than women to be exposed to other influences such as education. However, similar studies of women are very much needed. One study that did focus on the modernism of women, although from a somewhat different conceptual perspective, is the research in Turkey reported by Schnaiberg (1970a, 1970b). It is relevant to note his conclusion that ". . . the present findings are in considerable accord with those of investigations done in other societies (Smith and Inkeles, 1966; Inkeles, 1969a; Kahl, 1968), even though the previous studies dealt with male workers" (1970b, pp. 419–420). Most fertility surveys have been conducted with female respondents, of course, but these have generally not focused on the measurement and analysis of a sociopsychological pattern of individual modernity. A partial exception is the research carried out in Brazil by Rosen and Simmons (1971), which, while using rather limited psychological data, uncovered ". . . a set of

empirical linkages running from industrialization, through higher education and work status for women, modern female role attitudes and egalitarian
family structure to smaller family size" (p. 62).

Schnaiberg (1970*b*) discusses at length the issue of whether modernism
should be treated as a unitary or a multifaceted phenomenon, a point raised
earlier by Bendix (1967) and Gusfield (1967). In both the Harvard Project
and Kahl's study modernism is conceived as multidimensional, as evidenced
by the variety of scales used. However, the main analytic approach of both
investigations describes a syndrome of modernism and uses scores summed
across scales to relate modernism to other variables. Schnaiberg prefers to
look at each scale separately, stressing that modern and traditional elements
of attitudes and behavior can coexist in the same individual. A similar point
is made by Dawson et al. (1971), who argue also that the degree of dissonance and subsequent attitude change attributable to modern contacts
will differ according to the centrality of a particular traditional belief. It
seems to us that either the unitary or multifaceted approach may be
legitimately and profitably pursued, so long as the investigator is aware that
either choice entails certain benefits and drawbacks. Ideally, of course, the
same data will be analyzed in both ways and the results compared, which
Schnaiberg (1970*b*) attempted with less-than-clear results.

A different issue is whether what is "modern" can be defined by the
theoretical or empirical criteria devised by the investigator, or whether it
must be defined in terms of what the people in a culture themselves regard
as modern. This issue was raised in rather oversimplified terms by Stephenson (1968) and effectively answered by Inkeles (1969*b*), who pointed out
that both approaches are valid, but for different purposes. And just as with
the question of unitary or multifaceted analysis, it is useful to compare the
results of "outside" or "inside" criteria of modernism. This was in fact done
on a limited basis by Inkeles and his co-workers, resulting in additional
justification for the scale as used cross-nationally.

However, it must be stressed that the research on individual modernity
is not immune to the methodological issues that bedevil all cross-cultural
measurement (cf., Strauss, 1969), and comparative results must be interpreted with caution.

Three Themes Relating Individual Modernity to Fertility

In this section we will attempt to extract from the research literature
several clusters of modern traits that seem relevant to fertility change. We
are guided in our selection of traits both by the discussions in the population
literature of psychological components of fertility reviewed earlier, and by
the availability of pertinent data from studies of modernization and related
topics such as acculturation. The themes that stand out as important are
labeled here as subjective efficacy, orientation toward time, and openness
to change.

Subjective Efficacy. The traits discussed under this heading pertain to the perceived power relationship between man and his environment: specifically, to the belief that man can exert some control over his social and physical milieu. This aspect of psychological functioning has long been recognized as a significant variable for the differentiation of traditional and modern societies (Kluckholm, 1950) and more recently has become a focal point for measurement of individual differences (see Clifford, 1971). Kunkel (1970, pp. 225–240) provides a behavioralist perspective on the peasant's belief in a "capricious universe," pointing out the social and environmental conditions that reinforce this world view and discussing its implications for economic development. Back (1967), in a discussion of the relationship between fatalistic attitudes and fertility, notes that possibilities for volitional control in matters affecting family size are increasing and concludes that this trend enhances the relevance of sociopsychological research approaches to demographic phenomena.

Directly relevant for measurement in this area is the extensive research carried out with the I-E scale, derived from Rotter's conceptualization of internal and external control of reinforcement (Rotter, 1966; Throop and MacDonald, 1971). Related measurements that have been used extensively in international settings deal with the attribution of responsibility (Garcia-Esteve and Shaw, 1968; Heider, 1958), beliefs in the supernatural (Jahoda, 1970), and, of course, subjective efficacy (Williamson, 1970). In one way or another virtually all of the important studies of modernization have obtained measures of people's beliefs about their personal capacity to control what happens to them or the obverse, how much they feel controlled by fate, luck, supernatural beings, and the like (Doob, 1969; Kahl, 1968; Inkeles, 1969a; Lerner, 1958; McClelland, 1966).

In general the hypothesized social status and cultural differences related to these various dimensions have been confirmed: people who are more "modern," i.e., better educated, more literate, more urbanized, and more exposed to mass media, do exhibit a greater sense of personal efficacy and less fatalistic attitudes. However, there are exceptions to the expected cultural differences (Jahoda, 1970), and much of the I-E research has explored individual variations within social status categories. Studies in this area do not always differentiate between beliefs related to the controlling characteristics of the environment and the sense of personal mastery or ability to cope within confines of real environmental constraints (Gurin, Gurin, Lao, and Beattie, 1969; Smith, 1972). It must be kept in mind that more traditional peoples, lacking technology, are indeed less in control of their environment; moreover, modern urban man, overwhelmed by technology and "the system," also has reason to feel powerless. More complete knowledge might reveal an inverted-U shape relationship between subjective efficacy and modernization, but for our purposes we need only assert that research shows a direct relationship between modernizing influences and feelings of subjective efficacy for comparisons of selected groups.

Moreover, there is emerging evidence that subjective efficacy is linked both to preferred family size and to practice of birth control. The study by Williamson (1970) dealing with these three variables has already been reviewed. MacDonald (1970) reports that scores on the I-E scale differentiate significantly between users and nonusers of contraception among unmarried female college students in the United States. In a study designed to discover psychological differences between contraceptive users and nonusers among black working-class respondents in Chicago (Keller, Sims, Henry, and Crawford, 1970), significant differences were found on a scale of feelings of efficacy derived from TAT responses. In two studies that analyzed alienation in relation to fertility in the United States (Groat and Neal, 1967; Neal and Groat, 1970), the feeling of "powerlessness" was found to be related to fertility and ideal family size.

Orientation Toward Time. We will discuss here two distinctive aspects of orientation toward time: (1) time as a dimension running from the past to the future, and (2) time as a commodity to which a value can be imputed.

Orientation toward the time dimension is another of the elements considered by Kluckholm (1950) as functionally discriminating traditional and modern cultures. A classification of three types of societies based on time orientations is given by Useem and Useem (1968):

A tradition-oriented society is one which attempts to perpetuate its future out of its past by acting according to values which are implicit in its customs, rituals and traditions. . . . A modernizing society is one which creates its future rather than lives off its past, which continuously generates its culture both with respect to values and substantive content. A modern-oriented society is a complex society which states its values explicitly and does not so much reject its traditions as assess them along with other alternatives for expressing its values [p. 144].

This theme also appears in the reports of the Harvard Project, cited earlier. Back (1958) concludes from his study of the change-prone person in Puerto Rico that, ". . . the key ingredient in modernism is orientation toward the future" (p. 340).

The behavioral concomitant of orientation toward the future would seem to be planfulness, which appears as an important topic in most of the studies that have attempted to measure modernity (Back, 1958; Doob, 1969; Smith and Inkeles, 1966; Kahl, 1968; McClelland, 1961). Research evidence confirms that modern man is more flexible with respect to time, that he is as aware of the present and the future as he is of the past, and that he can more readily regulate his behavior in anticipation of future contingencies.

It appears also that modern man is more prone to be punctual and that he views time as a valued and useful commodity (McClelland, 1961). Hypotheses about the differential value of time have been confirmed not only by verbal survey responses but also by indirect measurements (McClelland, 1961) and by experiments assessing subjective judgments of time intervals under varying conditions (Doob, 1960; Meade, 1968).

As related to fertility, it is reasonable to postulate that planfulness and an orientation toward the future should enhance awareness and practice of birth control. The direct evidence on this point is not strong, although the study by Keller et al. (1970) did show a significant difference between users and nonusers of birth control on a scale of tendency to plan ahead. It should be recalled also that planfulness is among the core measures in the Kahl study and in the Harvard Project, both of which contain evidence for an inverse relationship between the modernity syndrome and fertility. In Clifford's U.S. study (1971) time orientation was one of the modern-traditional value dimensions measured and found to be related to fertility attitudes and behavior.

Openness to Change. We include under the category "openness to change" a number of concepts, including empathy, freedom from tradition and dogma, willingness to innovate, readiness for new experience, and change proneness. All of these concepts, used in slightly different ways by different investigators, are obviously integral components of modernity because modernity *is* change, innovation, and departure from tradition.

From a psychological viewpoint empathy is the most fully developed of these concepts. As noted by Lerner (1958), "The chronological transformation that accompanies modernization is psychic mobility, with empathy as an inner mechanism which enables newly mobile persons to *operate efficiently* in a changing world. Seeing oneself in the other fellow's position is an indispensable skill for people moving out of traditional settings." As conceived by Lerner, empathy is developed through a dual process of projection and introjection. The mass media are viewed as playing a crucial role in modernization as a "mobility multiplier."

The Harvard Project measured "readiness for new experience and openness to innovation and change," and Kahl investigated freedom from tradition in terms of "low integration with relatives." Other investigators have measured variables similar to "openness to change" for different countries, for example, Back (1958) in Puerto Rico, Schnaiberg (1970a) in Turkey, Bose (1962) and Joshi (1965) in India, and Yaukey (1961) in Lebanon.

If openness to new experience is to be related to fertility some intervening elements must be introduced. These might include the small family as a model in modern social strata, the availability of information about the benefits of birth control, and the accessibility of contraceptive services. The qualities of empathy and openness to new experience would facilitate the adoption of such modern ideas and practices (Rogers, 1962), but it is not necessarily true that these qualities are preconditions for adoption. Schuman et al. (1967) found that literacy was related to willingness to consider innovations and also that literate factory workers had a significantly higher contraceptive adoption rate in response to a family-planning advertising campaign. On the other hand, Freedman and Takeshita (1969) present evidence that a vigorous family-planning program in Taiwan had the effect of reducing preexisting modernity differentials in contraceptive practice, suggesting that a strong campaign can override "readiness to adopt" predispositions.

It seems clear that the concepts embraced here as "openness to change" reflect a significant alteration in personal style that is related to modernization, but measurement of these concepts has not been rigorous and more work is needed to delineate relationships with contraceptive practice and fertility.

Discussion

We have reviewed the relationship between modernization and fertility, described some of the research on individual modernity, and pointed out a few empirical linkages between modern personal characteristics and modern low-fertility patterns. But this is only a beginning. What have we learned that is new? What are the practical implications of the issues we have discussed? Where do we go from here?

We have learned that there are certain identifiable, measurable characteristics that differentiate modern and traditional individuals. This is hardly a momentous discovery since such a distinction has been discussed in the social-science literature for decades, but the systematic measurement of specific characteristics in a comparable way across many cultures is new and important.

The evidence we have cited to connect modern personality traits with fertility is scanty, but not unconvincing. Although little research of this kind has yet been done, the few carefully designed and executed studies that do exist tend to show the expected relationships. Research comparing personal characteristics of modern and traditional peoples is difficult to carry out, particularly if large samples are employed and multiple characteristics are assessed, so additional evidence will be slow in accumulating. But that kind of research is important, and we hope that the linkages between individual modernity and fertility that are indicated so sketchily in this chapter will provide some impetus and direction for further explorations. Recent efforts such as the Harvard Project demonstrate that measurement of personal attributes could feasibly and usefully be included in fertility surveys in the developing countries.

Inkeles (1966) has said that "it is only when a man has undergone a change in spirit—has acquired new ways of thinking, feeling and acting— that we can consider him truly modern." It is becoming possible to identify reliably those ways of thinking, feeling, and acting, which is a first step toward an understanding of the causes and consequences of being modern.

Causal explanations have centered on influences such as socialization practices (McClelland, 1961; Rosen, 1962), formal education and literacy (Inkeles, 1969a; Kahl, 1968; Schuman et al., 1967), work experience (Inkeles, 1969a; Kahl, 1968), experience in the city and modern culture contacts (Doob, 1960; Levine, 1970; Schnaiberg, 1970a), and exposure to mass media as a modernity facilitator (Lerner, 1958; Schramm, 1967). Few studies, however, have been designed in a manner to permit clear inferences about causality.

It is not surprising, but nonetheless interesting, to note the pervasive influence of formal education. It is not surprising because education is after all a preparation for modern life, and measures of individual modernity are bound to reflect that. There is a built-in relationship between education and some (but not all) of the items on modernity scales. The connection between education and modernity is of particular interest here because education has been shown in other studies to be a major factor affecting fertility. The effect of education on fertility is, of course, not direct; children are not taught in school to have smaller families, but rather the attitudes, values, and behaviors learned in school interact with subsequent life experiences to produce an overall trend toward lower fertility. The possibility exists then that analyses of the relationship between education and individual modernity will aid in understanding *how* and *why* education affects fertility.

It should be noted that there is a longstanding debate about the relative importance of changes in people or changes in socioeconomic settings as a prerequisite to modernization. Weiner (1966) summarizes the issues:

Although there are differences among social scientists as to *how* values and attitudes can be changed, it is possible to speak of one school of thought that believes that attitudinal and value changes are prerequisites to creating a modern society, economy, and political system. Other social scientists take issue with this rather fundamental assumption. As an alternative model, they suggest that the appropriate attitudes and, more importantly, the appropriate behavior will be forthcoming, once *opportunities* and *incentives* are provided. [Pp. 9–10]

In the context of societal modernization there are three major settings affecting the individual directly: the school, the city, and the factory. Each setting demands certain behaviors of the individual; each setting conveys certain information directly to the individual; and each setting increases the likelihood that the individual will be exposed to other stimuli, notably the mass media. Research on individual modernity is concerned with the non-transient effects on people of such influences and does not make any assumptions about whether personal change or institutional change deserves strategic priority in the modernization process. Societal modernization and individual modernity are, of course, interdependent and mutually reinforcing, and the important thing for development programs (including programs that aim to reduce fertility) is to understand the relationships and look for points where intervention may effectively accelerate change.

The major studies of individual modernity have focused on a syndrome, or pattern of traits, associated with indices of modernization. It is important to have this overall portrait of the modern person, but for some purposes it is important, too, to examine the component features, how they came to be, and what are their consequences. It is with this more detailed kind of analysis that one can begin to discern practical applications, for fertility limitation, of the study of individual modernity. From the multiple characteristics assessed in the Harvard Project, for instance, a limited number can be identified that seem plausibly related to family-size preferences or to effective practice of birth control. We have in fact attempted that in the preceding section of this chapter. Concentrating on those characteristics, one can then envisage a variety of efforts with practical import.

For example, it is only moderately useful for those concerned with population limitation to know that modernization tends to depress fertility. This knowledge may permit some projections of fertility trends based on the assumed pace of modernization, but acceleration of that pace is a political and economic problem of such immense dimensions that it seems beyond the reach of specific recommendations or actions. It is a bit more helpful for population planners to know that education is a component of modernization having a strong effect on fertility, since this permits specific recommendations about sectoral priorities—for example, that countries deeply concerned about excessive population growth might give special attention to the expansion of education in their development plans. Even here, however, practical action is limited because of economic and structural constraints and competing priorities in the developing countries. Another avenue, which has hardly been tried, would be to design educational programs related to the personal characteristics associated with fertility differences, attempting to alter those characteristics purposely rather than letting similar changes occur more slowly as a by-product of the modernization process.

The attitude of fatalism, for instance, seems clearly related to fertility. This attitude is in part a functional outcome of the peasant's real inability to control his own destiny, but it is also likely to be overgeneralized and to lag behind social change: fertility can be controlled even if local politics cannot, and better irrigation and seeds may provide predictable crop yields for the coming generation even though the weather was the major factor for this generation. It is not difficult to imagine educational programs, operating through the schools and the mass media, that would aim to decrease fatalistic outlooks (or at least differentiate the objects of fatalistic attitudes) and increase the sense of personal efficacy. Fatalism is, of course, but one example, illustrating that an increase in *individual modernity* could be a specific goal of some development programs, complementary to other efforts and in the long run presumably facilitating them.

Also in the communications sphere, but less ambitious in intent, would be efforts to use research data on modernism as guidance in the design of family-planning persuasive appeals. Current family-planning communications programs are linked only loosely to audience characteristics; they tend to use generalized appeals that are thought to be culturally appropriate. Research on individual modernity, comparing groups within a society, suggests ways in which messages might better be tailored to particular audiences. Profiles of modern and traditional persons, such as those provided by Inkeles and Kahl, provide some insight into the personal values that are salient for different segments of the society; the imaginative communications specialist should readily see ways in which the practice of family planning can be linked to fulfillment of those personal values.

Apart from such straightforward matters as recommendations for the content of communications and educational programs, research on individual modernity may help identify the microstructural elements in a society that are most closely linked to fertility. Again using as an example the connection between feelings of efficacy and fertility, one can ask a series of questions about the social conditions that facilitate the development of subjective efficacy. For instance, is literacy a major facilitator because it permits understanding of modern phenomena and increases coping ability in urban settings? What are the kinds of experience within a work setting that enhance a person's confidence in his ability to control future events? Which aspects of the experience of living in a city bring about alterations in a traditional fatalistic world view? Answers to questions like these will help fill the "understanding gap" about what accounts for the macroanalytic correlations between modernization and fertility indices and should be useful in the formulation of population-relevant priorities in development programs.

In addition to such potential long-term research outcomes, some immediate suggestions for research design may be discerned. An enormous mass of data on modern and traditional populations is being compiled via KAP and fertility surveys. These surveys typically do not attempt to assess the patterns of personal traits that are the focus of research on individual modernity, yet this could be done with relative ease. Smith and Inkeles (1966), for instance, have provided a short form of their OM-scale; this questionnaire taps the major dimensions of individual modernity and could readily be incorporated into a fertility survey. Fertility researchers should take advantage of the availability of such instruments to expand the content of their efforts, looking particularly for contrasts in patterns of personal traits that may emerge in comparison of high-fertility and low-fertility groups in the developing nations.

If this recommendation were followed, an important result would be increased understanding of the modernity of *women*, about which little is currently known. Some of the major modernizing influences that have been mentioned, such as work in a factory, are simply not available to women in much of the world. Urban living surely makes less of a difference for a woman, who is likely to be tied to the home by child care, than for a man, who is out working in the city, exposed to new things and interacting with different people. Education may have similar effects on men and women, but in most countries a female is likely to get less schooling. Yet if socialization practices are a key element in facilitating modern attitudes in children, a modern mother may be the central figure in bringing about societal modernization. Or if the woman's attitudes carry much weight in childbearing decisions, making her modern may be one of the most effective routes to a reduction in societal fertility. The emancipation of women from traditional restraints is, of course, a desirable goal on other grounds as well, and it is important to note that a reduction in childbearing is not only a result of modern attitudes but also an outcome that frees women from childrearing roles that inhibit participation in modern society.

That our understanding of individual modernity for both men and women is limited should be apparent from the material reviewed in this chapter. A hopeful beginning has been made, however, based upon the recognition that societal modernization brings about (and is dependent upon) changes in people. What those changes are, how they occur, and what are their consequences is knowledge potentially useful for accelerating the attainment of socially valued goals, including the goal of reduced rates of population growth.

REFERENCES

Adelman, I. and Morris, C. T. 1966. A quantitative study of social and political determinants of fertility. *Economic Development and Cultural Change* 14:129–157.

Back, K. W. 1958. The change-prone person in Puerto Rico. *Public Opinion Quarterly* 22:330–340.

———. 1967. New frontiers in demography and social psychology. *Demography* 4:90–97.

Bendix, R. 1967. Tradition and modernity reconsidered. *Comparative Studies in Society and History* 9:292–346 (cited in Schnaiberg, 1970).

Berelson, B. 1966. KAP studies on fertility. In B. Berelson et al., eds., *Family planning and population programs: a review of world developments.* Chicago: University of Chicago Press. Pp. 655–668.

———. 1969. Beyond family planning. *Studies in Family Planning* 38:1–16.

Blake, J. 1965. Demographic science and the redirection of population policy. In M. C. Sheps and J. C. Ridley, eds., *Public health and population change: current research issues.* Pittsburgh: University of Pittsburgh Press. Pp. 41–69.

———. 1968. Are babies consumer durables? A critique of the economic theory of reproductive motivation. *Population Studies* 22:5–25.

———. 1969. Population policy for Americans: is the government being misled? *Science* 164:522–529.

Bose, S. P. 1962. Peasant values and innovation in India. *American Journal of Sociology* 67:552–560.

Chilman, C. A. 1970. Probable social and psychological consequences of an American population policy aimed at the two-child family. *Annals of the New York Academy of Sciences* 175:868–879.

Clifford, W. B. 1971. Modern and traditional value orientations and fertility behavior: a social demographic study. *Demography* 8:37–48.

Coale, A. J. 1967. The voluntary control of human fertility. *Proceedings of the American Philosophical Society* 3:164–169.

Davis, K. 1967. Population policy: will current programs succeed? *Science* 158:730–739.

Davis, K. and Blake, J. 1956. Social structure and fertility: an analytical framework. *Economic Development and Cultural Change* 4:211–235.

Dawson, J. L. M. 1967. Traditional versus Western attitudes in West Africa: the construction, validation and application of a measuring device. *British Journal of Social Clinical Psychology* 6:81–96.

————. 1969. Attitude change and conflict among Australian aborigines. *Australian Journal of Psychology* 21:101–116.

Dawson, J. L. M.; Law, H.; Leung, A.; and Whitney, R. E. 1971. Scaling Chinese traditional-modern attitudes and the GSR measurement of "important" versus "unimportant" Chinese concepts. *Journal of Cross-cultural Psychology* 2:1–27.

Doob, L. W. 1960. *Becoming more civilized.* New Haven: Yale University Press.

————. 1969. Scales for assaying psychological modernization in Africa. *Public Opinion Quarterly* 31:414–421.

Duncan, O. D. 1966. Methodological issues in the analysis of social mobility. In N. J. Smelser and S. M. Lipset, eds., *Social structure and social mobility in economic development.* Chicago: Aldine.

Fawcett, J. T. 1970. *Psychology and population: behavioral research issues in fertility and family planning.* New York: The Population Council.

Freedman, R. 1962. Next steps in research on problems of motivation and communication in relation to family planning. In C. V. Kiser, ed., *Research in family planning.* Princeton: Princeton University Press. Pp. 595–604.

————. 1963a. The sociology of human fertility: a trend report and bibliography. *Current Sociology,* 1961–1962, Vols. 10–11. (Republished Oxford: Basil Blackwell, 1963.)

————. 1963b. Norms for family size in underdeveloped areas. *Proceedings of the Royal Society* 159:220–245.

————. 1967. Applications of the behavioral sciences to family planning programs. *Studies in Family Planning* 23:5–9.

Freedman, R. and Takeshita, J. 1969. *Family planning in Taiwan: an experiment in social change.* Princeton: Princeton University Press.

Garcia-Esteve, J. and Shaw, M. E. 1968. Rural and urban patterns of responsibility attribution in Puerto Rico. *Journal of Social Psychology* 74:143–149.

Gendell, M. 1967. Fertility and development in Brazil. *Demography* 4:143–157.

Goldberg, D. and Litton, G. 1969. Family planning: observations and an interpretive scheme. *Turkish Demography: Proceedings of a Conference,* Hacettepe University Publications, no. 7, pp. 219–240.

Groat, H. T. and Neal, A. G. 1967. Social psychological correlates of urban fertility. *American Sociological Review* 32:945–959.

Gurin, P.; Gurin, G; Lao, R. C.; and Beattie, M. 1969. Internal-external control in the motivational dynamics of Negro youth. *Journal of Social Issues* 25:29–53.

Gusfield, J. 1967. Tradition and modernity: misplaced polarities in the study of social change. *American Journal of Sociology* 72:351–362.

Hawley, A. H. and Prachuabmoh, V. 1966. Family growth and family planning in a rural district of Thailand. In B. Berelson et al., eds., *Family planning and population programs.* Chicago: University of Chicago Press. Pp. 523–544.

Hawthorn, G. 1970. *The sociology of fertility.* London: Collier-MacMillan.

Heer, D. M. 1966. Economic development and fertility. *Demography* 3:423–444.

————. 1969. Educational advance and fertility change. Paper presented at the London conference of the International Union for the Scientific Study of Population, September 1969.

Heider, F. 1958. *The psychology of interpersonal relations.* New York: Wiley.

Hill, R.; Stycos, J. M.; and Back, K. 1959. *The family and population control.* Chapel Hill: University of North Carolina Press.

Inkeles, A. 1966. The modernization of man. In M. Weiner, ed., *Modernization: the dynamics of growth.* New York: Basic Books. Pp. 138–150.

————. 1969a. Making men modern: on the causes and consequences of individual change in six developing countries. *American Journal of Sociology* 75:208–225.

————. 1969b. Comments on John Stephenson's "Is everyone going modern?" *American Journal of Sociology* 75:146–151.

Inkeles, A. and Smith, D. H. 1970. The fate of personal adjustment in the process of modernization. *International Journal of Comparative Sociology* 11:81–114.

Jahoda, G. 1970. Supernatural beliefs and changing cognitive structure among Ghanaian university students. *Journal of Cross-Cultural Psychology* 1:115–130.

Joshi, V. 1965. Personality profiles in industrial and preindustrial cultures: A TAT study. *Journal of Social Psychology* 66:161–180.

Kahl, J. A. 1968. *The measurement of modernisms: a study of values in Brazil and Mexico.* Austin: University of Texas Press.

Keller, A. B.; Sims, J. H.; Henry, W. E.; and Crawford, T. J. 1970. Psychological sources of "resistance" to family planning. *Merrill-Palmer Quarterly* 16:286–302.

Kirk, D. 1966. Factors affecting Moslem natality. In B. Berelson et al., eds., *Family planning and population programs.* Chicago: University of Chicago Press. Pp. 561–579.

Kluckholm, F. R. 1950. Dominant and substitute profiles of cultural orientations: their significance for the analysis of social stratification. *Social Forces* 28:376–393.

Kunkel, J. H. 1970. *Society and economic growth: a behavioral perspective of social change.* New York: Oxford University Press.

Lapham, R. 1971. Modernisation et contraception au Maroc central. *Population* 26 (special issue):79–104.

Lerner, D. 1958. *The passing of traditional society: modernizing the Middle East.* Glencoe, Ill.: Free Press.

———. 1968. Modernization: social aspects. In D. Sills, ed., *International encyclopedia of the social sciences.* New York: Macmillan and Free Press 10:386–395.

Levine, N. 1970. Old culture-new culture: a study of migrants in Ankara (Turkey). Unpublished manuscript.

McClelland, D. C. 1961. *The achieving society.* Princeton: Van Nostrand.

———. 1966. The impulse to modernization. In M. Weiner, ed., *Modernization: the dynamics of growth.* New York: Basic Books, Pp. 28–39.

McClelland, D. C. and Winter, D. G. 1969. *Motivating economic achievement.* New York: Free Press.

MacDonald, A. P. Jr., 1970. Internal-external locus of control and the practice of birth control, *Psychological Reports* 27:206.

Meade, R. D. 1968. Psychological time in India and America. *Journal of Social Psychology* 76:169–174.

Miro, C. A. and Rath, F. 1965. Preliminary findings of comparative fertility surveys in three Latin American cities. *Milbank Memorial Fund Quarterly* 43:36–68.

Mishler, E. G. and Westoff, C. F. 1955. A proposal for research on social psychological factors affecting fertility: concepts and hypotheses. In Milbank Memorial Fund, *Current research in human fertility.* New York: Milbank Memorial Fund. Pp. 121–150.

Mueller, E. 1970. Attitudes toward the economics of family size and their relation to fertility. Unpublished manuscript, University of Michigan.

Neal, A. G. and Groat, H. T. 1970. Alienation correlates of Catholic fertility. *American Journal of Sociology* 76:460–473.

Rainwater, L. 1965. *Family design: marital sexuality, family size, and contraception.* Chicago: Aldine.

Robinson, W. C. and Horlacher, D. E. 1971. Population growth and economic welfare. *Reports on Population/Family Planning,* no. 6, pp. 1–39.

Rogers, E. M. 1962. *Diffusion of innovations.* New York: Free Press.

Rosen, B. C. 1962. Socialization and achievement motivation in Brazil. *American Sociological Review* 27:612–624.

Rosen, B. C. and Simmons, A. B. 1971. Industrialization, family and fertility: a structural-psychological analysis of the Brazilian case. *Demography* 8:49–68.

Rotter, J. B. 1966. Generalized expectancies for internal versus external control of reinforcement. *Psychological Monographs* 80:1–28.

Ryder, N. B. 1959. Fertility. In P. M. Hauser and O. D. Duncan, eds., *The study of population: an inventory and appraisal.* Chicago: University of Chicago Press. Pp. 400–436.

Safilios-Rothschild, C. 1970. Toward a cross-cultural conceptualization of family modernity. *Journal of Comparative Family Studies* 1:17–25.

Schnaiberg, A. 1970a. Rural-urban residence and modernism: a study of Ankara Province, Turkey. *Demography* 7:71–85.

————. 1970b. Measuring modernism: theoretical and empirical explorations. *American Journal of Sociology* 76:394–425.

Schramm, W. 1967. Communication and change. In D. Lerner and W. Schramm, eds., *Communication and change in developnig countries*. Honolulu: East-West Center Press.

Schuman, H.; Inkeles, A.; and Smith, D. H. 1967. Some social psychological effects and noneffects of literacy in a new nation. *Economic Development and Cultural Change* 16:1–14.

Smith, D. H. and Inkeles, A. 1966. The OM Scale: a comparative socio-psychological measure of individual modernity. *Sociometry* 21:353–377.

Smith, M. B. 1972. "Normality"—for an abnormal age. In D. Offer and D. X. Freedman, eds., *Modern psychiatry and clinical research: essays in honor of Roy R. Grinker*. New York: Basic Books. Pp. 102–119.

Spengler, J. 1966. Values and fertility analysis. *Demography* 3:109–130.

————. 1969. Population problem: in search of a solution. *Science* 166:1234–1238.

Stephenson, J. B. 1968. Is everyone going modern? A critique and a suggestion for measuring modernism. *American Journal of Sociology* 74:265–275.

Strauss, M. A. 1969. Phenomenal identity and conceptual equivalence of measurement in cross-national comparative research. *Journal of Marriage and the Family* 31:233–241.

Stycos, J. M. 1968a. *Human fertility in Latin America*. Ithaca, N.Y.: Cornell University Press.

————. 1968b. Social class and differential fertility in Peru. In C. B. Nam, ed., *Population and society: a textbook of readings*. Boston: Houghton Mifflin. Pp. 181–184.

Stycos, J. M. and Weller, R. H. 1967. Female working roles and fertility. *Demography* 4:210–217.

Throop, W. E. and MacDonald, A. P. 1971. Internal-external locus of control: a bibliography. *Psychological Reports* 28:175–190.

United Nations. 1953. The determinants and consequences of population trends: a summary of the findings of studies on the relationships between population changes and economic and social conditions. *Population Studies*, no. 17.

Useem, J. and Useem, R. H. 1968. American-educated Indians and Americans in India: a comparison of two modernizing roles. *Journal of Social Issues* 24:143–158.

Weiner, M., ed. 1966. *Modernization: the dynamics of growth*. New York: Basic Books.

Westoff, C. F.; Potter, R. G.; and Sagi, P. C. 1963. *The third child*. Princeton: Princeton University Press.

Williamson, J. B. 1970. Subjective efficacy and ideal family size as predictors of favorability toward birth control. *Demography* 7:329–339.

Yaukey, D. 1961. *Fertility differences in a modernizing country, a survey of Lebanese couples*. Princeton: Princeton University Press.

————. 1969. On theorizing about fertility. *American Sociologist* 4:100–104.

PART II

The Social Context:
Two Countries

[5]

THE SOCIAL PSYCHOLOGY
OF FERTILITY BEHAVIOR
IN A VILLAGE IN INDIA

THOMAS POFFENBERGER
AND SHIRLEY B. POFFENBERGER

In 1901 the population of India was about 240 million; it is estimated that if the current growth rate continues, India will have a population of one billion before the end of the century. From the standpoint of density of population this would be equivalent to crowding everyone in the United States in 1970 into the state of Texas. But the population growth of India would not stop there. With a continuing growth rate of 2.5 percent a year the population will double every twenty-eight years. These figures make it obvious that either the birth rate must come down or the death rate must go up—or a combination of the two. It is clear that agricultural innovations, which are resulting in increased production of food grains, are not a solution to the population problem but will at most delay the time of crisis (Population Reference Bureau, 1970).

If the population of India is to level off by the time there are one billion people, which is a stated objective of the government, the birth rate will have to be cut in half by 1985. This would mean that married couples could not have on the average more than 2.4 children.

The Indian government officially recognized the problems that population growth posed for the country in 1951, and by the mid-1960s it had begun the development of a family-planning program. By the end of the 1960s the

NOTE: The authors wish to express their appreciation to the Ford Foundation, the Government of India, the University of Baroda, and the East-West Center, each of which provided part of the financial and institutional support for the project reported here. Special thanks go to Mrs. Amita Verma, Mr. Bihari Pandya and others in India who facilitated the study and participated in it. Useful comments on a draft of this manuscript were provided by Ronald Freedman, Reuben Hill, and Eugene Weiss.

program included 5,000 Family-Planning Centers and over 20,000 Subcenters whose personnel have endeavored to serve an increasing number of the nation's more than 500,000 villages. In addition a large number of government and private urban clinics have been developed throughout India.

In the last few years the program has depended largely on sterilization as a method of birth control; in addition an extensive project was begun recently to make condoms available by commercial channels at a subsidized cost. The absolute figures for sterilization are impressive, and there is evidence that the birth rate is declining (Agarwala, 1968). First reports from the 1971 Census are also regarded by the government as somewhat encouraging: the population was estimated to be 547 million, fourteen million less than the projection of 561 million. However, the growth rate for the decade 1961–1971 was still high, 24.6 percent compared with the previous decade's growth of 21.5 percent. Thus in spite of the government's massive effort to reduce population growth, there is full awareness that only a beginning has been made (Embassy of India, 1971).

Past studies have made it clear that even though a majority of people in India may know about various family-planning methods, few couples use any. For example, in a 1966 national probability sample (364 villages) it was found that although 60 percent of the nearly 6,000 men and women questioned said they knew about family planning, only 4.5 percent of the men and 3.2 percent of the women said they had ever used a family-planning method (Loomis, 1967,). A more intensive study of eight villages in three states in India found that most people knew about sterilization and the IUD and reported that they were favorable to the methods, but the report concluded: "The low level of adoption of vasectomy and the loop [IUD] indicate that the task of persuasion will not be easy" (Roy and Kivlin, 1968, p. 51).

Some critics believe that the fertility-control methods have not been adopted because the distribution system has not been adequate, or because methods of fertility control have not yet been developed that are acceptable to the people. Others take the position that regardless of the distribution system or the methods available, people will not adopt any method until they have four or five children; major changes in the culture and social structure will be necessary before two children will be the average desired number (Nag, 1969). Available data indicate a norm well above two. A large number of surveys conducted in various regions of the country, both rural and urban, covering most socioeconomic groups, have indicated that the range of stated desired number of children is from three to five, with the norm closer to three than to five (Agarwala, 1962; United Nations, 1961; National Sample Survey, 1963; Berelson, 1965). This apparent norm must be qualified, however, because of the importance of sons to the average Indian family. For example, in a survey conducted by the Indian Institute of Public Opinion, which asked an urban adult sample the number of sons and daughters they considered to be "ideal" for a family, the means were 1.7 sons and 1.2

daughters. The implications of this study may be of particular importance because the sample represented a relatively well-educated urban group that might be expected to take the lead in reduced fertility. All of the respondents were literate; 72 percent had completed secondary school, and more than 30 percent had obtained a college degree (Poffenberger, 1968*b*).

Because men and women who undergo sterilization are regarded as not wanting any more children (and to an extent this also seems to be true for women accepting the IUD in India), a further indication of the differential desire for sons and daughters may be obtained from clinic data on the number of living sons and daughters reported by those who have undergone sterilization. In a study in North India, of 892 rural men who had been vasectomized (1965–1966), the mean number of living sons reported was 2.9, and daughters, 1.9 (Poffenberger, 1967). In another study of clinic records of 1,395 IUD acceptors in New Delhi, 1965–1966, the mean number of living sons reported was 2.1, and daughters, 1.6.[1]

The Need for Intensive Studies of Small Groups

While reports of clinic data and surveys of knowledge, attitudes, and practices regarding fertility control are useful to determine regional and cultural differences. and variations relating to socioeconomic level, urban-rural residence, and sex, these studies lack the depth that is required for interpretation of differences in fertility behavior. There is need also for intensive studies. In-depth studies of small groups cannot, of course, be used to generalize about fertility behavior in all of India, but insights may be gained that have application to the interpretation of survey data, and the conclusions may be of some applied use to those who are concerned with population programs and family-planning work in modernizing societies.

The Problems

From the standpoint of government program implementation there are two interrelated problems. The first pertains to the number of children that individuals or couples desire; the second relates to the avoidance of unwanted children.

Freedman (1967) has asked why, when studies show that large numbers of women in developing countries say that they do not want any more children, they do not act according to their preference. The Indian government's family-planning program has been based on the assumption that people who say they do not want any more children will use a birth-control method if it is provided. It is probable that if every woman in India who wants to avoid having another child strongly enough to use indigenous (but often ineffective) methods adopted a method offered by the family-planning

---

[1] Unpublished data available from the authors.

program, a significant decline in the birth rate would result. The decline would be considerably greater if every woman who responded negatively to a question asking if she wanted any more children could be helped to avoid further pregnancies. It is clear, however, that attitude studies indicate a preference for an average of more than three children. Davis (1967) has made a strong case for the position that even if a national family-planning program enables each married couple to have the number of children they want, the resulting decline in fertility will be insufficient to stabilize population growth. In this chapter we will examine our data as it may have bearing on the goals villagers reach through having children and variables that cause them to have children beyond the numbers desired.

The Rajpur Village Study

In 1962 the village of Rajpur[2] in south-central Gujarat State was selected for an intensive study of socialization practices and social change. As data were collected during the first two years of the study in a series of intensive interviews and observations of village families, it became apparent that the research staff also had a unique opportunity to investigate certain aspects of the dynamics of fertility behavior that had relevance to the developing national family-planning program. As a result of exploratory questions related to family planning, it was decided that interviews might be facilitated by being focused on a family-planning educational program held in the village. This enabled the interviewing staff to broach the subject of family planning by asking if the husband or wife had attended a recent village film showing and exhibit of contraceptive methods. This was followed by questions about the respondent's evaluation of large and small families. Data on sexual behavior and experiences were also collected. Cooperation was possible to a greater extent with males than with females largely because the males could be interviewed in private, and they were cooperative in answering such questions. It was more difficult to interview females because they had to be interviewed in the home and were rarely alone. Although few women could discuss their own sex lives many of them supplied data related to traditional customs, which included sexual taboos, use of indigenous fertility-control methods, lying-in practices, superstitions relating to sex behavior and fertility, and other beliefs that had relevance to adoption or rejection of family-planning methods and to motivation to control fertility.

In order to collect these data the primary sample of sixty-six couples who had been interviewed in the childrearing study continued to be interviewed. A subsample of twenty-four couples, six from each of the major castes and judged to be most representative, were studied intensively in terms of

[2] The name of the village is fictitious.

variables related to social change.[3] The four major caste/community groups in the village were the Patidars (jati of Kanbi), Barias (Kolis), Bhils (Vasava jati), and Dheds[4] mostly belonging to the jati of Vanker. The Patidars were the traditional farmer-landowners' caste and made up 10 percent of the village population. The Barias, 46 percent of the village population, were for the most part tenant farmers though some owned land and a few were factory workers. The Bhils, 14 percent of the village population, were the descendants of tribal people who had originally been brought by the Patidars to serve as farm guards and laborers. The Dheds, who represented 6 percent of the village population, had traditionally been low-status weavers who also served as tenant farmers and laborers for the Patidars. Changes in status were taking place in all of these groups during the 1960s, notably a rise in status of the Dhed community, as a result of education and motivation to improve their standard of living. There was less change in the Baria and Bhil groups, which held more firmly to traditional values and farming roles.

It is not possible within the scope of a chapter to document adequately the complexities of variables that we believe relate to fertility and its control in the rural region of India where we have worked. We have therefore selected for examination those aspects we believe to be the most important from the standpoint of the national family-planning program. In the concluding section we will comment on possible research implications.

Desired Family Size and Advantages and Disadvantages of Large and Small Families

One aspect of the fertility-behavior study of the primary sample of mature married couples dealt with the identification of values regarding sex preferences and number of children desired by husbands and wives. A series of questions was asked to determine some of the motives behind the desire for a large or small family, including the benefits of having sons or daughters. Interviews were conducted individually by showing the husband or wife an 8 x 10 card divided into four line drawings, representing families having two, three, four, and five children. The children's figures were drawn with a minimum of lines, so that sex was not differentiated except in the interpretation of the villager. As the card was shown, the

---

[3] For background information on the village, see a preliminary report, Poffenberger, T., 1969.

[4] Members of this group were called untouchables and forced by high-caste villagers to carry away dead animals, especially cattle, until untouchability was outlawed by the Indian Constitution in 1950.

interviewer explained that each picture represented a particular size family. This procedure was used because previous interviews had shown that some village women lacked experience with numbers and abstract concepts. It was reasoned that the use of pictures of various-size families might facilitate awareness of the numbers to be discussed and that use of a picture card would increase attention to the questions. The interviewer made certain that the respondent understood the representations of families and then proceeded to ask which size family was preferred, what the ideal sex composition of the respondent's preferred number of children would be, and what alternative number of children would be acceptable, as well as the number of children the respondent would have in order to have a male child in case only females were born. In addition to these questions the respondent was asked the advantages and disadvantages of having a large or a small family. Although most of the respondents were not accustomed to thinking in terms of an ideal number of children, they did have opinions regarding a range of acceptable numbers of boys and girls and were able to mention advantages and disadvantages of the two ends of the range— two and five children. The following interview, which illustrates the kinds of questions asked, was taken with a woman considered to be representative of the lower-middle-caste Baria group. She was thirty-one years of age and had borne five children, all living at the time of the interview.

Q. Which family size do you like best?
A. One daughter and one son are best. [Then she pointed to the picture with five children.] But this looks like my family with many children.
Q. You said two children would be best. If you could not have that number, would you want one child or three children?
A. It is not good to have three children. Three is an unlucky number, so parents would have bad luck. I would prefer having four children.
Q. How many boys and girls are best?
A. You should stop after two . . . one boy and one girl . . . No! You should have four children, two boys and two girls, so each daughter would have a sister for company and each son would have a brother's company.
Q. What if all the children were girls? How many would you have to have a boy?
A. I would have more than five. There would definitely be a change of sex in the sixth delivery.
Q. What are the advantages of having two children?
A. Two children require less expenditure and are less of a burden on the parents. Parents will not have to work as hard to earn money to feed them.
Q. What are the disadvantages of having two children?
A. If there are only two children, one may be a girl. There is a saying, "One eye is no eye and one son is no son." [The respondent changed the subject.] Why did you not bring me the abortion tablets I asked for? [She teased the interviewer.] I am willing to pay fifteen rupees for them, but even so you did not bring them to me. [The interviewer had recommended that she visit a family-planning clinic several times before and again told the woman she could get advice there.] I do not approve of the tubectomy or the loop. I know a woman from this street who was operated on, and she does hard work, but hard work after the operation will cause poor health.

Q. What are the advantages of having five children?
A. It is good to have five children because then the family will be more enjoyable.
Q. What are the disadvantages of having five children?
A. You can see how hard we work to feed all the children!

In response to the question regarding the best number of children for a family to have, the mothers in the primary sample preferred larger families than the fathers did. The means indicated that the mothers wanted four (3.9) children, the fathers, three (3.1). When these parents were asked to state the advantages of "small" (two children) and "large" (five children) families, they could think of more advantages of the small family than of the large family. Tabulation of the fathers' responses revealed an average of nearly three (2.8) advantages of having a small family as compared with one (1.1) advantage of having a large family. The mothers' responses showed nearly as many (2.6) advantages of a small family, but (2.2) of a large family, indicating their ambivalence toward having few or many children.

The response to questions asking how many children a villager wanted and the advantages of relatively large and small families were sometimes misleading as a means of assessing a group family-size norm, however, because of the differential value assigned to sons and daughters. In a few cases a parent said that two or three children would be best, but it became clear in later remarks that he was actually thinking only of sons. Most parents thought that a family should have more sons than daughters, although this seemed to be more important to mothers than to fathers. The means for ideal family size and composition were 1.8 sons and 1.3 daughters for the fathers, and 2.5 sons and 1.4 daughters for the mothers.

Preference for sons was further indicated in the stated desire to keep having children until one had at least one son. Although some mothers remarked that a daughter would be helpful and sympathetic, it was not indicated that any parents would continue to have additional children to have a daughter once they had a sufficient number of sons. However, more than 62 percent of the mothers and 35 percent of the fathers said they would have six or more daughters if necessary in order to have at least one son.

We will now summarize the traditional need for a large family based upon our total village experience and then examine the responses of our sample to the questions regarding the goals reached through having a large family. We will then report on the comments regarding the advantages of having a small family.

The Traditional Need for a Large Family

In their fertility behavior the villagers were clearly motivated by the social and cultural milieu. Socialization practices were important; these determined not only role expectations but the degree of guilt or shame felt in violating expected behavior patterns. Both boys and girls were taught that their own desires must be secondary to those of parents and family members. A "good" son was characterized as one who remained with his parents in adulthood, obeyed them, contributed to the family's income, and took financial and social responsibility for family members when the father was deceased or too old to continue this responsibility. A "good" daughter was perceived as one who would never bring shame to her parents' family, or as a wife to the family of her husband. When a girl was eight to ten years of age she was told that she would soon go to her in-laws and must learn cooking and all the routines of the household so her mother would not be criticized for her lack of skill. She was told that she must obey and please her husband and her mother-in-law, or they might send her back to her parents. If a bride had difficulty in her husband's home she was not supposed to complain to anyone. She also knew as a result of this training that in order to fulfill her expected role successfully she must have a son.

A woman who did not have children or whose children died was referred to as a barren woman, and her future as a wife was uncertain. A wife who did not bear children or one whose children did not live past early childhood might be sent back to her parents' family. In a Baria family where the first wife did not have children for several years, a second wife was arranged for, and the first wife was assigned the role of a servant. A barren woman might also be thought to have an evil eye and to cause the illness or death of children in the community. The children in the Bhil community were warned not to go to the home of a woman who had lost all her children through illness.

There was also the desire to acquire the power and status that were accorded a mature woman with a family that included at least one son. The shy young bride who came to her in-laws' family in her early teens could become the powerful and dominating mother-in-law at a later stage of the family life cycle only through having a son live to maturity and remain with the family, contributing to its financial support and social prestige. Women in particular had very real personal and economic reasons for wanting to have mature sons. By the time a woman reaches age fifty to fifty-five in India (Census of India, 1961) it is likely that she will be a widow and be dependent on her son(s) for economic support.

While some villagers seemed to be aware that in India not as many children die now as in the past, this was not generally known, and there was still a sufficient number of deaths for women to consider it a risk to stop having children before her children reached a certain level of maturity. (Women hoped to avoid pregnancy as soon as it was apparent that an eldest son or daughter might soon have a child.) Several investigators (Heer and Smith, 1967; May and Heer, 1968) have examined the statistical problem of how many children are necessary in order that at least one son will live (to support parents in their old age) until the father is sixty-five years of age. Their model indicates that in a country where there is a life expectancy of fifty years, it will be necessary for the average mother to bear five children to insure that one son will survive. The model indicates this would result in an annual rate of population growth of about 2.5 percent, which was the estimated rate of growth in the Indian village studied during the middle to late 1960s. The village families seemed to be aware of the basic facts of the model. The "ideal" number and sex of children in a family, according to village parents, was two sons and one daughter, but understandably these children had to live to maturity for the parents to reach social and economic goals. For this idealized number to live to maturity it was necessary to have more than three children even though they might have two sons and a daughter. As one mother asked, "How can one have less than five children?"

The Advantages of Having a Large Family

The following comments are characteristic of the kinds of remarks that were made by villagers in relation to the advantages of having many (five) children:

Economic Factors. The importance of having sons for economic reasons was mentioned by 30 percent of the fathers and 56 percent of the mothers. For example, "More children can earn for the family . . . the father can also rest if there are more to earn for him. If there is only one son, then he has the whole economic burden—supporting the family and paying for all the ceremonies such as his sisters' weddings." "The advantage of having many sons is that they will have different occupations and earn more."

A point particularly stressed by the mothers (40 percent) but by only a few (12 percent) of the fathers was the fact that sons would provide them with economic security in old age. The presence of a number of widows in the village may have reinforced a woman's concern that if she did not have a mature son to carry on the family's business or farm work she might be left without support if her husband died. In making this point one mother said, "When there are five or six children, a parent can have a peaceful life in old age. Mothers can depend on their sons because they can rightfully claim anything from them."

Power and Status. Nearly 10 percent of the sample fathers and 23 percent of the mothers mentioned that having many sons was a means of achieving a position of strength, which discouraged anyone from trying to take advantage of the family, or that sons enhanced the family's status. The comments indicated that parents visualized situations where they might need a number of sons to protect them. For example, one mother said, "The biggest advantage of the large family is that when all the brothers unite, nobody dares bother them. They can live with power in their hands."

Other comments that related to status were:

If a woman has many children, others will look up to her. When someone asks a woman if she has children, she can say proudly, "I have many children."

It is a matter of pride to have many children. What would other people think of a person who has only two children?

Others envy the woman with a large family and say, "See that woman. She has five living sons."

If there are three married brothers living together and one wife has only two children, she will be looked down on by the other wives and people will talk about her and feel sorry for her because she has only two children.

Having many sons means more fame for the family. This way one's own surname group remains at the top.

Perpetuation of Family Lineage. About 10 percent of both mothers and fathers mentioned the importance of perpetuating the father's lineage: "A son is important for lineage. He keeps the 'door' open. I would not stop having children until a boy came." Another said, "At least one son is necessary to keep the lineage going."

Nurturance. It was clear that an important variable related to the births of children was the mothers' satisfaction in having infants and small children in the house. One-third of the mothers' responses but only one-tenth of the fathers' responses referred to the belief that large families are pleasant to have. The following comment was made by a mother: "If a family has five sons, there will be life and there will be pleasure in the house. Parents will enjoy seeing their children's children, but if parents have only one or two sons they will have to wait years to see many grandchildren, so if they have four or five sons they will not have to wait so long."

Another woman said, "If there are only two children in a family there will not be any pleasure in life. Life would be empty and without joy."

Salvation. A terminal Hindu religious goal is that of salvation, and one of the requirements for salvation is the performance of funerary rites by a son; however, only 1.6 percent of the fathers and 4.5 percent of the mothers mentioned the obligation of a son relative to the performance of rituals. One of these comments was: "Having many children is a hardship for the family but if a person does not have a son, then he will not get salvation. There should be someone who performs death rituals for the parents."

Fear of Infant-Child Mortality. The health of children was a major concern. Obviously if sons were to assume responsibility for the family and satisfy parental goals, it was necessary for them to live. The fear of death of children was mentioned by 34.8 percent of the mothers and 8.2 percent of the fathers. The high incidence of expression of this fear on the part of women was related to their uncertainty about economic support as well as to the low status that was assigned to childless widows who were referred to as *vanzani* (barren woman). One mother explained it this way: "Suppose a woman has a daughter and a son. If her son dies, then she has no one to look after her. This happens often. God may take away one child. Look at my son. He is my only son and he suffers from many diseases. He is thin and has boils. So, if a mother has five children, then at least two or three of the children will live."

Another mother said, "If there are only two children, a boy and a girl, and the boy dies, the mother is considered barren."

The Disadvantages of Having a Large Family

Although children were obviously necessary to achieve major goals the mothers and fathers were also aware of the disadvantages of having children.

Economic Costs. More than 90 percent of the fathers and 37 percent of the mothers said that an advantage of the small family was that it was easier to provide food, clothing, and shelter for fewer members. Also mentioned were the costs of such things as marriage ceremonies and education. As one father stated, "I have five children and they consume so much food that at present I am half-starved. They are like small snakes. They eat everything in the house. There is nothing good about having so many children."

The possibility of having a higher standard of living for members of a relatively small family was mentioned by 18 percent of the sample fathers and 9 percent of the mothers. One woman said, "With two children we could buy two sets of clothing for each child, whereas with four children we could buy only one set of clothing with the same money." Another said, "When there are two children in the family proper care can be given. My husband is an only child so he gets the best quality clothes. I too get good saris. Recently my husband had two 'tericot' shirts and a nylon shirt made for him. If he had other brothers and sisters he would not have had these high quality shirts."

A few parents (9 percent of fathers and 3 percent of mothers) mentioned that a family would face less expenditure on ceremonies if they had fewer children: "Parents would spend less money on marriage arrangements, and they could relax if they had fewer children." Another said, "Having many children means having greater debts. Parents have to spend much money on marriages and other social ceremonies such as those at the time of a daughter's pregnancy and childbirth and at the time she is sent back to her in-laws after her first delivery." These statements indicate a clear awareness of the relationship between family size and the cost of meeting ceremonial needs, which were defined by the social group as necessary to maintain or increase status.

In addition to expressions about the ceremonial costs incurred in relation to having children, the increasing need to educate children, particularly boys, was mentioned by nearly 25 percent of the fathers and by 6 percent of the mothers. As one father commented, "Having two children means that a better education is possible for them."

Division of Property. Seven percent of the fathers and 5 percent of the mothers mentioned a problem of both economic and social concern—the division of land. In the past if one son survived he would inherit the family's land. If there were two sons the land was shared or divided or one of the sons migrated, often out of the country. With more sons surviving than before, with almost no possibility of migration outside India, and with the cities offering few job opportunities, agricultural holdings have been divided into smaller units, making farming increasingly uneconomical. A farmer said, "If a father had four *bighas* (less than two acres) of land, two sons could share it and each would have two bighas, but if he had four sons each would get only one bigha."

Health. Many villagers, particularly women, expressed the concern that because children may not survive, a person needs to have more children than are actually wanted to insure that a certain number live. However, there was also clear recognition on the parents' part that having many children also increased the possibility of maternal and infant mortality. More than 70 percent of the mothers and nearly 50 percent of the fathers mentioned having less health problems as one of the advantages of having few children. Also more than 30 percent of the mothers and 12 percent of the fathers mentioned the physical strain on the mother that was the result of childbearing and care of many children. A typical mother's remark was, "Many children give trouble to the mother in rearing them. She has to work hard and cannot rest."

Specific reference to the strain on women in low-income families who had to do field work and had repeated pregnancies and childbirths without proper nutrition was mentioned by 8 percent of the husbands and 11 percent of the wives. A typical comment was, "Having many children means much hardship and the mother has lots of problems. This year three women died during delivery. If a mother has many children it is not good for her health." Others mentioned the relationship between the mother's health and the health of her children. One mother said, "If a woman has a child every year it is not good for the child's health because there is not enough breast milk and the child becomes weak."

Some also mentioned the greater care that might be given to two children. A few parents in the village have found in the last several years that by taking their children to doctors in the city, children who might have died now live. The cost of medical treatment, however, has often been too high for villagers and cannot be afforded if a family has many children who are ill. For example, one parent said, "If there are only two children in a family, they will be well cared for and will grow all right, but if there are many children they will grow in a rough way and will be poorly cared for. Children are just like plants. If they are close together, they do not grow well because their growth is hampered, but if they are spaced farther apart they will grow nicely."

Leisure. Some mothers (9 percent) mentioned the greater freedom that having fewer children makes possible. The following two comments illustrate the mothers' awareness of the relationship between childbearing and leisure time: "A family with two children can live happily. A woman is free to go wherever she likes and she has less work and can live comfortably." And in the case of a highly fecund woman, "A mother does not get time for her own pleasures. By the time one child grows up, there will be another and so on it goes. Mothers cannot go out and have any free time."

Proper Care and Responsibility for Parents. Some mothers believe that if they had fewer children these children would be more likely to take responsibility for aged parents than would children raised with many siblings. A typical remark follows: "If there are only two children in the family, one boy and one girl, then the only son will take proper care of the parents, because he knows he is the only son to look after them. The daughter can also sympathize with her mother knowing that she is the only one to share the mother's jewelry. It's good to have fewer children because they will be more intimate with their parents."

Family Status and Stability. We have seen that family status is perceived as being higher if there are many sons and that the family may be regarded as being more stable from both the standpoint of filial protection and economic security. However, it was obvious that a considerable number of villagers were aware of threats to the family from having many children. Nearly 40 percent of the mothers and 28 percent of the fathers expressed worries about family status and stability and the kinds of problems that could arise from many interpersonal relationships. While sons or daughters might bring recognition to the family, there was also the possibility that they might cause shame. One father said, "All members of a family are not good and some may spoil the family name. From this standpoint it is better to have a small family."

Another said, "Villagers should not have five sons because they will fight other people. They create problems for others by playing mischief. When youths turn into vagabonds it becomes difficult to control them."

It was not only sons who could lower family status. The parents feared that daughters might be sexually promiscuous. A typical remark was: "If a daughter is not of good character, then she will spoil the family name."

Family stability can be affected by conflict, and the likelihood of conflict increases with each additional family member. So while the large family was perceived by some as a happy family, it was also recognized that it might be an unhappy one. A father pointed out the conflicts that occur between sons, saying, "If there are two sons in the family, they will quarrel and there will be disputes." Another commented about the conflicts that can occur between sons' wives. "If there are many sons, then there will be many daughters-in-law and they will all quarrel among themselves. I would like just two sons." Children were also seen as a cause of husband-wife quarrels: "Many children create problems and one parent becomes unhappy with the other parent [over disciplinary measures]." A mother mentioned the possible internal family conflicts when property was divided: "Sons will think in terms of their share of property. It's difficult to keep good relationships among sons in a big family."

To summarize it was evident that both mothers and fathers were well aware of the problems presented by having a number of children in the early stages of the family life cycle. They knew they had difficulty in providing adequate food, clothing, and other needs, but they regarded this as a temporary stage and looked forward to the time when their sons would be old enough to do productive work and augment the family income. Some mothers and fathers preferred a small family, however, and there was obvious ambivalence in the minds of many others. In the final section we will examine these areas of ambivalence from the standpoint of possible implications in regard to attitude change.

Factors That Caused Villagers to Have Children beyond the Number Desired

Many of the couples in the sample who were still in their reproductive years had had a sufficient number of children, so that the perceived advantages of having an additional child were fewer than the disadvantages. Most of the women could be placed on a continuum from strongly wanting another child to strongly wanting to avoid having another child. There was not always agreement on the part of husbands and wives, and it was somewhat more difficult to rate the husbands. Our data give some support to the hypothesis that wives are more highly motivated to have children in the early stages of marriage than are husbands, but once they have the number they feel are necessary, they are more highly motivated to terminate fertility than are their husbands (Poffenberger, 1968a). It was, however, usually the husband's decision or the decision of the joint family that determined when the operation, either vasectomy or tubal ligation, would be performed.

Of the sixty-six sample couples sixteen of the wives or husbands had been sterilized by the time of the interviews regarding desired family size. These couples had an average of 5.1 living children, 3.4 sons and 1.7 daughters. An average of 1.5 children were said to have died, .5 sons and 1.0 daughters.[5] Seventeen of the couples were classified as wanting another child. These couples had an average of 3.4 living children, 1.3 sons and 2.1 daughters. An average of 1.8 children were said to have died, 1.0 sons and .8 daughters. The remaining couples seemed to fall in a group who indicated they did not want any more children, but who were resistant to accepting a sterilization operation or to the use of the IUD. However, some were using indigenous methods to prevent another birth. These resistant couples had an average of 5.2 living children, 2.9 boys and 2.3 girls. An average of 2.1 children were said to have died, 1.0 boys and 1.1 girls. It was evident that

[5] In the mothers' recollections of children who died there were indications of under-reporting of female mortality.

there were differences in the strength of desire to avoid having another child. These data indicate that the number of living sons and the number of sons who had died were important variables when a point was reached where one of the couple was willing to take what most husbands and wives regard as the extreme step of having a sterilization operation.

Reference-Group Influence

Another factor was the degree of willingness to try something new and unknown. In this regard the basic values of the reference group, e.g., caste and community, should be considered since they tended to determine the range of permissible behavior for individuals. Couples within the groups studied were constrained by commonly held mores since deviation might have resulted in some group sanctions. In terms of fertility behavior some couples did act counter to accepted practice, but it tended not to be until personal pressures became so great that there was a willingness to risk disapproval. The effect of group values was illustrated by two of the four groups studied, the Patidars and the Barias. While many members of the Patidar caste had adopted a terminal method of fertility control—either tubal ligation or vasectomy—few of the Baria caste had done so. The Patidars in this region, as pointed out by Nair (1961, pp. 170–178), have long been achievement-oriented and among the first to adopt innovations. Related to their modernized outlook has been their pragmatic approach to fertility control.

The Barias identified with a group who claimed to be descendants of warriors who had once conquered this area. Local Baria leaders who were influenced by members of the political reference group, *Kshatriya Sabha* (Kothari and Maru, 1965), influenced others to beware of limiting the size of their families, which would reduce their potential political power. Baria animistic beliefs also served as a restraint since local shamans claimed that the use of government-offered methods might offend deities of fertility and health, the mother goddesses.

Husband-Wife Communication

The lack of effective husband-wife communication also seemed to be a factor in delaying adoption of a government-approved family-planning method. While there obviously was always some communication between spouses, it seldom related to fertility control except in the later stages of the life cycle. There was usually little communication in the early stages of marriage because of the young wife's shyness and traditional submissiveness. In addition there was little reason for discussion since both husband and wife were strongly motivated to have children as soon as possible. However, with births of sons the status of the wife increased, and particularly after the death of her mother-in-law the wife became a significant person in her own right. Many women had long since overcome any fear of their husband, and as one retorted, "Why can't one talk of anything with her husband!" At this stage of the life cycle lack of husband-wife communication was of less significance as a deterrent to method adoption than at an earlier period, but by this time the couple may have had several more children than they really wanted.

Fatalism and Fertility-Control Methods

Fatalistic responses were more characteristic of women than of men. Fifty percent of the mothers in the sample and 20 percent of the fathers said that family size relates to the will of God. Fatalistic responses were also found to be more prevalent among the lower-caste Barias than among the higher-caste Patidars. A determinant of fatalism would seem to be previous experience controlling events. Lower-caste villagers and women traditionally were in a weaker position than higher-caste villagers and men in terms of their resources and their position to manipulate various aspects of their daily lives; in part because of their lower educational level they were more fearful of possible methods of fertility control that were available to them. The problems and fears faced by villagers in seeking effective modern medical treatment are still often great enough to make them rationalize that they do not need such help until a condition has progressed too far for effective treatment. In the case of fertility control fatalistic responses may be explained as evidences of rationalization to avoid taking unpleasant action to prevent a pregnancy or to take feared action such as an abortion after the event has occurred. With illness the motivation to take action increases as the disease progresses. The motivation to take some action to avoid another birth is greatest after a woman becomes pregnant. Before the event such comments as, "I have asked God to give my next child to my daughter," "I am now too old to have a child," or, "It is up to God," are common. However, once such women do become pregnant, if they are highly motivated to avoid another birth more often than not they make some attempt to avoid a birth by relying on a traditional abortifacient method. If the method fails the woman may again refer to the "will of God." But it is clear that villagers do make decisions and take action in regard to fertility matters.

In the early stages of the family life cycle if a wife does not have a child within a reasonable period of time, she will engage in various rituals and other behavior with the intention of effecting conception, to the extent that she may even have sexual relations with a male other than her husband. Many of the sample mothers said they tried to space births by avoiding sexual relations for one week immediately following menses, since there was a commonly held belief that this is the most fertile period. Prolonged sexual restraint may have had some effect on the spacing of births. A Baria woman said that she and her husband did not have sexual relations for seven months after delivery. Another Baria woman indicated she abstained for a year following delivery, saying, "If we had intercourse during that year it would spoil the breast milk. The semen contaminates the milk and will make the child sick." Another woman of the same caste said that she avoided intercourse for eighteen months after childbirth. She reasoned, "If abstinence is not observed, a woman will become fat and her whole body will suffer. People like me who are weak from so many pregnancies have to avoid sexual relations to keep our health."

In addition to various lengths of abstinence following birth, the infrequency of coitus may be important in delaying another pregnancy. A Baria woman confided in one of the female interviewers that she avoided sexual relations by not allowing her husband to find her alone in the house. A Bhil woman said that she and her husband had coitus infrequently until a baby began walking. She added, "We then have intercourse almost every day since it doesn't matter if I become pregnant again." Another Bhil woman said that daily sexual relations are not harmful for a woman with no children, but that after the birth of the first child intercourse should be limited to two or three times a week. After five years of marriage, she said, a couple should not have coitus more than once or twice a month.

A Patidar woman said, "The first few years, husbands demand to have sexual intercourse every day. After three children, they do not want it so often so there is wider spacing of children. An older husband is not demanding of sex. Two years' spacing is best. If the interval between children is less, it is bad for the child and he might die."[6]

Villagers have probably always resorted to some method of fertility control. The high-caste Patidar farmers in this region traditionally practiced female infanticide (Mehta, 1966). A Brahmin priest visited village homes occasionally and sold pills of his compounding that he said had been blessed by God and would prevent pregnancy if the woman took his course of treatment, but he cautioned that the pills would be effective only if God willed. One of the village medical practitioners was reported to have charged fifty rupees for several injections that he gave a woman to induce abortion when her husband requested it. (In spite of the injections the woman gave birth to a child.) The most commonly reported method used by villagers as an abortifacient was a homemade oral dosage of various ingredients, including pepper, crude sugar, oil, and sometimes liquor.

Fatalism then seemed less a factor in itself as a cause of inaction regarding fertility control than it was a justification for not taking feared action. This was particularly true in the case of the innovations offered by the govern-

---

[6] The declining interest in coitus on the part of husbands was supported by some of the males' responses. A Baria husband said, "After marriage, I went to my wife for intercourse four times a week. This continued for about seven years until my interest in sex decreased. Now my wife comes to me." An important cultural factor in the declining frequency of coitus reported by men seemed to be the belief that a drop of semen was equal to forty drops of blood and that one became weak if coitus was too frequent. A Bhil husband remarked, "I have reduced the frequency of sexual relations because I feel tired after intercourse and I think I lose my bodily strength."

ment. One Baria mother explained her resistance to the adoption of a government method, saying, "It is for God to give children and to take them away. Nowadays people talk about an operation, but why should one have an operation?" Her actual reason was found in another statement. "I do not like having so many children, nor did my husband want to have so many. He only wanted two or three, and now he tells me to go to the hospital to have an operation, but I am afraid of the operation. If I will not go, my husband said he would go, but a sterilization operation harms a person's health. One might even die. I am praying that I don't become pregnant again."

The lack of acceptability of methods offered by the government was clearly a major restraint upon fertility control. This was in part because each method had real disadvantages, but even more serious were the misconceptions about these methods and their effects. The rumors about the IUD were so adverse that few village women would consider having one. It was said to make a woman weak because of the bleeding it caused. There was some indication that women associated bleeding from an IUD insertion with menstruation, and there was a strong menstrual taboo in this area. A village woman was not able to perform her household duties or engage in religious rituals during periods of menstruation or postpartum uterine bleeding. In households where there was no other person who could take over the wife's duties, the tasks fell to her husband. In discussions with local clinic personnel it was pointed out that women were sometimes brought in by their husbands, who insisted that the IUD be removed because of the inconvenience it caused them. It was also rumored that the IUD caused ulcers and cancer, and stories were circulated that the terminal "wires" of the IUD would give the husband an electric shock and that one couple could not separate after intercourse because the husband's penis became entangled in the threads of the IUD. There was also misunderstanding as to the duration of an IUD's effectiveness. A Vanker woman who had an IUD inserted said that the doctor told her to return to the clinic in several years. This was interpreted by other village women as meaning that it was only effective for a rather short period of time, so that a woman might still become pregnant if she accepted an IUD.

Condoms that were offered by government clinics in the area during the 1960s were seldom used by villagers as a contraceptive method. Men rejected them, saying that they were only for use with prostitutes as a protection against venereal disease. One male leader pointed out that a woman would lose her strength if her husband used a condom. This belief also related to the equation of semen with blood, so if a man used a condom his wife "would not get her husband's power." A wife who reported that her husband had used a condom said, "We used it for two or three months before that baby (she pointed to a small child on the floor). Then one of my neighbors said that condoms cause disease so we stopped using it." Another woman complained that even though her husband had used a condom, she became pregnant, but she also revealed that he used the same condom repeatedly rather than purchase new ones.

The only government-offered methods that were seriously considered for adoption by the villagers were vasectomy and tubal ligation, but there were many reasons to fear these sterilization operations. Men in this area were fearful that if they had a vasectomy others might say they had been castrated (Poffenberger and Patel, 1964). One old man in a conversation with a younger husband who was interested in having the operation said, "You know those three Patidars that the Brahmin [a young village leader] took for the vasectomy . . . well they are now like *paviyas* [eunuchs]. Now where will their women go?" (One of the men who had a vasectomy complained that following the operation he was no longer able to have an erection, and another complained that he had lost his strength.)

A Baria who had told the female family-planning worker that he would have a vasectomy changed his mind when she came to get him. When asked why he said that he was afraid he would suffer from weakness and that a *bhuwa* (shaman) had told him the operation was against God's will. Another man said, "The operation will affect the health of a man or a woman. A woman may die during the operation or she will become fat afterward. A man will not be able to ride a bicycle. How would I get to work? I have decided not to have the operation."

Village women knew that many people who went to the hospital died, and this was a major fear of having a tubal ligation. The fear was reinforced by local rumors of deaths that were supposed to have resulted from the operation. Not only were village wives fearful that they might die as a result of surgery, but husbands and mothers-in-law were also resistant to suggestions that a wife should have a tubal ligation because they might be left with the extra household work and the care of the children during the wife's absence from the home or in case she died. A Baria wife complained that her mother-in-law would not permit her to have the operation, asking the wife, "Who will do the work for me?" Another Baria woman said, "I am tired of pregnancies and afraid of deliveries but my husband and mother-in-law will not let me have a tubectomy. They say that no one will take care of me in the hospital and that I will die. My husband does not have to suffer with childbirth, so I cannot change his mind."

Lower-caste men and women said that they had to work harder than the high-caste persons who were having operations and that they could not take the chance that they would be incapacitated because their life depended on their ability to do manual labor. They believed that their diet was inadequate to enable them to regain their strength after surgery. A Bhil woman said, "Sterilization is not good for poor people because we don't have good food to eat. The operation is all right for those who are healthy, but we poor people don't have enough money to buy the proper kind of food. We are laborers so we could not do our hard work after the operation." A Baria woman said, "After the tubectomy a woman has to rest at least six months. We women have to take care of a dairy buffalo, the house, children, and farm work, so we can't afford to rest that long."

Discussion and Research Implications

We have examined two basic questions raised in regard to Indian fertility—why people want the number of children they do, and why they do not act to terminate their fertility once they have achieved this number. An important question for research is the relationship between fertility attitudes and behavior. Villagers indicate a satisfaction with the ideal of two sons and one daughter, yet in terms of behavior they have an average of three sons and two daughters before having a vasectomy or tubal ligation.

Even a clear statement that another child is not desired does not predict adoption of an effective method. The reasons seem to lie in the fact that the question does not measure the degree to which a person wants to avoid having another child, the availability of an effective method, and if one is available, the degree of fear regarding the use of the method. If we are to understand behavior related to adoption of a birth-control method we must consider the strength of desire to avoid having another child compared with the fear related to the use of available methods to prevent conception or induce abortion. Questions asking why another child is not wanted and what the respondent's present behavior is regarding attempted control (i.e. the use of traditional methods) may give some useful attitudinal and behavior indices. Questions concerning fears regarding available government-recommended methods may indicate the degree of resistance. It is most likely then that adoption of a method may take place when the degree of desire to avoid having another child becomes greater than the fear of the use of the method. The family-planning program can approach individuals from both points—dealing with those variables that may increase desire to avoid having another child and with those variables that cause the individual to fear the use of modern, available, and effective methods.

There is evidence to support the position of Brewster Smith (Chapter 1) that since situational variables can be more easily modified than attitudes, more attention should be given to how peasants view innovations. It is evident that a significant increase in adoption would occur if villagers had a method of fertility control that when used would result in minimal dissonance. Because of the tendency to rationalize that a pregnancy will not occur and in view of the number of requests made to our research staff for some abortifacient pill, it seems that a culturally acceptable method for the villagers studied would be a pill that would bring on menses after a woman had missed a period or two. However, even with present government-offered family-planning methods, much could be done to reduce villagers' fears and aversions that relate to rejection of these methods.

There was an obvious lack of factual information upon which villagers' decisions were made—both regarding the number of children a couple needed to be reasonably sure of the survival of sons, and about ways in which fertility might be controlled. It is sometimes assumed that peasants are too irrational to make logical decisions. However, what seems logical or illogical is dependent upon what is *believed* to be the result of the decision, regardless of what the actual result may be. If there is a misconception regarding the probable consequences of an action, a decision may seem to be illogical from the point of view of one who is better informed. Since the vasectomy is a simple operation, usually having only minor aftereffects of short duration, extreme fear regarding it can be viewed as foolish. However, if one believes that he may become impotent or die as a result of this surgery, then considering having a vasectomy makes little sense regardless of the strength of a person's desire to avoid having another child. Therefore, the decision-making of the villagers may be quite rational and consistent with their beliefs, which relate to folklore and rumors as well as to hearsay about other villagers' postoperative complaints.

The mass media help to publicize family planning but are not effective in reducing anxiety about the various methods. To do this requires gaining the confidence of the people and then being able to explain each method in a way that can be understood in spite of the lack of socially acceptable terms related to reproduction in the local language. Perhaps more important is to determine ways to get those in the village who have adopted a method and are satisfied with it to tell others. There are such people, but they are reluctant to discuss the topic with neighbors. Persons who have undergone sterilization generally do not propagandize, even though their experience has been favorable, because in part they fear they may cause someone to have an operation that might have unfavorable consequences. As one woman remarked, "If I influenced someone and then that woman died, her relatives would say that it was my fault."

Although changes in attitudes are more difficult to bring about than changes in situations, it seems clear that the degree of fertility control required to achieve the goals of the government will not come about until attitude changes occur, both in terms of the available methods and in terms of the numbers of children regarded as necessary to reach culturally determined goals. In regard to desired family size it seems evident that the belief system is a complex of interrelated and conflicting values. In the intensive interviews with villagers, even though it was possible to elicit a response that the person wanted a specific number of children, further discussion indicated that the person usually did not have a strongly held belief regarding what a specific desired number should be. The villagers were usually uncertain, and it is this ambivalence that may have programmatic implications from the standpoint of attitude change. It is evident that they see advantages and disadvantages of having two children as well as of having four or five. (From a practical consideration no one would accept having only one child, and few want more than five.)

An area of research that might be useful for family-planning educational programs would be the testing of hypotheses about attitude change toward the desirability of having a small family. For example, a person might be confronted with inconsistencies that exist within his present value-attitude system regarding desired family size (e.g. Rokeach, 1968). Reviewed briefly below are some of the points of conflict and ambivalence at a cognitive level that might be used in changing attitudes, as well as relevant information of which villagers may not be aware.

Children are said to be gifts of God and fertility is not thought to be under human control, yet most village women eventually try to avoid having children once they have more than they want.

It is often said that a village wife cannot talk to her husband about such an intimate subject as fertility control, but many of the sample wives who had children reported they could talk to their husbands about anything.

It is said that extra children are required in order that some may survive to care for a mother in her old age; however, it is not generally known that children are not as likely to die now as in the past. When the subsample of forty-eight parents (twenty-four couples) was asked if they thought that there are more children alive now than in the past, there was general agreement that there are. When they were asked why they thought this was so, the most frequent response was that there is increased sex activity because this is the age of *Kaliyug* (a period of declining morality before the end of the world). One-half of these parents, however, said that more children die now than in the past; one-fourth indicated that more live; and the remaining parents were uncertain. Since many children still died in the village it was understandable that fear of children's deaths on the part of many parents was not in accord with the general trend toward lower infant and child mortality. Yet there was awareness on the part of some villagers of a decline in deaths. A few who said that not as many children die and some of those who were uncertain said they believed better health and medical care were the major reasons for the decline in child mortality. The high cost of medical care was mentioned by parents as a matter of concern, and some villagers who said that a family needs many children because they may die also said that proper medical care cannot be afforded if one has too many children.

A common criticism of youth made by middle-aged parents was that now sons are not as responsible as they were in the past and that parents cannot be certain that a son will take care of them in their old age. A frequently expressed remark was that it is necessary to have several sons to assure that at least one will be responsible, but some parents reasoned that an only son would be more considerate because he knows that his parents can only depend upon him.[7] Another common remark was that having many children gives a parent status, but it was also said that if children do not have good character they may also bring disgrace to the family, so it is better for parents to concentrate their attention on a few children and bring them up properly. While some parents said that the presence of many children brings joy to the household, others remarked that a large number of children is likely to result in tension and conflict.

Farmers wanted several sons to divide the work load, but it was recognized that having more than one son meant that the family's property might have to be divided. The presence of adult sons' wives and children often resulted in overcrowding of the village houses, which are usually small, and when a conflict developed the married sons and their families might move out or the house might be divided with a partition, so that family members would then have to live in less space and adult females would try to avoid each other in their daily activities.

It is our position then that village people have conflicting beliefs directly and indirectly related to fertility control and that this conflict has programmatic implications. The type of program and content would seem to be researchable areas. The problem would be to determine, for a particular group of people, the strength of antinatal factors and how they might be used in an educational program.

A recognized limitation of the government family-planning program in the area studied has been its female orientation. The village family-planning workers are women in spite of the fact that in the last few years the program has stressed male methods (the vasectomy and more recently the condom). The female worker in the village studied complained that the men did not want to talk to her and that the only way she could work was to talk to the women and hope that each would convince her husband to have the operation. Hill, Stycos, and Back (1959, pp. 372–373) have reported that one of the reasons for the modest achievements of the family-planning program in Puerto Rico was the fact that although the Puerto Rican family is traditionally male-centered, family-planning work was done only with the wife. In the Indian village, in spite of the strong patriarchal orientation and although husbands were often the major obstacle to effective family planning in all castes, a male family-planning worker never visited the village to talk with the men. How-

[7] Much attention has been given to consideration of incentives for having smaller families, such as providing social security payments to older people. A major problem is that the Indian government cannot afford the cost of a program covering all older people. Our data suggest that it is primarily the woman who is concerned that if her husband dies she will be left without a son to support her. A program that would insure the support of widows only if they did not have a living son would materially reduce the cost of such an incentive program. Even a small government-guaranteed income for widows might seem to have some advantage over the uncertainty of a son's support and perhaps reduce the pressure to have a sufficient number of sons so that one would be likely to survive.

ever, during the period of our investigation the male interviewers found that many of the husbands were concerned about having too many children. On the average the husbands wanted fewer children than the wives and reported fewer advantages of having a large family than did the wives. In addition male responses were judged to be less fatalistic. It was also the men who, in the last few years particularly, were feeling the economic pressure of having an increasing number of living children who had to be fed, clothed, and educated with a decreasing likelihood that the investment would pay off in economically rewarding work for sons when they were older. The husbands were interested and could be talked to about fertility-control methods, but a male approach was obviously needed in addition to the female worker's visits to the women.

Finally environmental and man-made situations in the past as well as at present have caused changes in belief systems consistent with behavior required for survival. Attention may be given to the rapid changes taking place in urban and rural areas. While it is true that individuals, if permitted, will give priority to their own interests over those of the group (e.g. Hardin, 1968), a point is reached in population growth where valued institutions and even one's own well-being are at stake. It is apparent that the increasing number of children in the village is putting pressure on both families and institutions. Changes in land usage and the introduction of agricultural innovations have caused fewer agricultural workers to be required at a time when more sons of the villagers live to maturity. Industries that have been developed adjacent to the city have provided jobs for some villagers but not nearly enough for all those who want and need them. Compared with agricultural work, male youths have found factory work attractive because of the regularity of cash wages and the shorter working hours. These advantages have enabled men to spend their free time in the city, in tea shops and cinemas, and have allowed them to purchase radios and consumer goods such as clothing of the type that is worn by men of the urban area.

The attraction of local industrial jobs has also caused a large number of immigrants to seek residence in this area. The result has been increasing serious unemployment and underemployment in the nearby villages and in the city. At a time of increasing living costs and consumer wants, farm laborers and menials in particular have often been forced to work for lower wages than they received in the past. At the same time factories have been able to select workers from the best educated and trained applicants. Villagers as well as urbanites are increasingly aware of the value of education as a qualification for employment.

Pressure on the educational system has resulted not only from the increase in the number of school-age children in the area each year but from the increasing percentage of children who attend beyond primary school from families that in the past did not consider an education necessary. While the population of the village studied increased at a rate of about 2.5 percent per year from 1961 to 1965, the total primary-school (Standards 1 to 7) enrollment increased nearly 10 percent each school year over the same period. Village leaders complained in Rajpur as well as in neighboring villages about the cost of adding classrooms and the increasing operating costs of schools.

The changes relating to modernization and increasing urbanization of this area do not seem to be bringing about any rapid change in the basic culture and social structure. Although there is evidence of an increasing desire on the part of youth for greater independence, strong forces hold the youth to traditional values. Socialization practices that psychologically bind the child to the mother and to the family remain largely unchanged. The values and goals of the extended family are still expressed by both male and female youth. Young men as well as women remain dependent upon family and caste members for marriage arrangements and educational opportunities, and male youths are dependent on relatives and caste-connected sources of employment for jobs once they complete their education. It seems that for some time in the future caste and the extended family will largely determine values related to fertility behavior as well as to other aspects of life. From our observations it seems that reduction in fertility may not take place by a breakdown of the family into nuclear units where the young couple is largely free to determine their own future, but because the growing population has resulted in forces that threaten the stability and traditions of the extended family itself. In this regard we believe it may be important to note that by the year 1969 a number of parents were telling their adult sons not to make the same mistake they did—that they should have a small family.

An example of the economic pressures felt as a result of declining child mortality was illustrated in the case of a high-caste Patidar landowner. As a result of his worries about financial problems due to difficulties he had in making marriage arrangements for his children, he had a nervous breakdown at the age of fifty and had to hospitalized. On one occasion the interviewer said that he overheard this man remark angrily to his sons, "Why don't you die? All my problems are because of you." He then told his sons to have no more than two children, and that one would even be better! He also had the government family-planning symbol—the red triangle—painted on the side of his village house with the program's slogan, "Two or three children— enough!"

We also had examples of the growing pressures of numbers of children on Rajpur village families of all social levels. The leader of the Bhil community told his married son to have a vasectomy after the son's wife had two sons and two daughters. The son, however, was afraid. The father then approached a male interviewer from the village research staff and asked him to convince his son that he should have a vasectomy, saying that when he was his son's age that it was possible to feed many children but that times had changed.

We may also cite some examples from a recent survey of Eleventh Standard students (final class in the secondary school with an average age of seventeen years) in a village near Rajpur in Baroda Taluka. Nearly all of the thirty-nine students made some reference to the problems created by having many children (Poffenberger and Sebaly, 1971).

One of the high-caste Patidar youths had three brothers and two sisters. The father was a landowning farmer who had a moderately high income by village standards. The youth's twenty-three-year-old brother lived with.the joint family and helped the father manage the farm. When the seventeen-year-old youth was interviewed he said he did not know what jobs would be available in the family for himself and his other brothers, ages twenty and fifteen years. He said he hoped to get a job in the city but knew that it would be difficult. He indicated that if he could not find a city job he would work on the family's farm. He explained why his family had financial problems, saying, "My family is in debt because my father had to borrow money on his land because of the dowry for my sister. We have enough earnings, but it is because of social costs that we must borrow. Things like a marriage or a naming ceremony make us borrow. If we did not have these expenses, then we could save some of our income. Because of all these expenses my father is trying to sell another part of our land." Then in response to a question that asked if his parents ever talked about family problems, he said, "My father and mother usually talk about our debt. They have often said to us that we should keep our families small or we will be in the same position."

In another family of middle-level caste there were five sons whose ages ranged from sixteen to thirty years. The three oldest sons were married, and all of them lived with the parents. The eldest had four children. The father's earnings as a clerk in a local factory were the main support of the joint family. One of the sons had a job as a hospital clerk in the nearby city, but the others were unemployed. The eighteen-year-old son who was interviewed commented, "Our family faces the problem of a money shortage because all of my brothers live with us. We have a large family to maintain. My parents always talk about the problem of money and the large size of our family, the cost of education and marriage." He added, "My mother was sterilized at the time of her last delivery, but family planning should have been used earlier."

The comments of one of the "scheduled-caste" youths were typical of the general economic problems faced by the families in lower socioeconomic levels. He reported that he was one of five living siblings—three brothers and two sisters. Two other sisters had died. The respondent was the eldest child. The father was an agricultural laborer but was not regularly employed. The mother apparently worked when she could. The youth said he hoped to become a teacher because it offered a steady income. He said that he would like to work in the city but would plan to live in the village with his parental family. He remarked, "We have a large family and a shortage of money. Seven of us are dependent on a monthly cash income of thirty rupees [less than $3]. Our family's size is a problem because sometimes my parents do not have work. My brother has completed SSC [secondary school examination] but cannot study further because there is so little money. There is nothing that can be done about our family size now, but the problem could have been avoided by family planning. Now my parents feel that a small family would have been better."

A study of the prevalence of the kinds of pressures that are created as a result of having more children live than did in the past and the reaction of villagers to these pressures would seem to be important for agents of change in planning and conducting family-planning training programs and village-level action programs.

In summary a researchable question is how local knowledge, beliefs, and changing environmental forces favorable to fertility control may be used to counteract misinformation and beliefs that result in continued high fertility. The potential for attitude-change exists, and in fact attitudes are already undergoing change both toward a smaller family-size norm and acceptance of presently available methods. We will close with a statement of a young Patidar bride. She said proudly, "In our caste we now have a tubectomy after three children."

REFERENCES

Agarwala, S. N. 1962. *Attitudes toward family planning in India.* Bombay: Asia.
———. 1968. Family planning targets in India for the next five years. In *Sixth all-India conference on family planning.* Chandigarh: Family Planning Association of India.
Berelson, B. 1965. KAP studies in fertility. In B. Berelson et al., ed., *Family planning and population programs.* Chicago: University of Chicago Press. Pp. 655–668.
Census of India 1961. Social and cultural tables. 1 (Part II–C[i]):19.
Davis, K. 1967. Population policy: will current programs succeed? *Science* 158:730–739.
Embassy of India (U.S.A.). 1971. *India News* 10:3.
Freedman, R. 1967. Application of the behavioral sciences to family planning programs. *Studies in Family Planning* 23:5–9.
Hardin, G. 1968. The tragedy of the commons. *Science* 162:1243–1248.
Heer, D. M. and Smith, D. O. 1967. Mortality level, desired family size, and population increase. Paper presented at the annual meeting of the Population Association of America, Cincinnati, Ohio, April 1967.
Hill, R.; Stycos, J. M.; and Back, K. W. 1959. *The family and population control, a Puerto Rican experiment in social change.* New Haven: Yale University Press.
Kothari, R. and Maru, R. 1965. Caste and secularism in India, case study of a caste federation. *Journal of Asian Studies* 25:33–50.
Loomis, C. P. 1967. Changes in rural India as related to social power and sex. *Behavioral Science and Community Development* (India) 1:1–27.
May, D. A. and Heer, D. M. 1968. Son survivorship, motivation and family size in India: a computer simulation. *Population Studies* 22:199–210.
Mehta, M. J. 1966. A study of the practice of female infanticide among the Kanbis of Gujarat. *Journal of the Gujarat Research Society* 28:57–66.
Nag, M. 1969. Can reproductive attitudes and behavior in a society change irrespective of the change in socioeconomic variables? Paper presented at the annual meeting of the American Anthropological Association, New Orleans, November 1969.
Nair, K. 1961. *Blossoms in the Dust.* London: Gerald Duckworth & Company, Ltd.
National Sample Survey. 1963. Report number 116/1, tables with notes on family planning, sixteenth round. Calcutta: Indian Statistical Institute.
Poffenberger, T. 1967. Age of wives and number of living children of a sample of men who had a vasectomy in Meerut District, U.P. *The Journal of Family Welfare* (India) 13:48–51.

————. 1968a. Husband-wife differences in attitudes toward fertility control innovations in rural India. *Indian Journal of Social Research* 9:36–42.

————. 1968b. Urban Indian attitudinal response and behavior related to family planning. *The Journal of Family Welfare* (India) 14:31–38.

————. 1969. *Husband-wife communication and motivational aspects of population control in an Indian village.* New Delhi: Central Family Planning Institute, Monograph Series 10.

Poffenberger, T. and Patel, H. G. 1964. The effect of local beliefs on attitudes toward vasectomy in two Indian villages in Gujarat State. *Population Review* (India) 8:37–44.

Poffenberger, T. and Sebaly, K. 1971. Population learning among secondary school students in an Indian village. Center for Population Planning, University of Michigan (mimeo).

Population Reference Bureau. 1970. India: ready or not, here they come. *Population Bulletin* 24:1–31.

Rokeach, M. 1968. *Beliefs, attitudes and values—a theory of organization and change.* San Francisco: Jossey-Boss.

Roy, P. and Kivlin, J. 1968. Health innovations and family planning. Hyderabad, India: National Institute of Community Development. Pp. 28–29.

United Nations. 1961. *Mysore population study* (ST/SOA/Ser. A/34). New York: Department of Economics and Social Affairs.

[6]

SOME PSYCHOLOGICAL ASPECTS
OF FERTILITY, FAMILY PLANNING,
AND POPULATION POLICY
IN THE UNITED STATES

CATHERINE S. CHILMAN

The United States faces a serious increase in the size of its population in the near future because of the baby boom that lasted from 1945 to 1957. These babies are now growing to maturity and are entering their prime childbearing years. Although the birth rate has been steadily declining since 1957, the sheer size of the youth population is a cause for grave concern. This concern is intensified by the recognition that a large U.S. population is a problem both to the United States and to other nations because it is bound up with the growing world-wide crisis in pollution and the possible exhaustion of the earth's natural resources.

In order to decrease the rate of population growth in the United States, a wide range of public policies and programs is needed. These policies and programs are far more likely to succeed if they are based on knowledge drawn from many disciplines, including the social and behavioral sciences. Reproductive behavior is related to a complex of causes rooted in the total life situation of a people and in the intricacies of human decision-making in an area of intense subjectivity and emotionality. Knowledge about population problems, contraceptive techniques, the advantages of a small family is not sufficient, by itself, to bring about sharp reductions in family size. Furthermore, experience here and in other countries has shown that making free family-planning services readily available does not bring about sufficiently widespread, continuously effective use of such services.

NOTE: Some portions of this chapter have been adapted from an earlier article by the author appearing in the *Journal of Marriage and the Family* 30, No. 2 (1968).

More knowledge is needed in the biological, social, and behavioral sciences to serve as guides to programs and policies that have a higher potential for success in reducing the rate of population growth. At present applicable knowledge derived from the behavioral sciences is particularly limited.

This chapter attempts to present a highly condensed (and therefore necessarily limited and overly simplified) summary of the social and psychological research findings in the United States that apply to our population problem. This summary includes the following: a brief sketch of today's demographic picture; the highlights of findings regarding the contraceptive knowledge, attitudes, and practices of American families; a somewhat more intensive analysis of the family-planning problems of low-income and black families; and a consideration of some frequently overlooked psychological factors that seem particularly likely to affect feminine contraceptive behavior. At the conclusion suggestions are made concerning further research and the development of population policies and programs.

Throughout this review the assumption is made that every effort should be made to resolve the population problem within a philosophical and political framework of humanistic democracy. Perhaps the central challenge facing this nation and other nations is whether the growing population and pollution crisis can be resolved by such an approach.

Population Growth in the United States

The U.S. birth rate has been declining steadily since 1957 to a present low of 17.5 per 1,000 population (Vital and Health Statistics, 1970). However, many demographers are concerned about the present size of the population and its potential for rapid growth in the future. The population of this country has increased from little over 100 million in 1920 to more than twice that number at present. Even if the relatively low present birth rate continues, the size of our population is bound to grow considerably (Miles, 1971).

A graphic picture of fertility trends in the United States over the past sixty years (see Figure 6–1) indicates a generally downward national trend from 1915 to 1935, with a trough during the Depression years. During World War II fertility rates rose, albeit somewhat unsteadily, and proceeded to spurt upward during the mid-1940s and into the late 1950s, with a peak in 1947 and a still higher one in 1957. Since 1957 the rate has generally declined, reaching a relative low of 86 per 1,000 by 1968 and rising slightly in 1970.

To those alarmed about the country's growing population, this generally downward trend of fertility rates in recent years could appear reassuring.

Figure 6–1. Live Births and Fertility Rates:
United States, 1910–1970.

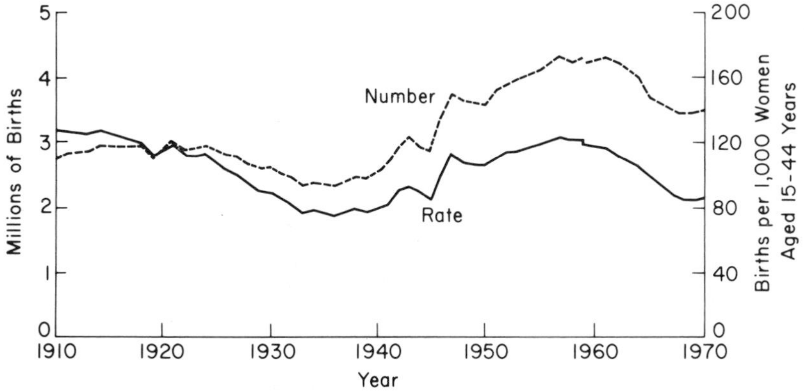

Source: Department of Health, Education and Welfare, Monthly
Vital Statistics Report, vol. 18, no. 11, supplement, January 30,
1970. (Updated by Monthly Reports through February, 1972.)

However, such reassurance may be without a solid base for the following
reasons:

1. Although the trend is downward, it is still over 20 percent higher than
that of the middle 1930s. An important aspect of the earlier decline in
fertility rates—the desire of some women to avoid childbearing altogether—
appears to be lacking now. Twenty-three percent of the ever married
women born between 1906 and 1910 and of childbearing age between 1925
and 1950 did not have children. As opposed to this, recent surveys of attitudes of younger women indicate that all but a very few of them want
children (Whelpton, Campbell, and Patterson, 1966).

2. The current decline in the fertility rate may be related to the possibility
that young people today, because of pressures for higher levels of education
and a higher youth unemployment rate, are not starting their families at
quite so young an age as their older brothers and sisters did in the middle
1950s. If this is the case the fertility rate may begin to rise again in the near
future, especially if employment opportunities for young people improve.

On the other hand, there is some hope that the rate of population growth
may decline if the present slight trend toward marriage at a later age is
strengthened. One of the reasons for the population spurt over the past
twenty-five years has been that men and women tended to marry young
and to become parents soon thereafter. However, it is unclear at present
whether this trend toward later marriage will become strong enough to
influence significantly population growth rates.

3. Population growth has been closely related to a sharp decrease in the
death rate, especially the infant death rate, which has been considerably

reduced over the past half-century. As of 1965, for instance, the national birth rate was still almost twice as high as the national death rate. Since, barring a major holocaust, it is very unlikely that the age-specific death rate will increase—in fact, vigorous efforts are currently being made to lower further the infant death rate—population stability can result only from a further lowering of fertility.

4. Even though the fertility rate may continue to decline—or remain at its present lowered levels—the number of babies born each year is almost certain to increase for at least the next fifteen years because of the baby boom of the mid-1940s and 1950s. For instance, between 1967 and 1980 the number of women of childbearing age will increase about 30 percent according to projections prepared by the U.S. Bureau of Census. In the ages that commonly account for the largest number of births (twenty to twenty-nine years), the increase will be even greater: about 48 percent.

This increase in the adult female population has led the Public Health Service (Vital and Health Statistics, 1970) to conclude that the total fertility rate must fall sharply and steadily over the next fifteen years if the annual *number* of births is to remain constant. According to the population growth projections of the Bureau of the Census, if American women continue to have about 2.5 children on the average, sixty-six million more people will be added to the population by the year 2000. Frejka (1970) estimates that the total fertility rate should be slightly over 1.00 if population is to be stabilized in the near future and notes that this is not a realistic prospect.

5. Studies using differing methods of assessment show that married women on the average want somewhere between 2.5 (Bumpass and Westoff, 1970) and 3.4 (Whelpton et al., 1966) children apiece. (These studies were conducted in 1965 and 1960, respectively.) It is clear that if these family-size values continue and women have the number of children they say they want, our population will continue to grow at a relatively rapid pace.

6. Although it is frequently claimed that the large families of the poor are the major cause for rapid population growth, this is fallacious. Because most families in the United States at present subscribe to the two- to three-child norm and because the poor make up only 15 percent of the population, it can readily be seen that the fertility behavior of the more affluent majority is the major source for the population problem (Blake, 1969).

Major Findings of Social Research Related to Family Planning

Many population and community resources experts see a continued upsurge in population growth as a threat to the national welfare. They forecast: a strain on the health, education, welfare, housing, and employment resources of the nation; a drain on natural resources; threats of air and water pollution; and pressure on other facilities such as the transportation system. They also point out that this nation, with its high standard of living and advanced technology, uses far more than its share of the world's resources, including the resources of pollution-free air and water. Continued population growth in the United States, therefore, offers a threat to the rest of the world as well as to this country.

Because of these threats there is an increasing advocacy of expanded family-planning programs or a firm population-control policy in the United States. Such programs and policies are far more likely to be effective if they are based on knowledge derived from many fields of research, including related social and psychological research. Despite the gaps and limitations in such research, much information is available that should be useful both to policy and program builders and to researchers as they seek to design further studies to enhance the range of knowledge needed in this field. Therefore, a summary of the major findings from related social and psychological studies is presented here.

1. The great majority of people in the United States (about 90 percent) reportedly approve of the concept of family planning (Whelpton et al., 1966; Westoff, Potter, and Sagi, 1963). High approval rates have been found for the majority of Catholics; still higher approval is found for other religious groups (Whelpton et al., 1966; Rainwater, 1965). Although most of the respondents in these investigations were married women, one small study of low-income Negro males revealed that three-fourths of them approved of family planning (Misra, 1967).

2. At all socioeconomic levels in this country and in most other countries studied—including some of the so-called disadvantaged nations—the average number of children that respondents say they desire is between two and four (Berelson, 1966).

3. The arrival of the fourth child seems to represent a critical point for a family. Even those relatively few families who had previously expressed a desire for more than four children revise their plans after the arrival of the fourth child (Berelson, 1966).

4. Evidence is beginning to emerge that families with more than four children, even when controls are established for differences in socioeconomic level, are less likely to be viewed by the children as happy (Moore and Holtzman, 1965) and are less likely to produce self-reliant, outgoing youngsters who achieve well in school (Douvan and Adelson, 1966; Clausen, 1966). There is also mounting, though not conclusive, evidence that children from large families have lower tested intelligence on the average and achieve less well occupationally (Duncan and Blau, 1967). An analysis of 1962 census data referring to the educational achievement of adult men in this country shows that almost twice as many men from one-child families (73 percent) complete high school as do those from families of four or more children (39 percent). Even when only low-income families are considered, this trend holds.

5. A higher level of authoritarianism and use of physical punishment is found among families of five or more children, even when socioeconomic and ethnic factors are controlled.

In a recent paper reviewing findings from earlier research and related theory, Nye, Carlson, and Garrett (1970) propose the following:

1. The larger the family, the more likely it is to be characterized by authoritarian parental practices.
2. The larger the family, the more likely the family will be characterized by father domination.
3. The larger the family, the less likely it will be characterized by a predominance of positive affect.
4. The larger the family, the more likely will the parental role-playing be characterized by severe stress (only very limited research support is available for this last proposition).

The authors conclude their analysis of available research evidence by commenting that in terms of the criteria of affect, stress, and interaction patterns, "the small family of one or two children is consistently found superior to either medium-sized or large families." However, further studies are needed, with careful consideration of possible associated variables, before one can be confident that family size alone plays such a crucial role in child development and family relations. (See also Chapter 7 of this book.)

6. Economic concern is most often cited by couples (usually female respondents) in the United States as the basic reason for limiting family size. It is closely tied to a desire to provide a better quality of life for one's children. Considerations of maternal and child health are rarely given by respondents.

Clues to motivation for large family size can be found in a study by Stolka and Barnett (1969). In a sample of young Catholic and Protestant women they found that strong pronatalist attitudes were associated with both being Catholic and having less than a high-school education. The reason given most often by all respondents for favoring having children was that "it is woman's role." This reason was given far more often than reasons relating to social prestige, religion, or marital happiness.

7. Recent studies reveal that on the average nonwhite wives say they want fewer children than white wives; some studies show this as particularly true for urban nonwhite women, in regions other than the South, and for nonwhite women who have more than an eighth-grade education (Whelpton et al., 1966; Misra, 1967; Hill and Jaffe, 1966; Blair, 1967).

8. Although it has been claimed frequently that parents have children to promote marital happiness, a recent study corroborating earlier findings indicates that marital happiness is not necessarily dependent upon the presence of children. Luckey and Bain (1970), in an analysis of a small sample of married couples, found that children were reported by parents as a major source of satisfaction only in those families in which the marriage relationship was poor. In marriages in which husbands and wives report an excellent

marital relationship, the children were not seen as being of primary importance to marital happiness.

These summarized findings are not necessarily synonymous with more basic motivations that play a part in actual behavior. In studies of the kind cited, problems of response bias and the role of underlying feelings are not likely to be effectively handled. Psychological theory, research, and observations stress the large part played in human behavior by the individual's drive for self-security, status, personal significance, and close human relationships. These factors, though generally not revealed in the findings, must surely have a strong effect on underlying motivation and overt behavior regarding timing of children, child-spacing, and family size.

Here and in other countries desire for small families and effective contraceptive practice is highly associated with urbanization, education (in the United States, more than an eighth-grade education), and high aspirations for one's children. In the United States, however, urbanization has failed to have the sharp, distinctive impact on desire for small families and related contraceptive practices that was anticipated by urban sociologists. These anticipations were based on the experience of Western European countries and Japan and on theories of urbanization. Urban and rural families in the United States are highly similar in that they generally want between two and four children—and for the most part have this number. The most distinctive deviation from the American pattern consists of families in the rural South and recent urban migrants from there, especially black families.

Among the reasons for the general lack of differences in desired family size between most urban and rural people in this country may be: the adequate level of income available to most families; the growing urbanization of rural areas through improved transportation facilities, the availability of mass media, and the mechanization of most farms; and the suburban and exurban living of many so-called urban families. It is well known that the suburban and exurban style of life is generally a family-centered one.

The relatively greater poverty, isolation, and racial segregation of the rural South probably play a large part in the different family-planning attitudes, information levels, and practices found in that region. The severe problems of the urban migrants from the rural South and their isolation in the poverty ghettos of the city (particularly in the case of blacks) probably contribute to their difficulties in family-size limitation.

In summary the major points emerging from social research are the following: the great majority of people in the United States reportedly approve of the concept of family planning; at all socioeconomic levels people apparently see a family of two to four children as being ideal; a family of four or more children *seems* to impose special strains on family life and to have adverse effects on the emotional and intellectual development of children; the chief reason parents give for wanting a small family are economic; acceptance of the small family norm and of contraceptives is generally associated with urbanization and higher levels of education; on the average, nonwhite families in the United States say they want smaller families (an ideal of three children) than whites; personality tests and related measures have failed so far to reveal psychological factors associated with the large or small family norm. In reference to the last point the difficulties in isolating significant, related psychological variables become apparent when one considers that reproductive norms and behavior are associated with a complex of biological, social, economic, experiential, and situational factors operating in the context of the total dynamics of the male and female mate relationship.

Comments on Female Psychology and Contraceptive Use

Failure to control family size effectively is associated to an unknown degree with the nature of the various available contraceptives. All methods have some disadvantages, and all have a margin of failure. In respect to such devices as the condom, diaphragm, and pill, the major focus of failure lies most obviously in human carelessness, low motivation, or resistance to "never taking a chance." Other reasons for failure may be lack of access to medical care and contraceptive supplies, basic desire for pregnancy to occur, psychological or cultural (including religious) conflicts over use of such contraceptives, and fear of the side effects of contraceptives.

Population planners and medical personnel tend to play down the importance of these side effects. Although these effects may offer very little or no risk to the basic health of the user, such symptoms as pain, nausea, dizziness, and bleeding (frequently associated with the early stages of using the pill and with using the IUD) are not to be lightly dismissed. Side effects such as these can be seen as serious obstacles, especially in the case of women with relatively low motivation, psychological conflicts regarding family planning, and cultural values that include contrary religious beliefs and skepticism and distrust of middle-class society.

The attitudes, feelings, and experiences of women are often overlooked by family-planning and population-control specialists. This is probably because such personnel (especially at policy-making and administrative levels) are male and because the great majority of them are either demographers or physicians. Their training and values stress heavily an intellectual and rational approach. Demographers, particularly, are trained to handle quantitative data as they apply to large groups and to think in highly logical, abstract terms. Yet the use of contraceptives is an intensely individual matter where the "logic of the emotions," rather than the logic of the intellect, where subjective attitudes and values, rather than objective data, play a very large part. Especially until safe and effective contraceptives (other than the condom) for men can be developed, particular attention should be paid to the "contraceptive" psychology of women, most particularly in relation to their interaction with men.

Although little formal research is available, theory and observations give a number of clues that can provide a basis for future studies. Probably the majority of women in our culture feel that the male should take the initiative in sexual relations. To a large extent an American female's sense of adequacy is derived from her sense of being sexually attractive to the male and ardently pursued by him.[1] This female desire to be sexually attractive and pursued affects her use of contraceptives—particularly the intercourse-connected ones such as the diaphragm and spermicidal jellies and foams. Both require planning in advance for intercourse at a specific time. As a result the woman's conscious or unconscious thought might be: "Does he really find me sexually attractive and does he want to have intercourse with me today—or tonight? If I am prepared and he doesn't seek me, then I will feel rejected and humiliated. I would rather take a chance on getting pregnant."

Somewhat the same line of subjective reasoning applies to oral contraceptives and the IUD, especially for unmarried or separated females. If these females are "perpetually contracepted" this implies that they are perpetually ready for intercourse. And the female asks, "Does he think he can have sex relations with me, with no marriage commitment, just because I am safe? If he knows I am on the pill or the IUD, does he think I am a 'loose woman'? I don't want to plan on seducing a man; I want to be swept off my feet by love and romantic passion" (see the report by Zelnik and Kantner, 1970).

For both married and unmarried women other attitudes may enter the picture such as: "He gets just as much—or more—out of sex as I do; why should *I* have to go through all this fuss?" "It isn't right that he can have me whenever he wants me, and *I* have to take the precautions—if I get pregnant, he'll have to pay for a change." Or "I love him, I want his baby, I want *our* baby—it's not sensible, but there is no greater sweetness in the world than a tiny baby; besides that's what women are for; I want to be a whole woman. Then, too, if I get pregnant, he will *have* to stay with me."

---

[1] It simply is not known whether such attitudes have a strong biological base or are largely induced by acculturation. From a biological viewpoint it is obvious that the man (but not the woman) must be sexually aroused if intercourse is to take place and that the fundamental nature of intercourse involves an aggressive act by the man and receptivity on the part of the woman. Biologically females can be almost constantly ready for intercourse, whereas males need periods of rest in between sexual acts, especially if an ejaculation is to occur. These biological factors probably play a part in cultural norms observed in most parts of the world that tend to emphasize male sexual aggression and female receptivity and relative passivity. These norms also include an emphasis on the female making herself sexually attractive to the man in order to stimulate his continuing, rather than sporadic, interest in her.

Although norms of this kind are being challenged, especially by the "liberated women," it is far from clear that their demand to be fully equal to men in all ways (including the sexual component) will gain widespread support among the majority of women (and men). Also it is not clear as to how deeply significant biological factors are in shaping the behavior of contemporary human beings.

All of the above expressed attitudes are associated with the identity and ego needs of the female as shaped by our culture (Rainwater, 1965; Hill, Stycos, and Back, 1959). Male physicians and family-planning researchers may never or rarely hear these attitudes expressed by their patients. It is noteworthy that females seldom overtly and frankly express their sexual feelings and attitudes to men (other than perhaps to husbands and lovers or through their writings). This reticence relates to the female's drive to subtly attract the male, to be pursued; it also relates to cultural norms that (until recently) have forbidden overt, frank sexuality to "good and lovable" women.

Assuming that these observations have considerable validity, a central implication is that the identity and ego needs of both women and men, particularly as expressed in male-female interaction, should be considered in family-planning programs. Family-planning programs deal with human beings, not population statistics. They seek to intervene with basic human functions in the sensitive areas of sex, intimate interpersonal relationships, reproduction, and parenthood. These functions are fundamentally related to powerful socializing factors that lie at the foundations of the human community. If these functions are treated in an obtuse, impersonal manner, further social-psychological problems of alienation, apathy, and despair may be the result (Chilman, 1970).

Poverty and Family Planning

There is a tendency in some quarters to view high fertility rates as a particular problem of the poor. Although this view is a somewhat inaccurate and myopic one, poor families are likely to differ from more affluent ones in terms of family formation, family size, and child-spacing. These problems in fertility control are important to consider because of the particular adverse effect they have on the economic state, health, and general well-being of low-income parents and children.

Poor People Have Larger Families on the Average

A larger proportion of low-income families have more than five children. As Orshansky points out, "Of the 15 million children being reared in poverty, 43 percent are growing up in a home with at least five youngsters under age 18. Indeed, the poverty rate among families rose sharply from 12 percent when there was one child in the home to 49 percent when there were six or more children. The poverty rate for all families with five or six children is 3½ times as high as for families with one or two children"

(Orshansky, 1965). The poverty aspects of this situation are emphasized when one considers what these figures mean in terms of average per capita income.

Another way of viewing family size and family income is presented by Campbell (1968), who shows that poor women (those below the "poverty line") have an average annual fertility rate that is almost twice as high as those who have incomes that are rated as adequate or higher.

To the rationalist, poor people "ought to have enough sense" to limit the size of their families. Such limitation, the rationalist argues, would provide poor people with an important opportunity to escape from poverty. From the rationalist's viewpoint poor people can be most effectively helped to control family size if: (1) free family-planning services are made readily available to them; and (2) information is provided regarding the importance and effectiveness of rational family-planning behavior, that is, matching family size and pregnancy timing to the economic, social, and health resources of the family and making consistent use of medically approved contraceptives.

Irrational components of family-planning behavior in general have already been discussed. These components are intensified for the poor person because of the defeating situation of poverty itself, which rarely yields to rational behavior; the consequent life styles of many of the defeated poor; low educational levels; and the isolation of the poor in urban ghettos or rural slums.

Early Marriage and Poverty

Alvin Schorr has analyzed certain family life patterns and their association with poverty (Schorr, 1966). Early age at marriage, early age of mother at birth of first child, large family size, children born more closely together, and a greater span of years of childbearing are behaviors more likely to occur for low-income families and are also one factor in the continuing poverty of many low-income families.

It is estimated that almost half of the white and over four-fifths of the nonwhite females who marry before the age of twenty are premaritally pregnant (Zelnik and Kantner, 1970). Very young marriages, when the bride is seventeen or younger, are apt to be more fragile than others. A number of studies show a close relationship between early marriage and later divorce (Burchinal, 1963), and a considerable body of research reveals that those who marry before age twenty-two or thereabouts are more likely than those who marry later to rate their marriage as unhappy by the time they have reached middle age (Burchinal, 1963). A very high proportion of the marriages of high-school students apparently involve premarital pregnancy (Schorr, 1966; Burchinal, 1963), so that the youthful bride and groom are likely to face leaving school, parenthood, and unemployment, or exceedingly low employment status, all in a short space of time.

Female Employment, Poverty, and Family Size

Working wives make a substantial financial contribution when they add their wages to those of the husband, often boosting poor families above the "poverty line." For instance, half of the families who were in the $7,000 to $15,000 a year income bracket in 1968 owed part of this higher income to the fact that wives, as well as husbands, were employed. Women who work during the early years of their marriage and defer pregnancy are more apt to have children spaced over a longer period of time and to belong to families that over the years achieve a better economic position (Schorr, 1966).

Although a small number of women may be working because they have few or no children due to sterility problems, in general families of working women tend to be smaller because of the motivation of these women to control family size. Working mothers tend to be upwardly mobile and to belong to the "working-class poor"—quite a different socioeconomic group from the long-term chronically unemployed or underemployed "very poor" (Chilman, 1966).

In the lowest income groups (family income under $2,000 a year) women tend to have an above average number of children, whether they work outside the home or not. Lack of educational preparation and vocational training, problems of poor physical and mental health, discrimination, high rates of marriage breakdown, child-care and transportation problems, and deficits in the job market combine to create severe and continuing employment problems for these parents at the bottom of the socioeconomic heap. Better family-planning practices alone would do little to help such families move out of poverty, even if both parents seek employment, unless the total life situation for such families is radically improved.

Education, Poverty, and Family Size

Although families with less education, lower employment status, rural origins, and lower incomes generally have larger families, women at these levels are similar to more advantaged women in terms of the number of children they say they would like to have. However, poor people are apt to have more difficulty in restricting family size and in spacing their children. Parents with an eighth-grade education or less have the most difficulties in effective family planning (Farley, 1965; Whelpton et al., 1966).

Studies show that while some form of fertility limitation is nearly universal in the United States, wives with little formal education are less likely to use contraceptives, especially in the early stages of family formation (Whelpton et al., 1966; Rainwater, 1965). It would be inappropriate, however, to equate difficulties in fertility control with lack of education beyond the eighth grade since the many factors that affect the level of educational attainment are also likely to affect contraceptive effectiveness. More immediate factors that adversely affect fertility control are, of course, lack of readily available free or low-cost family-planning clinics and contraceptive supplies plus ignorance about sex and reproduction.

Poverty, Family Size, and Race

The main reason for examining white-nonwhite fertility rates here is that there is a much higher rate of poverty for nonwhite (chiefly black) groups. According to analyses of 1960 Census data, 14 percent of white families and 47 percent of nonwhite families were found to be below the poverty line. (Poverty is defined in this instance as annual family income of less than $3,000.) Although the situation for nonwhites has improved somewhat since 1960, it is probable that 40 percent or more of these families are still below the poverty line.

The curve of fertility rates of nonwhite, compared to white, groups, as shown in Figure 6–2, reveals that nonwhite rates have been consistently higher since 1920, when data of this sort were first collected. Since 1947 the fertility rates of nonwhites have grown at a much more rapid rate than

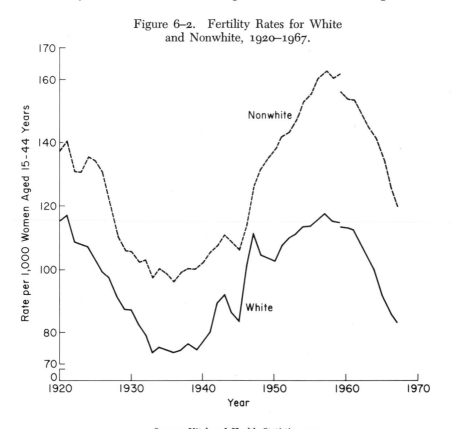

Figure 6–2.   Fertility Rates for White and Nonwhite, 1920–1967.

Source: Vital and Health Statistics, 1970.

those of whites, reaching a peak in 1958. Since that time nonwhite fertility rates have dropped somewhat more rapidly than white ones, although as of 1967 they were still consistently higher.

The following factors are among those primarily responsible for these fertility trends and differences: the higher proportion of nonwhites than whites of Southern rural background; the sharp drop in nonwhite infant and maternal mortality rates in the past forty-five years (because of increased attention given to adequate maternity and infant care for all members of the population); the lower average education of nonwhite groups; the lower average occupational and income status of nonwhites; a greater drop in sterility rates for nonwhites (partly related to better medical care); the greater proportion of nonwhite women who have five and six children; and a higher ratio of young women in their prime childbearing years in the nonwhite than in the white population (Lunde, 1965).

Contrasted to comparable white groups, nonwhites at most educational levels have less tendency to use contraceptives, especially at an early point in their marriages; this difference is strongest for those with a grade-school education, low occupational status, and current rural residence (Campbell, 1965; Hill and Jaffe, 1966; Blair, 1967; Bogue, 1965).

It is anticipated that nonwhite fertility ratios will become more similar to those of whites as nonwhites become increasingly acclimated to urban living and as their educational, income, and occupational opportunities improve.

Low-Income Life Styles

Low-income life styles, the so-called subcultures of poverty, arise out of the poverty situation itself. These life styles constitute an adaptive response to the deprivations and harsh constraints that are so frequently the lot of those at the bottom of the socioeconomic heap. Although the basic problems of the very poor are situational in nature, the poverty life styles that some of them adopt tend to interact with the poverty situation to tighten further the trap that prevents escape to higher socioeconomic levels (Chilman, 1966).

The poverty situation itself tends to lead to inadequate family-planning practices. As we have seen early family formation and large family size are associated with such situational factors as low occupational status, low income, little education, discrimination, isolation in rural slums or urban ghettos, and inaccessibility of contraceptive services. Large family size is one of the outcomes of this total situation; in turn this outcome tends to reenforce the poverty situation. And this situation tends to produce life styles that foster attitudes and practices inimical to effective contraceptive behavior.

The life styles include attitudes of fatalism, magical thinking, personalism, apathy, lack of long-range goal orientation, and hostile alienation from the more advantaged sector of society—especially its social institutions and authority figures. These life styles tend to stand in the way of actively planning (as compared to vaguely hoping) for a stable marriage, child-spacing, small family size, and positive future goals for one's self and one's children. For example, one study shows that less than one-third of those who trust to luck or fate approve of family planning, but of those who lack fatalistic attitudes, 80 percent favor family planning (Misra, 1967). A (frequently justified) lack of commitment to and faith in schools, clinics, social agencies, religious institutions, and the advice and services emanating therefrom often prevents or reduces the use of such services. These attitudes also tend to undermine a belief in the efficacy of contraceptive methods. Poor families who do use contraceptives tend not to start until they have had three or four children and then use them sporadically (Whelpton et al., 1966).

Other aspects of family life styles more prevalent among groups dwelling in long-term, severe poverty are likely to be associated with their problems in family planning. Various studies (Rainwater, 1965; Komarovsky, 1962; Herzog, 1963; Misra, 1967) indicate that:

1. A larger proportion of working-class and middle-class families than very poor families report happy marriages and mutually satisfying sex relationships.
2. Very poor men and women have a greater tendency to live in quite separate social and psychological worlds with little communication between husband and wife, whereas communication and shared activities are clearly related to marital happiness, and sex satisfaction, communication, and marital happiness are closely associated with effective family planning.
3. Hostile and mutually exploitative attitudes are more likely to occur between the sexes in poverty groups: the male tends to play an authoritarian role in the family; illegitimacy rates are higher; a larger number of marriages are broken by divorce, desertion, and separation; very poor people are likely to have extremely limited knowledge about sex, reproduction, and childbirth.
4. Sex relations are likely to be seen as proof of one's prowess as a man or woman rather than as a part of an interpersonal relationship. Peer group pressures for premarital and extramarital sex experiences are strong. These experiences are apt to be impulsively entered into and situationally determined. The male often sees little reason to protect the female from pregnancy in such relationships, and the female frequently sees little point in preparing herself in advance for sex relations that may or may not occur and a pregnancy that may or may not take place in consequence.
5. Parents are apt to fear giving sex education to their children in the belief that this may lead to "trouble." Misra's study (1967) provides clues to the relation between ignorance, shame and fear of sex, and lack of contraceptive effectiveness. Males in his sample who were shy and modest about sex were less likely to approve of family planning, less informed about it, and less apt to practice it.

Very poor people tend to adapt their values regarding sex to the conditions of poverty where jobs for men are scarce and wages are low, where public-assistance policies in some states forbid aid to families in which an able-bodied man is present in the home, and where the struggle for existence often breeds an atmosphere of fear, violence, and despair. The seeming impulsiveness of many of the very poor probably springs more from a depressed, powerless "can't care" attitude than from an irresponsible "don't care" approach. Apparent sex freedom is more likely to be a symptom of underlying loneliness and hopelessness about oneself and others than a positive search for pleasure. Such apparent freedom plus lack of effective contraception may frequently be associated with low self-esteem—a sense that one's own personal worthlessness precludes the relevance of aspiring to a "better life" through planning and self-direction. This is in line with formulations to the effect that impulse control is associated with strong self-esteem, a clear sense of identity, and a feeling of personal effectiveness.

In sum the sex-related and family-planning problems more prevalent among the very poor are apt to be an overt symptom of the more basic cluster of social, psychological, economic, and environmental deprivations that go with their disadvantaged life situation. In the case of nonwhite groups the deprivations imposed by poverty are expanded and intensified by the corrosive effects of racism. Thus it is to be expected that nonwhites would tend to have a correspondingly higher rate of problems in this area than whites.

Some Applications for Family-Planning and Population Policies

Poverty and Family Planning

The family-planning and population policies of the United States should not focus on poor people alone, who constitute a minority of the population and are not the source of our major population problems. A family-planning policy, by itself, is too narrow to either significantly aid low-income people or motivate them strongly to use contraceptives continuously and effectively. Effective family-planning policies must be part of a larger range of policies aimed at alleviating the conditions that undermine all aspects of the development and functioning of those who live in poverty.

It is an error to believe that economic need in the case of the very poor is a strong motivation for control of family size. Economic adversity during the Depression apparently served as a stimulus toward birth control on the part of the *general* population; it is likely that this general reaction was experienced by majority-group members who had earlier experiences orienting them toward an expectation that the Depression was a temporary setback: conditions would improve; their incomes would rise; they would be able to afford children later. This kind of future orientation had a part in the increased birth rate during the 1940s when economic conditions for the majority *did* improve. Thus economic security for the family as a strong motivation for effective birth control serves as a stimulus to those who have sound reasons to believe they can achieve it. Members of the long-term poverty-stricken segment of the population do not have cause to believe that real economic security can be theirs—either for themselves or their children.

Particularly for this group family-planning policies must be linked to income maintenance, educational opportunities, adequate housing, comprehensive medical and child-care services, and guaranteed employment policies—with jobs assured for women as well as for men.

The present federal policy that provides that free family-planning services be offered to the poor should be expanded to guarantee these services for all people, regardless of income. This is because population control and small family size are in the public interest at every socioeconomic level. Public policy also should include an emphasis on continuing research in all aspects of the family-planning field. Further studies are particularly needed concerning the relative effectiveness of a variety of program and policy approaches.

Psychological Sensitivity and Family Planning

Family-planning services should be based on a philosophy that includes an awareness of people as individual human beings who bring their total life experience to the matter of contraceptive use. The attitudes of people toward family planning are affected by their past life histories, their present situation, and their hopes and fears for the future. These attitudes are related to the dynamics of their family lives as well as to their interactions with the larger environment. Contraceptive use or nonuse affects the individual's sense of self in the very sensitive realms of sexual identity and competence. It most centrally affects the interaction between males and females as couples. Programs tend to be designed and administered by men for women. It would be more appropriate for them to be designed by male-female teams to reach both men and women as individuals and in a pair relationship.

More research is needed in this area, both in terms of basic and applied studies. It is important that these studies include single, as well as married, males and females. Research in the past has far too often included only married women in the study population.

Effective population control is seriously needed in this country. However, the goals might well become too narrow and specific. Programs that are focused only on controlling family size are apt to emphasize the technological and physical aspects of the problem. Such an emphasis can have a dehumanizing impact on both men and women. One adverse result may be negative social and psychological side effects in which people see themselves only as pawns in a numbers game: a life view that is already creating havoc in contemporary society (Chilman, 1970).

A Broader Approach to Population Policy

It is important to tie population policy to other related policies and to consider in advance the possible future consequences of policy alternatives.

One of the strongest arguments currently being made for a sharp reduction in the birth rate is that environmental pollution is creating a crisis of major proportions. It is frequently assumed that a larger population automatically means higher levels of such pollution; population control is sometimes advocated as *the* way to prevent further pollution of the environment.

A larger population will surely contaminate the environment further if we do not take drastic steps to harness the many major sources of such pollution, but chiefly solutions lie in a whole complex of actions besides those related to population size (Coale, 1970).

If we seek to stabilize population growth in the near future, this means that most couples must limit the size of their families to one child (assuming that we maintain our present high marriage rates of over 90 percent of the adult population). Consideration should be given to what effect such small family size would have on the age structure of the population in the next generation—and beyond. A relatively small number of children in the next generation would call for enormous adaptive changes in a society that has built so many of its values on nourishing and planning for the very young. "A better world for our children" has been a chief raison d'être for perhaps the majority of women. The dislocations in styles and goals of living occasioned by very small families should be anticipated now and, if possible, planned for in advance, especially in terms of new roles for women and new outlets for "human caring" activities for both sexes.

What kinds of children will we produce if most of them are raised in one-child families? What burdens might they carry in being *the* person to fulfill the hopes and fears of their parents? What "relationship deficits" might they develop unless ways are devised to provide them with many experiences with their peers from a very young age onward? And what of a generation twenty-five years hence that has an unusually small young adult population? What impact will this have on the liberalizing, creative forces young people are so apt to bring on the political, occupational, and social aspects of our society?

Although a reduction in the rate of population growth is obviously called for, stabilization of population growth in the United States in the near future may create at least as many problems as it solves. A population policy is needed that takes further account of the many related present and future aspects of the total social as well as physical ecology of our situation and prospects.

REFERENCES

Berelson, B. 1966. KAP studies on fertility. In B. Berelson et al., eds., *Family planning and population programs: a review of world developments.* Chicago: University of Chicago Press. Pp. 655–668.

Blair, A. 1967. A comparison of Negro and white fertility attitudes. In D. Bogue, ed., *Sociological contributions to family planning research.* Chicago: Community and Family Study Center, University of Chicago. Pp. 1–35.

Blake, J. 1969. Population policy for Americans: is the government being misled? *Science* 164:522–529.

Bogue, D. 1965. *The Westside fertility report.* Chicago: Community and Family Study Center, University of Chicago.

Bumpass, L. and Westoff, C. 1970. The perfect contraceptive population. *Science* 169: 1177–1182.

Burchinal, L. 1963. Research on young marriage. In M. B. Sussman, ed., *Sourcebook in marriage and the family.* Boston: Houghton Mifflin.

Campbell, A. 1965. The growth of American family studies. *Welfare in Review,* Vol. 3, no. 10:17–22.

————. 1968. The role of family planning in the reduction of poverty. *Journal of Marriage and the Family* 30:236–245.

Chilman, C. 1966. *Growing up poor.* Washington, D.C.: U.S. Department of Health, Education and Welfare.

————. 1970. Probable social and psychological consequences of an American population policy aimed at the two-child family. *Annals of the New York Academy of Sciences* 175:868–879.

Clausen, J. A. 1966. Family structure, socialization, and personality. In L. W. Hoffman and M. L. Hoffman, eds., *Review of child development research.* New York: Russell Sage Foundation 2:1–53.

Coale, A. J. 1970. Man and his environment. *Science* 170:132–136.

Douvan, E. and Adelson, J. 1966. *The adolescent experience.* New York: Wiley.

Duncan, O. and Blau, P. 1967. *The American occupational structure.* New York: Wiley.

Farley, R. 1965. Recent changes in Negro fertility. Paper presented at the Population Association of America, Washington, D.C., April 1965.

Freedman, R. 1966. Economic status, unemployment, and family growth. Final report to Division of Research, Welfare Administration, Project 10703–043, U.S. Department of Health, Education and Welfare (mimeo).

Freedman, R. and Slesinger, D. 1961. Fertility differentials for the indigenous non-farm population of the United States. *Population Studies* 15:161–173.

Frejka, T. 1970. United States: the implications of zero population growth. *Studies in family planning* 60:1–4.

Herzog, E. 1963. Some assumptions about the poor. *The Social Service Review* 36: 389–402.

Hill, A. and Jaffe, F. 1966. Negro fertility and family size preferences. In K. Clark and T. Parsons, eds., *Negro American.* Boston: Houghton Mifflin.

Hill, R.; Stycos, J.; and Back, K. 1959. *The family and population control.* Chapel Hill: University of North Carolina Press.

Kleegman, S. J. 1964. Contraception and the physician. In M. S. Calderone, ed., *Manual of contraceptive practice.* Baltimore: Williams & Wilkins. Pp. 35–44.

Komarovsky, M. 1962. *Blue collar marriage.* New York: Random House.

Luckey, E. and Bain, J. 1970. Children: a factor in marital satisfaction. *Journal of Marriage and the Family* 32:43–45.

Lunde, A. 1965. White-nonwhite fertility differentials in the United States. *Health Education and Welfare Indicators,* September 1965. Pp. 23–37.

Miles, R. 1971. The future population of the United States. *Population Bulletin* 27:4–31.

Misra, B. 1967. Correlates of males' attitudes toward family planning. In D. Bogue, ed.,

Sociological contributions to family planning. Chicago: Family and Community Study Center, University of Chicago. Pp. 161–266.

Moore, B. and Holtzman, W. 1965. *Tomorrow's parents.* Austin: Hogg Foundation, University of Texas.

Nye, I.; Carlson, J.; and Garrett, G. 1970. Family size, interaction, affect and stress. *Journal of Marriage and the Family* 32:216–226.

Orshansky, M. 1965. Whose who among the poor: a demographic view of poverty. *Social Security Bulletin,* Vol. 28, no. 7:3–32.

Population Reference Bureau. 1966. *Population profile.* Washington, D.C., April 15, 1966.

Rainwater, L. 1965. *Family design.* Chicago: Aldine.

Schorr, A. 1966. The family cycle and income development. *Social Security Bulletin,* Vol. 29, no. 2: 14–25.

Scommon, R. and Wattenberg, B. 1965. *This U.S.A.* New York: Doubleday.

Stolka. S. and Barnett, L. 1969. Education and religion as factors in women's attitudes motivating childbearing. *Journal of Marriage and the Family* 31:740–750.

U.S. Census Bureau. 1963. *Current population reports: consumer income.* P–60, no. 41, table 5; October 1, 1963.

Vital and Health Statistics. 1970. *Natality statistics analysis: United States, 1965–1967.* Public Health Service Pub. No. 1000, Series 21, no. 19. Washington, D.C.: U.S. Government Printing Office.

Westoff, C. F.; Potter, R. G.; and Sagi, P. C. 1963. *The third child.* Princeton: Princeton University Press.

Whelpton, P.; Campbell, A.; and Patterson, J. 1966. *Fertility and family planning in the United States.* Princeton: Princeton University Press.

Zelnik, M. and Kantner, J. 1970. United States: exploratory studies of Negro family formation—factors relating to illegitimacy. *Studies in Family Planning* 60:5–9.

PART III

Consequences of
Family Size and
Population Density

[7]

THE EFFECTS OF
FAMILY SIZE ON PARENTS
AND CHILDREN

JOHN A. CLAUSEN
AND SUZANNE R. CLAUSEN

Family size is the primary outcome variable with which fertility research and theory are concerned. The preceding chapters have documented the complexity of the social, psychological, and cultural influences upon fertility and resultant family size. The present chapter reverses this perspective and asks how family size itself influences the lives of parents and children. Family size is, then, our causal variable. If it is easier to measure than most variables of interest to behavioral scientists, we must not be deceived into thinking that its effects are easy to ascertain. They are not.

The reader of the foregoing chapters will already be aware that there are more components to the meaning of family size than merely the number of children in a family. Let us examine briefly some of the types of components that will have to be considered when one attempts to assess the correlates of increasing family size. One class consists of those normative and motivational features that are implicated in a given couple's fertility. Here the key consideration is that *wanted* children have a different value to parents than unwanted children. Cultural and subcultural norms set a general context of expectations as to the number of children desired. Individual experiences and motivations (or the absence of certain motivations) are likely to determine more specific expectations for the given couple, although some couples may not explicitly formulate their expectations. Efficient means of fertility control, competently undertaken, will permit some

NOTE: The preparation of this paper and especially the relevant analysis of data from the Oakland Growth Study were facilitated by services available through grant HD 04565 from the National Institute of Child Health and Human Development.

couples to achieve their fertility goals; other couples will be less successful. Discrepancies between desired and achieved family size not only modify the psychological meaning of a given number of children but may reflect parental characteristics; they are likely to be greatest when parents lack either the means or the competence to prevent conceptions.

It should be noted that if aspects of personality (motivational dynamics, attitudes, values) are related to the number of children desired and to actual family size, these same variables may be related to structural features of the family. Thus we might expect that men and women who have a traditional view of sex roles, with the husband and father being the authority figure and the wife and mother being the nurturant homemaker, are more likely to want a large family. If so we would find an association between family structure and number of children. In this instance, however, it would be quite wrong to interpret the greater role differentiation in larger families as being a consequence of family size; it would simply be a correlate, since both family size and role differentiation would be consequences of the initial orientations of husband and wife.

Another set of conditions influencing the meaning of family size involves the level and allocation of available resources. Insofar as larger families tend to be found among the poor, the most direct consequences of more children may be too little money for food, housing, and other necessities. But other resources are also involved; mothers and fathers are likely to be more fatigued and subjected to more stress, and inevitably they will have less time and energy for the care of each child. For each level of income and other resources available to parents, there may be a maximum number of children who can be cared for without undue stress and actual deprivation. In assessing the effects of family size it will be necessary to take into account available resources and also the patterns of their allocation as they affect role relationships and division of labor between husband and wife.

Just as motivations for having children are not necessarily closely tied to subsequent enjoyment of the children themselves, so the meaning and consequences of having a given number of children in the family will vary with each phase of the family cycle. The mother with four children under six and no help is likely to be extraordinarily hard pressed most of the time and perhaps overwhelmed when illness occurs. But a dozen years later she may be quite relaxed and pleased that her children are sufficiently grown for her to feel comfortable about taking a part-time job. Or again, if all the children want to go to college but are not outstanding scholars, the drain on the family budget may require that the mother work if the children are to be assisted to attend college. Although family-cycle phases would seem to exert important contextual effects, we shall have little adequate evidence on this score.

There is also a biological component to the meaning of family size. The first-born child inhabits a uterus unscarred by previous births, and he is nurtured within a younger organism than any of his later-born siblings. The larger the number of children born, in general, the more likely the mother is to have had damage to her reproductive system. Especially if births are closely spaced, large families may be expected to contain a higher proportion of children whose intrauterine life was in some sense problematic.

Finally there are those aspects of family size that derive directly from interactive processes within the family group. One would anticipate that the family, like any other group, would show structural differentiation such as increasing division of labor and formalization of role relationships as size increases. Role definitions and boundaries between the generations are likely to be more sharply drawn in the large than in the small family. Older children are likely to be delegated certain parental responsibilities, but one would anticipate that they would less often be treated like peers by their parents. Again, however, such features may also be influenced by social status and ethnic or religious background, so that size effects may be compounded with the effects of these other circumstances. We have already noted above the possibility that both patterns of role relationship and family size may be consequences of preexisting attitudes and values of the parents.

Before turning to an assessment of existing evidence, we might further note that family size is only one of a very large number of contextual variables that influence the socialization process. It would be startling if one found that family size accounted for a large proportion of the variance in the developmental histories of children. Indeed, it is reasonable to expect that the effects of family size will be modest enough so that variations in other contextual features or aspects of socialization will often obscure them, leading to inconclusive research results. There are very few studies that combine large samples of families with careful conceptualization and measurement. Despite this fact we shall find that a few of the effects of family size on both parents and children are found with sufficient frequency to be considered reasonably firm generalizations, at least within particular population segments.

Allocation of Resources and Style of Life

In countries that do not provide family allotments for children, increasing family size obviously means less money per child when income is allocated. Relatively more must be spent for food and housing, or the quantity and quality of food and housing provided must be less. At the lower end of the income scale the effects of family size on style of life are thus inexorable: fewer luxuries, more crowding, less margin of reserve for emergencies, coupled with a greater likelihood of emergencies, and in general an emphasis on "making do" with what one has.

This most obvious consequence of having a large number of children has received less research attention than have some relatively trivial aspects of large family size (such as those relating to position within the sibling order). Yet effects upon level and style of living and on the psychological atmosphere of the family deriving from pressures on resources of time, energy, and income are probably more potent than any other effects of large family size.

The Family Budget and Living Arrangements

In countries that provide substantial allotments to parents for each child, the pressures on income may not be quite so acute. Thus in France, where the size of family allowances rises as salary diminishes and number of children increases, the family of a blue-collar worker with five children may receive more than 50 percent of its income from the family allotment. Even in this case, however, the pressures on parental time and energy and on space available in housing tend to be much greater than in smaller families (Chombart de Lauwe, 1959, pp. 114–115).

Such research evidence as is available suggests that there are only modest shifts in the proportion of the family budget that goes to expenditures for housing, food, clothing, transportation, and medical care as the size of the family increases (Blood, 1962). The reason appears to be that there is not much leeway for major shifts in the proportionate allocation of funds for various necessities or presumed necessities when the quantity of funds is sharply limited, but there are marked *qualitative* changes in the allocation of funds. If there are more children, larger but less choice quarters are likely to be sought. Thus Douglas and Blomfield (1958), in their longitudinal study of a large cohort of children born in Great Britain in 1946, found that the quality of housing declined steadily as the number of children increased beyond two. At the same time crowding greatly increased, with more than half of the families having four or more children in the overcrowded category (more than 1½ persons per room). While housing in Great Britain in the early 1950s presented a rather grim picture generally because of the effects of World War II, the general relationship of family size to adequacy of housing available undoubtedly holds true for families in the United States today.

The family with many children must seek housing not in the most convenient place for husband and wife but in the place that will afford a maximum of space for the funds available and ideally will permit the children to play safely out of doors. While we are not familiar with any data bearing directly on the ways in which family size influences housing choices, the push toward peripheral or suburban living for the family with many children is likely to lead to more commuting time for the father and hence less time at home.

Similar considerations relate to the allocation of income to food. Cheaper cuts of meat and more starch will comprise the greater part of the diet of a six-child family than of a two-child family on the same budget. Again, medical care will be sought only when it appears that one is confronting serious illness or emergency. In the large family the wife and mother must plan more carefully and consistently if she is to manage.

Effects on the Parents

Pressures on space and funds clearly affect the whole family. Their psychological consequences are likely to be greatest on the parents, however, and they may well influence parental activity patterns and division of labor. The mother of several children is much less likely to take a job during their early years than is the mother of a single child.[1] She is, in a sense, more securely a captive of her family. Her husband, on the other hand, is under more pressure to earn extra money. Moonlighting on the part of the husband—that is, taking a second job—is most likely to occur when there are several children and very heavy pressures on income. As Wilensky (1963) has noted: "Moonlighting is most frequent among men caught in a life-cycle bind."

The costs imposed by having many children are not merely financial but psychological as well. Pohlman (1969) has discussed a number of the psychological costs, some deriving from the basic responsibilities of being a parent with even a single child and some increasing appreciably if not arithmetically with the addition of subsequent children. Especially during the early years, children connote broken sleep, noise, confusion, and particularly when there are several, congestion. Mothers of young children put in an inordinately long work week and tend to be confined to the home much of the time. The early years of motherhood are frequently remembered as the period when one constantly yearned for a full night's sleep and for a day free of demands. In our longitudinal data at the Institute of Human Development, mothers with three or more children fairly closely spaced, looking back at the early years of motherhood from the perspective of their late forties, are likely to recall those early years as years of extreme exhaustion and discouragement. The drain on their energies and the pressures on their span of control are undoubtedly a major factor in bringing about the routinization of rules and controls in child care.

[1] Thus a recent survey conducted among married respondents in large metropolitan areas found that the rate of employment dropped from 65 percent among women with no children, to 40 percent among those with one child, 30 percent among those with two or more children, and 22 percent among those with four or more children (Orden and Bradburn, 1969, p. 396).

Child-Care Practices and Parental Attitudes

In their exploratory study of the large family, Bossard and Boll (1956) suggested that parents in such families place high valuation on organization and leadership and stress cooperation and conformity for their children. They noted the tendency to delegate responsibility to older children for the care and control of younger siblings. In large families parents seemed less possessive and demanding in their interactions with their children. On the other hand, as we shall see, there is considerable evidence that parents in larger families are somewhat more authoritarian and, in certain respects at least, restrictive of the child's autonomy. For example, rules, often summarily imposed, are likely to replace individual attention when parents are confronted with the need to maintain order and peace among energetic youngsters confined to the house on a rainy day (Bartow, 1961).

Parental Values and Orientations. Rosen (1961) proposed that "in contrast to the small family, the large family is more likely to value responsibility above individual achievement, conformity above self-expression, cooperation and obedience above individualism" (p. 577). Our own expectations would accord with those of Rosen, yet in the largest, most careful study of the values parents hold for their children, Melvin Kohn (1969) found only a slight relationship between family size and values held by fathers.[2] There is a low but significant zero-order correlation between number of children and a factor score representing the valuing of conformity (as against self-direction), and sibship size is inversely related to the valuing of intellectual curiosity ("being interested in how and why things happen"). When social class and age of child are controlled, however, the correlation with conformity drops nearly to zero. Fathers with many children do appear to place a lower value on the children's being intellectually curious than do fathers of fewer children, but the partial correlation coefficient is only .07 (significant at less than < .01 because of the large sample size). If we take these data from a large, carefully selected and analyzed sample as a reasonably good estimate of relationships in the larger population, it is apparent that samples of 100 to 200 families are not likely to yield results that will do more than confuse the issue of how parental orientations relate to family size.

Parental Control and Discipline. Whether one relies upon parental reports or reports from children, there is rather consistent evidence that parental

---

[2] Kohn's research, based on a national sample of 3,101 fathers, touched only incidentally on the effects of family size (it being one of the control variables used). He has kindly provided us with additional tabulations, including both zero-order and partial correlation coefficients between the values fathers hold for their children and size of family (holding constant social class and age of index child in the partial correlations).

control tends to be more decisively exercised in the larger family. Parents are more often seen as autocratic or authoritarian and as less inclined to give explanations for the rules they invoke (Elder, 1962a; Elder and Bowerman, 1963). Nye, Carlson, and Garrett (1970) report that frequency of corporal punishment goes up and use of "discussion" as a control technique goes down as the number of children increases, and this finding accords with earlier reports of Elder and Bowerman (1963) and Clausen (1966). Nye and his associates also report a slight decline in permissiveness for adolescent boys and a marked decline for adolescent girls as family size increases. In families with six or more children, however, adolescent boys were actually allowed more autonomy than in smaller families. Girls, on the other hand, were more closely controlled in these very large families. As Nye and his associates note, this pattern would seem to derive from the greater difficulty of enforcing restrictions on boys, coupled with the potential costs of giving an adolescent girl a great deal of autonomy.

Relationships between the Parents

Companionship appears to be the most sought-after goal in marriage, but the chance to have children follows in second position among the various goals for marriage reported by husbands and wives in the United States (Blood and Wolfe, 1960, p. 150). To a degree the companionship of the couple may be enhanced by having children, but this will be so only if both want children and enjoy doing the things that children entail. Children place considerable constraints on the freedom and mobility of their parents, especially of the mother. If there is heavy pressure on economic resources, children may substantially cut down opportunities for companionship in other spheres than home and child care. Christensen (1968) and others have noted that as the number of children increases, husband and wife experience more interference with sexual activities. Both the effects of crowding and those of being continually "on call" would seem to enter into this association.

Role Relationships and Division of Labor. We have noted earlier the tendency to a sharper division of function between husband and wife in the large family. Mothers with three or four young children are far less likely to be employed outside the home than are those with one or two young children. Fathers, on the other hand, are likely to work more urgently and even to take extra employment to make ends meet. Several writers have suggested that the mother's power is at its lowest ebb in such families and that paternal domination is therefore more frequent (Heer, 1963). Blood and Wolfe (1960) also note that husbands highly successful in their occupations are likely to enjoy more power in family decision-making and also to be in a position to afford more children. Conversely, when wives exercise substantial authority they may choose to limit family size in order to work or pursue other activities of their own choice. Indeed, when husbands and wives wish to share many activities this may itself lead to family limitation. Rainwater (1965) found that wives who shared many activities with their husbands (joint conjugal relationship) were much more likely to want small or medium-sized families than were wives in marital pairs with more segregated role patterns. Thus it is extremely difficult to distinguish cause and effect when we examine relationships between family size and roles in the family.

Studies of personality in relation to fertility experience have consistently failed to show significant differences between personalities of parents with one or two children and those of parents with three or more children. To the extent that such differences do exist they are probably responsive to social and cultural emphases in particular populations at given times. In any event neither the personalities of the parents nor the patterns of dominance found in the families who made up the cohort studied intensively by Westoff and his associates bore any relationship to the number of children desired or to actual fertility performance (Bumpass and Westoff, 1970).

Insofar as differences in parental role relationships have been noted between small and large families, they have been modest. Elder and Bowerman (1963) found fathers a bit more likely to make final decisions on rules and discipline in families with four or more children than in smaller families, according to reports by the children. A more recent study by Campbell (1970) suggests that there may be some areas in which the mother's influence increases rather than decreases with increasing family size, most notably in decisions about social activities. Moreover, Campbell suggests that as the number of children increases, in some respects a "leveling process" may result rather than sharper role differentiation: "husbands tend to gain in the area which is most heavily wife-dominated, while wives gain in areas which are more subject to the husband's influence" (p. 48). But, again, Campbell notes that these relationships are not strong. Indeed, we are of the opinion that studies in different parts of the country, using slightly variant conceptualizations and measures, and not controlling for religion, social status, or stage of the family cycle, would show very little consistency in their findings. The techniques used to assess role relationships and division of labor have generally been crude and have almost always relied upon the reported perceptions of a single member of the family. All else being equal, one might expect to find a more clearly defined authority structure in the larger family that is functioning smoothly; it is not, however, clear that any particular pattern of parental role relationships is likely to emerge.[3]

[3] A recent dissertation analyzing patterns of authority and decision-making in the family found a greater tendency to centralization of authority in larger families and a greater tendency to semiautonomous relationships and individual negotiations in smaller families, though the differences were not statistically significant. See Pryor (1970).

Satisfaction with the Marriage

From the beginning of research on marital adjustment, it has been apparent that the relationship of marital satisfaction to number of children is not a simple one (Terman, 1938; Burgess and Cottrell, 1939). Among childless couples, those who desire children tend to report greater marital satisfaction than those who do not. In the early years of marriage childlessness may reflect the uncertainty of the husband and wife as to whether the marriage will last. Some unhappy wives may want children as a means of holding their husbands, but it would seem that more couples refrain from having children until they feel sure that the marriage will work out. During the early years of marriage divorces are substantially higher among the childless than among couples with children. They are even higher, however, among those whose pregnancies were of premarital origin (Christensen, 1968).

In general, women who have more children than they had wanted report lower marital satisfaction than those who have the number they had wanted, even when the actual number is the same (Michel and Feyrabend, 1969). In a not yet published study of Parisian couples, Andrée Michel (personal communication) found substantial negative correlations between excess fertility (the number of children beyond the wife's desired number) and several measures of the wife's satisfaction with the marriage—her general satisfaction, her assessment of her husband's affection and understanding, and her satisfaction with communication and with shared leisure-time activities. The measures of the wife's satisfaction were only minimally related to the total number of children, however. Several studies suggest that there may be an optimum number of children for marital satisfaction, based upon family resources and life style desired. Blood and Wolfe (1960) found marital satisfaction highest among wives with three children and lowest among those with five or more. The latter group of wives included a higher proportion who would have preferred fewer children. Very similar findings were reported by Farber and Blackman (1956).

Spacing of children is almost certainly relevant here, though the effects upon marital satisfaction may be limited to the years of infancy and childhood. As noted previously, a wife with many small children has few options. Unless her husband is exceptionally supportive and helpful, their relationship is likely to suffer the consequences of her feelings of powerlessness, especially as concerns with equality of the sexes become more general. On the other hand, marital satisfaction varies greatly from one phase of the family cycle to another, generally being highest in the early years and lowest in the period when the last child reaches late adolescence (Rollins and Feldman, 1970). Very few of the studies relating marital satisfaction to number of children have examined variations by family stages (though some have controlled for this variable by the nature of the cohort selected for study). Here again we must caution that available evidence suggests only weak relationships between family size and marital satisfaction, much less significant than the variations of marital satisfaction with family stage.

Effects on the Children

If the effects of family size upon the parents are largely to be understood in terms of the ways in which they respond to the demands and pressures put upon them by increasing numbers of children, effects upon the children are more diverse in origin. Among the sources of influence are the relative availability of parental care and responsiveness, the general circumstances deriving from the family's placement in the community and its style of life, the role of older siblings in the socialization of younger ones, and the general competition among siblings for scarce parental resources. We may note that studies of the effects of family size upon parents have been more largely undertaken by sociologists interested in the functioning of the family; studies of the effects upon children have been more largely undertaken by psychologists and physicians, especially as regards the effects in the early years.

Health and Physical Development

There are a number of respects in which the physical development of children from large families seems more problematic than that of children from small families. As noted in the introductory comments, the probability of intrauterine problems increases with parity of birth. For example, Passamanick and Lilienfeld (1956) report a tenfold increase in mental deficiency as one moves from the first child to the sixth child born to the mother. In general prematurity and its attendant problems and maldevelopment become more frequent with increasing parity of birth. A study by Benech, Mathieu, and Schreider (1960) found that height, weight, vital capacity, and strength all decline with increasing family size.

The association of shorter stature with larger family size was found in the Scottish Mental Survey (Scottish Council for Research in Education, 1953) and in the large longitudinal research of Douglas and Blomfield (1958) and obtains even when the father's occupation is controlled for. The Douglas research clearly supports the importance both of diet and of the circumstances under which the child eats. When there are few children the mother is able to give attention to how each is eating; when there are many she is likely to be preoccupied with the youngest.

Studies of the sucking rate and feeding patterns of infants, as related to parity of the mother, show inconsistent findings. Thus Waldrop and Bell (1966), in a study of neonates observed and rated an average of eighty hours after birth, noted greater lethargy as evidenced by sucking rate and crying among children from larger, more dense families (i.e., those in which children were closely spaced) than in smaller, less dense families. On the other hand, several studies have found that in general infants born to multiparous mothers take more milk at a feeding (bottle fed) and do so in a shorter period than do children born to primipara, presumably because more experienced mothers know how to present the nipple more effectively to the infant (Thoman, Turner, Liederman, and Barnett, 1970).

Apart from neonatal differences and the smaller stature of children from large families, it is difficult to know whether there are significant differences in the health histories of the children from large as against small sibships. Chen and Cobb (1960) concluded a very thorough review of the literature on family size in relation to health and disease with the statement that "on the whole, the study of the relation of sibship size to health and disease has been difficult and to date relatively unproductive because of the multitude of interacting variables which must be taken into consideration in interpreting the results" (p. 562). Those variables include not only the social and cultural correlates of sibship size in a given population but also the differential utilization of medical facilities by families of varying characteristics. A recent study by Petroni (1969) reports that the larger the family, the less likely are parents to regard a given degree of physical discomfort as a legitimate reason for taking the "sick role" or involving a physician. Parents with many children may also be less likely to report illness in a child.

The research of Douglas and Blomfield (1958) showed no relationship between family size and rates of medically attended accidents to the children, but did show marked differences in the utilization of health services by large families. A study of immunization practices among California households with preschool children conducted by Mellinger, Manheimer, and Kleman (1967) also attests to the relatively poor utilization of routine health services by parents in large families. Even with social status controlled, preschool children in families with four or more children were substantially less likely to have been adequately immunized. Mothers with several small children find it difficult to arrange to take their children for immunizations and other routine health care.

Intelligence and Cognitive Development

One of the earliest noted and most consistently reported findings relating to the effects of family size has been the decline in IQ as number of children increases.[4] Several of the early studies of large populations showed very substantial IQ differentials—as much as twenty-two IQ points be-

[4] A thoughtful discussion of the early studies and their interpretation is to be found in Anastasi (1956).

tween only children and children in families with six or more offspring (Scottish Council for Research in Education, 1949). In part these differentials were related to differential fertility among socioeconomic status groups, the largest families being far more numerous at the lower levels of status. But even when social class is held constant the decline in IQ with increasing family size is far from negligible, especially among working-class families. Among children whose fathers were in the professions the drop in IQ was not marked until family size of five or more children was attained; among boys from lower-middle-class families and both boys and girls from working-class families, however, IQ dropped appreciably even with three children.

When first observed in the Scottish studies, the association between family size and intelligence of the children led to the fear that less intelligent members of the population were reproducing at a much faster rate than the more intelligent. Some commentators announced that within a generation there would be an appreciable decline in level of intelligence as a consequence of such differential fertility. No such decline was revealed by subsequent studies, however, and except at the very lowest levels of status there does not appear to be a negative relationship between intelligence and unusually high fertility. Indeed, our own longitudinal analyses (unpublished) suggest the reverse. Among a cohort of 200 individuals followed from their early adolescence in the 1930s in Oakland, California, through the childbearing years, those with IQs above the median had significantly more children than those with IQs below the median. This group of subjects is now largely middle class and is much too small and atypical to serve as a basis for broad generalization, but the findings do suggest that within the middle class at least there appears to be no genetic basis for expecting lower IQs among children from larger families.

Attempts to account for this decline in IQ with increasing size of sibship have involved a variety of hypotheses. Dietary deficiencies, poorer parental care, poorer housing and schooling all seem implicated in the larger families except at the highest levels of status. In the Douglas study, it appeared that roughly a third of the IQ difference between children in sibships of one or two and sibships of four or more could be accounted for by the overlapping influences of poor housing, lack of parental interest, and poor schooling.

Several studies suggest that the deficit in tested intelligence with increasing family size is particularly great in the area of verbal skills (see especially Nisbet and Entwistle, 1967). Language skills seem to be most readily acquired by the first-born child, who has adult speech models much more available to him than do later-born children. The more siblings there are, the more likely it is that the children's speech will perpetuate constructions and codes that tend to be limited to the family circle. Both in the Scottish studies and in that of Douglas, the poorer performance of children from large families was as pronounced at age eight as at age eleven, suggesting that, insofar as there is a deficit in environmental stimulation (or in any other feature of the environment), it is operative in the early years.

Achievement Motivation and Educational Attainment. The decline in IQ with increasing size of sibship would suggest that children from large families would on the average be less successful academically. It would appear that they are in fact even more deficient in academic attainment than would be predicted on the basis of IQ alone (Douglas, 1964). In general, children from smaller families show both higher achievement motivation and superior academic performance than those from larger families (Elder, 1962b; Rosen, 1961). Parents with high educational and occupational aspirations for their children are likely to limit the number of their offspring to accord with their resources, especially among Protestants. They are also likely to set goals for their children and impose standards of excellence beyond those imposed by parents less ambitious for their children. It will be recalled that data relating to parental goals and practices suggest only modest support for the above proposition (intellectual curiosity does seem to be significantly more valued in the smaller family), but data secured from offspring themselves rather consistently attest to higher achievement motivation among children from small families, whether one assesses achievement motivation by the Thematic Appreciation Test (Rosen, 1961), an index of ambition (Turner, 1962), or educational aspirations and performance (Elder, 1962b).

Among Catholics it appears that achievement motivation and academic performance are less influenced by family size than they are among Protestants (Elder, 1962b; Floud, Halsey, and Martin, 1957). In large part this appears to be a consequence of the tendency of well-educated and occupationally successful Catholics to have larger rather than smaller families. The combination of parental motivations and adequate resources appears to offset the potentially negative influences of large family size on achievement motivation.

Apart from the decrements in intelligence and achievement motivation that are associated with larger family size, one would predict that fewer children from large families would be able to go to college simply because of the lesser resources available to any given child. A recent study by Adams and Meidam (1968) bears out this prediction, even controlling for father's occupation. The detrimental effects of increasing size of sibship appear earlier (i.e., at lower numbers) for children of blue-collar workers than for those of white-collar workers and earlier for females than for males. Moreover, children closely spaced together are somewhat less likely to attend college than those separated by longer birth intervals. Since closer spacing seems to be associated with increased lethargy and dependency in the infant and young child (Waldrop and Bell, 1966), with smaller stature (Grant, 1964), and with deficits in verbal intelligence (Nisbet and Entwistle, 1967), it is clear that something more than economic pressure is involved, but the causal mechanisms remain matters of conjecture.

Personality and Social Adjustment

To the extent that parental child-care practices and attitudes toward childrearing are influenced by the number of children in the family, one might expect that the personalities of the children would be influenced more generally, rather than merely in cognitive development. If parents are less available to their children, if they are more authoritarian in their interaction with the children, if they are more harried and less warmly accepting, one would expect the children to be less dependent upon their parents and to turn more to their siblings or to relationships outside the family for emotional support. Where and how a given child turns will depend upon his special talents and proclivities and upon his location among his siblings.

In a perceptive autobiographical account of the problems of a child in a very large family, René Durel (1971) recalls his school years and his search for a kind of self-confirmation that was not forthcoming from his parents and his dozen siblings:

> The scramble for attention in a large family often means that the only person one ever really listens to is oneself. . . .
>
> It was not really an unpleasant life, but a gradual sense of privation is inevitable, I think, in a large family. There are, in effect, no parents, since parental attentiveness and concern can be stretched only so far and no farther. When I recall my childhood now, I realize that very early I was searching elsewhere for (and very often finding) the attention I craved at home. [Pp. 30–31]

Durel's three older brothers were rough-and-ready outdoor types, not burdened by strong senses of conscience. He himself turned to academic pursuits and to fantasy. His autobiographical account makes clear the dangers of treating the large family as though it were the same environment for each of its members. Clearly it is not, and the varying constellations of identification and shared activities can have vastly different effects upon the developing personalities of the children. Even the grossly authoritarian behavior of the parents had quite different implications for the boys in Durel's family. The older ones grew in the image of their father—bigoted, sometimes brutal, a man who reveled in the vices of men. The younger boys apparently identified more closely with their mother, their older sisters, and women outside the family who responded lovingly and protectively toward them.

The larger the family size, the less attention any given child is likely to receive from his parents. One might assume, therefore, that children from smaller families would have higher self-esteem than those from large families. There is some evidence in support of this hypothesis, but it is not very strong. In Rosenberg's (1965) study of the adolescent self-image only children were somewhat overrepresented in the group having high self-esteem. On closer examination, however, only in the case of males was the difference significant. Effects beyond the first child were not at all consistent; a child with five or more siblings scored no lower on self-esteem than one with a single sibling. A more recent study by Sears (1970) shows small but significant correlations between a summary measure of the self-concept and the number of children in the family for both boys and girls aged twelve: the larger the family, the poorer was a child's self-concept.

In the course of preparing the present chapter, we have examined the relationship between sibship size and a number of personality measures for subjects of the Oakland Growth Study.[5] Among both boys and girls there was a significant tendency for those from smaller families to be less accepting of their peers and more likely to be seen as emphasizing the exclusiveness of their own "in-group." Girls from small families were rated much more sensitive to peer demands and less straightforward with their peers. Boys from small families perceived their parents as more fair and accepting of them than did boys from large families, supporting the previous report of Nye and his co-workers (1970). Among girls, perceptions of parents were not consistently related to family size in this sample except that girls from small families more often thought their parents old-fashioned. Boys from larger families were seen (by psychologists who observed them repeatedly) as more impulsive, tense, and excitable; the girls from larger families were rated more responsible. While all of these differences were statistically significant ($p < .05$) and seem to make sense, perhaps the most important generalization to be drawn is that the roles provided for boys and girls in larger families are clearly different, and they may have quite different implications for personality development.

Several researchers have attempted to assess the relationship of masculinity in boys to family size or to constellations of siblings. Strodtbeck and Creelan (1968) have assessed masculinity in several groups of adult males through the use of a measure of unconscious femininity, and they find such unconscious femininity at lowest ebb in males from sibships of size three. They hypothesize that in smaller families the home environment tends to be dominated by the values, techniques, and personality of the mothers, while in larger families the older siblings "adopt" younger ones. Unfortunately we are aware of no data on actual sex-role learning in families of different size.

The tendency of children from large families to seek social response from others has been frequently hypothesized and has been verified in a recent study by Masterson (1971) on need for approval. Gonda (1962)

---

[5] The number of subjects from sibships of four or more was roughly forty (out of a total of 160 subjects available throughout the adolescent years). Because of the small sample size, we report only those relationships that were found consistently for each sex in both the junior high and senior high years (independently assessed) and that reached at least the .01 level of significance overall, with social class controlled.

reports that persons reared in large families are more likely to be persistent complainers about pain than are persons from small families. He hypothesizes that they learned early in life to reduce tensions associated with pain by complaining and that in large families more opportunities (parental plus sibling) exist for such complaints to be effective in bringing tension-reducing responses. On the other hand, it might be argued that as a consequence of the greater pressures on parents in larger families, they tend to be less responsive to the child's needs and that the child in pain learns to shout about his problems in order to be heard.

Despite the evidence that parents of large families are less inclined to utilize medical services, several studies of clientele from child-guidance clinics suggest that children from large families are overrepresented. This was the finding of a systematic and well-controlled study of 3,000 children seen in clinics in France (Chombart de Lauwe, 1959) and of a more recent study of 1,581 children seen in a Philadelphia clinic (Tuckman and Regan, 1967). Differences in the problems presented by children from large and small families in the Philadelphia study are of some interest: children from large families less often showed anxiety and neurotic symptoms but more often had school problems or showed antisocial behavior. Since the social status of the family was not controlled, however, the symptom patterns undoubtedly reflect differentials in socioeconomic status as well as family size effects. Also one may assume that the school performance difficulties of children from larger families result in a higher proportion of direct referrals to clinics from the schools.

Although some studies have suggested that alcoholism may be more prevalent among men from large families (Smart, 1963), the distribution of size of family of origin among skid-row residents appears to be just about the same as that in the general population (Bahr, 1969). Again, there is no evidence that severe mental illness is in any way related to family size, although schizophrenic men tend not to marry or to have relatively few children if they do marry (Gregory, 1958).

Few of the studies that have sought to relate personality and social adjustment to family size have included an appreciable number of really large families, and it is possible that deleterious effects increase in the very large family. A study by Hawkes, Burchinal, and Gardner (1958) showed problems of adjustment, feelings of inferiority, and tendencies to daydream to be highest in families with five or more children. Nevertheless, the differences were only marginally significant. The most that one can say, then, is that characterizations of the large family as a closely knit, warmly accepting group producing happy, competent persons are not to be taken as descriptions of the typical larger family. Such happy families do, indeed, exist, but a greater proportion of large families appear to have more than their share of persons who have difficulties in the competitive realms of school and work.

Occupational Careers and Social Mobility

Since superior intelligence, high educational attainment, and high achievement motivation are among the major determinants of occupational success, one might expect children from small families to attain high occupational status more often than those from large families. The most thorough study relating social mobility to family size shows significant, consistent differences in mobility among individuals originating in all social strata (Svalastoga, 1959). Downward mobility from the occupational level of one's father is more frequent among children from large families and upward mobility more frequent among those from small families.

Size of Parental Family and Number of Own Children

Are children who grow up in large families themselves more likely to want more than an average number of children when they marry? A number of studies have addressed this question, and in general there is a positive correlation between the number of one's siblings and the number of one's own children. In large part, however, this relationship is attributable to continuities in the sociocultural attributes of one's family of orientation and one's family of procreation. Religion is an obvious case in point. Catholic families tend to be larger than Protestant families, for example. When one controls for religion, however, the relationship between size of sibship and number of own children proves to be a complex one.

Duncan, Freedman, Coble, and Slesinger (1965) note that women from large families tend to leave school at an earlier age, to marry earlier, and to begin childbearing at a younger age than do those from small families. Thus they are likely to be exposed to the risk of pregnancy over a longer period. Among Protestants especially, earlier school leaving and attendant lower social status seem very largely to explain the tendency of women *from* large families to *have* large families. As has been noted, however, among active Catholics the relationship between fertility and education is a direct one. Persons from smaller families, who again tend to achieve higher status, have *more* rather than *less* children. As a consequence, Bumpass and Westoff (1970) actually found a slight negative relationship between size of sibship and number of own children among active Catholics.

It has also been hypothesized that offspring are more likely to have about the same number of children their parents did if they were particularly well satisfied with their childhood family. On the other hand, if dissatisfied with their family of orientation, they might well idealize a family of different size. Thus the only child who desperately wanted siblings might tend to have a larger number of children, and the child with a half-dozen brothers and sisters who felt he never had enough of his parents' attention might well want only one or two children of his own. Hendershot (1969) found the relationship between number of siblings and number of own children highest among individuals who rated their families of orientation high in solidarity. Similarly Bumpass and Westoff (1970) report the same relationship among individuals who remember their childhood as happy or at least neutral, and the obverse relationship (i.e., a slight negative correlation) among individuals who remembered their childhood as unhappy. Again, it should be noted that the correlations are generally of modest magnitude.

Needed Research

Throughout this chapter we have noted gross inadequacies in much of the research bearing upon the effects of family size. From the discussion it will perhaps be apparent that no single research design will suffice to illuminate all of the effects of family size upon parents and children. Much of the data available was generated largely because family size is a convenient variable to assess. Neither theoretical premises nor considerations of adequacy of research design were paramount in most of these studies. This will undoubtedly continue to be true of much research to be carried out. And so long as the researcher analyzes his data with proper controls for socioeconomic status, family stage, and age of parents or children, valuable accretions of information on the effects of family size may result. Such analyses will not, however, greatly illuminate the ways in which family size exercises its effects.

In general, not only different populations of subjects but different research designs will be needed to assess the effects of family size on parents and on children. Despite the failure of past research to reveal personality as a significant source of differential fertility, the nagging thought that personality may be important persists. Most of the search for personality correlates of fertility has been carried out among women. Yet if such differences do exist, they seem more likely to be found among men. Mental disorder among men is much more often associated with failure to marry and with avoidance of sexual relations than it is among women. Data from one of the long-term longitudinal studies at Berkeley reveal significant correlations between several personality ratings of men at age thirty-eight and the number of their children, while revealing no significant relationships between these variables for female subjects.[6] Moreover, for men in this study group neuroticism assessed in adolescence is significantly related (negatively) to the number of children fathered, even when the analysis is limited to those subjects who married. These data come from a small and rather narrowly defined local population, so we would prefer to cite them as a reason for being unwilling to discard the personality hypothesis, not as adequate support for it. Most important, they came from a study in which personality has been carefully assessed, using many different methods in many different situations. None of the major studies of fertility experience has had comparable data on their subjects.

If the personalities of husbands or wives should be related to fertility experience, then personality assessments would have to be built into studies that seek to determine the influence of size of family on role relationships and on marital satisfaction. Even more important, expected levels of satisfaction at various stages of the family cycle will have to be taken into account in comparing families with differing numbers of children. If large families are, on the average, at a later stage of the family cycle, proper controls must be used. Since, however, there is much evidence that role relationships between parents and marital satisfaction are only minimally influenced by family size, one can hardly recommend a major study in this area.

Far more significant, in our opinion, would be attempts to assess the changes in life style and in parental socialization practices that occur as children are added to the family. Here short-range longitudinal studies might be most feasible, starting with cohorts of families that are not yet completed, some with one or two children and others with three or four, and collecting data on parental attitudes and practices, diet, housing, and other environmental circumstances over a period of perhaps five years. One would obviously want to assess the motivation for and meaning of

---

[6] We have examined both adolescent and adult personality ratings in relation both to the size of sibship and the number of own children. At age fifteen, males who subsequently fathered large families were rated (p <.05) more group oriented, happy, and content than those who subsequently fathered smaller families. Girls who subsequently had larger families were rated significantly more popular, well-adjusted, smooth functioning, and self-composed (p <.01 or <.05). When the men were rated at age thirty-eight, there were strong positive correlations (p <.01) between number of children and ratings of sexual adjustment, optimism, cheerfulness, relaxed style, self-acceptance, and unselfishness, and somewhat lower correlations (p <.05) between number of children and security, good adaptation to stress, and enjoyment of social activities. None of these personality ratings was significantly related to size of family for female subjects, despite the adolescent personality correlates of later family size.

The ratings in adolescence were based on intensive observation of the subjects in many situations; those at age thirty-eight were based on an average of eleven hours of interviewing, covering many phases of the individual's life experience. Since the interviewer knew how many children each subject had, ratings may have been biased by stereotypes of the happy, competent parent. In this instance, however, one would have expected ratings of mothers to show patterns similar to those of fathers.

additional children in the light of the goals and life style of the parents. It would be desirable to sample at least two and preferably three levels of socioeconomic status in order to assess the effects of differential economic pressures.

As regards the effects of family size upon the children, the need is again for data that will indicate how such effects come about. Most intriguing, because of the magnitude and consistency of differences found, is the question of influences on cognitive development. It would be helpful to have careful studies by students of psycholinguistics of children in small and larger sibships born to parents of comparable social status and linguistic practices. Also, the possibility of genetic differences needs to be dealt with definitively by studying children's IQs in relation to family size in samples of families matched on parental IQ.[7]

It is a fact that a variety of differences can be observed in studies comparing children from large and small families. That the differences are not always the same from one study to the next is not to say that these differences are chance phenomena. It is to say that family size in and of itself does not have an unequivocal influence. The consequences, for parents *or* children, will depend on motivations, on economic circumstances, on roles available in a given milieu, and on many transitory situational features. Studies that simply add further examples of influence will not markedly increase our understanding. The more interesting questions concerning the influences of family size are to be pursued through formulating how these variables interact in particular cultural groups or in families organized in particular constellations of authority and division of labor. Very few of the studies carried out to date have attempted such formulations. Only as family size is built into a theoretical perspective rather than being used as a handy background variable to include along with social class, age and sex—only as family size becomes genuinely problematic in certain developmental processes or relational networks—can we hope for real clarification of *how* family size makes a difference.

Summary and Conclusions

Insofar as family size and the spacing of children have significant effects on parents and children, what are their implications for family planning? In general the evidence quite consistently favors children from smaller families over those from larger families, and favors children born at least two years apart. Children from smaller, less dense families tend to be larger,

[7] The ongoing Intergenerational Study at the Institute of Human Development, University of California, Berkeley, will soon afford data to answer this question, since children of subjects tested a generation ago are currently being tested at comparable ages.

stronger, brighter, and more energetic, to get better medical care, to receive more education, to be better satisfied with their parents and with themselves, and to be more upwardly mobile in their occupational lives. Many of these tendencies derive from or are enhanced by the greater adequacy of available resources for family maintenance and child care in the small family. When parents want and can provide for a relatively large number of children, it does not appear that their children will be substantially disadvantaged, though advantages will still accrue to children from smaller families.

The effects of family size upon parental satisfactions are still more equivocal. While parents of larger families will often be under greater pressures and their role relationships and childrearing practices are likely to be affected by such pressures, they do not appear to differ appreciably from parents of small families in the values they hold for their children or in the satisfactions they derive from them. Marital satisfaction is slightly higher for parents of smaller families than for those with a large number of children, but this generalization holds only to the extent that the larger family results from unwanted children.

All of the above generalizations have been derived from research conducted among predominantly urban samples of families in Western Europe and the United States. They cannot, for the most part, be extended to farm families in Western society or to agrarian societies, to socialist countries with institutionalized day-care arrangements, or even to nations in the West that provide generous allotments for each child born. Certain of the effects of very large family size—especially those that stem from the finite capacities of parents to attend to the nonmaterial needs of their children— probably have wider validity, though they would not apply to extended families in which there are many parent surrogates.

Insofar as our findings can be generalized to Western urban families, do costs and consequences provide a cogent argument against having a large family? One's answer to this question will depend on personal values and circumstances. The psychological effects of family size can hardly be the primary rationale for limitation of births in any case, and it affords only a very modest rationale for couples who are in comfortable circumstances.

There is an aspect of small family size that we have not discussed but that needs to be considered. Parents who have only one or two children are in a sense far more vulnerable to tragedy than those with several children. An accident, a war, or the child's own failure or inability to achieve expected goals may deprive a couple in their middle years of the focus of their lifelong aspirations. The death or persistent unhappiness of one's child is a most difficult experience for any parent; it appears to be most devastating when that child is an only son or daughter. This then is another element to be weighed in the balance.

So many factors come into play in a couple's decision to have a given number of children that research findings on the effects of family size are not likely to determine that decision. However, since most prospective parents are only dimly aware of more than a few of these effects, a consideration of the prevailing tendencies of research findings may be helpful in arriving at a decision. It is with that hope that we conclude this review, although the most compelling reasons for limiting family size clearly lie elsewhere.

REFERENCES

Adams, B. N. and Meidam, M. T. 1968. Economics, family structure and college attendance. *American Journal of Sociology* 74:230–239.

Anastasi, A. 1956. Intelligence and family size. *Psychological Bulletin* 53:187–209.

Bahr, H. M. 1969. Family size and stability as antecedents of homelessness and excessive drinking. *Journal of Marriage and the Family* 31:477–483.

Bartow, J. A. 1961. Family size as related to child-rearing practices. Unpublished Ph.D. diss., Pennsylvania State University (abstract, *Journal of Home Economics* 54:230).

Benech, A.; Mathieu, B.; and Schreider, E. 1960. Family size and biological characteristics of the children. *Biotypologie* 21:4–36.

Blood, R. O. 1962. *Marriage.* New York: Free Press.

Blood, R. O. and Wolfe, D. M. 1960. *Husbands and wives: the dynamics of married living.* Glencoe, Ill.: Free Press.

Bonney, M. E. 1944. Relationships between social success, family size, socioeconomic home background, and intelligence among school children in grades III to V. *Sociometry* 7:26–39.

Bossard, J. H. S. and Boll, E. S. 1956. *The large family system.* Philadelphia: University of Pennsylvania Press.

Bumpass, L. L. and Westoff, C. F. 1970. *The later years of childbearing.* Princeton: Princeton University Press.

Burgess, E. W. and Cottrell, L. S. 1939. *Predicting success or failure in marriage.* Englewood Cliffs, N.J.: Prentice-Hall.

Campbell, F. L. 1970. Family growth and variation in family role structure. *Journal of Marriage and the Family* 32:45–53.

Chen, E. and Cobb, S. 1960. Family structure in relation to health and disease: a review of the literature. *Journal of Chronic Diseases* 12:544–567.

Chombart de Lauwe, M. J. 1959. *Psychopathologie sociale de l'enfant inadaptee.* Paris: Centre National de la Recherche Scientifique. Chap. 6.

Chombart de Lauwe, P. H. 1960. *Famille et habitation II Un essai d'observation experimentale.* Paris: Centre National de la Recherche Scientifique.

Christensen, H. T. 1968. Children in the family: relationship of number and spacing to marital success. *Journal of Marriage and the Family* 30:283–289.

Christensen, H. T. and Philbrick, R. E. 1952. Family size as a factor in the marital adjustments of college couples. *American Sociological Review* 17:306–312.

Clausen, J. A. 1966. Family structure, socialization and personality. In L. W. Hoffman and M. L. Hoffman, eds., *Review of child development research.* New York: Russell Sage Foundation 2:1–53.

Damrin, D. E. 1949. Family size and sibling age, sex, and position as related to certain aspects of adjustment. *Journal of Social Psychology* 29: 93–102.

Douglas, J. W. B. 1964. *The home and the school: a study of ability and attainment in the primary school.* London: MacGibbon & Kee.

Douglas, J. W. B. and Blomfield, J. M. 1958. *Children under five.* London: Allen and Unwin.

Duncan, O. D.; Freedman, R.; Coble, J. M.; and Slesinger, D. P. 1965. Marital fertility and the size of family of orientation. *Demography* 2:508–515.

Durel, R. 1971. Ut an don an al aron. *The New Yorker*, January 9, 1971, pp. 30–49.

Elder, G. H., Jr. 1962a. Structural variations in the child rearing relationship. *Sociometry* 25:241–262.

———. 1962b. Family structure: the effects of size and family, sex composition and ordinal position on academic motivation and achievement. In *Adolescent Achievement and Mobility Aspirations*. Chapel Hill: Institute for Research in Social Science. Pp. 59–72 (mimeo).

Elder, G. H., Jr., and Bowerman, C. E. 1963. Family structure and child rearing patterns: the effect of family size and sex composition. *American Sociological Review* 28: 891–905.

Farber, B. and Blackman, L. S. 1956. Marital role tensions and number and sex of children. *American Sociological Review* 21:596–601.

Floud, J. E.; Halsey, A. H.; and Martin, F. M. 1957. *Social class and educational opportunity*. London: Wm. Heinemann, Ltd.

Gonda, T. A. 1962. The relation between complaints of persistent pain and family size. *Journal of Neurology, Neurosurgery and Psychiatry* 25:277–281.

Grant, M. W. 1964. Rate of growth in relation to birth rank and family size. *British Journal of Preventive and Social Medicine* 18:35–42.

Gregory, I. 1958. An analysis of familial data on psychiatric patients: parental age, family size, birth order and ordinal position. *British Journal of Preventive and Social Medicine* 12:42–59.

Groat, H. T. and Neal, A. G. 1967. Social psychological correlates of urban fertility. *American Sociological Review* 32:945–959.

Hare, E. H. and Shaw, J. K. 1965. A study in family health: health in relation to family size. *British Journal of Psychiatry* 3:461–466.

Hawkes, G. R.; Burchinal, L.; and Gardner, B. 1958. Size of family and adjustment of children. *Marriage and Family Living* 20:65–68.

Heer, D. M. 1963. The measurement and basis of family power: an overview. *Marriage and Family Living* 25:133–139.

Hendershot, G. E. 1969. Birth order and fertility values. *Journal of Marriage and the Family* 31:27–33.

Higgins, J. V.; Reed, E. W.; and Reed, S. C. 1962. Intelligence and family size: a paradox resolved. *Eugenics Quarterly* 9:84–90.

Hoffman, L. W. 1963. The decision to work. In F. I. Nye and L. W. Hoffman, *The employed in America*. Chicago: Rand McNally.

Hoffman, L. W. and Wyatt, F. 1960. Social change and motivations for having larger families: some theoretical considerations. *Merrill-Palmer Quarterly* 6:235–244.

Hurley, J. R. and Palonen, D. P. 1967. Marital satisfaction and child density among university student parents. *Journal of Marriage and the Family* 29:483–484.

Kohn, M. L. 1969. *Class and conformity: a study in values*. Homewood, Ill.: Dorsey Press. P. 68.

Levy, D. M. 1937. Studies in sibling rivalry. *Research Monographs of the American Orthopsychiatric Association*, no. 2.

Masterson, M. L. 1971. Family structure variables and need approval. *Journal of Consulting and Clinical Psychology* 36:12.

Mellinger, G. D.; Manheimer, D. I.; and Kleman, M. T. 1967. Deterrents to adequate immunization of preschool children with special attention to families of lower socioeconomic status. Los Angeles: Los Angeles County Health Department, February 1967 (multilithed).

Michel, A. and Feyrabend, F. L. 1969. Real number of children and conjugal satisfaction in French urban families. *Journal of Marriage and the Family* 31:359–363.

Nisbet, J. 1961. Family environment and intelligence. In A. H. Halsey, J. Floud, and C. A. Anderson, eds., *Education, economy, and society*. New York: Free Press. Pp. 273–287. (Reprinted from *Eugenics Review* 45 [1953]:31–40.)

Nisbet, J. D. and Entwistle, N. J. 1967. Intelligence and family size, 1949–1965. *British Journal of Educational Psychology* 37:188–193.

Nye, I.; Carlson, J.; and Garrett, G. 1970. Family size, interaction, affect and stress. *Journal of Marriage and the Family* 32:216–226.

Orden, S. R. and Bradburn, N. M. 1969. Working wives and marital happiness. *American Journal of Sociology* 74:392–407.

Passamanick, B. and Lilienfeld, A. M. 1956. The association of maternal and fetal factors with the development of mental deficiency: II Relationship to maternal age, birth order, previous reproductive loss and degree of mental deficiency. *American Journal of Mental Deficiency* 60:557.

Petroni, F. 1969. Social class, family size and sick role. *Journal of Marriage and the Family* 31:728–735.

Pierce, J. V. 1959. *The educational motivation patterns of superior students who do and do not achieve in high school.* Report of U.S. Office of Education, Department of Health, Education and Welfare. University of Chicago, November 1959.

Pohlman, E. 1969. *The psychology of birth planning.* Cambridge, Mass.: Schenkman.

Pryor, C. G. B. 1970. Variations in children's roles according to birth order and family type. Unpublished Ph.D. diss., University of Michigan.

Rainwater, L. 1965. *Family design: Marital sexuality, family size, and contraception.* Chicago: Aldine.

Rehberg, R. A. and Westby, D. L. 1967. Parental encouragement, occupation, education and family size: artifactual or independent determinants of adolescent educational expectations? *Social Forces* 45: 362–374.

Rollins, B. C. and Feldman, H. 1970. Marital satisfaction over the family life cycle. *Journal of Marriage and the Family* 32:20–26.

Rosen, B. C. 1961. Family structure and achievement motivation. *American Sociological Review* 26:574–585.

———. 1964. Family structure and value transmission. *Merrill-Palmer Quarterly* 10: 59–76.

Rosenberg, M. 1965. *Society and the adolescent self-image.* Princeton: Princeton University Press.

Schachter, S. 1959. *The psychology of affiliation.* Stanford: Stanford University Press.

Scottish Council for Research in Education. 1949. *The trend of Scottish intelligence.* London: University of London Press.

———. 1953. *Social implications of the 1947 Scottish mental survey.* London: University of London Press.

Sears, R. R. 1970. Relation of early socialization experience to self-concepts and gender role in middle childhood. *Child Development* 41:267–289.

Smart, R. G. 1963. Alcoholism, birth order, and family size. *Journal of Abnormal and Social Psychology* 66:17–23.

Strodtbeck, F. L. and Creelan, P. G. 1968. The interaction linkage between family size, intelligence and sex role identity. *Journal of Marriage and the Family* 30:301–307.

Svalastoga, K. 1959. *Prestige, class and mobility.* London: Wm. Heinemann. Pp. 404–406.

Terman, L. M. 1938. *Psychological factors in marital happiness.* New York: McGraw-Hill.

Thoman, E. B.; Turner, A. M.; Leiderman, P. H.; and Barnett, C. R. 1970. Neonate-mother interaction: effects of parity on feeding behavior. *Child Development* 41: 1103–1111.

Tuckman, J. and Regan, R. A. 1967. Size of family and behavioral problems in children. *Journal of Genetic Psychology* 111:151–160.

Turner, R. H. 1962. Some family determinants of ambition. *Sociology and Social Research* 46:397–411.

Waldrop, M. F. and Bell, R. Q. 1964. Relation of preschool dependency behavior to family size and density. *Child Development* 35:1187–1195.

———. 1966. Effects of family size and density on newborn characteristics. *American Journal of Orthopsychiatry* 36:544–550.

Westoff, C. F.; Potter, R. G.; and Sagi, P. C. 1963. *The third child.* Princeton: Princeton University Press.

Wilensky, H. L. 1963. The moonlighter: a product of relative deprivation. *Industrial Relations* 3:105–124.

[8]

THE EFFECTS OF POPULATION DENSITY ON HUMANS

JONATHAN L. FREEDMAN

Despite the fact that population growth is one of the most serious problems facing the world today, despite the recognition that even if we are able to control our population growth we are for the moment stuck with huge numbers of people living in restricted spaces, and despite the fact that scientists in all fields are turning their attention more and more to problems of ecology and pollution, there has been surprisingly little research directly related to the question of how population density affects humans. One reason for this lack of research may be that all too many people, scientists included, assume that they know the answer to the question and therefore do not need to do research on it.

The popular press and even some scientific journals have tended to publish articles in which the clear assumption is that density is "bad." Zlutnick and Altman (1971) found the press to be a "veritable unending source of 'expert' opinions on the effects of crowding on human behavior." Crowding was reported to cause disease, physical malfunction, mental illness, crime, riots, war, drug addiction, alcoholism, family disorganization, psychological withdrawal, aggression, and a decreased quality of life. It is not surprising that nonscientists have developed opinions on this topic, but it is disheartening that scientists and responsible public officials have reached conclusions and made unequivocal statements without supporting evidence. Biologists and ethologists such as Lorenz (1966) and Leyhausen (1965) have also pronounced the judgment that aggression and violence are caused by high density. Although noting that crowding may sometimes

NOTE: The preparation of this chapter and the work by the author reported in it were supported in part by a grant from the Ford Foundation. The author is grateful to Simon Klevansky, Alan Levy, Stanley Heshka, Roberta Welte, Paul Ehrlich, and Judy Price with whom he has discussed many of the issues covered in the chapter.

be exciting, Proshansky, Ittelson, and Rivlin (1970) write that: "Some settings chronically contain excessive crowd densities that have immediate and long-range detrimental effects on individuals within them." Holford (1970) asserts that the lack of adequate space "leads very easily to neurosis, delinquency and violence.[1] And the Massachusetts Mental Health Commissioner, who is also a professor of psychiatry, was recently quoted as declaring that ". . . there is a toxic reaction caused in an individual when overcrowded by others" and that "now it is being increasingly observed among human beings that overcrowding caused alcoholism, psychosis and behavioral deviations apart from the influence of low income, inadequate food, and lack of education" (*New York Post*, January 19, 1971). Unfortunately in contrast to this plethora of opinions and statements, there is a paucity of hard data.

Before considering the available evidence in detail, let us be clear on two points concerning the focus of this chapter in terms of the definition of density. First, although there may be other ways of conceptualizing the problem, I shall generally define density simply as the number of individuals per unit of space. If there are ten individuals in 100 square feet, the density is greater than if there are five individuals or if there is 200 square feet of space. This definition distinguishes density from a number of potentially crucial variables such as the amount of privacy that is available, the necessity of individuals interacting, the absolute number of individuals present, and so on. These other factors may be important in determining the effect of density or in their own right, but they do not determine density per se. Sometimes there will be a question as to how to measure the available space. For example, in cities we could use population per residential acre or population per square foot of residential floor space. These would be quite similar for cities containing only one-story buildings, but quite different where high-rise apartment houses are present. Rather than choose between them, we shall use whatever measure or measures are employed in the research as long as it provides an indication of the amount of space available to each individual.

The second point is exceedingly important. I am concerned here with the effects of density itself, not density in conjunction with poverty, noise, malnutrition, filth, or any other factor that may tend to be associated with it. Obviously crowded slums should be eliminated even if crowding by itself is a positive benefit to human beings. Accordingly this chapter focuses on the question of how density, as distinguished from any other factor, affects humans. As we shall see throughout this review, it is often difficult to separate density from other variables, but by considering a variety of

---

[1] It is perhaps an indication of the strength of commitment to this negative evaluation of density that Holford implies that Jane Jacobs agrees with this position, even though the major point of her fascinating book on the city (1962) is that high concentrations of people have positive value.

approaches to the problem and many different kinds of data, we can get some idea what the evidence indicates.

The review is divided into several sections: research on nonhumans, demographic and survey studies of humans, field and observation studies of humans, laboratory and field experiments on humans, and a summary. There has been a great deal of work relevant to the question of how density affects nonhumans, and it is not reviewed exhaustively here. Rather, this section tries to summarize the current state of knowledge in this area, relying at times on reviews done by others. In contrast the review of research on humans does try to include all studies known to the author, although some selection has been made when there is a series of similar studies of tangential relevance, such as those on isolation. Purely theoretical or hypothetical papers have not been included since they seem to be of relatively little utility at the present time and since the purpose of this chapter is to assess what is known, not what is conjectured.

Research on Nonhumans

There is an extensive and distinguished body of research on the effects of population density and group size on nonhuman animals. Most of this work has used rodents as subjects, but a wide variety of other animals has been studied as well. The focus of the research has ranged from relatively gross responses such as population cycles, reproductive rates, and aggressiveness to detailed physiological reactions such as glandular changes and resistance to disease.

A number of studies, some done in the laboratory and some done in relatively natural field conditions, have demonstrated dramatic effects of overpopulation. In this work a population of animals is observed as it increases in size under benign conditions. The most famous laboratory study was conducted by Calhoun (1962a), and most of the other work has followed the same paradigm. A small number of animals, in this case rats, were placed in an enclosed area, given sufficient food and water, and allowed to increase freely. Under these conditions the population of the colony increased rapidly for a while, then began to level off, and finally decreased sharply. According to Calhoun, the maximum population achieved was considerably less than the space could have supported. Whether or not that is true, it is clear that the population did reach a maximum that was less than could actually fit in the available space and that this maximum was not maintained. Similar patterns have been observed in other laboratory studies by Calhoun and his associates (Calhoun, 1961, 1962b; Marsden, 1970), Louch (1956), Southwick (1955a, 1967), Chitty (1955),

Clark (1955), Snyder (1968); and in natural settings by Clough (1968), Deevey (1960), and Christian (e.g., Christian, Flyger, and Davis, 1960). These findings have included a wide variety of animals ranging from mice, voles, rats, and lemmings to hares, deer, chickens, and primates. That the population of animals will not continually increase, but will at some point stabilize or decrease even in benign environments seems to be well established. However, the causes of this phenomenon and the accompanying effects on the individual animals and on the social behavior of the animals are considerably less clear.

Calhoun and others have described breakdowns in normal social behaviors under conditions of high population density. There is a marked increase in aggressive behavior by some males, an increase in indiscriminate sexual behavior, invasion of nests by marauding males, attacks on pregnant females by these males, and a general increase in fighting and disorganized activity. In contrast some males became entirely passive, avoiding all social interaction, and some males clustered together in what Calhoun referred to as a "behavioral sink," which consisted of a large group of animals, more crowded than necessary, fighting on occasion and simply sitting idly at other times. Accompanying this behavior by the males was a breakdown in normal infant care by the females, a lack of adequate nestbuilding, and a consequent sharp rise in unsuccessful pregnancies and infant mortality. In an earlier study Southwick (1955b) also observed increased aggressiveness as population increased and noted that considerably more communal nesting (i.e., two or more parturient females in one nest) occurred. This communal nesting was associated with very low survival of the young. Clark (1955) and Snyder (1968) have made similar observations.

In all of these studies it appears that several quite distinct groups of animals emerge under high population density. Snyder (1968), working with mice, distinguishes among four classes of males: dominant animals who are large, relatively unscarred, and who roam freely; recluses who keep to themselves and are relatively healthy; huddlers who gather together in large undifferentiated groups; and withdrawn, hairless, wounded animals. Female animals appear to fall into three groups: healthy, unscarred animals capable of bearing young; small, unscarred animals who bear young, but the young generally die; and finally small, relatively unscarred huddlers who associate with the male huddlers in the "behavioral sink." Although the specific types of animals that have been observed vary somewhat according to which author is describing them, there is general agreement that different patterns of behavior emerge and that it is possible to identify relatively healthy, normal males and females, animals of both sexes that try to avoid social interaction, and a large group of animals that huddle together in an undifferentiated mass. Only animals in the first group seem to be capable of producing healthy offspring.

One immediate cause of the decrease in population appears to be the high rate of infant mortality caused by inadequate nests and maternal care.

This inadequate care is in turn caused by the breakdown in the social structure, the invasion of the nests by marauding males, and other disruptive activities. It is not clear, however, why this breakdown in social behavior occurs nor whether it is the sole cause of the population decline.

Several authors (e.g., Christian, 1950; Christian, Lloyd, and Davis, 1965; Wynne-Edwards, 1965) have proposed that population density is controlled by a more or less complicated interaction between certain physiological mechanisms and social behavior. In particular Christian and his co-workers have asserted that high population density produces social stress that in turn causes an overactivation of the pituitary-adrenal-gonadal system; that in turn leads to an increase in aggressive behavior, breakdown in normal social behavior, and more directly a decrease in fertility and normal sexual behavior. Christian stresses the endocrine control while Wynne-Edwards places greater emphasis on social behavior, but the theories have much in common. Whether or not this is the mechanism by which the size of the population is controlled, there is considerable evidence that the size of the population has effects on the endocrine system.

The relationship between population size and endocrine function has been reviewed in detail in a thoughtful article by Theissen and Rodgers (1961), and despite considerable work since that time, their basic conclusions still seem justified. I shall not, therefore, attempt a thorough review of this literature, but rather shall rely on their excellent paper supplementing it with some of the more recent experiments.

Although a few studies have been done on natural populations, most of the work in this area has dealt with animals raised under controlled laboratory conditions. The basic paradigm for virtually all of the experiments is to raise animals in individual cages until they reach a certain age (depending on the species) and then transfer them to cages containing a varying number of other animals. For example, Christian (1955) placed male white mice in groups of one, four, six, eight, sixteen, or thirty-two and after one week measured various physiological changes. In some studies, such as the one just mentioned, all of the cages are the same size, thus confounding the number of animals and the density. Other studies (e.g., Thiessen, 1964) compared mice in groups of one, ten, and twenty and equated the amount of space at 20.9 square inches per animal. And a few studies (e.g., Thiessen, Zolman, and Rodgers, 1962) varied number and density independently by varying the size of the cage while keeping number constant and also varying number while keeping density constant. This problem of separating density and size of the group will recur throughout this chapter, and it will be seen that there is no perfect solution to it.

What have these experiments shown on the effect of size and density on the endocrine system? It would be nice to be able to report that there are clear, consistent results. Unfortunately, although there are some strong trends in the findings, no single effect has been reported by all experimenters. The most well-established finding is that, as suggested by the social stress idea, animals living in larger groups tend to have larger adrenal glands. In a series of experiments Christian has consistently found this both in the laboratory and under natural conditions. It has also been reported by Brain and Nowell (1971), Morrison and Thatcher (1969), Siegel (1959), and others and has received indirect support from Louch (1956), who found greater adrenal cortical activity in larger groups. On the other hand, several authors (Southwick and Bland, 1959; McKeever, 1959) have found no relationship between size of the group and adrenal weight.

A possible explanation of the discrepancy was suggested by Southwick and Bland (1959), who found that only wounded animals had heavier adrenals, but Christian (1959) failed to confirm this. One possibility proposed by Barnett (1955) and Davis and Christian (1957) is that the effect on adrenal size is found only in subordinate animals. Since there is a high but not perfect correlation between dominance and amount of wounding, this might explain why some wounded animals show the effect more than others and would also explain why larger groups tended to have a larger mean adrenal weight; naturally there would be a higher percentage of subordinate animals in larger than in smaller groups (a single animal in a cage would obviously not be subordinate, and the major effects have been between animals raised alone and in groups). Thus although there is some inconsistency in the results, it does seem as if the bulk of the evidence indicates some effect of group size on adrenal weight. However, as Thiessen and Rodgers point out in their review, there is no evidence that population density per se is an important variable. They conclude that whatever effects have been found have been related to the size of the group rather than to the amount of space that is available per animal. They state that "mechanical restriction of living space appears to be unimportant within broad limits."

In addition to the research on adrenal size, there have been investigations of the effects of population size on related systems. Although once again the findings are not consistent, there is substantial evidence that the weight of the testes and seminal vesicles decreases as population size increases. Thiessen (1964) found a fairly consistent decrease in corrected testes weight (i.e., in relation to the total body weight) as the number of animals increased from one to ten and then to twenty, even with the amount of space equated. Christian (1955) found both vesicles and testes larger for animals raised alone than for animals raised in groups, although there was no difference according to the size of the group. Snyder reports a decrease in testes size and amount of spermatozoa for animals raised twenty to a cage versus those raised individually. And Southwick and Bland (1959) found a decrease in vesicle size as groups increased from one to four to eight to sixteen, even though they did not find any effect on either adrenal or testes weight. Despite some lack of consistency in these findings, it seems fair to conclude that increases in population tend to be associated with decreases in the weight of testes and vesicles and increases in male sterility. It should be pointed out, however, that most of the histological studies have found no gross pathologies of either adrenal or testes.

Closely related to this work on endocrine changes is a series of studies dealing with the effects of population on emotionality. The experiments cited earlier in which colonies were allowed to increase in population indicated that high population density produced increased aggressiveness and a general breakdown in social behavior. Several experimenters have attempted to demonstrate the effect of population density on emotionality under more controlled conditions. The typical effect, somewhat surprisingly, is that animals raised in groups are generally less emotional than those raised individually. For example, Morrison and Thatcher (1969) found less open field emotionality for animals raised in groups of sixteen or thirty-two than for animals raised individually or in groups of four. Ader (1965) found a similar effect and also a reduced startle response to a handling test for the group-raised animals. Ader, Kreutner, and Jacobs (1963) confirmed this result for emotionality, as did Thiessen (1964) and Thiessen, Zolman, and Rodgers (1962). In addition Conger, Sawrey, and Turrell (1958) found that animals who were tested in groups developed fewer ulcers in a conflict situation than those who were tested alone, although type of rearing had no effect. Thus contrary to the idea that being in a group is a stressful situation, it appears that group-raised animals are less emotional, at least under some circumstances, than those who are raised individually.

In general this work on endocrinal effects and emotionality has produced at best confusing results. It does seem as if group-raised animals display certain effects (particularly increased adrenal weight) that support the idea that population pressures produce stress. On the other hand, these results are inconsistent and are not supported by the findings regarding emotionality. It seems fair to say that animals placed in cages with a large number of other animals respond in part with increased adrenal activity and consequent increases in adrenal size and decreases in testes size, but that the animals apparently adapt to whatever stress the population pressure causes and do not become overly emotional or suffer a breakdown in their normal behavior. For purposes of this review two additional points are particularly relevant:

1. Whatever effects are found appeared to be due not to population density (i.e., not to the amount of space per animal) but to the number of animals in the cage.
2. The relatively mild and inconsistent effects found in the controlled experimental studies contrast sharply with the dramatic and destructive effects found when population increases greatly in the relatively uncontrolled conditions found in the studies of free-growing colonies. It may be that only the very large number of animals present in the colony situations or the long duration of the confinement in those studies will produce the social breakdowns that have been consistently reported under those circumstances.

There has also been some research on the effects of housing conditions on susceptibility to disease. The procedures followed in this research are similar to those described previously—animals are placed in cages either alone or with varying numbers of other animals—the major difference being that the animals are then injected with or exposed to a particular disease agent and their susceptibility and resistance to the disease is measured. A careful series of experiments by Plaut, Ader, Friedman, and Ritterson (1969) demonstrated that mice in groups were less resistant to malaria than animals raised individually. This effect was independent of the age and sex of the animals and also independent of how many of the animals in each cage were infected. More importantly the actual size of the cage and accordingly the actual density of the population had no effect—the only crucial variable was the number of individuals that were interacting. The experiment also showed that the critical element was the type of housing after rather than before the infection.

In contrast a study by the same group (Friedman, Lowell, and Ader, 1970) demonstrated exactly the opposite effect of group living on resistance to the encephalomyocarditis virus. Two different strains of mice were *more* resistant to the virus when housed in groups of five to twenty than when housed alone. The size of the group did not matter, but the animals housed individually were consistently more susceptible. And other studies (e.g., Tobach and Bloch, 1956) suggest that the effect of type of housing upon resistance to disease is dependent on a large number of factors, including the sex of the animal and the particular dosage used. In other words there is no evidence from work on nonhumans that grouped housing is consistently better or worse in terms of disease resistance than individual housing.

All in all, the work on animals, while suggestive, is somewhat inconsistent. Much of the work has been extremely well done, carefully thought out, and well executed. The inconsistency in the results does not, therefore, appear to be due to inadequate technique; rather it seems that the particular effects being studied are not consistent or depend on a variety of factors some of which are not yet specified. We seem to be left with the well-established fact that in enclosed colonies very large populations lead to social and eventually physical anomalies, including increased aggressiveness and poor maternal care.

More specific effects of the size of the group are increased adrenal activity and adrenal weight (although this may be limited to subordinate animals), decreased seminal vesicle and testes weight, and perhaps decreased amount of spermatozoa. Also, larger groups appear to produce a decrease in emotionality. The idea that the presence of other animals generally produces stress is not well supported, although the endocrinal effects are consistent with it. Most importantly none of the evidence suggests that density per se is associated with any consistent findings. Indeed, there is ample evidence that the crucial variable producing whatever effects are found is the number of animals in the cage, rather than the amount of space per animal.

Although these findings are fascinating and provocative, it is always difficult to generalize from research on nonhumans to humans, particularly when this involves complex social behaviors. As René Dubos has pointed out, "The readiness with which man adapts to potentially dangerous situations makes it unwise to apply directly to human life the results of experiments designed to test the acute effects of crowding on animals" (1970, p. 207). This means that although we can use this animal work as a starting point and as a source of ideas, we must turn to work on humans to understand how population density affects man.

Demographic and Survey Studies

One approach to this complex problem of discovering how density affects humans has been to assess the degree of relationship in actual communities between population density and measures of social, physical, and mental breakdown. Using census data, the density of various districts of a city or of various cities is measured; and this is correlated with rates of crime, juvenile delinquency, infant mortality, adult mortality, disease, mental illness, suicide, and anything else the author happens to be concerned with. This work varies widely in scope and methodological sophistication.

To begin with, there are a series of studies concerned with the patterns of crime and mental illness in and around cities, rather than with the question of the effects of density. The results of this research consistently indicate a higher incidence of crime, mental illness, and suicide in cities than in rural areas and in the center of cities than in the outskirts. Pollock and Furbush (1921) report a higher rate of mental disease in urban areas than in rural areas, and Landis and Page (1938) showed more specifically that cities with populations of less than 2,500 had a lower rate of mental disease than larger cities. Faris and Dunham (1939), Green (1939), and others have shown that the highest rates of mental illness occur in and around the downtown area of a city. Much of this early work is discussed in a widely quoted article by Queen (1940), who concluded that the data lend partial support to the hypothesis that "institutionalized mental patients come predominantly from areas of dense population. . . ." Similarly Schmid (1955) found a higher rate of completed and attempted suicide in downtown areas than in outlying districts, while Morris (1964) reports that bronchitis and lung cancer are much more common in urban than in rural areas.

Similar and even more dramatic differences occur in crime rates. Shaw and McKay (1942) and Schmid (1960) report much higher incidence of crime in the center of the city than in surrounding areas. And more recently the National Commission on the Causes and Prevention of Violence pointed out that violent crime in the United States is "primarily a phenomenon of large cities." Whereas there are 1,070 crimes per 100,000 people in rural areas, there are 2,376 in the suburbs, 3,430 in cities of 50,000 to 100,-000 population, and 5,307 in cities of over a quarter of a million population. Twenty-six cities with populations of half a million or more have 17 percent of the country's population and 45 percent of reported major violent crimes. The six cities with a million or more have 10 percent of the population and 30 percent of violent crimes. The rate of major crimes in the big cities is more than five times greater than in smaller cities, eight times greater than in the suburbs, and eleven times greater than in rural areas. There is little doubt that crime, mental illness, suicide, and even some physical illnesses occur more in areas of high population density.

As with most correlational statements, however, this relationship is diffi-cult to interpret. It would be a mistake to conclude on the basis of a rough overall correlation between density and these other variables that high population density was a causative factor in the relationship. There are many other factors associated with high density, such as economic level, to pick the most obvious example, that might be producing the effect. More careful analysis of these findings is necessary in order to try to ascertain the extent to which density per se is producing the relationship.

Although the rate of crime, for example, is greater in cities than in rural areas and within the city is greater in downtown than in outlying areas, it is possible to ask whether, holding the type of community constant, higher density is associated with higher crime. That is, do cities with higher den-sities have higher crime rates than cities of the same population with lower densities? Do downtown areas with higher densities have higher crime rates than downtown areas with lower densities? If the relationship does hold even when the type of community and the type of area is equated in this way, it would be much more convincing. Even then it would not constitute definitive evidence for a causative relationship between density and crime because, as will be seen later, other factors such as economic level must still be accounted for, but it would be more impressive than the simple correlations reported above.

Pollock and Furbush (1921) ranked twelve states in terms of rates of mental disease. Although the authors do not compute it themselves, a rough calculation of the relationship between these ranks and the relative densi-ties of the twelve states results in a rank order correlation of .4. While this is not a negligible relationship, it is clear that even in this gross measure only a small percentage of the variance is explained by population density. Although Massachusetts and New York rank near the top, Arizona, New Hampshire, and Maine do also. Schmid (1933) dealt only with large cities and found no relationship between the suicide rate and the size of the city (or for that matter its density). Landis and Page (1938) reported that the number of recruits rejected for army service because of mental disease in Holland bore no relation to the size of the city. In contrast Morris (1964) reports that the larger the community, the higher the rates of bronchitis and lung cancer. He attributes this primarily to the level of pollution in the larger cities, but at least the relationship does hold. A recent study by Pressman and Carol (1969) compared metropolitan areas that vary in density and are equivalent in terms of poverty level and other characteristics. They found no appreciable relationship between density and crime rate. Thus most attempts to find relationships between population density of roughly comparable communities and crime or illness have largely failed. What correlations have been found are generally low.

Obviously states or even cities differ in so many respects that the kind of comparisons just reported would be unlikely to produce strong relationships. Los Angeles has a much lower density than New York City and yet a much higher rate of major crime. But the two cities are so different in terms of living conditions, accuracy of crime reporting, poverty level, the use of cars versus public transportation, and so on that it is virtually impossible to conclude anything from this reverse relationship. Although high positive correlations between density and crime or mental illness would have been impressive and would have argued for the importance of density as a causative factor, the absence of such findings should be interpreted with caution. Similar arguments could be made for comparisons between areas within a given community, but at least parts of the same community have a tendency to share more characteristics. Accordingly let us now look at attempts to find relationships between density and other measures within one city.

The extensive study by Shaw and McKay (1942) found more crime in the central city and less as one goes outward. The authors divide the city into quartiles on the basis of the highest to lowest rates of juvenile delinquency for those areas and also provide figures on the percentage of population and area represented by those districts. Although the authors do not compute them it is possible to look at the relationship between rate of delinquency and density. With only four observations per city it makes little sense to compute correlations, but one can get a sense of the strength of the relationship between the two indicators. It is clear that this varied greatly from one city to another. The relationship between rate of delinquency and density appears to be high in Philadelphia, Richmond, and Denver, somewhat lower but still appreciable in Cleveland and Seattle, nonexistent in Birmingham, and actually negative in Chicago. Shaw and McKay devote most of their attention to Chicago and report that the highest concentration of juvenile delinquency occurs in areas of decreasing population and that in fact the correlation between delinquency and rate of population increase is —.54. Schmid (1960) also reports a higher crime rate in the central city and provides rates for the five major downtown districts. He does not concern himself with the relationship between density and crime in these districts, but does provide the appropriate figures. Within the downtown area there are low or negative correlations between density and crime depending on the particular type of crime that is selected.

Neither of these studies divides the cities into enough districts to provide a good indication of the actual relationship. This was done by Schmitt (1957, 1966) and Winsborough (1965). Schmitt computed five different measures of population density for the census tracts in Honolulu and correlated these measures with the rates of juvenile delinquency, adult crimes, suicide, mental hospital admissions, and other measures. In both studies, separated by approximately ten years, he found strong positive correlations between density and all measures of social, physical, and mental breakdown. The correlations with density as measured by population per net acre were .3 for infant death rate, .7 for tuberculosis rate, .83 for venereal disease rate, .74 for mental hospital rate, .50 for illegitimate birth rate, .63 for juvenile delinquency rate, .55 for prison rate, and, the one exception, .04 for suicide rate. In a similar study done in Chicago Winsborough (1965) also found positive correlations between population density and infant mortality, .32; death rate, .14; tuberculosis rate, .20; public assistance rate, .37; and public assistance to persons under eighteen, .45. Since these three studies constitute the most extensive attempt to assess the effect of density within a city and since they all obtain very strong correlations, it is important to consider them in some detail.

Population density within any one community tends to be highly correlated with many other potentially important factors. The most obvious of these are income, educational level, and migration rate, but one could also include the adequacy of police protection, availability of jobs, and so on. Any one of these factors might be the cause of the higher crime rate or rate of mental illness that is found in areas of greater density. For example, it is quite well established that socioeconomic class is highly associated with rates of mental illness (Hollingshead and Redlich, 1958). Thus in order to get a reasonable estimate of the actual relationship between density and mental illness, it is essential to equate areas on these other factors.

Unfortunately this is easier said than done. It is virtually impossible to find areas that differ in density but are identical in all other respects. Therefore, the technique that has been used is partial correlations that attempt to hold socioeconomic class and other factors constant by statistical technique and then compute the remaining relationships with density. This is what Pressman and Carol (1969) did in their study of metropolitan districts in the United States, and it will be remembered that they found no remaining relationship between density and crime rate.

Schmitt (1966) partialled out measures of education and income and still found a strong correlation between population per acre and his various measures of mental, social, and physical breakdown. For example, the simple correlation between density and tuberculosis rate is .72 and it was .65 after partialling out education and income; with venereal disease rate it went from .83 to .80, mental hospital admission rate .74 to .69, juvenile delinquency from .63 to .56, and so on. Except for suicide rate, which was low to begin with, the removal of education and income level produced only slight decrements in the correlations with density.

Since education and income are ordinarily so strongly correlated with both mental hospital rate and density, it is surprising to find such small differences between the simple and partial correlations. We would usually expect a substantial reduction in the correlation with density. This suggests that the measures of education and income may be somewhat questionable, and this is in fact the case. Education was measured as the percentage of persons twenty-five years or older with twelve or more years of schooling. This obviously divides the population into well-educated and not well-educated, but provides no indication of how many had very little schooling. Since the major effects of education on crime probably occur at the relatively low end of the continuum, this is a rather poor measure for our purposes. A much better and more typical measure of educational level would be median years of education, but for some reason this was not chosen. Similarly the measure of income is the percentage earning $3,000 per family or more. This line of demarcation splits the areas into lower class and the rest rather than providing distinctions between groups. Median income would obviously have been a much more sensitive measure.

It seems likely that both measures, while providing some indication of education and income, are inadequate as a means of controlling for these two variables and the partial correlations between population density and crime rate, for example, should not be interpreted as being totally independent of income and education. Nevertheless, it must be noted that Schmitt did get strong correlations between density and these other measures even while partialling out some indication of education and income.

Winsborough (1965) also used partial correlations to control for various factors that were themselves correlated with density and had much more sensitive measures for his control factors. He partialled out many factors, including percentage of workers in professional, technical, and kindred professions, median income of families, median years of school completed, percentage of population foreign born, median age, median rent, percentage of dwellings with no water, no bath, or dilapidated. The partial correlations with density were very different from the simple correlations. The correlation with infant death showed little change, going from .32 to .33, but correlation with overall death rate went from .14 to —.62, with tuberculosis went from .20 to —.67, with public assistance went from .37 to —.39, and for public assistance to persons under eighteen from .45 to .14. Thus three of the correlations went from moderately positive to strongly negative, and one went from substantially positive to close to zero. In other words, with economic, educational, and migrational levels partialled out, Winsborough found that density was actually associated with less morbidity, disease, and need for public assistance.

Although Winsborough used sensitive measures for his control factors, it is quite difficult to interpret partial correlations when this many factors are removed at once. Exactly what these negative correlations mean is unclear. It would certainly be a mistake to conclude that density actually has a strongly beneficial effect on tuberculosis rate. On the other hand, the lack of positive relationships when the factors are partialled out suggests that density is not an important factor in the variables that were measured.

This demographic work thus presents no clear picture of the relationship between density and crime, mental illness, or disease. Urban areas and the central districts of urban areas certainly have higher rates of crime and mental illness, but attempts to attribute this directly to density have been quite inconclusive. Cities have higher rates than rural districts, but densely populated cities do not necessarily have higher rates than less densely populated cities. Central districts and slums have higher rates than outlying residential districts, but once again this is not always associated with density. And even when there is a correlation with density, controlling for other factors sometimes removes the correlation with density, and sometimes it does not. The conflicting and generally weak results have led careful analysts of the situation to conclude that there is as yet no evidence of negative effects of high density. For example, Wilner and Baer (1970) conclude that "there is no body of convincing evidence that crowding in a dwelling unit contributes materially to mental disorder or to emotional stability." De Groot, Carroll, and Whitman (1970) conclude that ". . . the relationship between infectious phenomena and spatial variables is essentially spurious and specious. . . ." The data from the demographic studies that have been done thus far do not allow us to draw any definitive conclusions about the relationship between density and breakdown, but I think that on the whole the results from this line of work suggest at most a weak causative relationship between population density and crime, mental and physical illness, and other such variables.

Field and Observational Studies

A second approach to the problem has been to observe individuals who happen to be in situations that vary in density or who move from one level of density to another. These field studies do not have the firm controls that are present in laboratory experiments or the vast number of subjects that are present in the demographic work. On the other hand, they have the advantage of being done in relatively naturalistic settings and being on a small enough scale so that detailed measurements can be taken. Although there are countless anecdotal accounts of what happens under conditions of high density, there are unfortunately very few observational studies of a scientific nature. For example, Esser (1970) notes that autistic patients in a mental clinic respond negatively to crowding, and Leyhausen (1965) says that "nearly five years in prisoner-of-war camps taught me that over-crowded human societies reflect the symptoms of overcrowded wolf, cat, goat, mouse, rat, or rabbit communities to the last detail. . . ." These kinds of statements and observations are interesting as a source of ideas, but they do not constitute data in which we can have any confidence. The few careful field studies and laboratory experiments have generally not supported these intuitive notions gleaned from individuals' own experiences.

Mitchell (1971) conducted a detailed study of the effects of high-density housing on patterns of interaction among members of a family and on emo-tional strain manifested by the individuals. Although an earlier study by P. and M. Chombart de Lauwe (1959) suggested that density had an impor-tant effect on mental health, Mitchell found no evidence for this. His massive study conducted in Hong Kong interviewed thousands of people who lived in housing with densities ranging from below twenty-two square feet per person to over a hundred square feet per person. Except for families in the very lowest income brackets, there was no indication of a relationship between density and emotional strain. For the lowest-income families there was some effect on the amount of worrying that was reported by the respondents, with those living in less space reporting more worry-ing. But for all groups, including the lowest-income families, there was no relationship between density and symptomatic indices of emotional illness or of hostility. The author concludes that density in housing may have some effect on the kinds of interactions among members of the family, in partic-ular the amount of time that is spent in the house, but has no effect on emotionality or strain.

This does not mean, of course, that people should not have as much space as possible. There is a strong indication that given a choice people prefer larger rooms to smaller ones, larger apartments to cramped ones. That they prefer more living space, however, does not imply that the lack of space will have serious negative effects. All it means is that for aesthetic or social reasons they would like to have more space. It is perhaps surprising that given less space than they actually want, they do not seem to suffer appreciably—it does not even seem to affect their stated level of general happiness or satisfaction. On the other hand, throughout this chapter we should make the distinction between what people would like if they are actually asked and how they are affected by what they have.

Ittelson, Proshansky, and Rivlin (1970) have conducted a continuing study of behavior in psychiatric wards. They made careful observations of the behavior of the patients under varying conditions, among which were the size of the room and the number of people in it. In particular they focused on the percentage of the behavior that was social (i.e., interacting with another person). This was done in a number of hospitals, including public and private institutions, and, therefore, the findings can probably be generalized with some confidence. They report that with a few exceptions there is a higher percentage of nonsocial, passive behavior in larger rooms than in smaller ones. In other words, despite the presence of more patients, there is less social interaction.

Unfortunately, because this is not an experiment, it is difficult to interpret the finding. Patients in hospitals are not randomly assigned to rooms. To some extent assignment is based on ability to pay and the particular illness that the patient has, and the effects could be primarily or largely due to these kinds of variations. In addition the size of the room and the number of individuals in it are confounded as in most of these field studies. The larger rooms have not only more space but also more patients. Thus it is impossible to separate the effects of size from the effects of number. Since no data are given on the amount of square feet provided per patient, it is somewhat misleading to discuss the results in terms of density. Nevertheless, whatever the cause it is interesting that a smaller percentage of behavior is social in larger rooms containing more patients.

McGrew (1970) observed children at play in a nursery school in Scotland. In this study both amount of space and number of individuals being observed were varied. There were either sixteen or eight children playing in the room, and the amount of space available varied from 593 square feet to 778 square feet. Although the results were quite variable there was some suggestion that more aggressive behavior occurred when more children were present in the room. These effects are not large and are inconsistent, but they do suggest that the larger the number of individuals who have to interact, the more aggressive behavior occurs. In contrast the amount of space available had virtually no effect on the children's behavior. This is not surprising since even the highest density condition (i.e., sixteen children in the smaller room) provided thirty-seven square feet per child, which would hardly be considered crowded by most standards. In a follow-up study the author found that higher density did not increase the amount of physical contact between children, but once again this is not surprising given the amount of space available. A similar study by Hutt and Vaizey (1966) observed children at free play in either small or large groups and found that normal children were more aggressive and less social in larger groups.

The studies by McGrew and by Hutt and Vaizey both suffer from serious limitations because of the restricted sample of subjects observed. Unlike Ittelson, Proshansky, and Rivlin, who studied many different hospitals and many different subject populations, these other studies each involved only one group of children in one specific setting. This raises the possibility that the findings are specific to the particular individuals or situation. They thus must be considered more as case histories than experiments or observational studies in the usual sense.

At Columbia Judy Price and I have designed a study that is modeled closely after this work, but is not limited to one subject population. Just as in

McGrew's study children in school are observed during a free-play period under conditions of high and low density. Instead of observing only one group of children in one school, we are trying to use as many schools and groups as possible. Thus any findings must apply to at least a range of subjects and school conditions. Preliminary results based on about half the expected number of schools indicate no general effect of density on either aggressiveness or social behavior. The higher-density condition had more aggressiveness in just about as many schools as it had less aggressiveness. The study has, however, not been completed, so no final statements as to findings are possible.

Although observational studies suffer from lack of random assignment of subjects, from the lack of controls, from lack of differentiation between group size and density, and often from a concentration on only one group of individuals and therefore a lack of generalizability, this approach does strike us as a potentially fruitful one. It would be highly desirable to discover or to set up situations in natural environments in which density is varied and everything else is held constant as much as possible. Housing conditions are an obvious possibility, and classroom, playground, working conditions, and so on are also potential situations in which this might be arranged. At the present time there are very few such studies, but we can hope that many more will be done now that this is a problem of broader interest.

The existing studies have, as usual in this area, produced mixed results. Both McGrew and Hutt and Vaizey conclude from their work that high density produces an increase in aggressiveness, and Ittelson, Proshansky, and Rivlin suggest that it produces a decrease in social behavior. In contrast Mitchell, in a much longer duration study and with many more subjects, concludes that high-density housing conditions have little or no effect on emotional factors. Taking these studies at face value and ignoring whatever weaknesses they may have, this work does suggest that increasing the number of individuals who have to interact will sometimes increase the amount of aggressiveness that is expressed. On the other hand, there is no indication that the actual amount of space, that density per se, has any effect on behavior.

Experimental Studies

The lack of random assignment of subjects and the lack of control over the situation in demographic and field research make the meaning of the results ambiguous. If this kind of work had produced consistent effects of population density, it would have strongly suggested that density was the crucial variable, but other interpretations would always have been possible. The same is true, although perhaps less so, when consistent effects have not been discovered. It is always possible that the lack of consistent effects is due to the presence of other unspecified variables that are concealing or distorting the true effects of population density. In other words just as positive results would not have been definitive evidence in favor of the effect of density, so the absence of such results in relatively uncontrolled conditions does not constitute definitive evidence against it. The lack of consistent effects suggests, but by no means proves, that density per se is not a critical variable.

Some experiments have been specifically designed to test the effect of density on a number of variables. Although all of these experiments are limited to a greater or lesser extent in that they involve relatively small samples of subjects, relatively short duration of the density situation, and "unnatural" or atypical conditions, they do provide some indication of the effect of density under well-controlled conditions. Unfortunately there are very few such experiments.

One type of study that can loosely be called an experiment has been primarily concerned with the effect of isolation on individuals. Most of this research was conducted in cooperation with one or another branch of the United States Armed Forces. It was generally directed at questions involving air-raid shelters, submarines, and more recently space travel. The basic paradigm has been to put groups of two or three men in a room, isolate them totally from the outside world, and leave them there for some period of time. This work has typically and understandably involved relatively few groups of subjects. It is obviously a massive and expensive operation to isolate individuals for periods of time ranging up to three weeks, and very few researchers have the facilities to do it for even one group at a time. The other problem is that in most of the studies there is no adequate control group. For example, two men isolated in a 144-square-foot room for ten days are compared to two other men who simply live in a barracks during that period and work on the same kinds of tasks as the isolated men do. Obviously this is not the kind of control that we would like to see for purposes of assessing the true effect of isolation. Ideally the control would be as similar as possible to the isolated group rather than differing on so many dimensions. Perhaps an adequate control would be a group of two men who lived in an identical room for the identical period of time, but were allowed interaction with the outside world through windows or telephones and therefore differed only in the level of isolation they were enduring. Unfortunately, therefore, the research generally suffers from a number of serious methodological problems. Despite these weaknesses the research is interesting and closely related to problems of density.

An experiment by Haythorn, Altman, and Meyers (1966) compared groups of two men who were isolated for ten days with controls who were not isolated. The major emphasis was on the amount of stress felt by the various groups. There was a slight tendency for the isolates to report and manifest more stress, but the effects were generally quite small.[2]

Taylor, Wheeler, and Altman (1968) kept groups of two in a room for eight days and told some subjects that they would be in for four days and some that they would be in for twenty. Half of the groups were provided with two rooms, so that each of the members could have total privacy if he wanted it; half did not have the possibility of obtaining privacy. The subjects who were expecting a twenty-day period of isolation were generally more anxious throughout the study than those who were expecting only four. More important for our purposes is the difference between the privacy and nonprivacy conditions. The nonprivacy condition can be considered a high-density condition since the individuals had less space and were also forced into interactions more often. The results indicated that the privacy subjects were *more* anxious throughout the experiment than the nonprivacy groups. A second paper (Altman, Taylor, and Wheeler, 1971) reported that privacy groups performed less well on group tasks than nonprivacy groups.

These findings are especially interesting in the light of the emphasis that many writers have placed on the need for privacy. Many who are concerned about crowding and tend to attribute harmful effects to it have asserted that the key element is that privacy is difficult to obtain in situations of high population density. They have further stated that this lack of privacy produces severe negative effects (see Esser, 1970, for example). It is important to note that the results of these studies run exactly counter to this general notion. These may be special cases for one reason or another, but it is striking that this evidence on privacy indicates less anxiety and superior performance when privacy is *not* provided. While it seems likely that people do require some privacy and may be adversely affected if they do not get it, we have no evidence to support this, and it may be that privacy is less crucial than has been suspected.

Altman and Haythorn (1967) compared two-man groups isolated for ten days with nonisolated controls in their performance on three different tasks: a monitoring task performed by each of the men individually, and decoding and information processing tasks performed by the two men together. All of the differences between isolation and nonisolation groups were quite small, but there was some tendency for the isolation groups to do better than the controls on both of the group tasks and slightly worse on the individual task. In other words when they had to work together the groups that were isolated for ten days actually did better than did nonisolated groups. It might also be pointed out that the men were assigned to groups

---

[2] It should be pointed out that for all of this research the appropriate unit of analysis is the whole group rather than the individuals in it since obviously they are closely interrelated and not independent observations. Unfortunately the authors of this article, as well as other researchers in this field (e.g., Griffitt and Veitch, 1971, which will be described later), do the inappropriate analysis based on individuals. This distorts the strength of the result and makes it very difficult for the reader to assess their findings.

on the basis of tests that were supposed to choose compatible and incompatible groups. This group-composition factor was relatively unimportant, and the incompatible groups actually did slightly better on the tasks.

Finally in a recent unpublished study (Smith and Haythorn, 1971) density was varied explicitly. Two- and three-man groups were placed in either small (70 cubic feet) or large (200 cubic feet) rooms for twenty-one days. Thus the size of the group and the amount of space available were varied to some extent independently of each other. A great many measures of stress, anxiety, hostility, and annoyance were taken, but unfortunately only preliminary results are available at the moment. The major results for our purposes concern the effect of group size and density. The authors report the striking finding that two-man groups manifest more stress and more annoyance than three-man groups. This holds regardless of the amount of space that is available. The size of the room had no overall effect on the amount of stress manifested. Toward the end of the study there was some tendency for three-man groups to have more stress when crowded than when uncrowded, but this was somewhat reversed for the two-man groups and in any case was not consistent throughout the time period. The size of the room did, however, have a substantial and consistent effect on the amount of hostility expressed toward others in the group. There was less hositility expressed in the small than in the large room, regardless of the size of the group. In other words, in this study high density reduced rather than increased hostility.

This research on isolation is difficult to interpret. As we have said, there are not generally adequate controls, and the data analyses are often performed incorrectly. In addition, subjects who would volunteer or be required to serve in isolation studies may be quite different from the typical population. Nevertheless, it is impressive that the isolation groups show so little disruption and are sometimes even more efficient than nonisolated groups and that more space and the possibility of privacy do not necessarily have a beneficial effect—they may even produce more stress and hostility than less space or the absence of privacy. Once again, these findings must be considered suggestive rather than definitive, but there is certainly no evidence from this line of work that either isolation or density has strongly negative or aversive effects.

In addition to these experiments on isolation, there are a small number dealing with the use of space and more specifically with the effects of high density. Hall (1959, 1966) and Sommer (1959, 1961, 1969) have been concerned with how people use a given amount of space, how close they stand to each other, whether or not they move away from each other, what effects space has on social interaction, and so on. Although this work has not involved conditions that would ordinarily be considered "crowded" and does not vary density, it is certainly relevant to our concerns. Sommer in particular has conducted experiments and careful observations dealing with people's reactions to restrictions on their privacy, their territory, or more generally the space that they consider theirs. For example, he has shown that under most circumstances people will consider it an intrusion if someone sits down in a chair right next to them in a library when there are chairs available further away. Under these conditions the individual who is intruded upon will often move away. This work has also detailed some of the implications of spacing, such as the fact that seating arrangements are determined by and determine leadership in a group and how much interaction takes place. None of these experiments tells us anything specific about the effects of high density, but they do indicate that the amount of space available and its arrangement is an important factor in determining human behavior.

This brings us finally to experiments specifically designed to investigate the effects of density. In a recently published study Griffitt and Veitch (1971) put subjects in a sixty-three-square-foot room for about an hour. In half of the conditions three to five subjects occupied the room; in the other half of the conditions the number of subjects was twelve to sixteen. The subjects rated themselves on their subjective feelings of pleasantness, unpleasantness, comfortableness, uncomfortableness, and so on, performed a simple cancellation task, and rated how much they thought they would like a stranger who was described to them in terms of his responses to a series of issues. The subjects were run in either all-male or all-female groups. The results indicate that the larger groups report being less comfortable, that the experiment was less pleasant, and generally give more negative responses in describing their affective feelings. In addition they are more negative toward the stranger than are the smaller groups. There was no effect on performance of the simple cancellation task, nor do the authors report any sex differences. The statistical analysis of these data is done using the individual subject as the unit rather than the group, which, as noted earlier, is inappropriate and makes assessing the strength and reliability of the results difficult. In addition the density in the room is confounded with the size of the groups. Nevertheless, it does seem that this procedure produced some negative response to the combination of size and density.

One possibly important aspect of this experimental method is that the subjects are not interacting and are not in any sense a group. In fact they were placed in the room in such a way as to minimize face-to-face contact and did not talk throughout the study. In other words, rather than this being a group phenomenon, it is primarily a situation in which individuals find themselves either comfortably seated or uncomfortably crowded in a small room for no apparent reason and are then asked to perform a number of tasks and given a number of responses. This somewhat rarefied, unusual condition does produce negative responses, but it is difficult to interpret the finding.

A series of studies by the present author and his colleagues have investigated the effects of density on a number of different variables. The first group of experiments (Freedman, Klevansky, and Ehrlich, 1971) involved the effects of density on task performance. Density was varied by using rooms of 160, 80, and 35 square feet and placing either nine or five subjects in each room. The idea was that both number of subjects and the amount of space available were varied independently, and the effect of size of the group and density could then be assessed separately. In the first experiment subjects participated for three successive days four hours a day. They worked on six different tasks that were chosen to include simple mechanical operations, straightforward memory, concentration, and relatively complex creative manipulations. The tasks were:

1. A crossing-out task in which the subject was given a sheet containing random numbers and told to cross out all of a particular number that he could find.
2. A forming-words task in which the group was read six letters and told to form as many different English words as they could from these letters.
3. An objects-uses task in which a common object is described (e.g., a ten-gallon metal barrel), and each subject suggests as many different unique uses for it as he can.
4. A memory task in which twelve common words are read aloud at the rate of one per second, and the subject has to write down as many as he can after the reading is completed.
5. A concentration task in which clicks are sounded at the rate of about three per second at an unfixed rhythm, and the subject has to count them.
6. An object-uses task this time with the whole group working on it together.

The tasks were performed twice during each session in order to assess the effect of time spent in the room.

There were no effects whatsoever attributable to differences in density or group size. Subjects did as well when they were crowded as when they were not; high density neither facilitated nor interfered with their performance on either simple or complex tasks; and there was no indication that density produced greater effects over time.

Two additional experiments were conducted to verify this result. The second experiment was identical to the first except that only three of the tasks were used in order to maximize the likelihood of fatigue and boredom. The third experiment was identical to the second except that rather than high school students who served in the first, it involved women between the ages of twenty-five and sixty who were recruited through a temporary employment agency. In none of the experiments was there any indication that density affected performance. In all experiments for both populations and for all tasks, groups did as well under high-density conditions as they did under low-density conditions. This finding seems reliable at least for the conditions employed here.

Our second series of studies (Freedman, Levy, Price, Welte, Katz, and Ehrlich, 1971) indicated that interpersonal behavior *is* affected by crowding. We now have evidence that degree of density influences competitiveness, severity of sentencing, and liking for others. But the effects are not simple. The fascinating aspect of this work is that men and women seem to respond in opposite ways to the level of crowding we have used.

We placed high school boys or girls in either small or large rooms for four hours. During the first three hours they engaged in informal personal talk, in relatively normal discussions of complicated problems, and in a game requiring close cooperation. During the last hour the groups played a modified game of Prisoner's Dilemma in which each player could choose either a cooperative or competitive strategy on a series of trials. We were interested primarily in the number of cooperative choices as a function of crowding. Men competed more in the crowded room; women were less affected by room size, but competed somewhat less in the crowded room.

A second experiment used a different setting, different subject population, and different measures but obtained comparable results. Men and women over eighteen were recruited by classified newspaper ads in New York. The subjects ranged in age from seventeen to eighty and represented a wide variety of ethnic groups and educational and income levels. Once again, they were placed in either a large or small room for approximately four hours. During that time they first engaged in informal discussion and then listened to a series of taped courtroom cases for which they served as the jury. The group discussed some cases openly and did not discuss others, but for all cases each individual indicated his own decision separately and privately. In addition the subjects responded to a questionnaire on which they were asked how much they liked the other members of the group, how much they enjoyed the session, and other similar questions designed to measure their subjective reactions to the experience.

The pattern of results was similar to that of the previous experiment. Just as before, the men responded more negatively to the small room, while the women showed the opposite tendency. The men gave somewhat more severe sentences in the smaller room than they did in the larger room, while the women were more lenient in the smaller room. Unlike the previous result, however, this difference between rooms was much stronger for the women than for the men. Crowding had an even stronger effect on the individual's subjective reactions. The men in the small room found the experience less pleasant, liked the other members less, considered them less friendly, and thought they would make a less good jury than the men in the large room; whereas every difference was reversed for women, who rated the experience more pleasant, the other members more likable, friendlier, and a better jury in the small room than in the large room. When both men and women were included in a group, all effects of density disappeared. For mixed-sex groups there was no difference between crowded and uncrowded conditions, nor for the men or women in each group taken separately.

Thus the results are consistent for both studies. Apparently all male groups respond negatively to crowded conditions; they become suspicious and combative, almost as if they were showing the territoriality described in animals. Women respond positively; they seem to like the high density and become more intimate and friendly. And when men and women are mixed there are no effects of density.

As with the other kinds of research on this problem, the results of the experimental studies are somewhat inconsistent. Although our work agrees with that of Griffitt and Veitch and the isolation study by Altman and Haythorn (1967) in that density had little or no effect on task performance, the various studies disagree considerably in the effects they found on stress and interpersonal behavior. Griffitt and Veitch found that larger, more crowded groups were less comfortable, less happy, and manifested more negative interpersonal reactions. They also found no differences between all male and all female groups on these variables. In contrast Freedman et al. (1971) showed that all male groups were more competitive and aggressive and liked each other less when they were crowded than when they were not crowded, but all female groups generally reacted positively to the higher density conditions. And mixed groups showed no consistent responses to density. Smith and Haythorn (1971) actually report less hostility in crowded than in uncrowded conditions. In other words, if we take all of these results at face value and weight the studies equally, the one consistent result is the lack of effect on performance, while the negative result for males is found in several studies and not in another; the negative result for females is found in only one study, while positive results for females are found in two. I naturally have a tendency to trust the findings of my own research somewhat more than those of the others, and, therefore, it is probably inappropriate to try to differentiate among the various experiments at this point. It may, however, be useful to repeat that the Griffitt and Veitch study confounds the size of the group and density and involves a very unusual, nonsocial situation, while both the Smith and Haythorn and the Freedman et al. studies varied density independently of the size of the group and the latter studies involved considerably more realistic situations. Thus if one wanted to generalize from this work, it seems reasonable to lean somewhat more heavily on these latter studies.

All in all, despite the fairly consistent findings in the series of studies by the present author, the experimental research on the effects of density has produced mixed results. There is certainly no strong, consistent demonstration of either negative or positive effects of density on interpersonal or affective behavior, and there seems to be strong evidence that density does not adversely affect performance. The sex differences are intriguing, but perhaps more weight should be given to the finding that mixed groups show no effects at all. This line of research, therefore, suggests that density probably does not have overall negative effects on human beings, at least for the relatively short-term durations involved in the experimental studies. Instead, it suggests that whatever effects density does have will probably turn out to be quite complex, will depend in large part on the particular situation, and may also depend on characteristics of the individuals involved. This does not, of course, mean that density is unimportant; it merely means that short exposures to highly dense conditions do not have the strongly negative effects that some have feared.

Summary and Conclusions

There is strong and reasonably consistent evidence that high density, or perhaps the presence of large numbers of individuals that have to interact, produces negative effects in a wide variety of nonhuman animals. These effects include increased adrenal size, decreased testes size, and severe breakdowns in social and reproductive behavior. Many authors have been tempted to generalize from this work on nonhumans to human response to density, but this is a dangerous and questionable generalization. As this review of the literature has shown, there is in fact no substantial evidence that high density produces consistently negative effects on humans. Large-scale survey and demographic studies have generally failed to find an effect of density when other factors are controlled; observational studies in the field have produced mixed results; and controlled experimental studies have, with a few exceptions, found either no effects of density or complex, inconsistent effects.

It should be made clear that the amount of evidence available is far too little and much of it too confused for us to be able to draw any firm, definitive conclusions about the effects of density on human behavior. The crucial point is that statements about the negative effects of density on human beings are simply not justified by the data. As of now, the statement that coincides most closely with the results of the research is that within a wide range density is probably not a terribly important factor in determining human behavior and that what effects there are tend to be inconsistent and are therefore probably dependent on complicated and as yet unspecified variables in the situation. Additional research may, of course, warrant entirely different conclusions. Perhaps studies in the future will prove that density does have severe negative effects or that it does have these effects under conditions that can be specified. On the other hand, additional research may prove just the opposite—that density often has positive effects. All that we can say is that no such evidence exists now.

Based on my own research and the other available data, I would guess (and it is only a guess) that density per se is not particularly detrimental to humans. The other factors that tend to accompany crowding are, of course, very serious. High concentrations of people in one spot or too many people in the world as a whole cause problems in terms of food supply, strains on natural resources, pollution, and so on. But given a certain number of people in the world, we can ask whether it is harmful to have them concentrated in certain areas rather than having them spread more or less equally over the livable areas, and I suspect it is not.

I do think that the research may have been focusing on the wrong variable. Whereas density is not important, there is evidence from both animal and human research that substantial effects may be due to the absolute number of individuals who must interact. That is, assuming that the space available is small enough or arranged in such a way that individuals in it must interact, the sheer number of individuals is crucial. The effects need not be negative. I am simply suggesting that the number of individuals who must interact, rather than density, is the variable that produces substantial effects on human behavior.

Of course, the amount of space is not entirely irrelevant. Thirty children in a playground may fight, socialize, and even cooperate more than ten children; and the effect may occur equally in playgrounds of 200 square feet and 1,500 square feet. But a two-square-mile playground would probably eliminate the effect since the children might not interact at all. Nevertheless, within broad limits the amount of space and accordingly the population density would be relatively unimportant.

This is sheer speculation at the moment, but it does seem to fit much of the data reasonably well and also coincides to some extent with the generally held intuition that "something" about large numbers of people in one place has an effect. This intuition is often translated in terms of density, but given the results of the research, this seems unlikely. Instead, numbers may be the critical factor, for both good and bad, and perhaps the research should focus more on this in the future.

Finally the present review suggests to me that we should not be surprised to find our great cities continuing to function despite tremendous crowding; nor to find that the relative decrease in population in the cities that has occurred in recent years has not alleviated the problems that do exist. The monumental problems facing our cities do not seem to be caused by high densities. The problems would be just as great or greater if the cities covered twice as much area. Rather, the problems are due largely to economic and racial strains and to inefficient and sometimes irresponsible use of the available resources. It may well be that within the limits of the environment to supply their needs, high concentrations of humans are good rather than bad, or at least no more bad than good. Perhaps the positive effects such as interstimulation, feelings of intimacy, and excitement balance the difficulties in terms of the logistics of getting downtown and the problems of walking comfortably on crowded streets. This is, of course, highly speculative, and I say it as one who loves big cities; but I do think that the present findings and some others that are slowly appearing indicate that overpopulation should be worried about primarily in terms of its effect on the environment and the difficulties it causes in terms of supplying needs, rather than because of its psychological effects on humans. In particular, the problems of the cities should be seen in terms of poverty and bad transportation, in terms of logistics and supply, jobs and housing, resources and planning, rather than attributing the problems to the inherent evils of high density that may simply not exist.

REFERENCES

Ader, R. 1965. Effects of early experience and differential housing on behavior and susceptibility to gastric erosions in the rat. *Journal of Comparative and Physiological Psychology* 60:233.

Ader, R.; Kreutner, A., Jr.; and Jacobs, H. L. 1963. Social environment, emotionality and alloxan diabetes in the rat. *Psychosomatic Medicine* 25:60.

Altman, I.; Taylor, D. A.; and Wheeler, L. 1971. Ecological aspects of group behavior in social isolation. *Journal of Applied Social Psychology* 1:76–100.

Altman, I. and Haythorn, W. W. 1967. The effects of social isolation and group composition on performance. *Human Relations* 4:313–340.

Barnett, S. A. 1955. Competition among wild rats. *Nature* 175:126.

Brain, P. F. and Nowell, N. W. 1971. Isolation versus grouping effects on adrenal and gonadal functions in albino mice. 1. The male. *General and Comparative Endocrinology* 16:149–154.

Calhoun, J. B. 1961. Phenomena associated with population density. *Proceedings of the National Academy of Science* 47:428–449.

———. 1962a. Population density and social pathology. *Scientific American* 206:139–148.

———. 1962b. A "behavioral sink." In E. L. Bliss, ed., *Roots of behavior.* New York: Harper.

Chitty, D. 1955. Adverse effects of population density upon the viability of later generations. In J. B. Craig and N. W. Pirie, eds., *The number of man and animals.* London: Oliver & Boyd.

Chombart de Lauwe, P. and Chombart de Lauwe, M. 1959. *Psychopathologie sociale de l'enfant inadapte.* Paris: Centre National de la Recherche Scientifique.

Christian, J. J. 1950. The adreno-pituitary system and population cycles in mammals. *Journal of Mammology* 31:247–259.

———. 1955. Effect of population size on the adrenal glands and reproductive organs of male mice in populations of fixed size. *American Journal of Physiology* 182:292–300.

———. 1956. Adrenal and reproductive responses to population size in mice from freely growing populations. *Ecology* 37:258–273.

———. 1959. Lack of correlation between adrenal weight and injury in grouped male albino mice. *Proceedings of the Society of Experimental Biology and Medicine* 101:166–168.

———. 1963. Endocrine adaptive mechanisms and the physiologic regulation of population growth. In W. V. Mayer and R. G. Van Gelder, eds., *Physiological Mammology.* New York: Academic Press 1:189–353.

Christian, J. J. and Davis, D. E. 1956. The relationship between adrenal weight and population status of urban Norway rats. *Journal of Mammology* 37:475–486.

Christian, J. J.; Flyger, V.; and Davis, D. C. 1960. Factors in the mass mortality of a herd of sika deer *cervus nippon. Chesapeake Science* 1:79–95.

Christian, J. J.; Lloyd, J. A.; and Davis, D. E. 1965. The role of endocrines in the self-regulation of mammalian populations. *Recent Progress in Hormone Research* 21:501–578.

Clark, J. R. 1955. Influence of numbers on reproduction and survival in two experimental role populations. *Proceedings of the Royal Society* (London), B144:68–85.

Clough, G. C. 1965. Lemmings and population problems. *American Scientist* 53:199–212.

———. 1968. Social behavior and ecology of Norwegian lemmings during a population peak and crash. *Papers of the Norwegian State Game Research Institute,* Vol. 2, no. 28.

Conger, J. J.; Sawrey, W. L.; and Turrell, E. S. 1958. The role of social experience in the production of gastric ulcers in hooded rats placed in a conflict situation. *Journal of Abnormal and Social Psychology* 57:214.

Davis, D. E. and Christian, J. J. 1957. Relation of adrenal weight to social rank in mice. *Proceedings of the Society of Experimental Biology and Medicine* 94:728–731.

Deevey, E. S. 1960. The hare and the haruspex: a cautionary tale. *American Scientist* 48:415–429.

De Groot, I.; Carroll, R. L.; and Whitman, R. M. 1970. Human health and the spatial environment. Position paper for the First Invitational Conference on Health Research in Housing and Its Environment, Warrentown, Va., March 1970.

Dubos, R. 1970. The social environment. In H. M. Proshansky, W. H. Ittelson, and L. G. Rivlin, eds., *Environmental Psychology.* New York: Holt, Rinehart & Winston. Pp. 202–208.

Esser, A. H. 1970. Psychopathological aspects of crowding (human pollution). Talk delivered at the American Psychological Association Convention, Miami, 1970.

Faris, R. and Dunham, H. W. 1965. *Mental disorders in urban areas.* Chicago: University of Chicago Press, Phoenix Books (orig. ed., 1939).

Freedman, J. L.; Klevansky, S.; and Ehrlich, P. 1971. The effect of crowding on human task performance. *Journal of Applied Social Psychology* 1:7–25.

Freedman, J. L.; Levy, A.; Price, J.; Welte, R.; Katz, M.; and Ehrlich, P. 1971. The effect of density on human aggression and affective reactions. In preparation, 1971.

Friedman, S. B.; Lowell, A. G.; and Ader, R. 1970. Differential susceptibility to a viral agent in mice housed alone or in groups. *Psychosomatic Medicine* 32:285–299.

Green, H. W. 1939. Persons admitted to Cleveland State Hospital, 1928–1937. Cleveland: Cleveland Health Council.

Griffitt, W. and Veitch, R. 1971. Hot and crowded: influences of population density and temperature on interpersonal affective behavior. *Journal of Personality and Social Psychology* 17:92–98.

Hall, E. T. 1959. *The silent language.* New York: Doubleday.

———. 1966. *The hidden dimension.* New York: Doubleday.

Haythorn, W. W.; Altman, I.; and Meyers, T. I. 1966. Emotional symptomatology and stress in isolated pairs of men. *Journal of Experimental Research in Personality* 4: 290–306.

Holford, Sir W. 1970. The built environment: its creation, motivations and control. In H. M. Proshansky, W. H. Ittelson and L. G. Rivlin, eds., *Environmental Psychology.* New York: Holt, Rinehart & Winston. Pp. 549–560.

Hollingshead, A. B. and Redlich, F. C. 1958. *Social class and mental illness.* New York: Wiley.

Hutt, C. and McGrew, W. C. 1967. Effects of group density upon social behavior in humans. Paper presented in Symposium on Changes in Behavior with Population Density at Association for the Study of Animal Behavior meetings, Oxford, July 1967.

Hutt, C. and Vaizey, M. J. 1966. Differential effects of group density on social behavior. *Nature* 209:1371–1372.

Ittelson, W. H.; Proshansky, H. M.; and Rivlin, L. G. 1970. The environmental psychology of the psychiatric ward. In H. M. Proshansky, W. H. Ittelson, and L. G. Rivlin, eds., *Environmental Psychology.* New York: Holt, Rinehart & Winston. Pp. 419–439.

Jacobs, J. 1962. *Death and life of great American cities.* London: Cape, 1962.

Landis, C. and Page, J. D. 1938. *Modern society and mental disease.* New York: Farrar & Rinehart.

Leyhausen, P. 1965. The sane community—a density problem? *Discovery* 26:27–33.

Lorenz, K. S. 1966. *On aggression.* New York: Harcourt.

Louch, C. D. 1956. Adrenocortical activity in relation to the density and dynamics of three confined populations of *Microtus pennsylvanicus. Ecology* 37:701–713.

McGrew, W. C. 1970. Group density and children's behavior. Unpublished paper.

McKeever, S. 1959. Effects of reproductive activity on the weight of adrenal glands in *Mocrotus montanus. The Anatomical Record* 135:1–5.

Marsden, H. M. 1970. Crowding and animal behavior. Talk delivered at the American Psychological Association Convention, Miami, 1970.

Mitchell, R. E. 1971. Some social implications of high density housing. *American Sociological Review* 36:18–29.

Morris, J. N. 1964. *Uses of Epidemiology*. Baltimore: Williams & Wilkins. P. 29.

Morrison, B. J. and Thatcher, K. 1969. Overpopulation effects on social reduction of emotionality in the albino rat. *Journal of Comparative and Physiological Psychology* 69:658–662.

The National Commission on the Causes and Prevention of Violence. 1970. *To establish justice, to insure domestic tranquility*. New York: Praeger.

Plaut, S. M.; Ader, R.; Friedman, S. B.; and Ritterson, A. L. 1969. Social factors in resistance to malaria in the mouse: effects of groups vs. individual housing on resistance to plamodium berghei infection. *Psychosomatic Medicine* 31:536–552.

Pollock, H. M. and Furbush, A. M. 1921. Mental disease in 12 states, 1919. *Mental Hygiene* 5:353–389.

Pressman, I. and Carol, A. 1969. Crime as a diseconomy of scale. Talk delivered at convention of the Operations Research Society of America, Denver, Colo., June 1969.

Proshansky, H. M.; Ittelson, W. H.; and Rivlin, L. G. 1970. Freedom of choice and behavior in a physical setting. In H. M. Proshansky, W. H. Ittelson, and L. G. Rivlin, eds., *Environmental psychology*. New York: Holt, Rinehart & Winston. Pp. 173–183.

Queen, S. A. 1940. The ecological study of mental disorders. *American Sociological Review* 5:201–209.

Schmid, C. 1933. Suicide in Minneapolis, Minnesota, 1928–1932. *American Journal of Sociology* 39:30–49.

———. 1955. Completed and attempted suicides. *American Sociological Review* 20: 273–283.

———. 1960. Urban crime areas. *American Sociological Review* 25:527, 542, 655–678.

Schmitt, R. C. 1957. Density, delinquency, and crime in Honolulu. *Sociology and Social Research* 41:274–276.

———. 1966. Density, health, and social disorganization. *Journal of American Institute of Planners* 32:38–40.

Shaw, C. and McKay, H. D. 1942. *Juvenile delinquency and urban areas*. Chicago: University of Chicago Press.

Siegel, H. S. 1959. The relation between crowding and weight of adrenal glands in chickens. *Ecology* 40:494–498.

———. 1960. Effect of population density on the pituitary-adrenal cortical axis of cockerels. *Poultry Science* 39:500–510.

Smith, J.; Form, W.; and Stone, G. 1954. Local intimacy in a middle-sized city. *American Journal of Sociology* 60:276–285.

Smith, S. and Haythorn, W. W. 1971. The effects of compatability, crowding, group size and leadership seniority on stress. anxiety, hostility and annoyance in isolated groups. Unpublished data.

Smith, S. 1969. Studies of small groups in confinement. In J. P. Zubek, ed., *Sensory Deprivation: Fifteen Years of Research*. New York: Appleton-Century-Crofts.

Snyder, R. L. 1968. Reproduction and population pressures. In E. Stellar and J. M. Sprague, eds., *Progress in Physiological Psychology*. New York: Academic Press 2: 119–160.

Sommer, R. 1959. Studies in personal space. *Sociometry* 22:247–260.

———. 1961. Leadership and group geography. *Sociometry* 24:99–110.

———. 1969. *Personal space: the behavioral basis of design*. Englewood Cliffs, N.J.: Prentice-Hall.

Southwick, C. H. 1955a. The population dynamics of confined house mice supplied with unlimited food. *Ecology* 36:212–225.

———. 1955b. Regulatory mechanisms in house mouse populations. Social behavior affecting litter survival. *Ecology* 36:627–634.

———. 1967. An experimental study of intragroup agonistic behavior in rhesus monkeys (*Macaca mulatta*). *Behavior* 28:182–209.

Southwick, C. H. and Bland, V. P. 1959. Effect of population density on adrenal glands and reproductive organs of CFW mice. *American Journal of Physiology* 197:111–114.

Taylor, D. A.; Wheeler, L.; and Altman, I. 1968. Stress relations in socially isolated groups. *Journal of Personality and Social Psychology* 9:369–376.

Thiessen, D. D. 1964. Population density, mouse genotype, and endocrine function in behavior. *Journal of Comparative and Physiological Psychology* 57:412–416.

Thiessen, D. D. and Rodgers, D. W. 1961. Population density and endocrine function. *Psychological Bulletin* 58:441–451.

Thiessen, D. D.; Zolman, J. F.; and Rodgers, D. A. 1962. Relation between adrenal weight, brain cholinesterase activity, and hole-in-wall behavior of mice under different living conditions. *Journal of Comparative Physiological Psychology* 55:186.

Tobach, E. and Bloch, H. 1956. Effect of stress by crowding prior to and following tuberculosis infection. *American Journal of Physiology* 187:399–407.

Wilner, D. M. and Baer, W. G. 1970. Sociocultural factors in residential space. Environmental Control Administration, Health, Education and Welfare Department, 1970.

Winsborough, H. H. 1965. The social consequences of high population density. *Law and Contemporary Problems* 30:120–126.

Wynne-Edwards, V. C. 1965. Self-regulating systems in populations of animals. *Science* 147:1543–1548.

Zlutnick, S. and Altman, I. 1971. *Crowding and human behavior* (in press).

PART IV

Research on Methods of Birth Control

[9]

PSYCHOLOGICAL STUDIES
IN ABORTION

HENRY P. DAVID

Abortion is as old as humanity and probably universal in all cultures. Throughout history women have resorted to abortion to terminate unwanted pregnancies, regardless of religious or legal sanctions and often at considerable actual or psychological pain, physical risk, and financial cost (Devereux, 1955; Tietze and Lewit, 1969). An ancient Chinese medical text, said to have been written about 5,000 years ago, contains a recipe for the induction of abortion by mercury. Hippocrates recommended violent exercises as the best method (Tietze and Lewit, 1969).

As used by most physicians, the term "abortion" denotes the termination of a pregnancy before the fetus has attained viability; that is, before the fetus becomes capable of independent life outside the uterus. "Viability is usually defined in terms of duration of pregnancy and/or weight of fetus, or occasionally length of fetus" (World Health Organization, 1970, p. 6). A recent World Health Organization survey revealed considerable variation in the definitions used in different countries. Traditionally the twenty-eighth week of gestation has been identified with viability. More recently the twentieth week has gained the acceptance of the medical profession (Tietze, 1971). From a clinical point of view it is important to make a further distinction between abortions performed before and after the twelfth week of pregnancy. While there is general consensus that abortion continues to be the most widely practiced method of fertility control throughout the world, "the absence of records, which prevails to the present, makes

NOTE: Based in part on material gathered with grant support from the Center for Population Research (National Institute of Child Health and Human Development), the Ford Foundation, and the van Ameringen Foundation. I am pleased to acknowledge the continuing counsel of Christopher Tietze, who encouraged my initial interest, and the helpful suggestions made by Emily Moore.

any estimate of the extent of its practice almost entirely a matter of con-jecture" (Tietze, 1969a, p. 311).

The frequently cited figure of one million abortions per year in the United States cannot be readily substantiated. Effective procedures for centralized data collection, even for legal abortions, have not yet been extablished at the federal level or, with few exceptions, at the state level (Calderone, 1958; Gebhard, 1958; Bates and Zawadski, 1964; Lader, 1966; Niswander, Klein, and Randall, 1966; Smith, 1967; Beck, Newman, and Lewit, 1969; Tietze, 1970d). The limited verifiable American data suggest that until recently abortion by qualified practitioners has been most readily available to well-to-do white women (Gold, Erhardt, Jacobzinger, and Nelson, 1965; Tietze, 1969b). At this writing there is little basis for disagree-ment with Tietze's (1969a, p. 311) assertion that "induced abortion, and particularly illegal abortion, constitutes one of the major areas of ignorance within the scope of public health and population studies." At the same time, as Potts (1970a, p. 65) has noted, "no human community has ever shown a marked fall in the birthrate without a significant recourse to in-duced abortion." It is unlikely that presently available contraceptive procedures alone will suffice to reduce significantly population growth in developing nations wishing to lower their birth rate.

Abortion as a topic of systematic inquiry has been of special interest only to a small number of scientists. This is apparent from reviews of the world-wide abortion situation (Geijerstam, 1969; Callahan, 1970; David, 1970; Dourlen-Rollier, 1969; Hall, 1970a; Klinger, 1966; Mehlan, 1968; Muramatsu, 1967; Potts, 1970c; and Tietze, 1969a). It is a curious phenome-non that behavioral scientists have made rather limited contributions; for example, there are few well-designed studies of the effects of granted or denied abortions on the women concerned, their families, or society. In reviews of abortion research the same limited data tend to be cited repeat-edly, at times to support divergent opinions. However, interdisciplinary and transnational research approaches are increasing, stimulated by workshops, greater availability of funds, and a growing awareness among behavioral scientists of many nations of a social responsibility to contribute professional skills to an area touching the lives of so many individuals (Beck et al., 1969; Newman, Beck, and Lewit, 1970; David and Szabady, 1969; David and Bernheim, 1970).

Free association to the word "abortion" would probably yield a wide range of emotional responses, depending in part on age, marital status, religion, and nationality (Rossi, 1969). The many diverse "dogmas" and "beliefs" hovering around the concept of abortion have been dissected by Pohlman (1970) and by Sloane (1971). Blake (1971) extensively ana-lyzed the differences and changes in abortion views among representative groups of white Americans during the decade 1960 to 1970. She concluded that "it is to the educated and the influential that we must look for effect-ing rapid legislative change in spite of conservative opinions among important subgroups such as lower classes and women" (p. 548). It may well be decades before most Americans are willing to accept more neutral terms such as "pregnancy termination," which the British adopted in naming their 1967 abortion law, or the more recently suggested "postconception planning" (David, 1971a).

The purpose of this chapter is to present an overview of psychological studies in abortion, to cite major conclusions and weaknesses, and to suggest possible directions for future cooperative research. The term "psychological" is broadly defined; it includes psychiatric aspects. After a brief historical sketch of abortion legislation and practice, psychological sequelae of abortion are surveyed in terms of a perspective based on studies of pregnancy and spontaneous abortion, followed by a review of psychological effects of denied abortion. Subsequently psychological indications for abortion are discussed in relation to present practices in the United States, including the personal, ethical, and moral dilemma faced by many members of the medical and paramedical professions. Repeated abortion-seeking behavior is considered, along with the need for research on the decision-making process in pregnancy acceptance and termination. The potential impact of the prostaglandins on "postconception planning" is noted, along with the emerging opportunities for meaningful psychosocial studies and the complexities of behavioral research on the interrelationship of abortion and contraception.

Historical Sketch of Abortion Legislation and Practice

Under common law (that body of legal rules derived from decisions of judges based upon accepted customs and traditions) abortion was not considered an offense if performed with the woman's consent before she was "quick with child." Quickening marks the time of the first recognizable movements of the fetus, usually appearing around the sixteenth week of gestation. Except for a brief interlude in the sixteenth century, Christianity did not officially concern itself with pregnancy prevention or termination until 1869, when Pope Pius IX in his Constitution *Apostolicae Sedis* "made a sharp change in Church law by eliminating any distinction between a formed and unformed fetus in meting out the penalty of excommunication for abortion" (Callahan, 1970, p. 413). Diverse Catholic positions and other ethical issues have been sensitively reviewed by Callahan (1970), Means (1970), and Noonan (1967). Historical trends in psychiatry and abortion have also been summarized in the volumes edited by Hall (1970a) and Rosen (1954) and in the papers by Schwartz (1968), Levene and Ringney (1970), Sloane (1970), and others.

Surgical abortion before quickening was first prohibited in Britain by

Lord Ellenborough's Act of 1803 and subsequently in the United States by a section of the New York Revised Statutes of 1829 (enacted in 1828). The New York legislation was the earliest Anglo-American statute containing an express therapeutic exception, justifying abortion "if necessary to preserve the life of the mother" (Means, 1970). A careful review of documents contemporary with the passage of the legislation, as cited by Means (1970) and by Polsky (1970), demonstrates that the primary concern at the time was with the health of the woman, not with the life of the fetus before "quickening." This was the pre-Lister era of medicine when every operation endangered the patient's life through the grim possibility of infection, which physicians did not yet fully understand and could not control. In some hospitals one operation in every three ended in death. A hysterotomy (abortion by the abdominal approach) meant death to every second woman operated upon, whereas only 2 percent died in childbirth. Anesthesia, antibiotics, and blood banks were still to be developed (Hall, 1970b; Rosen, 1970).

By 1850 eleven more American states had followed the lead of New York. Only in New Jersey did one of the statutes receive a judicial construction by a contemporary court, explaining why the legislation had been passed: "The design of the statute was not to prevent the procuring of abortions, so much as to guard the health and life of the mother against the consequences of such attempts" (cited by Means, 1970, p. 140). Gradually the rest of the states followed suit, usually prohibiting abortion for any purposes other than to preserve the life of the mother. The last state to act was Mississippi in 1956.

Perhaps it was the temper of the times that persuaded the New York legislators in 1828 and their colleagues in other states to place the abortion statutes in the criminal code instead of in the medical practices or ethics acts where every previous and subsequent law governing medical and surgical procedures is to be found. The reasoning seems to have been that in all other operations a combination of a patient's natural caution and the practitioner's conscience sufficed to prevent unnecessary surgery. Only in the case of abortion did legislators add restrictive provisions to the penal codes (Means, 1970; Beck, 1970).

In 1920 the Soviet Union became the first country to legalize in-hospital abortion on request of the woman in the first trimester of pregnancy; the statute was repealed in 1936 but reintroduced in 1955. Interruption of pregnancy for economic as well as medical reasons was authorized in Japan in 1948. Most of the socialist countries of Central and Eastern Europe followed the post-Stalin Soviet lead in the mid-1950s. In the United States, however, it was just about impossible until recently to obtain a legal abortion for nonmedical reasons (Lucas, 1969; Roemer, 1971). A survey of abortion legislation in different countries has been compiled by de Moerloose (1971) for the World Health Organization.

The first American state to reform its law by broadening the conditions for permissible abortion was Colorado in 1967, followed subsequently by California, North Carolina, Maryland, Georgia, Arkansas, Delaware, New Mexico, Oregon, Kansas, South Carolina, Virginia, Hawaii, New York, Alaska, and Washington. Except for the last four states the so-called liberal state laws adopted since 1967 are based on the American Law Institute's Model Penal Code. In general these laws permit termination of pregnancy (1) when the life or physical or mental health of the mother is in danger, (2) when the child may be born with serious mental or physical defects, and (3) when conception is the result of rape or incest. In most states at least two physicians have to agree on the need for abortion, which must be performed in accredited hospitals by licensed physicians. Deficiencies of the model code, capriciousness in local administration, and the logistics of abortion services have fostered further attempts toward liberalization and/or repeal in several states (Heller and Whittington, 1970; Gold, 1971; Overstreet, 1971; Rockat, Tyler, and Schoenbucher, 1971; Tyler and Schneider, 1971).

The 1970 legislative reforms in Hawaii, New York, Alaska, and Washington have gone beyond the American Law Institute recommendations. Most liberal is the New York statute under whose terms abortion is a matter entirely between the patient and her physician. There is no requirement for state residency, mental health or other consultation, or performance of the abortion in a hospital. Termination, unrelated to the health or life of the mother, is permitted up to twenty-four weeks of pregnancy. There is a "conscience clause" for the physician morally opposed to abortion. New York, along with Hawaii, Alaska, Maryland, California, and Washington, also does not require the signature of a parent before a teenage girl can be aborted or of a husband before a married woman can be aborted.

The 1971 situation can best be described as dynamic. Induced abortions during the first trimester of gestation performed by trained personnel in hospitals are far safer than carrying pregnancies to term. A rate of around 2.8 deaths per 100,000 such abortions has been reported from several Eastern European countries, compared to a maternal mortality rate (excluding deaths from abortions) for white women in the United States during 1964–1966 of 18 per 100,000 live births (Tietze, 1969c, 1970a). Rapid, safe, and relatively low-cost terminations of early pregnancies can now be obtained in well-staffed out-of-hospital medical facilities in several American cities (David, 1971a); initial reports of morbidity and mortality compare favorably with those obtained in hospitals. The growing availability of legal abortion by trained practitioners is gradually supplanting the dangerous practice of induced abortion by untrained persons. The legal status of induced abortion may well be resolved if the Supreme Court rules that state laws restricting abortion are unduly vague and unconstitutional (Hall, 1970a, 1971a; Polsky, 1970). On the more distant horizon is the promise of the prostaglandins, a group of fatty acid compounds currently receiving much research attention in view of their seeming ability to terminate early pregnancy and induce menses. If eventually found safe, low cost, and suitable for self-administration, they offer women a new freedom, likely to reduce the need for surgical abortion as a method of "postconception planning" (David, 1971*a*).

Psychological Sequelae of Abortion

There is virtually no systematic research evidence on psychological or psychiatric sequelae of abortion. As noted by Callahan (1970):

> The compilation of data and reliable judgments on the psychiatric aspect of abortion is immensely frustrating. The literature on the subject is large, but marked on the whole by vagueness, an excessive reliance on the personal impressions of psychiatrists, a lack of empirical studies, and the absence of any systematic worldwide attempts to bring some methodological order into the whole area. [P. 48]

It may well be a truism that there is no psychologically painless way to cope with an unwanted pregnancy. While an abortion can elicit feelings of guilt, regret, or loss, an alternative solution, such as entering a forced marriage, bearing an out-of-wedlock child, giving a child up for adoption, or adding an unwanted child to an already strained marital situation, is also likely to be accompanied by psychological problems for the woman, the child, and society. It is curious how few papers there are in the literature on the emotional relief often seen after abortion and reported by the Osofskys (1971). The situation is compounded by the aura of controversy and illegality that continues to shroud abortion in many countries. To gain some perspective this section will begin by reviewing what is known from studies of pregnancy and spontaneous abortion before psychological sequelae of induced abortion are discussed.

Psychological Aspects of Pregnancy

No matter what the circumstances, pregnancy is a major biological and psychological event in the life of the woman, especially if it is her first pregnancy. It affects her attitude toward herself, her husband or lover, her mother, any children she may already have, her body, her sexuality, and her future life (Deutsch, 1945, 1948; Bibring, 1959, 1961; Grimm, 1967; and Chertok, 1969). The prevalence in normal women of anxiety, ambivalence, and stress associated with pregnancy has been well documented in the psychiatric literature (Pleshette, 1956; Tobin, 1957; Biskind, 1958; Robin, 1962; Jansson, 1965; Rheingold, 1964; Shainess, 1964, 1966, 1968, 1970; and others). If the child is unwanted by the woman or wanted despite societal pressures, "opportunities for conflict are multiplied and compounded" (Fleck, 1970, p. 43).

Erikson (1953) and Bibring (1959, 1961) view pregnancy as a developmental crisis. How a woman passes through this crisis depends upon the biological condition of her pregnancy and upon the whole social, psychological, and cultural context of her past, present, and projected future life. Deutsch (1948) suggests that the psychological experience of pregnancy is associated with the conditions under which the woman has conceived and the situation into which the child is born. The negative psychological impact of pregnancy on an unmarried woman can easily be matched in a married woman who already has several small children and lives in precarious socioeconomic circumstances. Just how a woman will respond psychologically is not easily predictable, but that pregnancy can become a maturing and growth experience even for young unmarried women is apparent from the pioneering studies reviewed by Fleck (1970) and more recent research by Payne (1970).

Spontaneous Abortion

It is widely believed that 10 to 20 percent of all pregnancies end in spontaneous abortion associated with abnormal development or death of the fetus, at times due to demonstrable chromosomal abnormalities or to maternal disorder (Taussig, 1936; Fisher, 1967; WHO, 1970). Tietze (1971) estimates the incidence of spontaneous abortion at about fifteen per hundred live births in the United States, with psychological causes being responsible for a minority of these. Dunbar (1967) suggests "that spontaneous abortion occurs more frequently in some women than in others . . . as a result, physicians are coming to speak of the abortion habit" (p. 23). Habitual abortions are defined by Clyne (1967) as three or more consecutive spontaneous abortions and are believed to have strong psychosomatic components in addition to organic causes.

The literature on spontaneous abortion has been succinctly reviewed by Pohlman (1969). A number of studies suggest that some spontaneous abortions may be psychologically produced, and that psychotherapy may be the treatment of choice when abortion is habitual. Pohlman cites Wengraf's (1953) suggestion that the existence of a fetus "antagonizes unconscious tendencies" with the result that the woman meets personal needs by expelling the fetus while presenting quite a contrasting picture at the conscious level. Wengraf and Dunbar conclude, from case study evidence, that it may be necessary for a woman with the abortion habit to keep trying to have a child as proof that she really wants one. Such ambivalent tendencies toward childbearing have been repeatedly noted by Clyne (1967) in his clinical practice.

Of course, it is not always easy to separate reports of spontaneous and illegally induced abortions, especially when legal codes are restrictive (Sadvokasova, 1967; David, 1971d). Perhaps, as Mann and Grimm (1962) suggest, only those women who tend to manifest their problems psychosomatically are good candidates for spontaneous abortion. However, as Pohlman (1969) concludes, there is

no controlled research that shows that abortion is more likely when conception is unwanted . . . one could always argue that women with psychosomatic problems were more "really" unwanting, even though they did not appear to consciously. Evidence is not available either to refute or confirm this hypothesis, and such evidence would be extremely hard to produce. [P. 282]

Adds a World Health Organization Scientific Report (1970, p. 24) "whilst emotional factors have often been incriminated in the causation of spontaneous abortion, this relationship must still be regarded as hypothetical and in need of further study."

Psychological Sequelae

After considering the problems encountered in psychological studies of pregnancy and spontaneous abortion, it becomes clearer why research on psychological sequelae of abortion is beset with complications. From a methodological view there is the additional difficulty that humanitarian considerations preclude establishment of randomly selected experimental and control groups for abortions denied and granted (Chilman, 1971).

As Janis (1958) observed, every surgical operation has psychological elements or sequelae that may leave psychological scars. Abortion is more complex "because pregnancy involves directly the core of femininity, a woman's creativeness in the most literal sense, her sexuality, her mothering capacities, and her family" (Fleck, 1970, p. 44). Much of the extensive psychiatric material on the alleged psychological trauma of abortion consists of impressionistic case reports. The 1934–1965 literature has been critically reviewed by Simon and Senturia (1966), who provide individual comments on twenty-four American and European studies. They note how sobering it is

to observe the ease with which reports can be embedded in the literature, quoted, and requoted many times without consideration for the data in the original paper. Deeply held personal convictions frequently seem to outweigh the importance of data, especially when conclusions are drawn. In the papers reviewed the findings and conclusions range from the suggestion that psychiatric illness almost always is the outcome of therapeutic abortion to its virtual absence as a postabortion complication. [P. 387]

Sloane (1969) and Walter (1970) have written a similar review. Callahan (1970) voices his distress more strongly:

In the light of contradictory professional judgments, the inadequacy of the data and a lack of anything approaching methodological refinement, one might almost feel justified in concluding that the surveys and the professional opinions are of little help. . . . One searches the literature in vain for the guiding hand of a sociologist in the preparation of the surveys or in interpreting their results. . . . Nor has anyone attempted to study the (poor) data in terms of a comparison of different cultures and what effect that would have on the meaning of the evidence. . . . Studies based on whole populations, those granted and those denied an abortion, are scanty; more are badly needed. Worst of all, there is hardly any attempt to clarify the meaning of the concepts employed. . . . The psychiatric literature is a conceptual desert, employing all sorts of common terms, but practically never telling us what they mean or ought to mean. Lacking such needed clarification, the survey results tell us too little of any value. No wonder, then, that the same data are read in contradictory ways and are easily used to justify the most divergent moral evaluations. [P. 71]

Simon and Senturia (1966) catalog the many deficiencies in sampling and in research design, including frequent failure to study preabortion psychological status, lack of clear definitions of psychiatric terminology, and the inability to compare studies within the same country, much less transnational samples. They suggest that ideally studies of the psychological effects of abortion

should contain the following elements: (1) the sample should be drawn to include a study group of women with therapeutic abortions for medical and psychiatric indications and a control group of women with spontaneous abortions; (2) a longitudinal study should include experimental and control groups evaluated as close to the time of abortion as possible. This should include preabortion evaluations of the therapeutic abortion group. The entire group should be followed with repeated evaluations over a period of years; (3) a retrospective study should include evaluations of women at varying periods of elapsed time since abortion; (4) data gathering should be standardized. Similar interviews, questionnaires, and psychological tests should be used in the various phases of the study. Data should be gathered in a systematic fashion about the mental status, physical health, and sociological and demographic variables. The data should make possible some reasonable estimate of the absence or presence of psychiatric illness, both prior to and following abortion; (5) criteria for judgments should be clearly defined prior to the actual data-gathering phase. The authors believe that studies so designed could answer many unsettled questions about the psychiatric sequelae of therapeutic abortions. [P. 388]

As Wolf (1970) has suggested, matching of groups should take into consideration age, parity, race, socioeconomic status, marital status, legality of abortion, stage of gestation, whether the abortion was for psychosocial or medical reasons, the type of operative procedure used, and psychological status and psychiatric diagnosis. Each of these variables may affect a woman's reaction to abortion differently.

There is some agreement that women with diagnosed prior psychiatric illness are more likely to have some difficulties after abortion (Meyerowitz, Satloff, and Romano, 1971). Most frequently cited is Ekblad's (1955) follow-up of 479 Swedish women who had terminated pregnancies for psychiatric reasons in Stockholm during 1949–1950. Only 1 percent of these women had postabortion psychiatric problems of sufficient severity to impair working capacity, but each of these cases had demonstrated some neurotic manifestations before abortion. Simon, Senturia, and Rothman (1967), in a retrospective study of all therapeutic abortions performed at the Jewish Hospital of St. Louis during 1955–1964, found that of thirty-two women who evidenced diagnosable psychiatric illness at follow-up after therapeutic abortions, thirty had experienced prior mental disorders. These researchers were particularly concerned with "the high incidence of sado-masochism, depression, and rejection of feminine biological role supports" (p. 657) among women requesting abortion, but they also noted that "a large number of women who were seriously disturbed before the abortion responded to the procedure well and improved following it."

It is seldom realized that postabortion psychosis is practically unknown (Jansson, 1965). Since there are some 4,000 documented postpartum psychoses requiring hospitalization in the United States per year, about one to two per 1,000 deliveries, there should be a sizeable number of hospitalized postabortion psychoses if abortion were as traumatic for some women as term delivery (Fleck, 1970). It would appear unlikely that a significant number of hospitalized psychoses related to abortion could be "hidden" in the records. Again, whereas "postpartum blues" are well known, typical depressive stress reactions to the end of pregnancy, "postabortion blues" have been observed to be generally brief and mild unless serious mental disturbance was apparent before abortion. Indeed, Kummer (1963) suggests that the whole concept of postabortion psychiatric illness may be a myth.

For many women abortion has a practical immediate value in eliminating the stress of an unwanted pregnancy (Kay and Schapira, 1967; Shainess, 1968; Walter, 1970; Whittington, 1970). This relief may be tinged with regret, at times followed by a brief period of remorse. Lee's (1969, p. 121) study of a select group of well-educated women whose pregnancies had been terminated by American physicians under illegal conditions suggests that reactions ranged along a continuum from "encapsulation" of the experience to "the development of a politicized concern with the fate of other women who seek abortions." She states that "the majority of the women reported that they were anxious to help others, even strangers, through the difficulties of abortion if they could" (p. 121). Emotional and psychological effects seldom lasted beyond a few months. Payne (1970) also noted "the impetus to further maturation and development that not infrequently results from the active resolution of a potentially disruptive crisis."

The liberalization of abortion statutes in Britain, the United States, and in other countries provides an opportunity to develop systematic studies and comparisons of the immediate and longer-term effects of differing abortion procedures by differently trained operators in diverse settings (Kessel, 1970; Pond, 1970; Tietze, 1970e). The role and training of abortion counselors needs to be more fully considered. Very useful would be the development of an easily administered psychological device for predicting with reasonable validity which women are at particularly high risk for psychological sequelae.

Discussions with colleagues in the United States and abroad reflect growing interest in conducting comparative psychosocial research in abortion-seeking behavior. A program of retrospective and prospective research exploring sociological, psychological, and gynecological variables has been initiated at Aberdeen (MacGillivray, 1971; McCance and McCance, 1970; Olley, 1970). Coughlin (1970) at Yale, Miller (1971) at Stanford, Notman, Payne, and Kravitz (1970) at Beth Israel in Boston, Smith, Steinhoff, Diamond, and Brown (1971) at Hawaii, and Osofsky and Osofsky (1971) at Syracuse have launched psychological studies of abortion, contraceptive behavior, and repeated abortion seeking, including psychiatric interviews and psychological tests. Additional studies are mentioned in the next sections of this chapter. It is likely that future research will lift the curtain of ignorance about abortion-seeking behavior and its sequelae.

Psychological Effects of Denied Abortion

The general hypothesis that "unwanted" pregnancies and births often have multiple and damaging consequences is hardly new. Reducing the number of unwanted children was one of the objectives motivating Margaret Sanger and the planned-parenthood movement (Lader, 1955). That "unwantedness" is a psychological handicap for children and their parents seems to be a widely accepted belief in the mental-health literature, typically based on and reinforced by individual case studies (Menninger, 1943). The circular relationship between excess fertility and conditions of poverty, and their relevance for mental health, has been well delineated (Lieberman, 1964; Rainwater, 1960).

The frequency of unwanted pregnancy is staggering. Despite the fact that 97 percent of fecund American women have used or expect to use contraception (Westoff and Ryder, 1969), more than half of all births were reported by married couples in 1965 as unplanned. One out of five births was said by the parents to have been unwanted at conception or any future time (Bumpass and Westoff, 1970a, 1970b). Only 26 percent of couples who did not intend to have more children (two-thirds of married couples) reported that they had been successful in planning both the number and timing of their children (Ryder and Westoff, 1969). Even with the most modern, effective methods of contraception, a significant number of unwanted births are produced by contraceptive failures. It was noted in the 1965 National Fertility Study, for example, that women using oral contraceptives reported a 5 percent failure rate, while IUD users reported an 8 percent failure rate (Ryder and Westoff, cited by Cutright, 1971). Extensive follow-up studies of operationally defined unwanted births, that is, children born to women denied abortion, are rare. Pohlman (1969) and Callahan (1970) cite the absence of objective research on the social and psychological cost of unwanted pregnancy to the child, family, and society.

There is no published evidence that the unexpected, unplanned, or even unwanted pregnancy is always "bad," or that a planned pregnancy more frequently produces a psychologically healthy child. The literature is sparse on the relationship of "unwantedness" or "wantedness" to specific, objective criteria of physical, mental, or social health and/or maladjustment (Pohlman, 1969). Little information has been compiled on psychological consequences for women whose requests for abortion have been approved or denied. With the myriad of difficulties associated until recently with abortion in most American states, it was rarely possible to follow the natural history of pregnancies in women who sought but were denied abortion (Beck et al., 1969; Tietze and Lewit, 1969; David, 1971b).

Beck (1970) cities a report by Caplan (1954) of his experiences in Israel with sixteen mothers. Each had several children and was in the main warm and generous with all except with the one child in psychiatric treatment. After many months of therapy each of these mothers was finally able to state that she had wanted to abort this particular pregnancy and had made numerous attempts to do so. Beck (1970) also writes movingly about the likely link between unwantedness and child abuse, citing data compiled in the United States by De Francis (1970), Haitch (1968), and Silver, Dublin, and Lourie (1969). The preventive effectiveness of abortion in mental-health practice is further delineated by Fleck (1964, 1970), who indicates that over 50 percent of children in foster care are either not adoptable because of some defect or are awaiting adoptions that fail to materialize. Resnick (1969), in reviewing the literature on child murders from 1751 to 1960, found that the number of filicidal mothers was twice as great as filicidal fathers. The most plausible and humane way to reduce the incidence of unwanted pregnancies is to permit couples to become parents only with their own informed consent (Lieberman, 1970).

Research designed to determine the significance of correlations between planned birth status and physical, psychological, and social outcomes is beset with a host of complicating factors. Inquiry about whether a child was desired at the time conception occurred is seldom made in medical or psychiatric centers, either during the diagnostic process or in therapy, despite its high relevance to the understanding of the parent-child relationship. Operational definitions of "unwanted child" and "wanted child" are difficult to establish for empirical research. Pohlman (1965) lists some of the problems facing the researcher:

1. Usually there are two or more family members whose feelings toward the child are important, and they may be in disagreement.

2. Any given individual may experience changes in feelings over time.

3. At any given time an individual may have a child whom he does not want at that moment, but whom he believes he would have wanted at a later time.

4. A parent may have wanted some children, especially those born first, but not all; in some cases feelings toward an unwanted "extra child" may generalize to other children.

5. Individuals are influenced by many factors, some of which may tend to make him "want" and others to "unwant" a given child.

6. An individual may repress certain feelings, so that at the "conscious" level he "wants" a child, and at the "unconscious" level he does not, and vice versa.

7. The individual may conceal from others even those feelings of which he is conscious; the statements he makes to them may vary, depending on who "they" are.

8. A child may be wanted for unhealthy or superficial reasons; not all wanting is emotionally healthy.

9. In some cultures and in some families there may never be any particular decision as to whether a child is wanted; the term may be almost meaningless, particularly if having children is part of a conventional or traditional institutional pattern.

In addition to Pohlman's categories there are still other considerations that compound the problem, such as pregnancy due to incest or rape or contraceptive failure, the psychobiological need of some women to assure themselves that they are capable of conceiving without, however, wanting the child, and deliveries of live infants following unsuccessful efforts to induce abortion.

Reviews of the literature (Tietze, 1965; Forssman and Thuwe, 1966; Geijerstam, 1969; Kasdon, 1969; and Pohlman, 1969) yield only one attempted matched control study of children born to women denied abortion. Forssman and Thuwe (1966) report a twenty-year follow-up study of 120 children born to Swedish women whose requests for abortion on psychiatric grounds had been denied. The control children were same-sexed babies born in the same hospital immediately after delivery of the "unwanted" child. The authors report that an examination of available records twenty years later showed that many more of the unwanted than the control children "had not had the advantage of a secure family life during childhood." They were registered more often with psychiatric services, had engaged in more antisocial and criminal behavior, and had received more public assistance. The results obtained pointed to the unwanted children "being born into a worse situation than the control children." Matching of the experimental and control children was limited primarily to sex, age, and place of birth. There were, however, some major differences between the two groups. For example, 26.7 percent of the unwanted children were born out-of-wedlock, compared to 7.5 percent of the control children. Eight of the unwanted children were adopted by others, compared to none of the control children. Similar differences existed on such variables as mother's age and parity and the family's socioeconomic status.

Now in progress in Prague, Czechoslovakia, is a follow-up study of the first seven to nine years of life of approximately 200 children born during 1961–1963 to women denied abortion both on initial request and on subsequent appeal (Potts, 1967; Schüller and Stupková, 1969; Matejcek, 1970). The control children were carried to term by mothers who knowingly stopped some form of contraceptive practice or else accepted an unplanned pregnancy and did not seek abortion. In comparing the pioneering Forssman and Thuwe study with the Czech project, it is worth noting these differences:

1. The Swedish women applied for abortion on psychiatric grounds and were refused once, whereas the Czech women applied for interruption of pregnancy on social and general health grounds and were refused twice.
2. The Czech control children are matched with the experimental children for sex, age, number of siblings, birth order, and attendance in the same class in the same school, while the mothers are matched for age, marital status, parity, and education and occupation of the father (insofar as possible).
3. In addition to the availability of extensive chronological medical and educational records, all the Czech children and their parents are participating in individual social, psychological, psychiatric, and medical assessment procedures.
4. Whereas the Swedish study focused primarily on later stages of social development, the Czech study will concentrate on earlier stages, particularly the prenatal and natal periods, infancy, early childhood, and the first two years of school.
5. In addition to testing for statistical differences between the two groups, subgroups will be considered in terms of reasons for denial of abortion and demographic variables.

Particularly unique in the Czech study is the wealth of objective data available on both the experimental and control children beginning with the prenatal period. For example, a total of eleven different routinely prepared reports exists for each child from the prenatal period to his current school year. Forms are completed jointly by medical and educational personnel. Even the original abortion commission records with stated reasons for requested abortions are available for review. At this writing the selecting and matching of experimental and control children has been completed with sufficient precautions so that none of the research staff studying and interviewing the children and the parents will have prior knowledge whether a given child was "wanted" or not.

The Prague study holds the promise of providing, perhaps for the first time, objective data comparing the physical, mental, social, and educational development of a group of children meeting an operational definition of "unwanted" with a matched control group of children operationally defined as "wanted" or "accepted." The results are likely to be of significance, regardless of outcome, advancing the present state of knowledge in child development and the psychology of pregnancy, as well as providing some evidence of the consequences over time of denied abortion.

Psychological Indications for Abortion

With the rapid progress in medical care many more pregnancies are being carried to term than in earlier years. Health hazards have decreased, and as one consequence, "psychiatric indications" have become the major "reason" for performing legal abortions. For example, of the 2,194 terminations of pregnancy under the first year of the liberalized Maryland abortion statute, 94 percent were performed on the basis of psychiatric indications (Cushner, 1970). However, according to Wolf (1970), most of these recommendations were not strictly psychiatric, if that term is defined as indicative of the presence of deeply ingrained neurotic or psychotic traits or the certain danger of suicide.

The symptoms presented by patients usually consist of a variety of personality disorders, impulsive behavior, misjudgment, or excessive use of certain defenses (denial, forgetfulness, etc.), interacting with environmental problems and resulting in severe, often transient, emotional problems. [P. 4]

It is apparent that "psychiatric indications" are really more psychological, socioeconomic, and humanitarian than exclusively medical. According to Sloane (1969), "There are no clear-cut psychiatric indications for therapeutic abortion." Suicidal threats constitute the most frequent reason for psychiatric referral, but Rosen (1967) holds that "there are no data to support a view that suicide for refused abortion, or as a result of pregnancy, is significant anywhere." Still, no clinician can simply ignore such threats. This view is supported by Whitlock and Edwards (1968), who reviewed the literature and concluded that "suicide in pregnancy is not so uncommon as widely believed." But they also found in their study of 483 women who attempted suicide in Brisbane, Australia, that the incidence of pregnant women in their group was about the same as in the female population at large. Marcus (1965) suggests that when a woman assumes the risks of an illegal abortion, she may be unwittingly desirous of suicide. The literature yields little, if any, cogent data on what happens over time to a woman who threatens suicide but does not follow through when abortion is denied, or the eventual impact of her distraught attitude on her subsequent behavior as a mother.

In April 1970 the American Medical Association Council on Mental Health noted that the "criterion to preserve the health or mental health of the woman is such that almost any psychiatric illness can be interpreted to meet the test." Psychiatric consultation is particularly difficult, even odious, in those states where it is a mandatory requirement for legal abortion (Peck, 1968). No other surgical procedure anywhere requires by law prior consultation by another medical specialist. As Eisenberg (1970) admits: "I write letters recommending abortion that are frankly fraudulent, because I am satisfied to be used so that someone may obtain what our society would otherwise deny her" (p. 62). Small wonder that many psychiatric recommendations are *pro forma*, based on a brief interview with patients well primed in advance on what to say. Numerous psychiatrists chafe about their awkward position in being asked to evaluate the "risk to mental health" of a specific pregnancy, which requires interpreting legal terms and in a sense granting "dispensation" from the law's restrictions (Levene and Ringney, 1970). Referral as a legalistic routine, rather than as consultation on the basis of individual need, is very likely to add to the already heavy psychological burden of the woman seeking to terminate an unwanted pregnancy.

While it is apparent that pregnancy and childbearing can precipitate or intensify psychological disorder, particularly in interaction with a stress-inducing socioeconomic or cultural environment, there is no present body of data "to help us determine, with any degree of certainty *which* women with unwanted pregnancies will succumb to major psychiatric illness as a result of that stress and which will be able to cope with pregnancy and childbearing satisfactorily" (Whittington, 1970, p. 62). Adds Callahan (1970): "In the absence of systematic empirical studies and in the presence of a vast difference of opinion among psychiatrists themselves, it is unlikely that anything approaching consistency of practice, necessary clarity and definition can be at present achieved" (p. 66). It is a disturbing commentary that, according to Beck et al. (1969), no information has ever been compiled on the psychosocial characteristics or motivations of women whose requests for abortion were denied in the United States.

Another approach is suggested by Simon (1970) following his earlier surveys of the literature and continuing research (1966, 1967). Agreeing that "psychiatric diagnosis as such is usually not a major issue," Simon (1970) recommends that

therapeutic abortion should be considered when the woman displays a deep-seated conviction arrived at on her own and not through pressure of spouse, family, friends, or physician, that the pregnancy is unwanted and intolerable, and she wishes to interrupt it; when the possibility exists that the woman would injure or kill herself; when the possibility exists of the woman injuring or killing others, particularly the newborn; when the problems related to management of the continuing pregnancy (hospitalization, restraint, care of the newborn) are so overwhelming, complicated and noxious in their own right that they make interruption a more therapeutic and practical choice; when continuation would result in extreme anguish as seen in a situation in which there is high risk of serious pathology in the child due to hereditary or congenital defect; when the psychiatric illness that might result would be of great length, difficult to treat and difficult to reverse; and when the pregnancy has been forced upon the woman through rape, or the woman's lack of awareness as in pregnancy of the very young, or in mental defectives. [P. 299]

The Doctor's Dilemma

Abortion represents a personal, ethical, and moral dilemma not only for mental-health consultants but for many other physicians, paramedical personnel, and public-health administrators. It may well be, as White (1970, p. 57) has suggested, that some male physicians fear giving a woman the freedom to decide about abortion: "Pregnancy symbolizes proof of male potency. If men grant women the right to dispose of this proof whenever they want to, we men feel terribly threatened lest women rob us of our potency and our masculinity at will."

Another obstacle is the abortion committee, a time-consuming and expensive procedure, very vulnerable to individual prejudices (Hammond, 1964). After abortion law reform in 1967 the Colorado Medical Society set "guidelines" for interpretation of the statute. In many instances these guidelines were more restrictive than the law implied (Dafoe, 1970). It might well be useful for psychologists to join with anthropologists in exploring the cultural blocks existing on the level of administrative bureaucracies, medical organizations, and decision-making agencies (Polgar, 1971; Hall, 1971b; Walter, 1970).

Should U.S. abortion laws be declared unconstitutional, many physicians will be forced to develop and act on personal standards for performing or not performing an abortion. Medical training, with its emphasis on life-giving and life-promoting functions, may contribute to a disinclination to participate in life-rationing activities (Peck, 1968). There is considerable need to study in depth the attitudes of medical and paramedical practitioners to sexuality, pregnancy, family planning, contraception, and abortion (Hern, 1971; Lerner, Arnold, and Wassertheil, 1971). It is essential to determine not only expressed attitudes but also likely behavior in given circumstances (Cushner, 1970).

Another serious barrier to progress is the still frequently encountered attitude that sex is sinful outside of marriage, that women should be punished for having played and been caught, and that pregnancy termination should not be made easy. It is difficult for many practitioners to develop genuine empathy with a woman enmeshed in the psychological morass of an unwelcome pregnancy or to accept abortion as a "therapeutic socio-medical obligation" (Hall, 1971a, p. 44). Numerous physicians support but are reluctant in their own practice to accept the right of a woman to determine for herself how many children she wishes to have and when she wants to have them. Self-determination is sharply reduced in abortion "for reasons that are primarily referable to sociopolitical considerations, the economic and social status of the woman requesting the abortion, the personal and religious convictions of physicians and abortion committee members" (Beck, 1970, p. 263). And yet the evidence is persuasive that many abortions are being performed by licensed, competent, and often highly conscientious physicians practicing under illegal conditions infrequently challenged by law-enforcement officials.

Numerous studies reflect the scant attention to human sexuality in traditional medical education and the inner conflicts and ambivalence of a considerable segment of the health professions in diverse parts of the world (Herndon and Nash, 1962; Lief, 1963; Peck, 1968; Mehlan, 1968, 1969; Leban, 1969; Sadvokasova, 1969; Dalsace and Dourlen-Rollier, 1970). Sensitive research is required to help develop educational programs designed to enhance awareness and skill for dealing adequately and appropriately with abortion and other fertility-related problems (Gendel and Gleason, 1971).

Repeated Abortion-Seeking Behavior

With the increasing liberalization or repeal of abortion statutes in the United States, and the rapid shift from self-induced or illegal abortion by untrained persons to legal abortion at reasonable cost in medical centers, American public-health concerns are gradually shifting to problems associated with repeated abortion-seeking behavior. Is there a likelihood that a significant number of women will rely on abortion as a preferred method of family planning? Is it feasible to identify at first abortion those women who are at particular high risk for repeated abortions? If so, is it possible to provide intensive counseling and motivate such women to shift to effective contraceptive practice? There are no ready answers. The nearly 1,200 annotated references to the 1960–1967 world literature on induced abortion compiled by Geijerstam (1969) and the 217-item bibliography on international family planning, 1966–1968, compiled by Kasdon (1969), make no index references to studies of repeated abortion-seeking behavior. Research on the psychological dynamics of the abortion decision-making process, particularly in repeated abortion seeking, is rare.

The incidence of repeated abortion seeking is increasing in Hungary, Japan, and the Soviet Union, the only countries where abortions on request of the woman have been legally available during the first trimester of pregnancy and often more readily accessible than modern contraceptives. In Hungary the percentage of women having had three or more abortions rose from 12 to 17 percent among those requesting abortions between 1960 and 1965 (Szabady, 1969). In a 1970 study of 279 women interviewed by physicians in six Budapest health centers, sixty-six women (24 percent) admitted having three or more previous abortions, and 73 percent indicated that they might again resort to abortion to terminate a future pregnancy (Szabady and Klinger, 1970). Callahan's (1970) review of studies in Japan cites the trend toward an "abortion habit." Repeated abortion seeking is an acknowledged public-health problem in the Soviet Union (David, 1971c). In a recent survey of 1,000 Armenian women coming for an abortion to a Yerevan hospital, a frequency of 4.7 previous abortions was noted per woman interviewed (Arutyunyan, 1968).

The Demographic Research Institute of the Hungarian Central Statistical Office has initiated a study of demographic and psychosocial aspects of repeated abortion-seeking behavior in situations where contraceptives are equally readily available. Two matched groups of women are being interviewed. Those in the first group will have had an abortion, instruction in contraception, another abortion, further instruction, and at least a third abortion. The second group will consist of women who after their first abortion successfully practiced oral contraception and had no further abortions during the subsequent two years. Psychological items have been included in the extensive questionnaire. Following the completion of pilot studies, it is anticipated that representative national samples of "repeaters" and "nonrepeaters" will be surveyed.

One of the few American studies of illegal abortion seeking to include information on repeated abortion-seeking behavior is Lee's (1969) report on sixty-nine "well-educated, intelligent, and sophisticated women," who had obtained medical advice on contraception after their first abortion, which had been performed by a physician under illegal circumstances more than a year before data collection. Of these sixty-nine women, twenty-eight, or 43 percent, had had a second abortion; and of these twenty-eight repeaters, nine, or 32 percent, had a third abortion. Lee indicates that the repeated abortions observed may be an artifact of the study design and indicative of the difficulties unmarried women had in obtaining and using effective contraceptives in the United States during the late 1950s and early 1960s. She concludes that "it is contraceptive use or nonuse which is the best predictor of multiple abortions, along with the time of exposure" (p. 119).

An effort to develop better understanding of the dynamics of repeated abortion-seeking behavior has been initiated at the University of Geneva (Kellerhals and Pasini, 1970). Among a group of 3,000 women interviewed for a psychosocial research project on contraceptive behavior, about 500 women admitted having had one legal abortion, and 107 women (3.5 percent) indicated having had more than one previous abortion. The women having had no abortion, one abortion, and two or more abortions are being compared in terms of social and psychological variables, including social status and level, social norms of abortion, integration, degree of social disorganization, occupational aims, and contraceptive behavior. The study will also endeavor to seek answers regarding psychological acceptability of abortion versus contraception, degree of character stability, sadomasochistic tendencies, and other psychodynamic aspects, provided suitable assessment instruments can be developed. Of special interest in the Geneva study is the concept of conflict and ambivalence in the decision-making process related to abortion.

Efforts to identify women who are particularly high risks for repeated abortion-seeking have been initiated with the assistance of Gough and his colleagues at the Institute of Personality Assessment and Research at the University of California in Berkeley (see Chapter 12). A twenty-minute kit using the femininity, modernization, and socialization scales of the California Psychological Inventory is being administered in several centers in the United States and abroad. The objective is to determine whether such women can indeed be identified and then be given special counseling to encourage more effective use of contraceptives. Similar exploratory studies are planned in Yugoslavia (Kapor-Stanulovic, 1971).

That the effectiveness of contraceptive methods can be influenced by subtle psychological factors has been amply demonstrated by Lehfeldt (1959, 1969). He noted "errors and omissions" in the use of contraceptives among couples who were highly motivated, intelligent, and fully familiar with contraceptive methods. Concluding that failure experienced by such couples must be due to subconscious factors, Lehfeldt termed this syndrome "Willful Exposure to Unwanted Pregnancy" (WEUP). "The exposure to pregnancy is called willful rather than accidental, for, in the Freudian sense, it seems to betray an emotional desire for pregnancy that is neither conscious nor rationally sound." These couples have ambivalent feelings about pregnancy; neither contraception nor pregnancy offers a solution, so they alternate between protection and exposure. Male WEUP can be diagnosed in such "accidents" as omission of the condom or wrong technique in practicing coitus interruptus. Female WEUP is more apparent in "forgetting" to take the pill or to insert the diaphragm.

The unconscious meaning of contraception and its exploitation in neurotic acting out was further suggested by Devereux (1965) in his report of thirty-eight mostly psychoneurotic cases. His findings indicate that the adequacy or inadequacy of contraceptives is only marginally determined by rational considerations and by proper instruction, and that the prime motivating factors in inadequate use of contraceptives are "masochistic brinkmanship, unconscious wishes to become pregnant, and aggressive impulses toward the partner." The "forgetting" of contraceptives is very likely overdetermined by a whole array of unconscious motives that have very little to do with the rational problem of avoiding pregnancy for practical reasons.

The importance of psychological factors is also apparent from a study of 100 unmarried teenagers who had given birth at the Yale New Haven Hospital in 1959 and 1960 (Sarrel, 1967). Within five years less than 10 percent had married, while 95 percent had again become pregnant and delivered 340 additional babies. Subsequently all unmarried girls under age nineteen who came to the hospital for prenatal care were registered in a teenage-mother clinic established by Sarrel. Within the next two years only seven of 100 girls became pregnant again. Systematic studies of repeated unwanted pregnancies and repeated abortion-seeking behavior are very much needed for a better understanding of the dynamics of human fertility.

The Prostaglandins

In discussions of evolving psychological research related to abortion, consideration must be given to the prostaglandins, a form of naturally occurring fatty acid compounds, several of which may emerge as the family-planning agents of the future. Although the prostaglandins have been known since the mid-1930s, research on their contributions to fertility regulation dates from 1965 when Sultan M. M. Karim, Professor of Pharmacology at Makerere University in Kampala, Uganda, discovered that prostaglandins stimulated the uterus to contract. Subsequently Karim and Filshie (1970), a group of Swedish researchers (Roth-Brandel, Bygdeman, Wigvist, and Bergström, 1970), and others have reported on various dosages and methods of applying prostaglandins to terminate pregnancies ranging in duration from nine to twenty-eight weeks (Embrey, 1970; Magil, 1970; Potts, 1970b). Work is in progress to develop derivatives and analogues that may be more selective, potent, and free of side effects (Speroff and Anderson, 1971).

Particularly promising was Karim's (1970) announcement of the development of suppositories and tampons containing prostaglandin crystals. Self-administration of prostaglandins through the vaginal route, as suggested by Speidel and Ravenholt (1970) and others, is a giant step toward attaining an "ideal means of fertility control . . . a nontoxic and completely effective substance which, when self-administered by women on a single occasion, would insure nonpregnancy at the completion of one monthly cycle" (p. 565). While initial results with prostaglandins are encouraging, large-scale trials will be necessary before recommendations can be made for routine clinical use. Prostaglandins have not yet been approved by any national drug-regulating authority. Under the strict rules developed by the Food and Drug Administration (in part because of criticisms encountered after the relatively rapid approval of oral contraceptives) permission for marketing prostaglandins in the United States is probably some years away. But it is not too early to envisage the social impact of the potential availability of prostaglandins in the form of medicated tampons or vaginal suppositories, offering women, if they so choose, the revolutionary freedom of inducing menses after a period has been "missed" and the prospect of an unwanted pregnancy becomes apparent.

For perhaps the first time in the history of contraceptive technology and reproductive physiology, behavioral scientists have an opportunity to join with medical colleagues in exploring the social, epidemiological, psychological, motivational, and cultural impact of a new birth-prevention procedure on women of childbearing age *before* that method becomes widely available. If prostaglandins prove to be safe, effective, and low cost, it is essential that social scientists be prepared with practical recommendations for policy-makers and for family-planning educators ready to launch large-scale information campaigns to spur voluntary control of fertility at the postconception level. Much more needs to be known about the psychosocial meaning of menstruation in diverse cultures and about how different women respond to the first suspicion of pregnancy. Might once-a-month self-administration of a prostaglandin-impregnated tampon become an accepted way of assuring cycle regulation, less encumbered with the religious strictures, social taboos, or psychic conflicts now associated with contraception and abortion? Are prostaglandins more likely than other coitus-independent procedures to meet the aspirations of families for a better life? And if so, how? Would "postconceptive contraception" be perceived as an euphemism for abortion? What will be the social and societal effects of ability to terminate early unwanted pregnancies and postpone parenthood in complete secrecy, without medical involvement or public registration? Plans for cooperative studies need to be developed now to coordinate evolving field experience, to move from "hypothetical" to practical research conducted under actual field conditions, and to assure availability of internationally comparable data.

Abortion and Contraception

The notion of conception prevention is historically far more recent than the ancient practice of birth prevention by abortion. Where readily available, abortion requires little prior educational effort; a missed period and anxiety about an unwanted pregnancy usually provide sufficient motivation. Effective contraceptive practice, however, usually means acceptance of a new level of shared responsibility in sexual behavior, exposure to and acceptance of contraceptive information and education, and conscious precoital planning. In Kessel's (1970) view, acceptance of contraception seems to require a prolonged community educational effort "of at least a generation." An orderly progression from abortion to contraception over the years cannot be assumed.

The relationship between abortion and contraception in a given population is difficult to assess, particularly when the situation is a highly fluid one. While questions are being raised about the presumed deleterious effects of readily available abortion on effective contraceptive practice, the hope is also expressed that improvements in contraceptive technology, greater access to contraceptives, and widespread family-planning educational campaigns will gradually reduce the incidence of abortions, especially repeated abortions. However, the relationship of abortion to contraception under diverse circumstances of relative availability and legality has not been widely studied. As Moore (1970) has noted,

> From the personal point of view, induced abortion in general, unlike most contraception, is 100 percent effective, coitus-independent, a one-time operation, based on a certainty rather than a probability and the only method (currently available) to terminate an existing pregnancy voluntarily. [P. 7]

In some countries of Eastern Europe the economic cost of a legal abortion is cheaper for some women than are oral contraceptives or the insertion of a loop. While induced abortion is medically simple and safe when performed early and under proper circumstances, social, psychological, and economic costs of repeated abortions have not been sufficiently studied to permit reasoned judgment.

In a recent review of public health aspects of abortion on request, Tietze (1970c) concludes that

> greater availability of legal abortion tends to increase the total frequency of induced abortion, which includes legal and illegal abortion, for three obvious reasons: first, some pregnancies are aborted which otherwise would have been carried to term; second, these women are able to conceive again earlier than after term delivery; and third, the motivation to practice contraception is reduced. While the last effect appears to have been of some importance in a few countries of Eastern Europe, there is no way to predict the response of a population accustomed to the use of modern contraceptive methods or if effective contraceptive services are provided [p. 380].

While it is possible to speculate that the rate at which a country or community accepts effective contraceptive practice might have been more rapid in the absence of abortion on demand, it is not feasible to obtain hard evidence. The Hungarian, Soviet, and Japanese experience is difficult to interpret accurately because abortion on request was legalized in these countries long before modern contraceptives became widely available. There is impressionistic evidence, however, of laxity of contraceptive practice, coupled with a slowly evolving medical commitment to modern contraception (Callahan, 1970; David, 1970, 1971c; Szabady and Klinger, 1970; Potts, 1970a, 1970c; Tietze, 1970c).

So far there is not sufficient information to state with confidence what the effect of liberalized abortion is on an already contraceptive-oriented society, such as the United States, where abortion is widely considered to be a "hindsight" method, reserved primarily for "accidents" or contraceptive failure, and is not usually a planned procedure. It should be recalled that even if twenty-five million women of childbearing age in the United States used the pill regularly, an annual 1 percent failure rate would result in about 250,000 unwanted pregnancies per year (Hardin, 1967). British experience, compiled since the liberalized abortion act was implemented in 1968, suggests that repeated abortions are becoming a problem, especially among younger single girls (Hendell and Simms, 1971). In the Aberdeen studies Olley (1970) found that repeated risk taking and repeated out-of-wedlock pregnancy were not associated with any intellectual pattern. Informal personal inquiries suggest that contraceptives are still not easily obtainable for unmarried women in some parts of Britain.

An example of the complementary rather than competitive relationship between abortion and contraception in total fertility control is provided in the countries of Latin America where abortion has always been illegal and modern methods of contraception are only gradually becoming more widely available, filtering down from the sophisticated elite to the large masses of urban poor. Clandestine abortions as a means of spacing children or terminating unwanted pregnancies are performed mostly for socioeconomic reasons. As the pressure for small families mounts, couples are more likely to resort to whatever means of birth prevention are available. In some sections of Latin America an increase in illegal abortion and in contraceptive practice appears to be accompanying a gradual decrease in fertility, with distinctive patterns noted in diverse socioeconomic groups in different countries (Mertens, 1970).

On the basis of his epidemiological research in Santiago, Chile, Requeña (1969, 1970) noted that women in the higher socioeconomic stratum of society, with the lowest birth rate, tended to rely primarily on contraception backed by abortion. Women in the middle stratum, with an intermediate birth rate, used abortion as the major method for limiting family size while moving gradually toward wider acceptance of contraceptive methods. Women in the lowest stratum, with the highest birth rate, generally did not practice contraception or abortion. The socioeconomically most backward women, comprising the largest population segment, are increasingly turning to abortion, which may herald an eventual acceptance of contraception. Through this model Requeña and his colleagues explain the decline in fertility in Chile accompanied by a "temporary" increase in illegal abortions. Similar trends of rising abortion rates following the introduction of government-sponsored family-planning programs have been termed transitional in Korea, Taiwan, and other developing countries (Potts, 1970a; Moore, 1970).

The notion of using contraceptives as a "preventive" measure in fertility control, and as a substitute for the "curative" of abortion, takes time to filter through socioeconomic-cultural substrata of society. This is another reason for recommending that family-planning education programs be closely attuned to local cultural values, while making certain that an adequate supply of contraceptives is physically available and "psychologically accessible" to all segments of the population. The success of intensive efforts to foster acceptance of contraceptive practice after abortion has been demonstrated in Yugoslavia by Mojic and Gold, as summarized in David (1970). Studies in Taiwan and in selected areas of Japan show that "educational efforts to increase use of contraception can be successful and that they are followed by a decline in abortion rates in situations where such rates had risen following introduction of family-planning programs" (Moore, 1970, p. 7).

There is one other situation that must be considered. What happens when a previously liberal abortion law suddenly becomes restrictive, as happened in the Soviet Union in 1936 and in Rumania in October 1966? Predictably the Rumanian birth rate soared from a monthly low of 12.8 per 1,000 population in December 1966 to a high of 39.9 in September 1967. Since that high-water mark the birth rate has gradually receded to a monthly low of 17.9 recorded in December 1969. The annual birth rate rose from 14.3 per 1,000 population in 1966 to 27.4 in 1967, but subsequently declined to 26.7 in 1968 and 21.1 in 1970 (David, 1970, 1971d). The incidence of "spontaneous abortion" has increased significantly, and the impression prevails that illegal abortion is again being practiced in greater numbers. Similar trends were noted in the Soviet Union before abortion was relegalized in 1956 (Sadvokasova, 1969). While modern contraceptives are not being produced in Rumania, their sale is not prohibited. Rumanians seem to have adjusted to the new restrictive abortion law by resorting to traditional contraceptive practices, probably importing modern contraceptives from other Eastern European countries, and procuring non-legally induced abortions. The evidence is persuasive that when couples are highly motivated to limit family size, they will find a way to do so.

After reviewing the world literature on the complex and sensitive interrelationship of abortion and contraception, Moore (1971) offers the following *tentative* conclusions:

(1) poor use of contraception, or use of poor contraceptives, promotes abortion use; (2) good use of contraception, or use of good contraceptives, reduces abortion use; (3) abortion is probably an essential, if undesirable, interim measure between no fertility control at all and preventing births by contraception; (4) abortion should not be seen as the preferred method; it can be used initially as an emergency measure in the absence of contraceptives, and eventually as a back-up measure when contraceptives are in general use; and (5) while abortion is only one means by which a population already disposed to limit family size can do so, its ready availability (legally or with little fear of prosecution) probably serves as a stimulant to resorting to it.

The very liberal New York State abortion law offers some American women, for the first time, a choice between reliance on abortion or on contraception, or, perhaps more realistically, the choice of a medically safer but less than 100 percent effective contraceptive backed by easily available abortion. This situation opens the door to a kind of psychosocial research that was not previously feasible. Variables related to contraceptive practice or laxity can now be studied in greater depth, with potential practical contributions to family-planning education programs (Huntington, 1970).

Summary

The world literature is replete with clinical observations and assumptions about psychological aspects of abortion, but systematic studies are few and far between. Following a brief historical sketch of abortion, this chapter has attempted to present a critical overview of research, including previous and current studies, on the psychosocial effects of pregnancy terminations performed and denied. The dilemma of psychiatric indications and the ethical problems of the professions are reviewed. Consideration is given to needed transnational psychosocial research on the interrelationship between abortion and contraception and on the decision-making process in pregnancy prevention, acceptance, or termination. Also noted are psychosocial aspects of repeated abortion-seeking behavior and research related to the potential acceptance of self-administered prostaglandin vaginal suppositories, which may reduce dependence on surgically induced abortion to terminate early unwanted pregnancies.

Efforts to educate large groups of women of childbearing age to take precautions against the possibility of pregnancy have not been as successful as originally hoped when the coitus-independent pill and intrauterine devices became available on a mass basis. Most women throughout the world, and especially in the developing countries, have found it easier to postpone action until faced with the urgent need for coping with the reality of a missed menstrual period and the threat of an unwanted pregnancy. Surgical abortion is not, however, the preferred method of birth limitation, and every effort should be made to substitute self-administered procedures for preventing an unwanted pregnancy or for early "postconception planning" if some form of menses-inducing procedure proves to be safe, effective, and low cost. Now is the time for behavioral scientists to join with colleagues in other professions in planning and conducting practical, systematic, and internationally comparable psychosocial research in abortion-seeking behavior in diverse cultures.

REFERENCES

Arutyunyan, L. A. 1968. Some characteristics of family planning in the Armenian SSR (according to materials from a special survey). In *Proceedings of the All-Union Scientific Conference on Problems of Population of the Trans Caucasus.* Yerevan: Scientific Research Institute of Economics and Planning, Gosplan of Armenia.

Bates, J. E. and Zawadski, E. S. 1964. *Abortion: a study in medical sociology.* Springfield, Ill.: Charles C Thomas.

Beck, M. B. 1970. Abortion: the mental health consequences of unwantedness. *Seminars in Psychiatry* 2:263–274.

Beck, M. B.; Newman, S. H.; and Lewit, S. 1969. Abortion: a national public and mental health problem—past, present, and proposed research. *American Journal of Public Health* 59:2131–2143.

Bibring, G. L. 1959. Some considerations of the psychological processes in pregnancy. *The psychoanalytic study of the child,* Vol. 14. New York: International Universities Press. Pp. 113–121.

Bibring, G. L.; Dwyer, T.; Huntington, D.; and Valenstein, A. 1961. A study of the psychological processes of pregnancy and of the earliest mother-child relationship. *The psychoanalytic study of the child,* Vol. 16. New York: International Universities Press. Pp. 9–24.

Biskind, L. H. 1958. Emotional aspects of prenatal care. *Postgraduate Medicine* 24: 633–637.

Blake, J. 1971. Abortion and public opinion: the 1960–1970 decade. *Science* 171: 540–549.

Bumpass, L. and Westoff, C. 1970*a*. Unwanted births and U.S. population growth. *Family Planning Perspectives* 2:9–11.

———. 1970*b*. The perfect contraceptive population. *Science* 169:1177–1182.

Calderone, M. S., ed. 1958. *Abortion in the United States.* New York: Hoeber-Harper.

Callahan, D. 1970. *Abortion: law, choice and morality.* New York: Macmillan.

Caplan, E. 1954. The disturbance of mother-child relationship by unsuccessful attempts at abortion. *Mental Hygiene* 38:67–80.

Chertok, L. 1969. *Motherhood and personality.* London: Tavistock.

Chilman, C. 1971. Draft chapter of forthcoming book, *The family and public social policy.*

Clyne, M. B. 1967. General practitioners forum. Habitual abortion: a psychosomatic disorder. *Practitioner* 199:83–90.

Coughlin, P. M. 1970. Personal communication.

Cushner, I. 1970. Report in *American Medical News,* June 8, 1970.

Cutright, P. 1971. Illegitimacy: myths, causes, and cures. *Family Planning Perspectives,* Vol. 3, no. 1:25–48.

Dafoe, C. A. 1970. Thoughtful action needed now to find middle ground on abortion. *American Medical News,* June 8, 1970.

Dalsace, J. and Dourlen-Rollier, A. M. 1970. *l'Avortement.* Paris: Casterman.

David, H. P. 1970. *Family planning and abortion in the socialist countries of Central and Eastern Europe.* New York: The Population Council.

———. 1971*a*. Abortion: public health concerns and needed psychosocial research. *American Journal of Public Health* 61:510–516.

———. 1971*b*. Mental health and family planning. *Family Planning Perspectives,* Vol. 3, no. 2:20–23.

———. 1971*c*. Observations on abortion and family planning in the Soviet Union. Notes on a 1970 visit to Moscow. Washington, D.C.: American Institutes for Research (Memo).

———. 1971*d*. Abortion legislation: the Romanian experience. Paper presented at Population Association of America, Washington, D.C., April 1971.

David, H. P. and Bernheim, J., eds. 1970. *Proceedings of the Conference on Psychosocial Factors in Transnational Family Planning Research*. Washington, D.C.: American Institutes for Research.

David, H. P.; Szabady, E. et al. 1969. *Proceedings of the Research Planning Conference for Transnational Studies in Family Planning*. Washington, D.C.: American Institutes for Research.

De Francis, V. 1970. Child abuse—preview of a nationwide survey (1963). Cited in M. B. Beck, Abortion: the mental health consequences of unwantedness. *Seminars in Psychiatry* 2:263–274.

de Moerloose, J. 1971. Abortion legislation throughout the world. *WHO Features*, March 1971, no. 3.

Deutsch, H. 1945. *Psychology of women*. New York: Grune & Stratton.

———. 1948. An introduction to the discussion of the psychological problems of pregnancy. In M. J. E. Senn, ed., *Transactions of the Second Conference [on] Problems of Early Infancy*. New York: Josiah Macy, Jr., Foundation. 2:11–17.

Devereux, G. 1955. *A study of abortion in primitive societies*. New York: Julian Press.

———. 1965. A psychoanalytic study of contraception. *Journal of Sex Research* 1: 105–134.

Dourlen-Rollier, A. M. 1969. *Le planning familial dans le monde*. Paris: Payot.

Dunbar, F. 1967. A psychosomatic approach to abortion and the abortion habit. In H. Rosen, ed., *Abortion in America*. Boston: Beacon Press. Pp. 22–31.

Eisenberg, L. 1970. Comment on abortion and psychiatry. In R. Hall, ed., *Abortion in a changing world*. New York: Columbia University Press. 2:61–62.

Ekblad, M. 1955. Induced abortion on psychiatric grounds: a follow-up study of 479 women. *Acta Psychiatrica et Neurologica Scandinavica*, Supplementum 99, pp. 3–238.

Embrey, M. P. 1970. Induction of abortion by prostaglandin E_1 and E_2. *British Medical Journal* 2:258–260.

Erikson, E. H. 1953. Growth and crisis of the healthy personality. In C. Kluckhohn, H. A. Murray, and D. Schneider, eds., *Personality in nature, society and culture*. New York: Alfred Knopf.

Fisher, R. S. 1967. Criminal abortion. In H. Rosen, ed., *Abortion in America*. Boston: Beacon Press. Pp. 3–11.

Fleck, S. 1964. Family welfare, mental health, and birth control. *Journal of Family Law* 3:241–247.

———. 1970. Some psychiatric aspects of abortion. *Journal of Nervous and Mental Disease* 151:42–50.

Forssman, H. and Thuwe, I. 1966. 120 children born after therapeutic abortion refused. *Acta Psychiatrica Scandinavica* 42:71–78.

Gebhard, P. et al. 1958. *Pregnancy, birth, and abortion*. New York: Harper.

Geijerstam, E. K. 1969. *An annotated bibliography of induced abortion*. Ann Arbor: University of Michigan Press.

Gendel, E. S. and Gleason, J. A. 1971. Education about abortion. *American Journal of Public Health* 61:520–529.

Gold, E. M. 1971. Abortion—1970. *American Journal of Public Health* 61:487–488.

Gold, E. M.; Erhardt, C. L.; Jacobziner, H.; and Nelson, F. G. 1965. Therapeutic abortions in New York City: a 20 year review. *American Journal of Public Health* 55:964–972.

Grimm, E. R. 1967. Psychological and social factors in pregnancy, delivery and outcome. In S. A. Richardson and A. F. Guttmacher, eds., *Childbearing: its social and psychological aspects*. Baltimore: Williams & Wilkins. Pp. 1–52.

Haitch, R. 1968. Orphans of the living: the foster care crisis. *Public Affairs Pamphlet*, no. 418.

Hall, R. E. 1970a. *Abortion in a changing world*. New York: Columbia University Press. 2 vols.

———. 1970b. The abortion revolution. *Playboy*, September 1970.

———. 1971a. Widening frontiers of legalized abortion. *Medical World News*, Obstetrics and Gynecology Issue, pp. 44–52.

———. 1971b. Abortion: Physician and hospital attitudes. *American Journal of Public Health* 61:517–519.

Hammond, H. 1964. Therapeutic abortion; ten years' experience with hospital committee control. *American Journal of Obstetrics and Gynecology* 89:349–355.

Hardin, G. 1967. A scientist's case for abortion. *Redbook*, May 1967, p. 62.

Heller, A. and Whittington, H. G. 1970. The Colorado report. *Seminars in Psychiatry* 2:361–374.

Hendell, K. and Simms, M. 1971. *Abortion law reformed.* London: Owen, 1971.

Hern, W. M. 1971. Is pregnancy really normal? *Family Planning Perspectives* 3:5–10.

Herndon, C. N. and Nash, E. M. 1962. Premarriage and marriage counseling. *Journal of the American Medical Association* 180:395–401.

Huntington, D. S. 1970. Summary report of workshop. In H. P. David and J. Bernheim, *Proceedings of the Conference on Psychosocial Factors in Transnational Family Planning Research.* Washington, D.C.: American Institutes for Research.

Janis, I. 1958. *Psychological stress.* New York: Wiley.

Jansson, B. 1965. Mental disorders after abortion. *Acta Psychiatrica Scandinavica* 41: 87–110.

Kapor-Stanulovic, N. 1971. Personal communication.

Karim, S. M. M. 1970. Paper presented at Conference on Prostaglandins, New York Academy of Science, September 1970.

Karim, S. M. and Filshie, E. M. 1970. Therapeutic abortion using prostaglandin 2 alpha. *Lancet* 1:157.

Kasdon, D. L. 1969. *International family planning, 1966–1968; a bibliography.* Chevy Chase, Md.: National Institute of Mental Health.

Kay, D. W. K. and Schapira, K. 1967. Psychiatric sequelae of termination of pregnancy. *British Medical Journal* 1:299.

Kellerhals, J. and Pasini, W. 1970. Studies in abortion-seeking behavior. In H. P. David and J. Bernheim, eds., *Proceedings of the Conference on Psychosocial Factors in Transnational Family Planning Research.* Washington, D.C.: American Institutes for Research. Pp. 44–54.

Kessel, E. 1970. Pregnancy termination program. Unpublished paper.

Klinger, A. 1966. Abortion programs. In B. Berelson, ed., *Family planning and population programs.* Chicago: University of Chicago Press. Pp. 465–476.

Kummer, J. 1963. Post-abortion psychiatric illness—a myth? *American Journal of Psychiatry* 119:980–983.

Lader, L. 1955. *The Margaret Sanger story and the fight for birth control.* New York: Doubleday.

———. 1966. *Abortion.* Indianapolis: Bobbs-Merrill.

Leban, J. ed. 1969. *Teaching family planning.* New York: Josiah Macy, Jr., Foundation.

Lee, N. H. 1969. *The search for an abortionist.* Chicago: University of Chicago Press.

Lehfeldt, H. 1959. Willful exposure to unwanted pregnancy (WEUP). *American Journal of Obstetrics and Gynecology* 78:661–665.

———. 1969. Psychological factors in contraception. *Journal of Contemporary Psychotherapy* 1:109–114.

Lerner, R. C.; Arnold, C. B.; and Wassertheil, S. 1971. New York's obstetricians surveyed on abortion. *Family Planning Perspectives* 3:56.

Levene, H. I. and Ringney, F. J. 1970. Law, prevention psychiatry, and therapeutic abortion. *Journal of Nervous and Mental Disease* 151:51–59.

Lieberman, E. J. 1964. Preventive psychiatry and family planning. *Journal of Marriage and the Family* 26:471–477.

———. 1970. Reserving a womb: case for the small family. *American Journal of Public Health* 60:87–92.

Lief, H. I. 1963. What medical schools teach about sex. *Bulletin of Tulane University Medical Faculty* 22:161–168.

Lucas, R. 1969. *Analysis of abortion laws in the United States.* New York: Association for the Study of Abortion.

McCance, C. and McCance, P. F. 1970. Abortion or not? Who decides? An inquiry by questionnaire into the attitudes of gynecologists and psychiatrists in Aberdeen. *Seminars in Psychiatry* 2:352–360.

MacGillivray, I. 1971. Abortion in the north-east of Scotland. *Journal of Biosocial Science* 3:89–92.

Magil, B. 1970. Prostaglandins. *Medical World News*, August 28, 1970.

Mann, E. C. and Grimm, E. R. 1962. Habitual abortion. In W. S. Kroger and S. C. Freed, eds., *Psychosomatic gynecology*. Hollywood: Wilshire. Pp. 153–159.

Marcus, H. 1965. Symposium on "The social problem of abortion." *Bulletin of the Sloan Hospital for Women* 11:76.

Matejcek, Z. 1970. Report from Prague: A study of unwanted children. In H. P. David and J. Bernheim, eds., *Proceedings of the Conference on Psychosocial Factors in Transnational Family Planning Research*. Washington, D.C.: American Institutes for Research. Pp. 26–28.

Means, C. C. 1970. A historian's view. In R. E. Hall, ed., *Abortion in a changing world*. New York: Columbia University Press. 1:18–24; 2:137–142.

Mehlan, K. H. 1968. The abortion situation in worldwide perspective. In K. H. Mehlan, ed., *Arzt und Familienplanung*. Berlin: Verlag Volk und Gesundheit. Pp. 69–99.

————. 1969. Teaching family planning in Eastern Europe: the significance of the high abortion rate. In J. Leban, ed., *Teaching family planning*. New York: Josiah Macy, Jr., Foundation. Pp. 61–76.

Menninger, K. 1943. Psychiatric aspects of contraception. *Bulletin of the Menninger Clinic* 7:36–40.

Mertens, W. 1970. Fertility and family planning research in Latin America: an overview of recent developments. Paper presented at the Conferencia Regional Latinoamericano de Poblacion, Mexico City, August 1970.

Meyerowitz, S.; Satloff, A.: and Romano, J. 1971. Induced abortion for psychiatric indication. *American Journal of Psychiatry* 127:1153–1160.

Miller, W. B. 1971. Personality and ego factors relative to family planning and population control. Stanford University Medical School. Unpublished paper.

Miller, W. B. and Weisz, A. E. 1971. A brief summary of a study on the psychosocial aspects of unwanted pregnancy. Stanford University Medical School, unpublished paper.

Moore, E. C. 1970. Induced abortion and contraception: theoretical considerations. *Studies in Family Planning* 53:7–8.

————. 1971. Draft of forthcoming monograph on abortion, prepared for The Population Council.

Muramatsu, M., ed. 1967. *Japan's experience in family planning—past and present*. Tokyo: Family Planning Federation of Japan. P. 78.

Newman, S. H.; Beck, M. B.; and Lewit, S. 1970. Abortion, obtained and denied: research approaches. *Studies in Family Planning* 53:1–8.

Niswander, K.; Klein, M.; and Randall, C. 1966. Changing attitudes toward therapeutic abortion. *Journal of the American Medical Association* 196:1140–1143.

Noonan, J. T., Jr. 1967. Abortion and the Catholic Church: a summary history. *Natural Law Forum* 12:85–131.

Notman, M. T.; Payne, E. C.; and Kravitz, A. R. 1970. Therapeutic abortion and mental illness: implications of the positive value of illness. Unpublished paper.

Olley, P. C. 1970. Age, marriage, personality, and distress: a study of personality factors in women referred for therapeutic abortion. *Seminars in Psychiatry* 2:341–351.

Osofsky, J. D. and Osofsky, H. J. 1971. The psychological reactions of patients to legalized abortions. Paper presented at the meetings of the American Orthopsychiatric Association, Washington, D.C., March 1971.

Overstreet, E. W. 1971. Logistic problems of legal abortion. *American Journal of Public Health* 61:496–499.

Payne, E. C. 1970. Fertility control, pregnancy, and abortion. Unpublished paper.

Peck, A. 1968. Therapeutic abortion: patients, doctors, and society. *American Journal of Psychiatry* 125:797–804.

Pleshette, N. et al. 1956. A study of anxieties during pregnancy, labor, the early and late puerperium. *Bulletin of the New York Academy of Medicine* 32:436.

Pohlman, E. W. 1965. "Wanted" and "unwanted": toward less ambiguous definition. *Eugenics Quarterly* 12:19–27.

————. 1969. *The psychology of birth planning*. Cambridge, Mass.: Schenkman.

————. 1970. Abortion dogmas needing research scrutiny. *Seminars in Psychiatry* 2:220–230.

Polgar, S. 1971. Culture, history, and population dynamics. In S. Polgar, ed., *Culture and population: a collection of current studies*. Chapel Hill: Carolina Population Center, Monograph no. 9.

Polsky, S. 1970. Legal aspects of abortion. *Seminars in Psychiatry* 2:246–257.

Pond, D. A. 1970. Therapeutic abortion in Great Britain. *Seminars in Psychiatry* 2: 336–340.

Potts, D. M. 1967. Legal abortion in Eastern Europe. *Eugenics Review* 59:232–250.

———. 1970a. Termination of pregnancy. *British Medical Journal* 26:65–71.

———. 1970b. The prostaglandins—a new factor in fertility control. *IPPF Medical Bulletin*, Vol. 4, no. 5:1–4.

———. 1970c. Postconceptive control of fertility. *International Journal of Gynecology and Obstetrics* 8:957–970.

Rainwater, L. 1960. *And the poor get children*. Chicago: Quadrangle Books.

Ravenholt, R. T. 1970. Abortion and public health. In R. E. Hall, ed., *Abortion in a changing world*. New York: Columbia University Press. 2:49–51.

Requeña, M. 1969. Chilean program of abortion control and fertility planning: present situation and forecast for the next decade. In S. J. Behrman, ed., *Fertility and family planning: a world view*. Ann Arbor: University of Michigan Press. Pp. 478–489.

———. 1970. Abortion in Latin America. In R. E. Hall, ed., *Abortion in a changing world*. New York: Columbia University Press. 1:338–352.

Requeña, M. and Monreal, T. 1968. Evaluation of induced abortion control and family planning programs in Chile. *Milbank Memorial Fund Quarterly* 46(Part 2):191–218.

Resnick, P. 1969. Child murder by parents: a psychiatric review of filicide. *American Journal of Psychiatry* 126:325–334.

Rheingold, J. C. 1964. *The fear of being a woman*. New York: Grune & Stratton. P. 518.

Robin, A. A. 1962. The psychological changes of normal parturition. *Psychiatric Quarterly* 36:129.

Rockat, R. W.; Tyler, C. W., Jr.; and Schoenbucher, A. K. 1971. An epidemiological analysis of abortion in Georgia. *American Journal of Public Health* 61:543–552.

Roemer, R. 1971. Abortion law reform and repeal: legislation and judicial development. *American Journal of Public Health* 61:500–509.

Rosen, H., ed. 1954. *Therapeutic abortion*. New York: Julian Press.

———, ed. 1967. *Abortion in America*. Boston: Beacon Press.

———. 1970. Abortion in America. *American Journal of Psychiatry* 126:133–135.

Rossi, A. S. 1969. Abortion and social change. *Dissent*, Vol. 16, no. 4:338–346.

Roth-Brandel, U.; Bygdeman, M.; Wiqvist, N.; and Bergström, S. 1970. Prostaglandins for induction of therapeutic abortion. *Lancet* 1:190.

Ryder, N. B. and Westoff, C. F. 1969. Fertility planning status: United States, 1965. *Demography* 6:435–444.

———. 1971. Contraceptive efficacy in the U.S., 1965. Unpublished paper, 1970. Cited in P. Cutright, "Illegitimacy: myths, causes and cures," *Family Planning Perspectives* 3:25–48.

Sadvokasova, E. A. 1969. *Social-hygienic aspects of the regulation of family size*. Moscow: Meditsina.

Schüller, V. and Stupková, E. 1969. Legal abortion and the possibilities of studying its psychosocial consequences. In H. P. David, E. Szabady et al., *Proceedings of the Research Planning Conference for Transnational Studies in Family Planning*. Budapest, Hungary, September 1969. Washington, D.C.: American Institutes for Research. Pp. 12–16.

Schwartz, R. A. 1968. Psychiatry and the abortion laws: an overview. *Comprehensive Psychiatry* 9:99–117.

Sarrel, P. M. 1967. The university hospital and the teenage unwed mother. *American Journal of Public Health* 57:1308–1313.

Shainess, N. 1964. Feminine identity and mothering. In J. Masserman, ed., *Science and psychoanalysis*. New York: Grune & Stratton. Vol. 7.

———. 1966. Psychological problems associated with motherhood. In S. Arieti, ed., *American handbook of psychiatry*. New York: Basic Books.

———. 1968. Abortion: social, psychiatric, and psychoanalytic perspectives. *New York State Journal of Medicine* 68:3070–3073.

————. 1970. Abortion is no man's business. *Psychology Today*, May 1970.

Silver, L. B.; Dublin, C. C.; and Lourie, R. 1969. Does violence breed violence? Contributions from a study of the child abuse syndrome. *American Journal of Psychiatry*, Vol. 126, no. 3:404–407.

Simon, N. M. 1970. Psychological and emotional indications for therapeutic abortion. *Seminars in Psychiatry* 2:283–301.

Simon, N. M. and Senturia, A. G. 1966. Psychiatric sequelae of abortion. *Archives of General Psychiatry* 15:378–389.

Simon, N.; Senturia, A. G.; and Rothman, D. 1967. Psychiatric illness following therapeutic abortion. *American Journal of Psychiatry* 124:59–65.

Sloane, R. B. 1969. The unwanted pregnancy. *The New England Journal of Medicine* 280:1206–1213.

————, ed. 1970. Psychiatric aspects of abortion. *Seminars in Psychiatry* 2:211–382.

————. 1971. Emotional difficulties of therapeutic abortion. *Medical World News*, Obstetrics and Gynecology Issue 12:56–59.

Smith, D., ed. 1967. *Abortion and the law*. Cleveland: Western Reserve University Press.

Smith, R. G.; Steinhoff, P. G.; Diamond, M.; and Brown, N. 1971. Abortion in Hawaii: the first 124 days. *American Journal of Public Health* 61:530–542.

Speidel, J. J. and Ravenholt, R. T. 1970. Ideal means of fertility control. *Lancet* 1:565.

Speroff, L. and Anderson, G. 1971. The promise of the prostaglandins. *Medical World News*, Obstetrics and Gynecology Issue 12:59–61.

Szabady, E. 1969. *Hungarian fertility and family planning studies*. Budapest: Demographic Research Institute.

Szabady, E. and Klinger, A. 1970. Report from Budapest: Pilot survey of repeated abortion-seeking. In H. P. David and J. Bernheim, *Proceedings of the Conference on Psychosocial Factors in Transnational Family Planning Research*. Washington, D.C.: American Institutes for Research. Pp. 31–43.

Taussig, F. T. 1936. *Abortion, spontaneous and induced: medical and social aspects*. St. Louis: Mosby.

Tietze, C. 1965. *Bibliography on fertility control, 1950–1965*. New York: National Committee on Maternal Health.

————. 1969a. Induced abortion as a method of fertility control. In S. J. Behrman et al., eds., *Fertility and family planning: a world view*. Ann Arbor: University of Michigan Press. Pp. 311–337.

————. 1969b. Legal abortion in industrialized countries. In N. Sadik et al., eds., *Population control*. Islamabad: Pakistan Family Planning Council.

————. 1969c. Mortality with contraception and induced abortion. *Studies in Family Planning* 45:6–8.

————. 1970a. Somatic consequences of abortion. *Studies in Family Planning* 53:2–3.

————. 1970b. Abortion laws and abortion practices in Europe. In A. J. Sobrero and L. McKee, eds., *Advances in planned parenthood V*. Amsterdam: Exerpta Medica Foundation, International Congress Series. 207:194–212.

————. 1970c. Abortion on request: its consequences for population trends and public health. *Seminars in Psychiatry* 2:375–381.

————. 1970d. United States: therapeutic abortion, 1963–1968. *Studies in Family Planning* 59:5–7.

————. 1970e. *Joint program for the study of abortion*. New York: The Population Council (mimeo).

————. 1971. Personal communication.

Tietze, C. and Lewit, S. 1969. Abortion. *Scientific American* 220:21–27.

Tobin, S. M. 1957. Emotional depression during pregnancy. *Obstetrics and Gynecology* 10:677–681.

Tyler, C. W., Jr. and Schneider, J. 1971. The logistics of abortion services in the absence of restrictive criminal legislation in the United States. *American Journal of Public Health* 61:489–495.

Walter, G. S. 1970. Psychologic and emotional consequences of elective abortion. *Obstetrics and Gynecology* 36:482–491.

Wengraf, F. 1953. *Psychosomatic approach to gynecology and obstetrics*. Springfield, Ill.: Charles C Thomas.

Westoff, C. F. and Ryder, N. B. 1969. Recent trends in attitudes toward fertility control and in the practice of contraception in the United States. In S. J. Behrman, L. Corsa, Jr., and R. Freedman, eds., *Fertility and family planning*. Ann Arbor: University of Michigan Press. Pp. 388–412.

White, R. B. 1970. Comments on abortion and psychiatry. In R. E. Hall, ed., *Abortion in a changing world*. New York: Columbia University Press. 2:54–57.

Whitlock, F. A. and Edwards, J. E. 1968. Pregnancy and attempted suicide. *Comprehensive Psychiatry* 9:1–12.

Whittington, H. G. 1970. Evaluation of therapeutic abortion as an element of preventive psychiatry. *American Journal of Psychiatry* 126:1224–1229.

Wolf, S. R. 1970. Therapeutic abortion: a liaison psychiatrist's perspective. *Studies in Family Planning* no. 53:4.

World Health Organization. 1970. Report of a scientific group on spontaneous and induced abortion. *WHO Technical Report Series*, no. 461. Geneva: World Health Organization.

[10]

PSYCHOLOGICAL FACTORS IN THE ACCEPTANCE AND USE OF ORAL CONTRACEPTIVES

JUDITH BARDWICK

The psychological literature on oral contraception reveals a research area still searching for the important variables. The papers are easy to list and difficult to summarize, as this area is characterized by diverse measuring instruments applied to different populations who were using biochemically varied contraceptives. Without a coherent psychological theory or an adequate physiological model the basic variables that need measuring—much less the techniques to measure them—are uncertain. While psychologists emphasize motives, most studies measure effects. While we assume that underlying the observed differences in contraceptive behavior there are differences in beliefs, values, or knowledge, we do not have the data to support the assumption. While psychologists can conceive of demographic phenomena as the sum of the behavior of individuals, we know very little about the psychodynamics of contraception responsibility. One of the disconcerting truths is that most of the literature on contraception seems preoccupied with family; it is as though the use of a neutral phrase like "family planning" encourages investigators to forget that sex is part of the process, ignores the probability of anxiety and defenses, and takes as data only the conscious, verbalized self-reports of subjects.

It is important and interesting that the large-scale survey studies have not revealed differences in contraceptive behaviors in correlation with psychological variables. Both the Indianapolis study (Whelpton and Kiser, 1946–1958) and the Princeton study (Westoff, Potter, Sagi, and Mishler, 1961; Westoff, Potter, and Sagi, 1963; Bumpass and Westoff, 1969) were based upon structured interviews with large samples in their childbearing years, and neither study showed significant correlations between psychological variables and fertility behavior. Admittedly the Indianapolis study is an old one (1941), but still, the same kinds of variables were assessed as in recent studies—status and security, community and family background, interest in home and children, personality characteristics, marital adjustment, and husband-wife dominance. The size of the planned family did relate to economic factors but not to those psychological variables. The Princeton study used a more diverse sample and was longitudinal, assessing attitudes over roughly a ten-year period. Sociocultural environment, social-psychological variables, and personality characteristics were measured. Kiser (1967) has summarized the results, noting that the study had contributed information about religion and socioeconomic status, but "as with the Indianapolis Study, its failure to yield much association of psychological factors to fertility behavior suggests that the relevant psychological attributes either were not chosen or were inadequately measured" (p. 394). Similarly the major national surveys, the 1955 and 1960 Growth of American Families surveys (Freedman, Whelpton, and Campbell, 1959; Whelpton, Campbell, and Patterson, 1966) and the 1965 National Fertility Study (Westoff and Ryder, 1969), did find relationships between contraceptive behavior and socioeconomic variables like religion, education, urban or rural residence, but did not find differences in fertility or fertility attitudes in terms of psychological dynamics. Assuming that psychological characteristics are important, one may hypothesize that the relevant psychological variables were not measured. While people seem to be able to talk about sex, family size, or contraception, in our experience the explanatory or predictive variables seem to be the use of denial, the level of sexual anxiety and/or guilt, the level of interpersonal dependence and passivity, and the origins of vulnerability or self-esteem. These variables are not generally observable at the conscious interview level when adequate defenses are operating in a nonpathological population.

In addition when we measure psychological variables related specifically to oral contraception, the task is made even more complicated because the contraceptive effects a systemic body change that results in physical symptoms especially in the reproductive system. The systemic effect of the oral contraceptive seems to include effects upon the central nervous system and a general reaction tendency, which we can measure as affect changes. Since the reproductive system is affected responses to the pill can also reflect attitudes about these particular body parts, anxiety about body integrity or the body image, and ideas about fertility, masculinity, and femininity. While the pill normally creates physical changes, we can observe a wide range of psychological and psychosomatic responses to these changes and can hypothesize psychological causes. Psychology is not the only factor involved; pills vary in their effect according to their progestin or estrogen level, the ratio between the steroids, and perhaps the normal circulating levels of the endocrines in the woman. Most studies have *asked* women to *remember* their physical and psychological responses with the responses of women on different pills lumped *together*. Much of the research has been done by physicians, and they have logically been concerned with the effectiveness of the contraceptives and with the occurrence of side effects. Even within this essentially medical or physiological literature we find that the incidence of side effects differs markedly between preparations and with the same preparation studied by different investigators. The differences in the incidence of side effects with the same preparation have been reported to be as great as those obtained with different pills (Nilsson and Sölvell, 1967). Many of the studies have been clinical reports by psychiatrists or obstetricians with all of the problems of subjective reporting. Studies with more experimental ambitions have tended to assess conscious recall of the more obvious kinds of psychological variables, using an incredible diversity of instruments (suggesting that after reviewing previous results each investigator tried something else), but generally using tests that have been designed to be stable and reliable in order to measure psychological change. Fortunately this is an area of relevance from both social and theoretical perspectives and lends itself to the needs and interests of many researchers; we can reasonably expect an increase in sophisticated studies.

In this chapter we will first discuss the emotional cycle of women as it relates to the endocrine phases of the menstrual cycle, and what happens to the emotional cycle when endocrine levels are changed by oral contraceptives. The next section is a discussion of biochemical factors underlying emotional responses and changes of women using pills. In the second half of this chapter psychological factors involved in the use of rejection of the oral contraceptives and in psychosomatic responses to the pill are discussed.

Affect Changes Associated with Oral Contraceptives

In addition to the methodological problems just discussed, it seems likely that there has been an underreporting of undesirable effects because of the perceived need for population control. Difficulties in the dispassionate and full evaluation of these drugs (Kane, Treadway, and Ewing, 1969) adds to the difficulty of trying to explain why studies have reported increased feelings of well-being and mild to moderate euphoria—as well as elevated levels of tiredness, depression, and irritability. In this part of the literature survey we will review the effects of the pills on menstrually related affects, depression, libido, and other changes.

Glick's (1967) survey of twenty-six studies in the medical literature prior to 1966 reported six studies that had mentioned that premenstrual tension was alleviated in their patients taking the pill. None of the studies had comparative data on premenstrual complaints prior to pill use, and none reported symptom frequency at other phases of the cycle. In a survey of four reports on drug use in psychiatric populations, Glick (1967) found that psychiatric patients whose symptoms worsened in association with the menses generally improved under pill medication, but these studies lacked controls. Jackson (1966, p. 158) has also reported that when women are on steroid contraceptives, nervousness, premenstrual tension, irritability, and dysmenorrhea disappear. Bakker and Dightman (1966) studied 100 women over four years and noted that norethynodrel relieved premenstrual tension. When the women went off the pill for a month they complained of higher levels of premenstrual tension, and the authors attributed this to a fear of pregnancy. Moos (1968) administered a questionnaire to 450 women using an unspecified oral contraceptive and 298 not using the pill. He asked the women to rate a variety of symptoms for the menstrual, premenstrual, and intermenstrual phases of their recent cycle and their worst cycle. He found fewer symptoms in the oral contraceptive group, who reported shorter menstrual cycles, less heavy flow, less tension, restlessness, depression, irritability, pain, disruption of concentration, and behavioral change during the premenstrual and menstrual phases of their cycle. He found that most women reported a slight decrease in menstrual symptoms, but 10 percent reported a significant increase. Unlike our data which I will report, Moos found that cyclic mood fluctuations occurred whether or not women were using oral contraceptives. While there was a difference in the severity of the periodic mood change, with pill users reporting less severe changes, both pill users and nonusers reported a significant increase in moodiness, depression, irritability, and physical symptoms at premenstruation and menstruation. These results may be influenced by the research method, because expectations of cyclic mood changes can alter perception and recall.

Reports of the frequency of depressive responses to oral contraceptives range from a frequency of zero to over 50 percent. In Glick's (1967) survey nineteen of the studies, done primarily by obstetrician-gynecologists, sporadically reported emotional distress, and the highest frequency of depression was 5 percent. Thus Glick noted that "if depression does occur during drug use, it occurs rarely. It is not clear that this is related to drug administration." Nilsson and Almgren (1968) saw women early in pregnancy and then six to seven months postpartum. In the postpartum period 104 subjects were not using the pill and fifty-four were. During pregnancy and the second day postpartum there had been no significant psychiatric differences between the groups. Six months postpartum, pill users had 12.5 percent more psychiatric symptoms than nonpill users, and the incidence of both depression (15.3 percent) and neurasthenia (18.3 percent) was significantly increased. Nilsson's and Almgren's results suggest a causal connection between the use of oral contraceptives and an increase in psychiatric symptoms, largely due, they feel, to hormonal factors. In a study of thirty-nine women Huffer, Levin, and Aronson (1970) found that on oral contraceptives, eleven had depressive reactions and five reported a loss of sexual interest that was not related to depression. Their subjects developed these symptoms while on the oral contraceptives, and when they stopped using them the symptoms stopped. They suggest that those women who become depressive (and possibly frigid) while on hormonal contraceptive agents may represent a biochemically distinct group. Kane, Treadway, and Ewing (1969) found that unfavorable responses to the oral contraceptives occur more frequently than the literature suggests (in twenty-eight of their fifty subjects), and mild to moderate depression, irritability, and lethargy occur most often, especially in a psychiatric population. Chernick (1965) reported that almost 40 percent of his 166 gynecological patients complained of increased irritability, tension, and depression while on the oral contraceptives. Wearing (1963) found that depression occurred in 16 percent of his sixty-two patients, and when women became depressed the depression became more severe the longer the patients remained on the drug. Similarly when Lewis and Hoghughi (1969) compared pill users with a control group, considerably more women on pills experienced depressive symptoms, and only women on pills suffered severe, intense symptoms. Women whose pills had a high progestin level tended to be the most depressed and were more depressed the longer they had been on the pill. In addition depressive reactions were more frequent among women who had experienced depression before they had used the pill. (Two factors begin to loom in importance: the steroid effect per se and a psychological predisposition.)

In contrast Zell and Crisp (1964) found no increase in emotional distress among their 250 patients after the initial anxiety about a new medication had declined. Both Murawski et al. (1968) and Bakker and Dightman (1966) studied women who were using Enovid. Murawski et al. studied seventy-two women over a fifteen-month period, measuring emotions with the Clyde Mood Scale and the Mirror Picture Test, and found no increase in depression. Actually they not only reported that they "did not detect enough depression to change mean depression scores," but also said, "Exogenous override of an intrinsic hormonal cycle does not appear to exert any systematic effect on a woman's emotional life or change her self-image or self-esteem in any observable fashion." (Measurements of greater sensitivity seem to lead to quite different conclusions;- this assertion by Murawski et al. reflects, I think, premature certainty.) Bakker and Dightman (1966) tested 100 women five times with the Minnesota Multiphasic Personality Inventory (MMPI) and concluded that depression was a "scapegoat" side effect in which women could blame other problems on the pill while the pill itself did not cause depression. This may be true for their sample because Enovid is an estrogen-dominated pill, and it is progestin that seems to be responsible for depressive side effects. It might be worth noting that Slugett and Lawson (1967) studied eighty-six women who were using Norinyl (1 mg. norethisterone and .05 mg. mestranol), and they reported that after six months depression was found in none of the subjects although 23 percent had had depressive symptoms before pill use. At that time, however, there was a dropout rate of 50 percent of the women, for reasons that were not analyzed!

Women on the pills have also been reported to be more irritable or tense in general (not premenstrually) (Kane, 1968; Chernick, 1965; Wearing, 1963; Grant and Pryse-Davies, 1968), to get more headaches (Grant, 1970), to gain weight on the progestin-dominant compounds (Chernick, 1965; Behrman, 1969), and to become more aggressive, especially on pills that combine norethindrone acetate with ethinylestradiol (Grant and Pryse-Davies, 1968). Sexual arousability or orgasmic capacity (which are usually called "libido" in this literature) has been reported to increase, decrease, and remain unaffected (Grant and Pryse-Davies, 1968; Bakker and Dightman, 1966; Kane, 1968; Glick, 1967).

The variability of response is illustrated when we look at the study by Kane, Daly, Ewing, and Keeler (1967) where fifty women were studied using clinical interviews and personality tests. Undesirable effects were reported by twenty-eight women, eleven felt better on the drugs, and eleven reported no change. Symptomatically, depression and a deceased sexual interest were most often reported. In their second study (1969) 139 women were interviewed. Depression (34 percent), irritability (29 percent), and lethargy (23 percent) were the most common complaints, and while 15 percent of the women reported a decrease in sexual interest, 7 percent reported an increase. Increases and decreases in the capacity for orgasm were equal in frequency. Kane feels that the pill does not result in unusual stress, but rather the development of an increased susceptibility to stress, so that while there is no definitive fixed change in the way the women feel, there is an increase in emotional responsivity and greater affect variability. Relevant to the high dropout rate of pill users, it is important to note that 64 percent of Kane's sample perceived changes in themselves as a consequence of pill use. More than 50 percent of the women studied reported adverse reactions, and at least one-fourth of those women felt badly enough to want to stop using this form of contraception. Resistance to pill use may reasonably be expected to be high when feelings of depression, irritability, and lethargy are common, and disturbances in the desire for and the enjoyment of sex also occur frequently. Kane (1969), Ideström (1966), and Sturgis (1968) have reported psychotic episodes with the use of, or the withdrawal from, combination or sequential contraceptives. While rare and in opposition to studies reporting amelioration of menstrually related symptoms in psychiatric populations, these extreme responses suggest that there may be particular risks when these drugs are used by people with known psychiatric illnesses.

Measurement and memory seem to confound these data, so that generally speaking retrospective studies report a larger number of mental and sexual side effects than do predictive studies. For example, in 1967 Nilsson was a co-author of two studies. In the Nilsson, Jacobson, and Ingemanson (1967) paper they reported a study of the responses of 281 women using Anovlar (4 mg. norethistosterone acetate and .05 mg. etinyloestradiol) after the women had used the pill for one to two years. While 45 percent said that their sexual adjustment had improved mostly because they felt more secure, 26 percent reported an impaired sexual adjustment, and there was an increase in psychiatric symptoms in 17 percent of the respondents. In the paper that Nilsson published with Sölvell (1967) for a prospective double-blind study of four different preparations, tiredness and/or depression increased significantly only during the first month, and there were no significant changes in libido over the twelve months of observation.

Traditionally and as an important control, drug studies have used control groups on a placebo. That not too many placebo studies exist in the literature on oral contraceptives is understandable. But there are a few: Bakker (1965) has reported a double-blind crossover study of an estrogen-progestin combination, estrogen, and a placebo. Of their twenty-seven women twenty preferred either the estrogen or the combination contraceptive, reporting that they felt marvelous. Negative responses, including complaints about moodiness, fatigue, changes in sexual arousability, weight gain, and insomnia, were most frequent among those using the estrogen-progestin pill. Actually it was quite difficult to evaluate responses during the placebo period because withdrawal effects were so common. What I found most interesting was the observation that among twelve women who reported an increased sexual drive, six who were glad about the increase stayed on the pill, while the other six rejected the pills because of the very same change. Grounds, Davies, and Mowbray (1970) compared ten subjects on Ovulen and ten who were given an inert substance. The two groups were initially matched, and the significantly greater number of symptoms reported by those on the active substance would seem to relate to the effects of the drug rather than to levels of neuroticism. An interesting detail of the findings was that the number of symptoms within the control group did relate to levels of neuroticism but were independent of neuroticism for those on an active drug. In contrast Aznar-Ramos et al. (1969) gave a placebo to 147 women who had just had a spontaneous abortion and were interested in becoming pregnant. There were a total of 424 months of observation since patients were seen every month when they came for their supply of what they were told was a contraceptive tablet. In 141 of the treatment months there were no complaints, but in the remaining 283 months there was a large variety of side effects reported. In the months of observation the most frequent symptom was a decrease in libido (29.5 percent), followed by headache (15.6 percent), pain and bloating in the lower abdomen (13.7 percent), dizziness (11.1 percent), lumbar pain (8.0 percent), nervousness and an increase in libido (6.4 percent), dysmenorrhea (6.1 percent), abdominal pain (5.2 percent), and nausea (4.2 percent). Some infrequent symptoms were more exotic: paresthesia, postcoital bleeding, hirsutism. In brief, with the exception of nausea there were no significant differences in the frequency of undesirable side effects between this population who were on a placebo and those effects reported in the literature as the result of oral contraception administration.

An understanding of the psychodynamics of contraception must include the effects of the steroids themselves since they effect physiological changes and an appreciation of those changes within the psyche of individual women. In the next section I will report a series of three studies of moods in correlation with endocrine levels. To our surprise, generally speaking, individual differences made no difference in these studies.

Moods and Endocrine Level

Because of our interest in the psychology of women, my students and I have become interested in the underlying physiology of mood changes especially during the menstrual cycle. Correlational studies have demonstrated predictable affective fluctuations in correlation with the ovarian hormone activity that regulates ovulation. During the first half of a normal menstrual cycle estrogen production gradually increases and reaches a maximum level at midcycle or ovulation. At this point the corpus luteum begins to produce progesterone, and during the second half of the cycle large quantities of both estrogen and progesterone circulate until a few days before menstruation, when endocrine levels decrease swiftly. Estrogen and progesterone levels are negligible throughout the premenstrual and menstrual phases of the cycle.

There are two types of oral contraceptives, combination and sequential. The combination pills include estrogen and progestin together, while the sequential pills are composed of an initial sequence of pills composed of only estrogen followed by pills combining estrogen and progestin. When women use *combination* oral contraceptives both the quantity and the pattern of the circulating steroids are changed. Use of the pill results in the inhibition of estrogen and progesterone production by the ovaries, and instead large quantities of synthetic estrogen and progesterone (progestin) are taken for twenty or twenty-one days. Now neither estrogen nor progestin are as variable as they normally are, since high levels of progestin are circulating throughout the entire cycle instead of only during the second half, and a fixed quantity of estrogen is circulating that is some three to six times ovulation levels. In comparison with normal menstrual-cycle physiology endocrine levels on a combination regime are elevated and stable. Women who use *sequential* pills have estrogen administered for fifteen to sixteen days, followed by five days of both estrogen and progestin. While the steroid levels are higher than normal, the sequence of endocrine activity on sequential pills is like that of the normal menstrual cycle.

The quantity of hormones that are metabolized when women are using oral contraceptives is substantially higher than at any phase of the normal menstrual cycle (Goldzieher and Rice-Wray, 1966; Drill, 1966). During the days when women take a pill the circulating level of estrogen remains constant. About two days after the last pill is taken there is probably a slight decrease in estrogen, but the decrease is far less severe than occurs premenstrually during a normal cycle. When combination pills are used progestin circulation is relatively stable throughout the cycle, although the quantity circulating depends upon the dosage of that particular brand. During a sequential cycle progestin levels are high between days 21–27. Progesterone increases for six to seven days after ovulation in a normal cycle (days 15–21) and decreases during the last few days of the cycle (days 24–27). The exact amount of estrogen or progesterone (progestin) circulating depends upon the woman's normal production of hormones and the dosage level of the pill. Pills may be either estrogen or progestin dominant (Behrman, 1969), and since these steroids are antagonistic to each other in physiological effects, physiological and psychological reactions of women may vary accordingly.

In 1939 Benedek and Rubenstein published a classic study of the correlation between menstrual-cycle phase and psychodynamic processes. Based upon the psychoanalytic material of fifteen women they found that when estrogen levels were increasing during the first half of the cycle, the general mood was one of alertness, well-being, activity, outward direction, and heterosexuality. A high level of ego integration was achieved at ovulation, but as progesterone levels increased the mood changed and was characteristically passive-receptive, relaxed, narcissistic, and often reflected wishes for impregnation. Premenstrually, they found, women were tense, and the psychological material reflected aggression and anxiety (Benedek, 1939a, and Rubenstein, 1939b). When the menstrual flow started tension abated, and with the return of estrogen production there was a return to a more positive mood.

Experimental investigation of menstrual mood changes has been largely in the form of an interview or a self-report questionnaire. Another approach is the analysis of five-minute samples of spontaneous speech, using the Gottschalk and Gleser (1969) method of content analysis. In 1962 Gottschalk, Kaplan, Gleser, and Winget used this method while they studied five women over the course of two or three menstrual cycles. In four of the five subjects they found statistically significant affect changes during the cycle. Ivey and Bardwick (1968) applied the Gottschalk-Gleser technique to twenty-six undergraduates for two successive menstrual-cycle phases at ovulation and premenstruation. The anxiety level at premenstruation was strikingly higher than that at ovulation ($p < .0005$). When the samples of speech were analyzed for themes, hostility was high at premenstruation while self-esteem, or the feeling of ability to cope, was high at ovulation. The Ivey and Bardwick data were thus similar in theme to the Benedek and Rubenstein data.

The Gottschalk-Gleser technique proved sensitive to mood change and corroborated clinical or anecdotal evidence of a mood cycle in correlation with the endocrine cycle. Since oral contraceptives alter the endocrine cycle we hypothesized that the affect cycle of women on oral contraceptives ought to be different from those with normal menstrual cycles. Paige (1969) then used the Gottschalk-Gleser anxiety and hostility scales on the verbal samples of 102 married women on the fourth day of menstruation, the tenth and sixteenth day of the cycle, and two days preceding the next menstrual period. Thirty-eight women were not using the pill and never had, fifty-two subjects were using the combination pill, and twelve women were using sequential pills. We hypothesized that women on the combination pill, whose endocrine levels were stable, would not experience the cyclic affect fluctuations found in normal women. We also hypothesized that women on sequential pills, whose endocrine pattern is like that of nonpill women, would, like normal menstruating women, experience high levels of anxiety and hostility premenstrually and low levels of these negative moods at ovulation.

These hypotheses were supported; in general the results of nonpill women replicated the Ivey and Bardwick data. Women who were not using oral contraceptives experienced an affect cycle in correlation with the menstrual cycle (hostility = $p < .001$; anxiety = $p < .05$). Women using sequential pills experienced the same pattern in level of anxiety as did nonpill women. But women who were using the combination pill experienced no significant change in the level of anxiety or hostility through the cycle (hostility = $p < .95$; anxiety = $p < .25$). In this study women using combination pills did not have the same wide swing in affects as did nonpill women and those using sequential pills. This was a change in affect pattern and not quantity, since the total anxiety and hostility scores for those using and not using pills were not significantly different. In this study—and the next one—we found that when hormone levels are held fairly constant, as occurs with the use of a combination oral contraceptive, anxiety and hostility levels are also rather constant. The attitudinal and demographic variables of age, education, social class origin, parity, religion, menstrual history, predisposition to complain about physical or emotional symptoms, and prior expectations about the effects of oral contraceptives did not distinguish between those who did and did not use an oral contraceptive and therefore did not account for the difference in affect patterns. Thus the hypothesis that physiological factors are involved was sustained.

The preceding studies measured moods but not behavior. Oakes (1970) conducted a study designed to replicate the work of Ivey and Bardwick and Paige and to extend their findings with a measure of game-playing behavior. Using the two-person, non-zero-sum game of Prisoner's Dilemma (see Rapoport and Chammah, 1965, for details) we expected to find that game-playing behavior would differ according to menstrual-cycle phase for those not using a combination oral contraceptive, while those on combination pills would show no variation at different cycle phases. Oakes did replicate Paige's finding that for women on combination pills there were no significant differences in anxiety, hostility, or total negative affect scores between midcycle and premenstruation. Surprisingly Oakes did not replicate the Ivey and Bardwick and the Paige data for nonpill women—that is, Oakes did not find significant affect variability for nonpill women in conjunction with menstrual-cycle phase. We suspect that this lack of variability may be due to the very sensitivity of the Gottschalk-Gleser technique. Both the Ivey and Bardwick and the Paige data were taken at the convenience of each woman in her home; Oakes collected her data at the Mental Health Research Institute, an institutional building filled with computers and other potentially threatening evidences of technology. It is possible that constraints were induced by this place, and this may have precluded the expression of powerful negative emotions to a stranger, especially by premenstrual nonpill women who should be experiencing the highest levels of negative effects. Like Paige, Oakes found no significant differences between her populations of young married women who were using pills or another contraceptive on variables including age, religion, social class origin, education of the woman, education of her father, parity, and menarchal history. But those using combination pills were more anxious, and this suggests the possibility that different kinds of psychological variables might differentiate between the populations, and secondly, perhaps the endocrines of the pill exert an effect themselves.

One can approach the latter idea by examining the psychological differences within the self-selected population of oral contraceptive users, comparing those on estrogen and those on progestin-dominated pills. Oakes compared the Gough Adjective Checklist responses of those eighteen women on a progestin-dominant pill (Orthonovum, Norinyl, Ovral, Norlestrin, and Provest) with those twelve women on Ovulen, an estrogen-dominant pill. One might expect to find women using estrogen-dominant contraceptives higher in irritability and premenstrual tension, while those on a progestin-dominant compound would be lower in libido and higher in premenstrual depression (Grant and Pryse-Davies, 1968; *British Medical Journal*, 1968; Behrman, 1969). Women whose pills were high in estrogen concentration scored significantly higher in self-descriptions of aggression, assertiveness, and hostility. Those on progestin-dominant pills scored significantly higher in self-descriptions of deference, nurturance, and affiliation. These self-descriptions are similar in quality to what was predicted and are very like those menstrual-phase descriptions by Benedek and Rubenstein (1939*a*, 1939*b*).

Oakes found that nonpill women played the Prisoner's Dilemma game somewhat less cooperatively (or more competitively) than did those using the pill, which makes sense because nonpill women expressed higher scores on the Gough Adjective Checklist and the Buss-Durkee Assault measure on aggressive, outward-striving, active, assertive qualities, which were radically different from the more hesitant, self-effacing, and defensive postures of those on pills. Nonpill women cooperated less than did pill women, and while pill women played the same at both midcycle and premenstruation, nonpill women were significantly less cooperative at midcycle. Thus nonpill women, who were in general less dependent than pill users, were able to act more assertively at midcycle when we expect self-esteem to be high.

We have found then that there may be personality qualities that differentiate pill users from nonpill users, and that will be discussed further in the last section of this chapter. Additionally the data are fairly consistent in suggesting that active or assertive qualities may be associated with higher estrogen levels. When the game-playing behavior of Oakes's subjects was examined it was found that nonpill women at midcycle played less cooperatively than pill women at both cycle phases or nonpill women at premenstruation. While the data are quite tentative the personality measures also tended to divide between nonpill women at midcycle and the other three groups. Nonpill women experience a peak in estrogen level at ovulation, while progesterone levels are negligible. Pill women at midcycle have high levels of both estrogen and progestin. Because some of the synthetic progestins are antiestrogenic (Kistner, 1966), it is possible that estrogenic effects may be negated by the progestins. Oakes has suggested that while the absolute levels of circulating estrogens and progestins differ in women who do and do not use oral contraceptives, it may be the relative rather than the absolute concentration that determines the estrogen or progesterone effect. Thus premenstruation, when both hormones are low, may be similar to that period when both are high. Nonpill women at premenstruation, combination pill users at midcycle, and pill users at premenstruation are all similar in the sense that their estrogen levels are countered by circulating progesterone. Only the midcycle women who were not on pills had high estrogen levels uninfluenced by progesterone, and these were the women who played more competitively and scored high in measures of dominance, self-confidence, and aggression.

Some of our data suggest that there may be personality variables that differentiate between pill users and nonpill users, and we will explore personality qualities within that self-selected population of pill users. The sequence of studies just discussed, on the other hand, suggests that the hormone levels may contribute to differences between populations, and it seems reasonable to suggest that further studies of oral contraceptives take into consideration dosage levels and the ratio of estrogen and progestin levels.

Biological Origins of Steroid-Related Affects

Crude correlational studies involving estrogen and progesterone levels and associated affects and behaviors are not adequate. Understanding of these correlational relationships and the frequently contradictory data would seem to require a sophisticated understanding of the biochemical relationships involved. Because a great deal is unknown, and because the steroid effects are complex, interactive, systemic, and specific, the main thrust of this section will be to evoke awareness of physiological underpinnings of psychological phenomena but without that elegant simplicity that emerges when even complex phenomena are well understood. Since we do not know the etiology of menstrual-cycle symptoms, it is not surprising to find that the mechanisms by which oral contraceptives produce some symptoms and alleviate others are not clearly understood. Since the oral contraceptives affect many different tissues and enzyme systems, explanations of symptoms will include the chemical composition of a pill and the physiological characteristics and psychiatric history of individuals.

The pharmacologic and metabolic effects of estrogen and progesterone have an impact not only on the reproductive tract but also on general body functions such as fluid and electrolyte status, hematologic condition, and the status of extragonadal endocrine structures (Wallach and Garcia, 1968). Estrogen affects sodium and water retention, premenstrual tension, mucorrhea and irritability, and increased vascularity of various parts of the body. Progestogens have been related to the development of acne and seborrhea, sodium loss, and depression. It is also possible that levels of estrogens and progestogens affect cerebral blood flow, which could lead to altered behavior (Wallach and Garcia, 1968). Kane, Lipton, and Ewing (1969) have summarized some of the animal research demonstrating significant interaction between catecholamine and gonadal hormones, with the hormones probably influencing the sensitivity to catecholamines of receptors in the central nervous system. It is also possible that women who experience depression (and other significant emotions?) while on the gestagens may form a biochemically different subgroup, so that their hormonal system becomes altered in such a way as to produce depression (Huffer, Levin, and Aronson, 1970). Similarly Michael, Saayman, and Zumpe (1967) have demonstrated that sexual receptivity in rhesus monkeys is inhibited by progesterone, and it is conceivable that a biochemical basis for the loss of sexual arousability in some women on oral contraceptives will be found. Aside from the possible interaction of psychological variables, this research will be complicated because the effects of the oral contraceptives are not simply due to circulating quantities of estrogen and progestin, but probably also to interactions between them and exogenous hormones (Sölvell and Nilsson, 1968).

If the endocrine organization is to be understood it is necessary to move from the study of single endocrine systems in isolation to studies of pattern changes in the total hormonal balance (Mason et al., 1966). In addition to effects upon one reproductive system the gonadal hormones may also affect norepinephrine metabolism in the brain as well as cerebral monoamine function (Janowsky and Davis, 1970).

Indirect evidence from changes in emotional behavior when significant changes in estrogen and progesterone levels occur in women suggests that monoamines in the brain may be related to these mood changes. Janowsky and Davis (1970) have concluded that estrogen and progesterone, like reserpine and monoamine oxidase inhibitors, affect mood states and alter in vivo monoamine levels. Thus there is a growing body of evidence that the gonadal hormones do cause changes in the metabolism of catecholamines, and this may be important in understanding affective changes in women.

Grant and Pryse-Davies (1968) studied 794 women, each of whom received one or more of thirty-four types of combination and sequential contraceptives. In general the combination pills increased depression and lowered libido more than the sequential pills did. When the pill level of estrogen was low a woman was more likely to experience depression—just as women not on pills are more likely to experience depression premenstrually, when estrogen levels decline. Similarly Lewis and Hoghughi (1969) found a trend toward higher depression scores the longer a woman remained on the pill.

Grant and Pryse-Davies feel that the emotional changes associated with the oral contraceptive may be the result of changes in the levels of monoamine oxidase. In a normal menstrual cycle there is a strong increase in monoamine oxidase activity during the late secretory stage, but women on combination contraceptives experience this rise at about the twelfth day of the cycle. Grant and Pryse-Davies found that depression and loss of libido was highest with those strongly progestogenic compounds containing small amounts of estrogen, which caused high monoamine oxidase activity for most of the cycle. The lowest levels of depression were associated with the use of strongly estrogenic sequential pills, which have weak monoamine oxidase levels during most of the cycle, because progestin is not introduced into the body until the twenty-first or twenty-second day of the cycle. When the combination pill has a high dose of estrogen, even though it may be strongly progestogenic and activate strong monoamine oxidase activity early in the cycle, the high level of estrogen seems to protect against the depressant effect. It is possible that progestogens produce generalized changes in monoamine oxidase metabolism, in the hypothalamus as well as the endometrium, and this may be a factor in the occurrence of depression and a loss of libido in women (Grant and Pryse-Davies, 1968; Grant, 1970). Marcotte, Kane, Obrist, and Lipton (1970) report that changes in the gonadal hormones seem to effect changes in the metabolism of catecholamines, which results in changes of behavior, including changes in sexual behavior, sleep patterns, and depression levels.

Lest the reader think that things are clear we might note that West (1968) responded to the Grant and Pryse-Davies paper (1968) with a report of 1,000 women in a five-year follow-up study. As far as the combination pills were concerned, West did not confirm the Grant and Pryse-Davies observation; West did not find that depression or loss of libido was dosage specific. Dr. West wonders if the specificity of response lies in the pill or the patient. Waxman (1968) also responded to the Grant and Pryse-Davies paper and reports that he has been using injections of progesterone for the treatment of premenstrual depression with excellent results! Similar results have been reported by Bower and Altschule (1956) and Keeler, Kane, and Daly (1964).

On the other hand, Kane (1968) notes that there are data indicating that progesterone is a central nervous system depressant, and it is likely that this is also true of progestins.

Another area of research activity, especially in relation to depression, concerns the possibility that changes in the metabolism of tryptophan and its subsequent metabolism to a serotonin (5-hydroxytryptamine) may be important in the evolution of depressive reactions. Depressed patients excrete less tryptamine when they are depressed and, when they recover tryptamine excretion is increased. Steroids, including oral contraceptives, appear to influence tryptophan metabolism. Their effect may be the creation of a functional deficiency of pyridoxine; pyridoxine is a co-enzyme in the conversion of tryptophan to nicotinic acid ribonucleotide and to 5-hydroxytryptamine. There is some evidence that premedication with pyridoxine may prevent the disturbance of tryptophan metabolism; a contraceptive pill incorporating pyridoxine is being marketed in Spain, and a few cases of pill-induced depression have responded to pyridoxine (*British Medical Journal,* 1969). (Further discussion will be found in Winston, 1969*a,* 1969*b*; Baumblatt and Winston, 1970; Nistico and Preziosi, 1970; Rose and Braidman, 1970.)

The physiological effects of normal steroid levels, much less the changed levels induced by oral contraceptives, are not well known, and the mechanisms are not well understood. Clearly the idea is emerging that not just the gonads or reproductive end organs but the entire body including the central nervous system is affected when women use oral contraceptives. While the implication of that idea is there when we observe consistent and significant mood changes associated with endocrine levels, the potency, complexity, or frequency of central nervous system change is highlighted when we read the biochemical papers. Freud noted that "sometimes, a cigar is only a cigar." Sometimes an affect may be less symbolic than metabolic.

Psychological Factors in Contraceptive Responses

This section is embarrassingly short. There have been very few studies of responses to oral contraceptives that are primarily psychological, and there have been even fewer attempts to understand the psychodynamics of contraceptive responsibility and psychological responses or psychosomatic complaints as they are related to the needs, conflicts, goals, and defenses of women. Would research be improved if perspectives changed and we looked less specifically at responses to contraceptives per se, but rather considered contraception within the context of the total psychodynamic ecology?

Bakker and Dightman (1964), Rock (1965), and Murawski et al. (1968) found that women who were skeptical about the effects of the oral contraceptives, or women who suffered chronic psychosomatic complaints, were more likely to experience psychological and physical side effects when they used the pill. Bakker and Dightman used empirical test data (i.e., depression scale of the MMPI; Edwards Personality Preference Schedule, and the 16 Personality Factor Questionnaire), historical information, and inquiries into somatic complaints and a record of pill omissions. They did not find consistent correlations between personality traits, as they measured them, and the tendency to complain about side effects. They felt that those women who forgot their pills were unable to assume responsibility, to control impulses, and to strive for long-range goals. Kroger and Peacock (1968) reported that the anxiety scores of women who were chronically emotionally distrubed were more likely to increase when oral contraceptives were used than were the scores of well-adjusted women.

Zell and Crisp (1964) studied 250 private patients who had used Enovid for one to three years and found that most of their patients experienced an improvement in their sexual adjustment, attributed by the investigators to the fact that oral contraception is clearly separated in time and body part from coitus. I found it notable that this adjustment occurred with no increase in emotional conflicts or "sexual acting out" (or promiscuity) even though Zell and Crisp reported that the latter was a frequent fear of their patients. (One wonders about the origin, the meaning, of this particular anxiety.) Similar results—of enhanced sexuality or no significant change in the patients' own evaluation of libido as the result of pill use—have been reported by Bakker and Dightman (1964), Pincus et al. (1959), Wallach, Watson, and Garcia (1967), Ziegler and Rodgers (1966), and Ringrose

(1965). Ringrose, for example, reported that 53 percent expressed an improvement in sexual satisfaction, 4 percent experienced decreased gratification, and 35 percent reported no change. Increased arousability has been reported in frequencies of 1.4 to 50 percent and decreased libido in frequencies of 1 to 25 percent (Hauser and Schubiger, 1965; Ringrose, 1965; Mears and Grant, 1962). Nilsson, Jacobson, and Ingemanson (1967) found that while sexual responses were not related to the women's psychiatric history, there was a strong association between a high number of psychiatric symptoms and a decrease in sexual arousability. They also reported that those women who experienced an impairment in their sex lives discontinued use of the pills significantly early. It seems likely that relationships between psychological variables and pill responses, as well as an underestimate of negative responses, are significantly influenced by the high dropout rate of those who respond negatively. We may note that these studies have not analyzed sexual or depression responses in correlation with steroid levels.

There is some evidence that psychological variables may be predictive. Marcotte et al. (1970), in a systematic double-blind study of three patients, found an interaction between pill use and personality so that those who seemed most in conflict about their femininity experienced the most symptoms. Herzberg and Coppen (1970) compared the responses of 152 women on the pill and forty controls. After eleven months thirty-one women (20.4 percent) stopped using the pills because of depression and irritability (9), headache (13), loss of interest in sex (6), swelling of hands and feet (6), unacceptable weight gain (11), extreme tiredness (5), plans for pregnancy (5), breathlessness (1), breast cancer (1), rash (1), and nausea (2). They found that the composition of the combination contraceptive did not influence the frequency of side effects. Among their subjects those who developed moderate or severe irritability and/or depression had higher neuroticism or extraversion scores on the Maudsley Personality Inventory. And of those who got depressed 47 percent of them had experienced moderate or severe premenstrual depression before pill use, compared with 27 percent of the pill group as a whole. (Of course, that doesn't tell us whether this is primarily a psychogenic, psychosomatic, or steroid-change effect.)

While some studies (Hauser and Schubiger, 1965; La Gravinese, 1965) have found a relationship between the use of oral contraceptives and psychoneurosis or depression, other studies (Zell and Crisp, 1964; Bakker and Dightman, 1966; Linthorst, 1967) have found no such relationship. Nilsson et al. (1967) had the clinical impression that there is a relationship between the frequency of neurotic symptoms and the use of oral contraceptives. In 1966 they sent a questionnaire to the 281 women who had received Anovlar from the Department of Obstetrics and Gynecology at Lund. About 15 percent stopped using the pill because of psychiatric or sexual changes, and another 20 percent stopped because of weight gain, nausea, and other somatic symptoms. About 17 percent reported a marked increase in psychiatric symptoms, and another rather large group experienced a small or moderate number of symptoms. The most frequent symptoms were neurasthenic or depressive, quite like the symptoms Nilsson found in early pregnancy. In this study there was a tendency for women who had those symptoms in pregnancy to have the same kind of symptoms on oral contraceptives. Interestingly Kutner and Duffy (1970) found that women who were less feminine (based on scores from the MMPI) reported more instances of swollen and sore breasts, which the women believed was a foremost symptom of pregnancy, and those women continued to fear pregnancy although they were using the oral contraceptive. In the Nilsson et al. (1967) study those who had a history of psychiatric symptoms did report a high level or increase in psychiatric symptoms, but the frequency of psychiatric symptoms was only slightly lower in women with no such history. About 9 percent of the women reported an improvement in psychiatric symptoms, which seemed related to feeling more sexually secure, and overall about half of the subjects felt an improvement in their sexual adaptability because they felt more secure. But these results do suggest that psychiatric side effects are almost as common as more purely somatic symptoms and are often intense enough for women to discontinue pill use. The frequency of psychiatric side effects was related to a previous history of psychiatric symptoms and to responses during pregnancy, but was not related to age, parity, marital status, or social class. Again, we have the impression that these sociodemographic characteristics are not the important variables.

Orchard (1969) feels that the inability to tolerate oral contraceptives is frequently evidence of psychological problems in the patient, irrespective of whether the complaint is specifically a somatic side effect, a nonspecific somatic change, or a psychiatric disturbance. He feels that these complaints reflect the anxiety of those many women who have sexual problems for which they are reluctant to accept responsibility. Reviewing the evidence, he concludes that reports of a diminished sexual feeling because of the contraceptive is the acting out of a scapegoat reaction by a woman not prepared to accept her sexual anxiety. Orchard believes that the psychiatric health of the patient and her increased self-observation are important determinants of her responses. Edwards (1969) responded to Orchard's paper with a severe critique, pointing to the data that steroid levels do correlate with libidinal and depressive reactions (e.g., Grant and Pryse-Davies); he notes, for example, that depression and a loss of libido are more common with strongly progestinic compounds with low dosages of estrogen. Edwards asks whether psychotherapeutic intervention would be as effective as a change to a less progestinic compound.

Several papers have examined the dynamic meaning of observable fears. Zell and Crisp (1964) found three important fears expressed: (1) fears about bodily damage, which represented legitimate concern and sometimes castration anxieties and penis envy; (2) fear that one would lose control of one's sexual impulses with latent fantasies of prostitution, which were often defenses against feared sexual impulses that had been controlled by acknowledgment of a fear of pregnancy; (3) fears about one's future fertility, which was often an expression of anxiety about the ability to bear children, perceived as the most important source of self-esteem. Gluckman (1969) finds that about half of the women seen in psychiatric practice who are using oral contraceptives attribute some aspects of their psychiatric complaints to the pill. He points out the important difference between the somatic symptom like weight gain or breakthrough bleeding and the patient's response to the somatic phenomenon. The importance of contraception within the total dynamics of the individual is illustrated clinically. For example, some of his patients use contraceptives in order to please their husband or mother, but while they deny it secretly they want to be pregnant. Because the husband does not want a child, the wife subjugates her needs but retaliates with physical and emotional symptoms. It is important to remember that obesity, temper, depression, and frigidity all have a punishing quality. Many of his patients complain bitterly of a nightly ritual where the husband inquires whether or not she remembered to take the pill; they feel as though the pill has removed their privacy, they resent both the pill and the husband, and they feel reduced to a sexual object. Murawski et al. (1968) found that the depression some patients experienced was not linked to steroid effects but was understandable as a disappointment because the magical fantasies of what the pill was expected to do were not fulfilled.

Because of the need to perceive oneself as sexually adjusted, liberated, or spontaneous, awareness of sexual anxiety or inhibition may often invoke defenses that are threatened when a contraceptive is used. When, for instance, fears of pregnancy can no longer be used to justify infrequent coitus or low arousability, individuals are confronted with sexual inadequacy. Because of the dynamics of the culture it is more threatening to self-esteem to acknowledge sexual inadequacy than almost any other kind of inadequacy. It may then become imperative for the psychological stability of the individual, as well as the relationship between the couple, to cease using an effective contraceptive and reintroduce a real possibility of pregnancy. In the Cullberg, Gelli, and Jonsson study (1969) it was found that those who were initially anxious about contraception and who had a low interest in sex are least likely to adjust to the pills. This may occur because fears about contraceptives reflect fears within the sexual relationship; moreover, when sexual demands increase because of the low pregnancy risk, the sexual problem becomes manifest. In addition to psychopharmacological effects there are concurrent psychological dynamics; research in the psychology of oral-contraceptive responses must become more complexly psychosomatic and psychodynamic. (It is astonishing that a review of this literature did not reveal a single psychological study of attitude change.)

Several methodological problems seem critical: while there is a need for population-size changes in contraception so that population growth will be reduced, large-scale research methods have not been productive. It is possible that understanding population responses to the oral contraceptive (as well as any other contraceptive) may require a model developed from the more clinical study of individuals and their anxieties and defenses in interaction with those social-psychological variables like peer acceptance and sources of role satisfaction, as well as characteristic susceptibility to endocrine change, the clinical effect of steroid levels and ratios, and the long-term effects of steroid medication. Difficulties are compounded when one realizes that it is difficult just to define some of the important dependent variables—what, for example, is libido or sexual adjustment? Inconsistency in the data probably reflects a failure to control for dosage levels as well as nonreplication of methodologies between studies used on quite different populations. There has been no recognition that tests designed to measure stable personality traits may be insensitive to personality change. There has been little cognizance of the psychodynamics evoked when sexual anxieties are aroused, little awareness of the distortion that occurs when conscious verbalization is the measure and individuals resort to stereotyped responses in order to please the researcher and maintain their self-esteem. Understanding contraceptive responses in context will be enhanced when a more adequate model of the psychology of women has evolved; current models, whether psychoanalytic or not, are largely assumptions derived from studies of men (Bardwick, 1971).

A Predictive Study of Psychological and Psychosomatic Responses to Oral Contraceptives

In the years 1967–1969 Joan Zweben and I interviewed 107 women before they began using an oral contraceptive in an attempt to predict psychological and psychosomatic responses to pill use (Bardwick, 1969; Bardwick, 1970). Physicians' impressions that an easy tolerance of the pill or severe discomfort and rejection were essentially psychological phenomena seemed a logical hypothesis, and we tried to explore these dynamics with measures that assessed variables that had been important in psychosomatic studies of the female reproductive system. The three most important variables seemed to be passivity, or the inability to express aggression directly; dependence, or the need to perceive oneself as valued by others because that is the major source for feelings of self-esteem; and denial, which is a primitive psychological defense in which reality is simply not perceived. Women who cope with anxiety by expressing it in psychosomatic symptoms tend to be dependent upon others for feelings of esteem, are very vulnerable to being rejected by others, are fearful of expressing anger because it may alienate others who would then reject them, and are very likely to use the immature and vulnerable defense of denial (Bardwick, 1971).

This model, although logical, proved too simplistic; the coding of responses had to be more specific. Denial was important as a mechanism, but it was really best understood as a defensive attempt at coping by an immature personality who does not have more adequate and sophisticated defenses. The best single predictor was the specific denial of sexual anxiety rather than a general use of denial. We had to distinguish between a feeling, a conflict, and the defense. Thus denial was important as it related specifically to a particular conflict, such as sex, anger, dependency, and guilt. Similarly passivity in general was indicative of a psychological structure or a maturity level, but the association between passivity level and pill responses emerged when passivity was divided into an inability to overtly express anger and an inability to assume responsibility. Also, we had to distinguish between a developmentally normal level of anxiety about sex and pregnancy and a sex anxiety that was not developmentally appropriate and expressed fears about body integrity.

We tried to measure the woman's psychological relationship to her body, feelings of trust or mistrust toward her sexual partner, her goals, her self-perceptions, what made her happy, angry, or depressed, attitudes about contraception in general and the pills in particular, and her sexual experiences, responses, and motives. Before the woman started to use the oral contraceptive she was seen for two hours by Joan Zweben or myself. We gave her the Franck Drawing Completion Test (a measure of unconscious body relationships), the Nichols Subtle Scale (a questionnaire that measures passivity), the Cornell Medical Index for Women (a detailed health questionnaire), and a standardized interview. Three months later each woman received a four-card Thematic Apperception Test (with cards selected to measure unconscious attitudes toward heterosexual relationships, sex, maternity, dependence, and passivity), and a detailed questionnaire about her response to the pills. The Franck, the TAT, and the two questionnaires were coded and scored by two clinicians.

The subjects were volunteers from a Planned Parenthood clinic in Ann Arbor and University of Michigan students recruited through advertisements in local papers. The age range was from seventeen to thirty-five and the mean age was twenty. While only four girls did not feel some level of commitment to their sexual partner, only fifteen were married, thirty-two were engaged, and fifty-five had a regular boyfriend. Eighty of the subjects were undergraduate or graduate students; among those married many were the wives of students. Thus almost all of this sample were extremely motivated to use the pills successfully because there was no choice about pregnancy in their lives. Only 10 percent of this sample had previously assumed responsibility for contraception, having used a female contraceptive like the diaphragm, foam, or IUD; while 7 percent had used rhythm and 28 percent relied on condoms, 41 percent of this educated group had used nothing. These data reinforce our observation that the assumption of responsibility for contraception by young women is an extraordinarily important decision.

Body Changes

The follow-up questionnaire revealed that all of the women reported body changes as the result of pill use. What emerged as interesting was the type of body change reported and the psychological response to that reported physical state. We divided the body changes into normal, unusual, and beneficent.

Normal body changes are probably directly related to steroid levels, ratios, and changes in levels. These symptoms include larger and more tender breasts, shorter and more regular menstrual cycles with reduced flow and reduced cramps, some breakthrough bleeding and vaginal discharge, weight gain and water retention, nausea, diarrhea, less acne or other skin changes, headaches, varicose veins, nose bleed, leg cramps, sweating, and some fatigue.

In general girls who are not psychologically healthy do not report these body changes—they report others. These changes are reported by psychologically healthier girls, and each girl reports a limited number of changes. Healthier women do not report *unusual* or *beneficent* body changes (which are discussed below). That is, when psychologically healthier women report body changes they cite those that are linked to the physiological changes caused by pill use, and each woman does not report many of these changes. Acknowledgment of these changes is accompanied with nonpathological levels of anxiety or hostility, and similarly there is no attribution of a magical beneficence to the change. Those who are psychologically healthy are not generally passive, they do not externalize responsibility and can deal with anger, they are not anxious about sex, they do not use denial, they do not normally have gynecological symptoms, and they did not report psychosomatic or anxiety symptoms before they began using the pills.

Unusual body changes are characteristically antithetical to the pharmaceutical effects, and most important they are not only distressing to the woman, they ought to be distressing to the partner, too. These symptoms are: smaller breasts, less regular cycle, increased menstrual flow, increased cramps, and increased acne. The major characteristic of women who presented these symptoms was passivity in the sense of difficulty in expressing anger. The passivity variable was more important than the level of sex anxiety, but the anger in this context was about being "sexually used" in the relationship. It is as though the woman is expressing her anger somatically in a way that may force her partner to become responsible for contraception because they are both unhappy about these changes and because he ought to care for her welfare. Not only is she likely to induce guilt in her partner, she has also "made" herself less sexually desirable and less sexually available (e.g., increased flow and cramps). A woman following this pattern is characteristically low in guilt, and not only does she report unusual body changes, she will also report negative psychological changes. Women who were similarly highly passive, but also high in guilt, did not report unusual body changes and negative psychological changes. Those who were high in guilt internalized their anger, while those who didn't feel guilt externalized their anger and manipulated the relationship.

Beneficent body changes do not seem linked to steroid levels, are not normal statistically, and unlike unusual changes are characterized by very beneficent results. These symptoms are: more energy, decreased appetite, and loss of weight. These women were not necessarily passive—the major characteristic of those subjects who reported beneficent body changes was their high level of dependency, which in this context means dependence upon the heterosexual partner for feelings of self-esteem. The beneficent symptom assures the continued use of the contraceptive and the assumption of contraceptive responsibility because the pill has positive effects that enhance the value of the girl (i.e., loss of weight, increased energy).

Psychological Changes

We also analyzed the follow-up questionnaires for self-reported psychological changes. Negative psychological changes include (but are not limited to): less acceptance of the menstrual cycle, feeling that the body is less attractive, feeling less feminine, increased depression, increased anxiety, feeling moodier, having less energy and less ability to cope, increased premenstrual tension, less interest in one's appearance, less enjoyment of sex, decreased sexual arousability, and decreased frequency of orgasm. We should note that these responses were generated by the subjects; we did not offer a checklist of symptoms.

Negative psychological changes were reported by a group of healthier subjects and a group who were less healthy. We suspect that the healthier girls are experiencing appropriate (i.e., normal) levels of sexual anxiety and anger because they are responsible for contraception, and their negative sentiments express these dynamics as well as a recognition of normal body changes. It is likely that these negative feelings will be verbally expressed to the heterosexual partner because these women characteristically do not use denial, are not passive about expressing anger, can accept responsibility, do not generally feel guilty, and see words as a way of resolving conflict. That is, these women experience some appropriate level of anxiety or resentment that can be verbalized to the interviewer. The motives of the healthier girl to continue to use the contraceptive outweigh her irritation, but she expresses her negative feelings and acknowledges body changes that she does not like—these are normal body changes, pharmacologically related. The psychological data support the idea of frequent resentment or ambivalence within the sexual relationship for this population, and the healthier girl seems able to tolerate awareness of her ambivalence and vulnerability.

Negative psychological responses were also reported by those women who were passive in the sense of being unable to accept responsibility. These women often had experienced psychosomatic symptoms before pill use, use denial, are sex anxious (but characteristically report that their sex life is good), report unusual body changes, and characteristically do not see words as a medium for resolving conflicts. The women do not feel guilt because of their hostility and seem to project their negative feelings onto somatic changes, attributing the responsibility for the negative somatic or psychological changes to the pill, the doctor, or the partner. That is an indirect form of hostility with the cause attributed to someone or something other than the self. This is not a general use of denial but the specific denial of sexual responsibility and involvement. Although she also feels negative about the situation, the healthier girl is able to accept her responsibility, involvement, and ambivalence and may cope with reality in a more mature manner.

Positive psychological changes—which are the opposite of the negative changes—are often reported by women who have a history of body symptoms. They tend to be women who characteristically experience psychosomatic symptoms and who, at least for a short time, experience tremendous relief when pregnancy is not possible because pregnancy is an enormous threat to their body integrity. The dynamics here involve denial and are not healthy. There are at least two general kinds of sex anxiety. One is an expression of a relatively mature conflict, sexual in content, often Oedipal in dynamics. The other kind of sex anxiety, and the one that is germane here, is a much more primitive anxiety that is related to the threat of body damage, boundary vulnerability, and a lack of a strong body image. In this case the threat is less sexual than it is the destruction of body integrity through penetration and mutilation. Like beneficent body changes, the citing of positive psychological changes is linked with high levels of dependency —as well as sex anxiety, passivity, and denial. In vulnerable women the dependence seems to result in a transformation of what are normally ambivalent or somewhat negative experiences to extraordinarily positive ones, so that their responses cannot endanger the heterosexual relationship through unpleasant physical changes or less pleasing personalities. These are the subjects who most often report high levels of self-esteem at the follow-up.

We really did not find a clear cluster of healthier subjects reporting only positive psychological changes, and we feel that this is because the report of only positive changes is an expression of psychological defenses. The pill does affect the body, and ambivalence about those changes, fear of possible physical damage due to pill use, and ambivalence about sexual participation and responsibility are normal. The absence of these normal ambivalences seems to be due to the use of denial and other defenses.

Therefore, a moderate number of negative responses is often associated with a healthier personality who has more mature coping techniques and a sounder perception of reality.

Implication of This Study

This was a predictive study, and in a general sense it was successful. The personality variables that we assumed to be the critical ones do seem to be associated in meaningful ways with the dependent variables, and the use of dynamic models, projective techniques, and clinical judgments in addition to more conscious data was critical. But I would like to add a note of caution: in addition to the very real possibility that there are other very significant variables operating that we did not measure, the specific psychological or psychosomatic outcome seemed to be the result of the net balance of these psychological variables, and the prediction of individual responses becomes very complicated.

While we had set out to study psychosomatic responses we found that we also had studied morals, ambivalence, anxiety, and motives. While sexual mores have been changing since the 1920s, liberal sexual morals coexist with more traditional conservative ones. Similarly girls' traditional primary motive to achieve heterosexual success and marriage has been challenged by the women's liberation movement, but data indicate that this traditional goal has not really changed. Characteristically during adolescence the pressure to attract boys becomes crucial to self-esteem, and academic achievements become less important as affiliation needs become preeminent. Our data are consistent with the traditional idea that girls achieve identity within the affiliative relationship and are anxious within the relationship. This period of uncertain morality has increased their feelings of psychological vulnerability.

The most frequently cited reasons for choosing the pill as a contraceptive were its safety, convenience, low cost, and the fact that it seemed least mechanical. At another level, however, motives for using the pill revealed hopes and anxieties about sex. Among our subjects 42 percent hoped that the pill would reduce fears about pregnancy and *therefore* would enable them to become sexually aroused.

> This makes sex spontaneous. The other way it's too premeditated.
> I find I don't resent taking the pill like I did having to use the diaphragm and am not put off so much as I don't feel like I'm preparing for sex when I take the pill.
> I expect the pill to make me able to reach orgasm.
> The pill will make sex spontaneous.

Before they started to use the pill, some subjects denied any fears at all, and those who did express worries tended to list negative consequences that were widely publicized in the media: "I expect things like morning sickness"; "about blood clotting, the danger is less than pregnancy, both psychologically and physically"; "I'm a bit afraid of changing hormones, cancer, and varicose veins"; "I'm afraid they won't work"; "I'm afraid I'll forget to take them."

Responses at the time of the follow-up tended to reveal higher levels of fear than had been expressed at the initial interview:

I refuse to be scared. I won't have to worry. It's too easy.

Sometimes when I take the pill in the evening, I think I'm doing something against my body which isn't natural—like I would take away something of my femininity.

Before I took the pills I was kind of scared that I couldn't have as much control over myself as before.

I feel that to males the pill is kind of mystical because it prevents pregnancy.

I dislike feeling that I cannot control my body but a pill can.

Premarital sex I can justify, but you take the pill when you're alone, not romantic—whether you like him today or not.

I have the feeling that the menstrual cycle is now mechanical, something I caused, not a part of me.

The pill is not a tangible contraceptive.

In answer to the question, "If there was a pill for men like the pill for women, who would you prefer to be responsible for contraception?" 72 percent said they wanted control, 16 percent preferred male responsibility, and 12 percent said both should be responsible. Responses to this question tended to indicate levels of trust or mistrust in the relationship, some resentment and envy that the male can enjoy sex without feeling responsible, and the idea that contraception threatens the male ego.

It doesn't matter, but I'm so frightened of pregnancy, then let me know I've taken the pill.

I think I trust him better than myself. Maybe me—because if anything happens, it happens to me.

Me. Because the girl would take pregnancy more seriously than the boy.

Women, because the man is more excited and he'd be less responsible.

My boyfriend wants me to take the pill because he sees it as a commitment to the relationship.

Men should. It's bad enough they . . . I feel funny—taking all the responsibility and he's not doing anything. They should.

Men. Women have enough problems. Women have to have kids, take care of it, stay home. Men want sex—women do it because they love him.

Theoretically him—but pills don't bother me. Men would be better, more successful—women have to take them continuously. Hits the source with men.

Him—because I'm more moral—it bothers me more than it would him. And it would give him more of a commitment than me.

Women—because it's her baby and it would take away the masculinity of the boy.

I'm afraid, psychologically, that a man would feel impotent if he took a pill—and I don't care for myself.

We asked our subjects, "Why do you make love?" The responses tended to be stereotyped, part of the cultural milieu, but not true for the individual. In this population probably the most frequent response was that sex was a way of communicating love in a relationship that they hoped was mutual or the observation that if they didn't participate sexually, he would leave the relationship. For most, physical sex was important because the male made it important; for these women sex tended not to be important in its own right. Thus sexual attitudes tended to reveal the dynamics of the hetero-sexual relationship.

Because it's a means of getting closer to him.

With him it's a giving, sharing, relaxing experience. If I say that I don't feel like it, he'll just hold me instead. The ultimate is being together.

The emotional commitment resulted in my having orgasm.

I enjoy it and it makes the other person happy.

Right now to please him.

A very social thing to do—a way of reaching people.

I don't know. I think it's really necessary as a symbol of the involvement.

It's pleasurable I guess. It's expected.

It seems natural and because at this point it would harm the relationship not to. He demands it.

I hate to deny my husband although he's very good.

Very few of our subjects experienced orgasm, and while they expressed some disappointment it really wasn't terribly important because their major gratification from sex was the enhancement of closeness in the relationship. But when one is not certain that the commitment to the relationship is mutual, when one participates in sex primarily to secure love or because of fear of losing love, the psychological vulnerability overburdens the sex act. The assumption of contraceptive responsibility adds to the psycholog-ical burden because it means that the woman has to acknowledge her sexual decision. Thus taking the pill, at least in this population, can arouse anxiety about morality, and this anxiety and guilt is strongly defended against. In spite of any "sexual revolution" sex (and therefore contracep-tion) is emotionally threatening because this population of young women derives little physical pleasure from coitus and because they are afraid that they have degraded themselves and will be abandoned by their part-ners because they are immoral. These anxieties were clearest in the TAT themes that were collected at the time of the follow-up. The most frequent themes were:

Repetitive themes of men walking out

Men are argumentative, even violent

Fear of rejection by men; very mistrustful of men

Guilt in sex and the need to expiate it

Sees the male as using the women uncaringly for his own pleasure

Denial of hostility to men

Men leave her behind. Very afraid of being left alone and helpless

A view of sex as guilt-ridden and illicit

Prostitution fantasy with much shame and guilt

Sees self as constantly rejected, perpetually two-timed, deceived by men whom she serves loyally and trustingly

Guilt about premarital sex

We were shocked by the extremely high levels of anxiety, hostility, and what looked like general pathology centering on sexual themes in the TAT protocols, and we tested an additional 100 young women, most of whom were students at the university. Their responses were basically identical to those of the first sample, and these data reinforce the idea that sexual anxieties and ambivalence are generally characteristic of this population. The young women whom we saw were logically preoccupied with the achievement of important heterosexual relationships and with their identity within the relationship. Participation in sex as well as the assumption of contraceptive responsibility seemed to increase powerful negative emotions.

While some girls could talk about guilt feelings or fears that men would leave the relationship if they refused intercourse, on an unconscious level prostitution anxieties and fears of abandonment were the consequences of sex. Without an independent identity and self-esteem this becomes an unresolvable conflict. Women whose self-esteem is high are better able to participate in sex as free agents, less vulnerable to feelings of being used. But young women of the age and status of our sample are characteristically dependent upon others' acceptance, fearful of being rejected, defining and esteeming themselves in terms of the responses of others—especially their male partner.

Based upon the subjects we have seen, we think that conflict about the sexual use of the body has not diminished in this college generation in spite of safe contraception and an evolving sexual freedom in the culture. The origin of the conflict lies in the girl's ambivalence toward her reproductive system, her vulnerability in interpersonal relationships, her difficulty in experiencing sex as a physical rather than a psychological involvement, and the residues of an older morality that are still powerful and that have been internalized as a standard of behavior.

Some Final Remarks

It is possible that the particular contributions that psychologists might make to the understanding of contraceptive and family-planning behaviors will evolve from intensive studies of the sexual, parental, and role concepts, of the needs, fears, expectations, and contradictions in the psychosocial ecology of individuals, couples, and families. It would seem that hidden under the rational and stereotyped responses typical of survey data, potent, ambivalent, contradictory, emotional psychodynamics operate in the area of "family planning"—which really refers to sex, trust, life style, adulthood, virtue, creativity, responsibility, femininity, masculinity, normalcy, and most of the rest of the things that are important. An enormous assumption in this discussion, clearly untested, is that population-sized phenomena can be understood as the sum of the psychological dynamics and behaviors of individuals at different stages of life.

One of the realities that seems to be missing from the oral contraceptive literature is the fact that the change in steroid levels really and truly results in changes in one's body. The research also indicates that endocrine levels affect psychological functioning. Not only might these changes be resented, but it seems appropriate that women experience fear. While one might recommend that psychologists innovate attitude change studies and/ or laboratory experiments in fear reduction, or remind physicians to explain the mechanics of the pill to patients, it seems much more logical to exert efforts to develop techniques that are not so physiologically radical. (Why is most of the psychological research and contraceptive techniques directed to the female?)

It seems obvious that we have problems of measurement. Worse, we have problems of knowing what to measure. What one measures is a function of one's theory, of the experimenter's perception of what might be going on. The explanatory concepts, the variables that you assess, change as general theory evolves. It makes an enormous difference, for example, when one understands that a high "femininity" score on most standardized psychological instruments is not a measure of an internalized ego quality, but is usually an assessment of a verbalized conformity to a visible social norm. Understanding contraceptive dynamics will require sophisticated theory including the psychology of women, the psychology of the family, the value of children to parents, fears of death, and dimensions of responsibility, control, and time perspective.

It would seem premature to come to a conclusion. It does seem likely, however, that psychologists will be able to contribute toward understanding motivations for contraception, ambivalence and resistance to contraception, and dynamics underlying contraceptive behavior. Perhaps the most important ideas that emerge from a review of this literature are the need for an understanding of oral contraceptive behavior within the context of a more adequate psychology of women, a recognition that data are a function of how they are measured, and an awareness that the pill works because it changes the body.

REFERENCES

Aznar-Ramos, R.; Giner-Velazquez, J.; Lara-Ricalde, R.; and Martinez-Manautou, J. 1969. Incidence of side effects with contraceptive placebo. *American Journal of Obstetrics and Gynecology* 105:1144–1149.

Bakke, J. L. 1965. A double-blind study of progestin estrogen combination in the management of the menopause. *Pacific Medical Surgery* 73:200–205.

Bakker, C. B. and Dightman, C. R. 1964. Psychological factors in fertility control. *Fertility and Sterility* 15:559.

——. 1966. Side effects of oral contraceptives. *Journal of Obstetrics and Gynecology* (British Commonwealth) 28:373–379.

Bardwick, Judith, M. 1969. An interim report on the results of a study of the psychological and psychosomatic consequences of using oral contraceptives (mimeo).

——. 1970. Psychological and psychosomatic responses to oral contraceptive use. *Women on Campus; a Symposium*. Ann Arbor: Continuing Education for Women.

——. 1971. *The psychology of women*. New York: Harper & Row.

Baumblatt, M. J. and Winston, F. 1970. Pyridoxine and the pill. *Lancet* 1:832–833.

Behrman, S. J. 1969. Which pill to choose? *Hospital Practice* 4:34–39.

Benedek, Therese and Rubenstein, B. 1939a. The correlations between ovarian activity and psychodynamic processes: I. the ovulative phase. *Psychosomatic Medicine* 1: 245–270.

——. 1939b. The correlations between ovarian activity and psychodynamic processes: II. the menstrual phase. *Psychosomatic Medicine* 1:461–485.

Bower, W. H. and Altschule, R., M. D. 1956. Use of progesterone in the treatment of post-partum psychosis. *New England Journal of Medicine* 254:157.

British Medical Journal. 1968. Today's drugs: oral contraceptives—choice of product. 1:690–692.

——. 1969. Oral contraception and depression. 4:380–381.

Bumpass, L. and Westoff, C. F. 1969. The prediction of completed fertility. *Demography* 6:445–454.

Chernick, Beryl. 1965. Side effects of cyclic therapy with norethindrone and mestranol. *Fertility and Sterility* 16:445–454.

Cullberg, J.; Gelli, M. G.; Jonsson, C. O. 1969. Mental and sexual adjustment before and after six months' use of an oral contraceptive. *Acta Psychiatrica Scandinavica* 45: 259–276.

Daly, R. J.; Kane, F. J., Jr.; and Ewing, J. A. 1967. Psychosis associated with the use of a sequential oral contraceptive. *Lancet* 2:444.

Dennis, K. J. and Jeffery, J. d'A. 1968. Depression and oral contraceptives. *Lancet* 2: 454–455.

Drill, V. A. 1966. *Oral contraceptives*. New York: McGraw-Hill.

Edwards, I. S. 1969. Psychiatric aspects of oral contraceptives. *Medical Journal of Australia* 1:1054–1055.

Freedman, R.; Whelpton, P. K.; and Campbell, A. A. 1959. *Family planning, sterility, and population growth*. New York: McGraw-Hill.

Glick, I. D. 1967. Mood and behavioral changes associated with the use of the oral contraceptive agents. *Psychopharmacologia* 10:363–374.

Gluckman, L. K. 1969. Psychiatric aspects of failure with oral contraceptives. *New Zealand Medical Journal* 70:10–13.

Goldzieher, J. and Rice-Wray, E. 1966. *Oral contraceptives*. Springfield, Ill.: Charles C Thomas.

Gottschalk, L. A. and Gleser, G. C. 1969. *The measurement of psychological states through the content analysis of verbal behavior*. Berkeley: University of California Press.

Gottschalk, L. A.; Kaplan, S. M.; Gleser, G. C.; and Winget, C. M. 1962. Variations in magnitude of emotion: a method applied to anxiety and hostility during phases of the menstrual cycle. *Psychosomatic Medicine* 24:300–311.

Grant, Ellen, C. G. 1970. Metabolic effects of oral contraceptives. *British Medical Journal* 3:402–403.

Grant, E. C., and Pryse-Davies, J. 1968. Effect of oral contraceptives on depressive mood changes and on endometrial monoamine oxidase and phosphatases. *British Medical Journal* 3:777–780.

Grounds, D.; Davies, B.; and Mowbray, R. 1970. The contraceptive pill, side effects and personality: report of a controlled double-blind trial. *British Journal of Psychiatry* 116:169–172.

Hauser, G. A. and Schubiger, V. 1965. Nebener scheinungen der Ovulation Shemmenden Präparate. *Archiv fur Gynaekologie* 202:175–182.

Herzberg, B. and Coppen, A. 1970. Changes in psychological symptoms in women taking oral contraceptives. *British Journal of Psychiatry* 116:161–163.

Huffer, V.; Levin, L.; and Aronson, H. 1970. Oral contraceptives: depression and frigidity. *Journal of Nervous and Mental Disease* 151:35–41.

Ideström, C. M. 1966. Reaction to norethisterone withdrawal. *Lancet* 1:718.

Ivey, M. E. and Bardwick, J. M. 1968. Patterns of affective fluctuation in the menstrual cycle. *Psychosomatic Medicine* 30:336–345.

Jackson, H. 1966. *Antifertility compounds in the male and female.* Springfield, Ill.: Charles C Thomas.

Janowsky, D. S. and Davis, J. M. 1970. Progesterone-estrogen effects on uptake and release of norepinephrine by synaptosomes. *Life Sciences* 9:525–531.

Kane, F. J., Jr. 1968. Psychiatric reaction to oral contraceptives. *American Journal of Obstetrics and Gynecology* 102:1053–1063.

Kane, F. J., Jr. 1969. Psychosis associated with the use of oral contraceptive agents. *Southern Medical Journal* 62:190–192.

Kane, F. J., Jr.; Daly, R. J.; Ewing, J. A.; and Keeler, M. H. 1967. Mood and behavioral changes with progestational agents. *British Journal of Psychiatry* 113:265–268.

Kane, F. J. and Keeler, M. H. 1965. Use of Enovid in post-partum mental disorders. *Southern Medical Journal* 58:1089.

Kane, F. J.; Lipton, M. A.; and Ewing, J. A. 1969. Hormonal influences in female sexual response. *Archives of General Psychiatry* 20:202–209.

Kane, F. J.; Treadway, C. R.; and Ewing, J. A. 1969. Emotional change associated with oral contraceptives in female psychiatric patients. *Comprehensive Psychiatry* 10:16–30.

Keeler, M. H.; Kane, F.; and Daly, R. 1964. An acute schizophrenic episode following abrupt withdrawal of Enovid in a patient with previous post-partum psychiatric disorder. *American Journal of Psychiatry* 120:1123.

Kiser, C. V. 1967. The growth of American families studies: an assessment of significance. *Demography* 4:388–396.

Kistner, R. W. 1966. Oral contraceptives—safety factors in prolonged use of progestin-estrogen combinations. I. *Postgraduate Medicine* 39:207–216.

Kroger, W. S. and Peacock, J. F. 1968. Psychophysiological effects with an ovulation inhibitor. *Psychosomatics* 9:67–70.

Kutner, J. S. and Duffy, T. J. 1970. A psychological analysis of oral contraceptives and the intrauterine device. *Contraception* 2:289–296.

La Gravinese, N. 1965. Psico-nevrosi Pseudogravidiche da gestageni. *Policinico* (Prat) 72:1639–1644.

Lewis, A. and Hoghughi, M. 1969. An evaluation of depression as a side effect of oral contraceptives. *British Journal of Psychiatry* 115:697–701.

Linthorst, G. 1967. Menopauze en postmenopauze. Het võor en tigen van een preventie. *Nederlands Tijdschrift voor Geneeskunde* 111:769–773.

Marcotte, D. B.; Kane, F. J.; Obrist, P.; and Lipton, M. A. 1970. Psychophysiologic changes accompanying oral contraceptive use. *British Journal of Psychiatry* 116: 165–167.

Mason, J.; Wherry, F. E.; Brady, J. V.; Tollener, G. A.; Goodman, A. C.; and Beer, B. 1966. Psychological influence on plasma insulin levels in the monkey. *Psychosomatic Medicine* 28:767–768.

Mears, Eleanor and Grant, Ellen. 1962. "Anovlar" as an oral contraceptive. *British Medical Journal* 2:75–79.

Michael, R. P.; Saayman, G. S.; and Zumpe, D. 1967. Inhibition of sexual receptivity by progesterone in rhesus monkeys. *Journal of Endocrinology* 39:309–310.

Moos, R. H. 1968. Psychological aspects of oral contraceptives. *Archives of General Psychiatry* 19:87–94.

Murawski, B. J.; Sapir, P. E.; Shulman, N.; Ryan, G. M., Jr.; and Sturgis, S. H. 1968. An investigation of mood states in women taking oral contraceptives. *Fertility and Sterility* 19:50–63.

Nilsson, A. and Almgren, P. E. 1968. Psychiatric symptoms during the post-partum period as related to use of oral contraceptives. *British Medical Journal* 2:453–455.

Nilsson, A.; Jacobson, L.; and Ingemanson, C. A. 1967. Side-effects of an oral contraceptive with particular attention to mental symptoms and sexual adaptation. *Acta Obstetrica et Gynecologica Scandinavica* 46:537–556.

Nilsson, L. and Sölvell, L. 1967. Clinical studies on oral contraceptives—randomized, doubleblind, crossover study of 4 different preparations (Anovlar Mite, Lyndiol Mite, Ovulen, Volidan). *Acta Obstetrica et Gynecologica Scandinavica* 46(Suppl. 8):1–31.

Nistico, G. and Preziosi, P. 1970. Contraceptives, brain serotonin, and liver tryptophan pyrrolase. *Lancet* 2:213.

Oakes, Merilee R. 1970. Pills, periods, and personality. Unpublished Ph.D. diss., University of Michigan.

Orchard, W. H. 1969. Psychiatric aspects of oral contraceptives. *Medical Journal of Australia* 1:872–876.

Paige, Karen E. 1969. The effects of contraceptives on affective fluctuations associated with the menstrual cycle. Unpublished Ph.D. diss., University of Michigan.

Pincus, G.; Garcia, C. R.; Rock, J.; Paniagua, M.; Pendleton, A.; Laraque, F.; Nicolas, R.; Borno, R.; and Pean, V. 1959. Effectiveness of an oral contraceptive. *Science* 130:81.

Rapoport, A. and Chammah, A. 1965. *Prisoner's dilemma*. Ann Arbor: University of Michigan Press.

Ringrose, C. A. D. 1965. Emotional responses of married women receiving oral contraceptives. *Canadian Medical Association Journal* 92:1207.

Rock, J. 1965. "Let's be honest about the pill!" *Journal of the American Medical Association* 192:401–403.

Rose, D. P. and Braidman, I. P. 1970. Oral contraceptives, depression, and amino acid metabolism. *Lancet* 1:1117–1118.

Slugett, J. and Lawson, J. 1967. Side effects of oral contraceptives. *Lancet* 2:612.

Sölvell, L. and Nilsson, L. 1968. A clinical study on a sequential oral contraceptive-ovisec. *Acta Obstetrica et Gynecologica Scandinavica* 47(Suppl. 6):3–25.

Sölvell, L.; Nilsson, L.; and Westholm, H. 1968. Amount of menstrual blood loss during sequenial oral contraceptive therapy-ovisec. *Acta Obstetrica et Gynecologica Scandinavica* 47(Suppl. 6):27–32.

Sturgis, S. H. 1968. Oral contraceptives and their effect on sex behavior. *Medical Aspects of Human Sexuality* 2:4–9.

Swanson, D. W.; Barron, A.; Floren, A.; and Smith, J. A. 1964. Use of norethynodrel in psychotic females. *American Journal of Psychiatry* 120:1101.

Wallach, E. E. and Garcia, C. R. 1968. Emotional factors in oral contraception. *Clinical Obstetrics and Gynecology* 11:684–697.

Wallach, E. E.; Watson, F. M., Jr.; and Garcia, C. R. 1967. Patient acceptance of oral contraceptives. II. The private patient. *American Journal of Obstetrics and Gynecology* 98:1071.

Waxman, D. 1968. Mood and the "pill." *British Medical Journal* 4:188.

Wearing, M. P. 1963. The use of norethindrone (2 mg.) with mestranol (1 mg.) in fertility control. *Canadian Medical Association Journal* 89:239.

West, Joy. 1968. Mood and the "pill." *British Medical Journal* 4:187–188.

Westoff, C. F.; Potter, R. G.; and Sagi, P. C. 1963. *The third child*. Princeton: Princeton University Press.

Westoff, C. F.; Potter, R. G.; Sagi, P. C.; and Mishler, E. G. 1961. *Family growth in metropolitan America*. Princeton: Princeton University Press.

Westoff, C. F. and Ryder, N. B. 1969. Recent trends in attitudes toward fertility control and the practice of contraception in the United States. In S. J. Behrman et al., eds., *Fertility and family planning*. Ann Arbor: University of Michigan Press. Pp. 388–412.

Whelpton, P. K.; Campbell, A. A.; and Patterson, J. E. 1966. *Fertility and family planning in the United States*. Princeton: Princeton University Press.

Whelpton, P. K. and Kiser, C. V., eds. 1946–1958. *Social and psychological factors affecting fertility*. New York: Milbank Memorial Fund. 5 vols.

Winston, F. 1969a. Oral contraceptives and depression. *Lancet* 1:1209.

————. 1969b. Oral contraceptives and depression. *Lancet* 2:377.

Zell, J. R. and Crisp, W. E. 1964. Psychiatric evaluation of the use of oral contraceptives. A study of 250 private patients. *American Journal of Obstetrics and Gynecology* 23:657.

Ziegler, F. J. and Rodgers, D. A. 1966. Vasectomy, ovulation suppressors, and sexual behavior. Paper presented at American Ortho-Psychiatric Meeting, April 15, 1966.

[11]

PSYCHOLOGICAL REACTIONS
TO SURGICAL CONTRACEPTION

DAVID A. RODGERS
AND FREDERICK J. ZIEGLER

This chapter deals with psychological reactions to the male operation of vasectomy and the female operations of salpingectomy and hysterectomy when these are done at the voluntary request of the subject primarily for purposes of contraception. We will contend that the usual custom of calling these operations sterilization is arbitrary and not really appropriate. For the procedures of vasectomy and salpingectomy or tubal ligation we suggest the alternative description of surgical contraception rather than sterilization. The present chapter will not deal with psychological reactions to castration (orchidectomy or oophorectomy), which is a sterilizing procedure that is almost never used as a voluntary procedure of contraception per se.

No accurate data are available on the incidence of surgical contraception in most countries of the world, although survey information does suggest that there has been a sharp increase in frequency during the last decade. These forms of birth control are highly favored by many population-planning experts as well as by many individual couples. Official government policy in India has stimulated widespread use of vasectomy there. Salpingectomy is most widely used for contraception in Puerto Rico. Presser (1970) summarizes the available incidence data from various countries. The number of people involved is far from trivial. For example, she cites 32 percent incidence of salpingectomy among ever married women in Puerto Rico in 1965. She cites 5 percent incidence of surgical contraception among a 1965 sample of women ages eighteen to thirty-nine in the United States, with an additional 6 percent having been sterilized for remedial purposes. She cites a 3 percent incidence of vasectomy among husbands of this 1965 sample of U.S. women.

Definitive studies of psychological reaction to surgical contraception are lacking in spite of the many millions of persons who are utilizing these procedures. Some studies have nevertheless been done and will be reviewed in the present chapter. The most comprehensive of these studies have dealt with middle-class or lower-class American couples, and the extent to which the results can be generalized validly beyond the groups studied remains unknown. We suggest that the assumption that these results cannot be generalized, in the absence of other evidence, is no more warranted than is the alternative assumption that the results can be generalized.

Psychological Characteristics of Surgical Contraception

The normal reproductive sequence requires the production of male gametes or sperm in the male testes and of female gametes or ova in the female ovaries; the transportation of the sperm from the testes through the vas deferens and seminal vesicles and urethra of the male into the female vagina and subsequently into the uterus and fallopian tubes of the female; and the meeting of sperm with ova released from the ovaries as the ova move through the fallopian tubes toward the uterus. Following fertilization by union of a sperm and ovum, the resulting zygote attaches itself to the wall of the uterus, where it grows into a fetus and, after a period of gestation and subsequent birth, a neonatal child.

All contraceptive procedures are directed toward disrupting this sequence of events at some point prior to implantation of the fertilized ovum on the wall of the uterus. Procedures that disrupt the sequence after implantation are considered to be abortion rather than contraceptive procedures. Oral contraceptive pills either prevent release of the ova from the ovaries or prevent implantation of the fertilized ovum on the wall of the uterus, or both. Intrauterine devices (IUDs) prevent implantation on the wall of the uterus. Condoms and diaphragms impose a mechanical barrier in the normal passageway along which the gametes ultimately unite. Foams and jellies impose a chemical barrier in this same passageway. Various behavioral contraceptive procedures such as the rhythm method, coitus interruptus, and nonintercourse procedures of sexual contact utilize either time factors (as in the case of the rhythm method) or mechanical factors (as in the case of the other procedures) to avoid conjunction of viable male and female gametes. Surgical contraception imposes a mechanical barrier to the passageway along which gamete union might otherwise occur. In the case of vasectomy this barrier is imposed at the site of the vas deferens in the male. In the case of salpingectomy or tubal ligation and of hysterectomy this barrier is imposed at the location of the fallopian tubes of the female.

In addition hysterectomy would also obviously prevent implantation and subsequent gestation.

Since from a contraceptive point of view surgical contraception functions on the same basis that a condom or a diaphragm does, mechanically blocking the passageway through which the gametes ultimately might join, the question can be raised as to why special attention should be given to psychological reactions to these surgical procedures over and beyond psychological reactions to mechanical contraception. Data indicate that there clearly is greater reaction to surgical than to nonsurgical mechanical contraception, and the source of this reaction can be sought in two alternative directions. First, nearly all contraceptive procedures have some side effects that are inevitably associated with the procedure but somewhat extraneous to contraception per se. For example, use of the condom requires interrupting other ongoing activity after an erection has been obtained in order to apply the sheath. This interruption itself is usually annoying and not part of the contraceptive function. Similarly changes in sensation along the penile shaft secondary to covering it with a sheath are also irrelevant to the contraceptive function of a condom, but they often constitute another basis for disliking it as a contraceptive procedure. In a similar sense psychological reactions to the surgical contraceptive procedures may depend on side effects that are extraneous to the contraception itself. The nature of these procedures will therefore be briefly reviewed for what light might be shed on the reaction of users to these procedures.

An alternative direction for understanding psychological reaction to the operations, which will be explored later in this chapter, is the informational meaning of the procedures, apart from otherwise unrelated consequences. If a vasectomy or tubal ligation imposed an entirely nonannoying and subjectively nondetectable barrier to passage of the gametes, such that the only subjective basis for responding to the operative effects would be the personal knowledge that the operation had been performed, these procedures would still have significant psychological effects on the users. It is these effects with which the present chapter is primarily concerned, but these effects can best be understood after careful consideration of the physiological nature of the procedures.

Salpingectomy or Tubal Ligation

Salpingectomy consists of interrupting and tying a woman's fallopian tubes, the small tubes that run from the ovaries to the uterus, through which the ova pass. After the operation ova are still released and probably move down the proximal end of the fallopian tubes, but are eventually resorbed when they cannot go beyond the blocked passage. The female hormone production of the ovaries is normally released into the blood supply to the ovaries and is not logically affected by surgical contraception. The fallopian tubes are located deep in the abdominal cavity, which must be surgically entered during the operation. It can be entered either through an abdominal wall incision or through the vagina. The vaginal approach is less traumatic generally, but it may be associated with some increased risk of accidental injury to, or ligation of, other structures such as the blood supply to the kidneys. As with any abdominal procedure some risk exists that subsequent scar tissue or adhesions will develop following salpingectomy and will produce some associated symptomatology. While this is not a common occurrence, it may result in an adverse reaction to the operation when it does occur; and knowledge that it is possible may provide a conceptual basis for conversion reaction abdominal complaints in women who do not actually develop this condition. There is a period of general debility following salpingectomy, secondary to the abdominal surgery itself, which also may result in some adverse reaction to the procedure. This period of debility is often no greater, or not much greater, than debility from delivery itself when the operation is performed immediately postpartum, a common time for a tubal ligation. In any event psychological reaction to contraception resulting from the operation is inevitably confounded with any psychological impacts that may have resulted from debility associated with the operative procedure itself. Data on differential contributions of such debility or reaction to the operation as a contraceptive procedure are not available to our knowledge and probably await research that has not yet been done.

Hysterectomy

If a woman no longer wishes to become pregnant, the uterus becomes an essentially superfluous organ. Since uterine cancer is a small but real risk in women and becomes an increasing risk with advancing age, removal of the uterus has been recommended by some authorities and is often used as an alternative to tubal ligation for surgical contraception. It is a more certain contraceptive procedure, in that perhaps as high as 1 percent of tubal ligations are followed by spontaneous reanastomosis or reopening of one of the fallopian tubes, often resulting in pregnancy. Side effects from a hysterectomy are much more pronounced than are those from a tubal ligation. First, the operative procedure itself is more major, usually involves a larger abdominal incision, involves more trauma to the abdominal cavity at the time of the operation, is followed by more risk of subsequent adhesions or postoperative complications, and may result in a somewhat longer period of postoperative debility. With removal of the uterus menstruation is also terminated. Termination of menstruation, with associated termination of menstrually associated cramps and other symptomatology, would seem to constitute a positive practical gain of this procedure. On the negative side the absence of menstruation is a reminder of permanence of contraception, may be psychologically associated with postmenopausal "over the hill" status as a woman or more directly with loss of femininity. Thus hysterectomy as a contraceptive procedure carries with it as a side effect all of the psychological reactions that may be associated with menstruation and the relationship of menstruation to femininity.

As an illustration of the complexity of this side effect contribution to the meaning of sterilization, some women may utilize menstruation as an excuse for avoiding sexual relations for a period of perhaps one week a month, and often longer if premenstrual tension is exploited as an excuse for avoiding intercourse. This bargaining power concerning sexual relations is, of course, retained following tubal ligation, even though risk of pregnancy is avoided. What on the surface may be complained about as a debilitating experience (menstruation) can thus covertly or "psychologically" be utilized by some women as a positive and highly valuable pawn in the heterosexual marriage game. This is but one of many dimensions that would need careful evaluation before our knowledge of psychological reactions to this particular contraceptive procedure would be complete.

Details of the hysterectomy procedure will not be reviewed here, since this procedure is generally well known. The operation consists of removing the uterus, an organ about the size of a small pear, that is attached to and located immediately above the vagina. The vagina itself is not altered significantly, and the intra-abdominal contents easily readjust to the absence of the uterus such that no residual subjective sensations are associated with this surgical alteration of abdominal content. As far as is known, subjective sensations associated with intercourse (for both partners) are essentially unaffected following complete recovery from the operation.

Vasectomy

Vasectomy consists of cutting and tying the two cut ends of each vas deferens that transports sperm from a testis to the seminal vesicles in the male. These small tubes pass from the scrotum into the abdominal cavity. The operation is performed in the scrotal area. Surgically the procedure is a simple one, usually done under local anesthetic through one or two small incisions in the scrotum. It normally takes from ten to twenty minutes and is usually done as an in-office procedure. In the hands of a competent and experienced surgeon the procedure is seldom associated with serious medical complications. For example, in a series of fifty vasectomies performed in North Carolina, forty-seven of the fifty patients reported almost no pain in the postoperative days, and thirty-one of the fifty patients lost no time from work as a result of the operation. Only one patient lost more than three days from work (Garrison and Gamble, 1950). These data are typical of findings in other studies reported.

The testicular contribution to ejaculate volume amounts to from 5 to 10 percent (Phadke, 1964; Lee, 1966). Since ejaculate volume fluctuates considerably with time since previous intercourse and other variables, it is unlikely that a 10 percent reduction in volume significantly alters subjective sensations associated with ejaculation—sensations that are not likely to be precisely discriminating of volume parameters in any event. In one direct comparison Lee (1966) did not find statistically significant difference in ejaculate volume of vasectomized versus nonvasectomized subjects. Concerning subjective experience of ejaculate volume, Lee found that in one group of approximately 1,000 Japanese men who had undergone vasectomy 9 percent subjectively felt semen volume had decreased, whereas 4 percent felt that semen volume had increased. In another series of 130 patients 4 percent reported sensation of decreased volume, whereas 3 percent reported sensation of increased volume. These data suggest that change in ejaculate volume is not likely to be a major stimulus parameter following vasectomy.

As would be expected from the nature of the operation, hormone levels are not altered following vasectomy (Phadke, 1964). Hormones from the testes are released directly into the blood supply to the testes and do not depend on patency of the vas deferens.

One rather consistent sequel to the operation is an expansion of the testicular section of vas under pressure of the testicular secretion of sperm and associated fluid. According to Schmidt (1969), the resulting engorgement of the epididymis tubules and the vas can result in temporary discomfort and can lead to rupture of a tubule and resultant formation of a spermatic granuloma that in some cases can result in a spontaneous rechannelization to the distal end of the vas and spontaneous circumvention of the vasectomy; in other cases it can result in permanent proximal obstruction of the vas such that subsequent vasovasostomy would be ineffectual in restoring fertility unless it were also associated with a successful epididymovasostomy as well. It is thought by some that these or associated processes may also result in development of autoimmunity to the man's own sperm, which would result in temporary or permanent sterility via an immune mechanism. Frequency of circulating antibodies against own sperm has been reported to be higher in postvasectomized men than in nonvasectomized men, tending to support this hypothesis (Phadke and Padukone, 1964; Rümke and Hellinga, 1959; Wolfers, 1970). These side effects to vasectomy may result in some physiological sensations (associated with congestion at the proximal end of the vas) and autoimmune or mechanical sterility other than that associated with the surgical blocking of the vas deferens itself. An additional complication is a failure rate of probably in excess of 1 percent (Presser, 1970), in which spontaneous rechannelization of the vas, as described above, takes place to circumvent the surgically induced sterilization. Often the first knowledge of this surgical failure is pregnancy of the wife or partner.

Technically the term "vasectomy" is a misnomer since the vas deferens is merely severed and tied or only partially removed. This distinction is important, because reanastomosis of the two ends of the vas is a not uncommon surgical procedure, that may result in successful restoration of reproductive capacity. Phadke (1964) reported successful reanastomosis of the vas deferens, with demonstration of sperm in the semen postoperatively, in 90 percent of a series of forty-nine operations one to sixteen years postvasectomy. Of this series of forty-nine cases thirty-one reconstructions were followed by pregnancies, conclusively demonstrating a restoration of fertility in a minimum of 63 percent of his series. In contrast Presser (1970) reports that successful reversal of tubal ligation has occurred in from 17 to 29 percent of cases on the average. This percentage might, of course, be considerably higher if enough such operations were performed for surgeons to gain experience and skill, since reversal of tubal ligation is a rather uncommon procedure.

In terms of surgical risk vasectomy is considerably safer than either tubal ligation or hysterectomy. No deaths have been reported secondary to vasectomy as an operative procedure, whereas Tietze (1960) has estimated that mortality rate for tubal sterilization is about one per 3,000 operations, corresponding roughly to the risk of death from childbirth in the United States. The mortality rate for hysterectomy would probably be comparable or slightly higher. Surgical reversal of vasectomy is also simpler and more successful than is surgical reversal of tubal ligation.

Psychological Reactions to Tubal Ligation and Hysterectomy

It seems reasonable to infer that the primary psychological reaction to the surgical contraceptive procedures of tubal ligation and hysterectomy is to the self-knowledge that these operations have been performed rather than to the noncontraceptive physiological side effects of the operation. Little research work has been done on these differential considerations, but there apparently are few subjective complaints that can be attributed to physiological changes per se after full recovery from the operative procedures. For example, Sacks and LaCroix (1962) stated that in a series of 100 patients, 89 percent denied any change of pelvic consciousness, except for some changes associated with menstruation that might be expected with advancing age. The remaining 11 percent noted symptoms such as pain in their ovaries, backaches, constipation, and related symptoms. These kinds of complaints in this percentage of women are not unusual in the normal population, and we are inclined to doubt that they indicate postoperative physiological side effects to the operative procedures.

Several studies have been done of psychological response following gynecological surgery and especially following hysterectomy. Most of these studies, however, concern hysterectomies done for medical reasons other than contraception; therefore they are not directly relevant to the present review. For example, Melody (1962) reported occurrence of severe depressive illness in approximately 4 percent of a series of 267 hysterectomized women. Apparently other severe complications were relatively rare. It is difficult to relate these findings and findings of similar studies to surgical contraception, however. As Fischer (1962) has pointed out, gynecological surgery for reasons of medical necessity can be reacted to by some patients as constituting "a kindly rescue in which a 'bad' organ that is causing pain and suffering, is 'poisoning,' or is slowly destroying the patient and killing her is removed by a friend or god. . . . On the other hand, she can view the removal of organs as detrimental, making her worse than she was before by making her defective and removing valuable things. In this fantasy, she may also fear or hate the surgeon. Sometimes her reactions are mixed." Presumably reactions would be different in procedures voluntarily sought to achieve personally desired goals.

Even when the operative procedures are for purposes of contraception, they are not always voluntarily sought by patients and may be done for medical rather than personal reasons. Sacks and LaCroix (1962), for example, reported eighteen patients out of a study series of 100 patients who regretted having permitted tubal ligation. In 60 percent of this group either the husband or the wife, or both, voiced objection to sterilization at the time the operation was recommended.

One fact that is clear from the reported studies of women following gynecological surgery is that the uterus and other pelvic organs can be invested with much psychological meaning over and beyond their direct physiological functional utility. This potential psychological meaning of the pelvic organs is documented by Drellich and Bieber (1958) and by Fischer (1962). Some of their findings would probably apply to at least some women obtaining either tubal ligation or hysterectomy for contraception. These studies found some women who, even though they desired no more children, viewed the loss of childbearing ability as rendering a woman something less than a complete female. Drellich and Bieber also found many women who expressed regret over loss of the uterus because of the specific feminine functions that they attributed to this organ. In their series a majority of the women looked upon menstruation as a necessary and valuable function whose termination was viewed with regret. Many felt that menstruation was a way of ridding the body of harmful wastes. Others felt that it was a timing device that regulated bodily functions and to some degree regulated social functions. Others felt that the uterus was a sexual organ somewhat akin to the male penis, removal of which would destroy their sexual desire and pleasure. These latter concerns about the uterus itself would, of course, apply only to hysterectomy as a contraceptive procedure and not to tubal ligation, which does not remove the uterus and which leaves unaffected the associated processes of menstruation. Their particular study concerned total hysterectomy, with a removal of the ovaries as well as the uterus, and it would be difficult to assess the differential effect of hysterectomy alone. Nevertheless, it seems apparent that there is, indeed, much potential for psychological reaction to hysterectomy, depending on the specific personal meaning that the uterus has to the particular subject involved. It is difficult to draw general conclusions from their study, since apparently there were wide individual differences in attitudes and since much of the information about the meaning of the uterus was obtained from women prior to the operation rather than postoperatively. On follow-up study of these women the investigators did find rather marked differences in response to the operation. Several patients had no decrease in their sexual desires or effective sexual functioning. Several others believed themselves to be raw, tender, and vulnerable inside postoperatively, an opinion that was sometimes shared by their spouses. Somewhat limiting the generality of results from this study is the fact that no general response was abstracted from this series of women: "It is apparent that while the sex life of many of our patients was very decidedly affected by the hysterectomy, the manifestations of change were in no way uniform" (p. 327).

Fischer's report (1962) further documents individual reactions to hysterectomy but also indicates the potential of therapeutic intervention for changing the negative emotional impact of anticipated gynecological surgery. He thus suggests that the psychological reaction to the operation may be ameliorated by appropriate psychotherapeutic intervention, a finding that would suggest that the psychological reactions are not inevitable and are subject to modification.

Of somewhat more relevance to the psychological import of contraceptive surgery per se, independent of additional factors associated with hysterectomy, are the studies of Barglow and his co-workers and of Sacks and LaCroix. Barglow (1964) found that conscious pregnancy fantasies or symptoms and signs were observed in 152 women out of a series of 190 patients followed several months or years after sterilization surgery. These women apparently were not a random selection of surgical contraceptive patients, so generalizations to the population at large are not possible. Barglow's data, nevertheless, indicate that loss of potential for pregnancy was regarded by many women as a significant personal loss. For many patients (45 percent of his sample) the pregnancy fantasies seemed to serve the function of the working through of a loss, with a resulting healthy acceptance of their postoperative state of permanent contraception. Thirty percent of his sample showed more immature response, consisting of hysterical conversion symptoms and vicarious dependent-need gratification through identification with their own children or similar mechanisms. Some of these women apparently sought alternative ways of coping with some aversion to sexual relations once fear of pregnancy was removed. For example, one patient, who had avoided intercourse with her husband presumably through fear of pregnancy preoperatively, joined a fanatical religious cult postoperatively that justified disinterest in sexuality subsequently. Patients of this group apparently were not able to accept the loss of childbearing function and showed evidence of guilt and shame that was accompanied with a conscious sense of disappointment with the operation, yearning for another pregnancy, and occasional attempts to have a rechannelization procedure. Some of these women even persisted in the use of contraceptive measures postoperatively, continuing to manifest an intense fear of conception. A third group of women (25 percent of this particular series) showed initial total acceptance of the loss of fertility; nevertheless, they often showed delayed recovery or minor surgical complications and subsequently reported feelings of inferiority, weakness, and emptiness and a sense of being a damaged and changed person. Subsequent misfortunes of life such as accidents, obesity, frigidity, marriage failure, and other physical illnesses tended to be blamed on the operation. Many of the women in this group also showed manifestations of pseudopregnancy, apparently in an unconscious rejection of their state of permanent contraception. Both in this series and in a subsequent series (Barglow, Gunther, Johnson, and Meltzer, 1965) the most severe postoperative reactions were much more frequent among hysterectomy patients than among tubal ligation patients. In this systematic series differentiating the two procedures, in which a group of twenty-two high-parity patients were randomly assigned to either tubal ligation or hysterectomy for contraception postpartum, only three of twelve hysterectomy patients had a good outcome postoperatively, whereas eight of ten tubal ligation patients had a good outcome. Thus it would seem that psychological reaction to tubal ligation is much less profound than psychological reaction to hysterectomy when these procedures are done for purposes of contraception. These investigators also found a significant relationship between preoperative anxiety about the procedure and long-term response to the procedure, with nine of twelve patients who had high preoperative anxiety showing a poor response and only two of ten women with low preoperative anxiety showing a poor response. These data are somewhat confounded with the fact that more women anticipating hysterectomy showed high preoperative anxiety than did those anticipating tubal ligation. A further confounding and perhaps related finding was that nine of the original twelve women rated as high in preoperative anxiety also experienced difficult or complicated immediate postoperative courses. Difficult postoperative experience thus also related to a poor outcome, albeit confounded with hysterectomy and high preoperative anxiety, with eight of eleven patients showing a poor outcome following postoperative complications.

One interesting finding of the Barglow et al. group was that successful emotional adjustment postoperatively seemed to be correlated in a majority of the women with the presence of the strikingly unrealistic fantasy that they may have retained the ability to become pregnant again. This fantasy was most common in the tubal ligation group. This subjective concept that the tubal ligation may not be a permanent procedure suggests the importance of our recommendation that these procedures be considered surgical contraception rather than surgical sterilization, since contraception seems to be a much more tolerable self-conception than is permanent sterilization.

Since the Barglow et al. series did concern women that presumably wanted surgical contraception, the high percentage of poor outcomes—as reflected by expressed dissatisfaction with the procedure, exacerbation of physical or psychological symptoms, and deterioration of sexual or social relationships—suggests that the psychological response to these procedures needs considerably more assessment than it has received to date. Eleven of the twenty-two patients, or exactly 50 percent, were rated as having a poor outcome. Two of ten, or 20 percent, of the tubal ligation patients were rated as having a poor outcome, and nine of twelve, or 75 percent, of the hysterectomy patients were so rated. This is a small series, of course, and it is unfortunate that to date we do not have careful study of a larger series. This particular group consisted of multiparous women, with an average of eight living children among women with a history of vaginal deliveries, and of five living children among women with a history of Caesarean deliveries. They were drawn from a population composed mostly of southern-born, economically deprived Negro women, seen in a public clinic in Chicago. The degree to which these data can be transferred to other populations is, of course, unknown.

Psychological Response to Vasectomy

Much more systematic study has been done of psychological response to vasectomy as surgical contraception than of response to the female contraceptive surgeries. Several retrospective studies have been done on populations in Europe (Hinderer, 1947; Hauser, 1955), the United States (Laidlaw and Bass, 1964; The Simon Population Trust, 1969), North Carolina (Garrison and Gamble, 1950), California (Popenoe, 1929; Poffenberger and Poffenberger, 1963; Landis and Poffenberger, 1965), India (Dandekar, 1963), Korea (Lee, 1966), and England (Wolfers, 1970). Such retrospective studies almost invariably report a high percentage of subjects (in excess of 90 percent and as high as 99 percent) who are favorably inclined toward the operation and state they would have the operation repeated. A generally small percentage, usually 1 to 3 percent, state that they have suffered some deterioration in their sexual lives and would not have the operation repeated. A slightly larger percentage, but less than 10 percent, may report that they would not repeat the operation because of changes in life circumstance, but deny any significant deleterious emotional or sexual impact from the procedure.

In contrast to these highly favorable postoperative survey findings, a few investigators have raised more serious doubts about how benign vasectomy is. Wolfers (1970), in her somewhat more penetrating survey in England for example, found evidence of psychological impairment in 12 percent of her sample and felt that most survey approaches underestimated negative postoperative reaction. Johnson (1964) reports on a series of men seen at a veterans' hospital who showed marked emotional deterioration following vasectomy operations. These reactions were sufficiently severe to result in hospitalization within one year following surgery in eleven men out of a sample of eighty-three patients. Seventeen of the eighty-three men apparently regretted having had the operation. This sample was drawn from psychiatric patients, so could be expected to contain a high percentage of negative reactors. Nevertheless, the severity of the reactions of these patients does suggest considerable potential for negative reaction to the procedure.

Perhaps more disturbing is the report of Erickson (1954), giving several case histories of therapy with men for whom vasectomy clearly had a rather profound psychological impact, but in whom the impact was often disguised both from the patient himself and from his family. In several cases the full extent of the pathology resulting from the operation was manifest long after the operation had been completed, following a period of apparently unproblematic adjustment. While this was a short series of cases and is subject to the usual questions about case-history reports, nevertheless, it clearly raises the possibility that some of the primary impact of the contraceptive surgeries may be manifest indirectly and without awareness of the subject.

Ziegler, Rodgers, and associates used a prospective design to study psychological reactions of two groups of men to vasectomy. One group was followed a year after the operation, the initial data having been obtained a few weeks preoperatively (Rodgers, Ziegler, Altrocchi, and Levy, 1965; see also Rodgers, Ziegler, Rohr, and Prentiss, 1963). Thirty-four of these thirty-five men expressed satisfaction with the contraceptive procedure, as in other survey studies; but seven reported decreased sexual functioning, and psychological test analysis (primarily Minnesota Multiphasic Personality Inventory) indicated increased psychological disturbance in fifteen of this group, with only two of the thirty-five showing some improvement on the tests. These results thus suggest that there is more negative emotional impact from the operation than retrospective survey results would indicate. In a second study couples were followed for four years postoperatively and were studied more intensively by interview, questionnaire, and testing procedures (Ziegler, Rodgers, and Kriegsman, 1966; Ziegler and Rodgers, 1968; Rodgers and Ziegler, 1968; Ziegler, Rodgers, and Prentiss, 1969). Forty-two couples were followed in this study, and data were compared to a group of thirty-nine couples using oral contraceptives. While no traumatic postoperative effects were found, careful comparison against the couples using oral contraceptives demonstrated adverse changes in marital satisfaction and in overall adjustment of the husbands and their wives two years after vasectomy. The data were interpreted as suggesting that the vasectomy operation was generally responded to as though it had demasculinizing potential. The behavior of the man after vasectomy was more systematically scrutinized by himself and by his wife and possibly by others for evidence of unmasculine features. As a consequence, the range of acceptable behaviors was narrowed for each subject on a rather individualized basis, reflecting each person's circumstances and each person's interpretation of "unmasculine" behavior. In some cases the result was a favorable decrease in immature and indecisive behavior, with improvement in occupational, parental, and husband role enactments. In other and perhaps more characteristic cases the result was a decrease in flexibility that reduced personal effectiveness, that heightened personal anxiety, and that produced some increased marital disharmony and dissatisfaction of the wife.

An example of the threat to masculinity that the operation seemed to impose was the change in sexual behavior in the vasectomy group as compared to the oral contraceptive group. Frequency of intercourse increased somewhat in both groups, but more markedly in the vasectomy group, probably because of an initial depressed frequency in that particular group. For the oral contraceptive group sexual problems were most often associated with low frequency of sexual intercourse, rate of intercourse being reduced if impotency or other problems existed. The inverse relationship was found in the vasectomy group four years postoperatively, with impotency being most likely in the high frequency of intercourse group. It was inferred that these men were overreaching their sexual capacity in order to confirm their own masculinity, with resulting deleterious effects on sexual performance. The study did not find an increase in promiscuous behavior or a decrease in noncoital sexual activity, suggesting that these other aspects of sexuality were not markedly affected. On other assessment parameters no significant differences between the vasectomy-using and the oral-contraceptive-using couples were demonstrable in the areas of marital satisfaction and emotional upset after four years.

It was felt that the extensive research contact with these subjects probably minimized adverse reactions, so that the first study done by this team was viewed as a better estimate of the general population response to vasectomy. This apparent effect of the study team in preventing more overtly disturbed psychological functioning leads us to recommend routine counseling of men and their wives prior to vasectomy and several times subsequent to it to try to eliminate or minimize any potential individual or marital problems.

One explanation suggested for the paradoxically high stated enthusiasm for vasectomy postoperatively, in association with evidence of the apparent negative impact of the operation, was that a process of dissonance reduction might take place in which men overemphasized their enthusiasm as a way of denying the discrepancy between their own attitudes and a condition that they could not easily alter. This affirmative arguing for the procedure might in fact have created some problems for these subjects by advertising to the public that they had had vasectomy operations. In a study of cultural attitudes toward vasectomy Rodgers, Ziegler, and Levy (1967) found that both a Protestant couples group and a college student group rated much more unfavorably a couple who was identified as having had a vasectomy than they did an otherwise identical couple who was identified as using oral contraception. Thus in the United States there would appear to be a rather strong negative cultural attitude toward vasectomy and couples who utilize this procedure, which might further negatively affect men who have had the operation and might be especially troublesome for men who seek to quell their own anxiety by publicly declaring their enthusiasm for the procedure.

Sterilization versus Contraception

From the studies so far done we would conclude that both vasectomy and tubal ligation or hysterectomy are subjectively experienced as posing a threat to the masculinity and femininity, respectively, of at least some of the subjects undergoing these procedures. The present research data are by no means comprehensive, and much more definitive work must be done before adequate understanding of psychological reaction to these procedures can be obtained. Nevertheless, several tentative issues can be suggested on the basis of present data. A major issue is one raised at the beginning of this chapter: why is there so much more profound psychological reaction to surgical contraception than to other forms of contraception? We would like to consider this issue at somewhat more length at this point.

Sterilization technically means rendering incapable of reproduction. For at least the duration of a given intercourse experience, the goal of all contraceptive use is, of course, functional sterility. Nonetheless, we do not normally describe a woman wearing a well-fitting diaphragm as sterile. Presumably the capacity for reproduction is still retained as a potential if not a current state by such a woman. If distinctions are to be made between potential and current capability of reproduction, between what might be called temporary and permanent sterility in the definitional sense, then other considerations immediately come to mind. A man with a vasectomy (assuming that he has not developed an autoimmune response to his own sperm) is still producing sperm and still has the potential of impregnating a woman if the vas deferens is rechannelized. Similarly a woman with a tubal ligation is still producing ova and still has an intact uterus, so she is potentially able to become pregnant if the fallopian tubes were rechannelized. While altering these surgical mechanical barriers to impregnation may be somewhat more complicated than removing a diaphragm, condom, or IUD or than ceasing to take pills, the basic principle is no different and the potential for reproduction remains. Sterility would thus be, we feel, a misnomer for these operative procedures.

At a somewhat more complex level we can even raise the question of what is meant by reproduction, and then we can break the reproductive process itself into at least four distinct steps. The first step is the production of male or female gametes. Capacity to produce one or the other of these gametes is the most common biological conception of capacity to reproduce, or of nonsterility. In the human such capacity is dependent on retention of functional ovarian or testicular tissue. Removal of the ovaries or testes, called castration, is thus the most definitive sterilizing procedure in this conventional sense. In addition to destroying capacity to produce gametes, the castration procedures also destroy capacity to produce male and female hormones, hormones that have physiological functions other than merely those of reproduction per se. These procedures are seldom resorted to for contraceptive purposes, therefore, except in some quasi-punitive situations, even though the hormones themselves could be supplied exogenously such that primary and secondary sexual capacities other than reproduction would not necessarily be altered. It may be of technical interest that simpler species of animals and plants can now be reproduced by an asexual process called cloning, and that potentially this process of reproduction may be extended to humans as well. If such were the case sterility in the strict sense of incapacity to reproduce one's own kind literally could not be induced since almost any cellular material can be utilized for cloning. Such capacity for reproduction through cloning does not currently exist for the human species, however, and castration remains the definitive sterilizing procedure by effectively preventing the production of gametes that are necessary for sexual reproduction.

A second step in the reproductive process is the passage of the gametes from their respective sites of origin to a point of union. For humans this usually means that the sperm pass from the testes, through the vas deferens, seminal vesicles, and urethra, into the vagina during intercourse, from thence into the host uterus and into the fallopian tubes. The egg passes from the ovary into the fallopian tube, where it is fertilized by a sperm and subsequently migrates to the wall of the uterus. As has been discussed previously, mechanical contraception consists of disrupting the channels along which egg and sperm travel to unite. While patency of these channels is necessary for reproduction, we would argue that infertility accomplished by disrupting the mechanical patency of these channels should be called contraception rather than sterilization. If such were the case then vasectomy and tubal ligation would clearly be contraceptive and not sterilization procedures. In this sense we feel that Barglow's women are conceptually correct in fantasizing that they retain the potential for pregnancy even though their tubes are tied.

The third step of the reproductive process consists of growth of the fertilized egg (the zygote) once it is implanted on the wall of the uterus, during the period of gestation, until the baby is born. This requires an intact female uterus, at least until such time as "test tube" babies become a reality. In many species fertilized ova are routinely transplanted from the biological mother to a host uterus in another female, where gestation and delivery take place. That is, gestation need not occur in the biological mother in these species. Presumably this process of implantation and gestation in a host uterus is possible in the human species as well, although to our knowledge it has not actually been accomplished. This potential for utilization of a host mother for gestation raises the question of whether even a hysterectomy should be regarded as a sterilizing procedure. Potentially, at least, a hysterectomized woman can still contribute as much to sexual reproduction as can a man—namely, a gamete that once fertilized can grow into a child if implanted in a suitable host uterus. Since potential for pregnancy is clearly a feminine function, hysterectomy would reduce this component of femininity, but perhaps technically should not be regarded as a sterilizing procedure per se.

The fourth step in reproduction of one's own species would consist of nurturing a newborn infant to maturity in a hospitable social environment. Species reproduction does not, of course, end with the birth of an infant, which is nonviable if left entirely to itself. Many people seem capable of generating biological offspring without being capable of providing satisfactory social or psychological support for the subsequent maturation process. Perhaps it would be meaningful to talk about social sterility in such individuals or couples, although discussion of such a concept is beyond the scope of the present chapter except to suggest that the concept of sterility should either include any stage of reproductive capacity, including social sterility, or should be restricted only to the capacity to produce gametes, which is the interpretation we would favor. In the latter case we would again repeat that the present chapter deals with psychological reaction to surgical contraception and not to sterilization. If our interpretation of the research literature is correct, we feel that consistent emphasis on this point might well make these operative procedures both more acceptable and less psychologically hazardous to the population for whom they are useful.

Sexual Behavior and Surgical Contraception—
Theoretical Considerations

With apologies to Freud we suggest that one problem with studies of contraception, which is directed toward preserving intercourse without resultant fertility, is a relative absence of a good psychological theory of sexual behavior. Why, for example, does not removal of fear of pregnancy result in marked increase in satisfaction with sexual behavior following surgical contraception? Why is partial impotency often associated with increasing frequency of sexual relations following vasectomy? These are but two of many questions that might be clarified with a more adequate theory of the psychology of sex. The present section is a brief attempt to outline rudimentary aspects of such a theory.

We suggest that sexual arousal or erection for the male depends on a degree of novelty or pleasurable unusualness in the sexual situation, combined with a relative absence of fear of sexual inadequacy. We suggest that women prefer an absence of the unexpected in the sexual situation, rather than novelty, before they can relax and become sexually responsive. The basis of response of men and women is thus somewhat discordant (see Masters and Johnson, 1966). The slow working out of this discordance, with the husband pushing for new approaches or techniques or repeatedly pursuing a "conquest" against the resistance of a reluctant wife, may provide the interesting novelty that makes possible a long experience of potency for the husband within a monogamous relationship. Other uncertainties, such as the risk of pregnancy, might also contribute to the arousal of the male but detract from the responsiveness of the female (although an unconscious desire for pregnancy might result in an unexpected female receptivity at times when the risk of pregnancy was high). Women in turn may adapt more quickly to new sexual experiences than do men, so that experiences remain arousingly novel for men long after they have become comfortably familiar for women. These periods during which techniques have "comfortable novelty" for a couple should be ones of orgasmic compatibility.

If a given female partner is always available on demand or on a fixed schedule for essentially a routine and unvarying pattern of intercourse, the situation should lose its uncertainty and therefore in time its capacity to be arousing to the male partner. This may be the basis for many impotency problems following ten or fifteen years of marriage, impotency that often vanishes in the novelty of an extramarital affair. The Don Juan syndrome of impotency following thorough exploration of all parameters of sexuality that the subject can think of would represent a similar adaptation to sex in which the possibility of the unusual was essentially exhausted. This same syndrome may account for Marshall's recent report (1971) that Mangaians "probably are far more subject to impotency in later years than is the American male." In the Mangaian culture the men are encouraged to be very active sexually from an early age, with a large number of partners both before and during marriage.

Men who demand frequent sexual intercourse following vasectomy, as evidence to themselves of their own continuing potency, may thereby more quickly reduce the novelty in their relations with their wives. In turn, their wives may be more routinely sexually available to them postoperatively than preoperatively, further reducing the "challenge" and novelty of the situation. This combination would predictably, and apparently does, result in increased impotency problems. The fear of performance failure, added to the lack of novelty, would contribute further to the impotency syndrome, which in turn might lead to redoubled efforts at a high rate of intercourse to disconfirm any loss of masculinity from the vasectomy, resulting in the combination of increase in frequency with increase in impotency that we observed. Contributing still further to shifting the balance more toward fear of performance failure and away from novelty for the male would be the relative certainty of contraception and the relative unalterability of the surgical procedures as compared to the nonsurgical ones.

If these speculations are correct then they suggest that the initial sexual response to male surgical contraception should be reasonably good, with the novelty of "does it still work?" contributing interest and the fear of failure being readily disconfirmable, while the wife's participation would be sufficiently unchanged as not to create problems in her responsiveness. Long-range effects, however, might be more negative, as has been discussed above, as a high frequency of intercourse to disconfirm operative effects could reduce novelty and produce some failure experiences, with a shift of focus from seeking pleasure to concern about disproving inadequacy. The initial sexual response to female surgical contraception might be more problematic, with the woman being even more in need of confidence that nothing unexpected would happen while she is recovering from the operation. This might be counteracted in part by the "deprivation syndrome" of her husband and the novelty that her surgery would introduce for him, leaving him arousable by even the safest and gentlest of routines until his wife regained confidence. Unless an initial hesitancy of the woman to renew sexual behavior became stabilized as an enduring phobia, long-term sexual adjustment after female surgical contraception should be satisfactory, in terms of this theorizing.

For both men and women long-term personal adjustment might follow a different course from their sexual adjustment following these surgical procedures and would depend on how successfully they came to terms with the factually unrealistic but psychologically important threat to their or their spouse's masculinity or femininity that the operations apparently pose.

Conclusions and Summary

Frequency of surgical contraception has been increasing rather rapidly during the last decade. The procedures, vasectomy and salpingectomy, impose mechanical barriers that prevent ultimate union of the gametes. In mode of action, therefore, they are similar to a condom or a diaphragm. Salpingectomy involves abdominal surgery and is subject to the risk and side effects associated with such surgery. Surgically vasectomy is a minor procedure, usually done in ten or fifteen minutes in an office visit. Physiological side effects from vasectomy are usually minor. With both procedures there is a small risk, approximately 1 percent, of rechannelization of the obstructed passages. The operations do not alter hormone levels, ejaculate volume, physiological potential for sexual arousal, or other physiological parameters to any important degree. The procedures can be surgically reversed in approximately 60 to 90 percent of vasectomies when done by an experienced surgeon and in a much smaller percentage of salpingectomies. Except for operative risks with salpingectomies, the primary hazards of surgical contraception are psychological ones. There is evidence that Americans respond emotionally to the operations as though they had the potential for demasculinizing or defeminizing the person operated on, with the result that postoperatively, the person operated on may respond in a more rigidly masculine or feminine manner to disprove that the operation had such an effect. This "disconfirmation of loss of masculinity or femininity" may result in increased stresses in the marriage as well as, at times, improvement in vocational or similar role functioning. The issue of whether or not the husband should and does get a vasectomy is often a pawn in the marriage interaction game, with the husband feeling that he has given up something significant if he gets the operation and is therefore entitled to a significant payoff in return. The exact manifestation and effects this bargaining has will vary from family to family. Apparently the best predictors of favorable or unfavorable response to vasectomy, as well as to other forms of contraception, are comparisons of the husband's and the wife's characteristics rather than the characteristics of either taken alone. To what extent these dynamics generalize beyond the American culture, or even beyond middle-class American culture, is not known.

No adequate data are available on severity of emotional response to surgical contraception. Some available data can be interpreted as indicating that almost all subjects show some negative postoperative emotional response. Other data indicate that even severe negative responses may be ostensibly unrelated to the operations and may therefore go undetected. The vast majority of subjects claim to be satisfied with the procedures postoperatively, nevertheless, and there is no compelling evidence to indicate widespread severe negative emotional sequelae. To our knowledge there are no data available to indicate relative emotional response to surgical contraception versus response to an unwanted pregnancy, often an alternative to effective contraception. The procedures are highly favored in family-planning circles for their effectiveness.

Much of the emotional reaction to these operative procedures apparently results from their association with castration or true sterilization. Therefore, we suggest that these procedures be called by the more accurate title of surgical contraception rather than by the more common title of sterilization. We also suggest that much of the negative emotional response to the procedures can be avoided by thorough discussion with the subjects, preoperatively and postoperatively, of the nature of the particular operation and their expectations, anxieties, and distortions concerning it. The only utility of the operations as regards sexual parameters appears to be prevention of conception. They do not appear to improve impotence or premature ejaculation or frigidity problems. Conversely on the average they do not appear to worsen these problems or to increase the risk of extramarital activity.

REFERENCES

Barglow, P. 1964. Pseudocyesis and psychiatric sequelae of sterilization. *Archives of General Psychiatry* 11:571–580.

Barglow, P.; Gunther, M. S.; Johnson, A.; and Meltzer, H. J. 1965. Hysterectomy and tubal ligation: a psychiatric comparison. *Obstetrics and Gynecology* 25:520–527.

Dandekar, K. 1963. After-effects of vasectomy. *Artha Vijnana* 5:211–224.

Drellich, M. G. and Bieber, I. 1958. The psychologic importance of the uterus and its functions. *Journal of Nervous and Mental Disease* 126:322–336.

Erickson, M. H. 1954. The psychological significance of vasectomy. In H. Rosen, ed., *Therapeutic abortion*. New York: Julian Press. Pp. 57–86.

Fischer, H. K. 1962. Emotional problems associated with gynecologic surgery. *Clinical Obstetrics and Gynecology* 5:597–614.

Garrison, P. L. and Gamble, C. J. 1950. Sexual effects of vasectomy. *Journal of the American Medical Association* 144:293–295.

Hauser, E. 1955. Die Sterilisation des Mannes zur Verhutung von Schwangerschaften. *Praxis* 44:477–484, 500–506.

Hinderer, M. 1947. Uber die Sterilisation des Mannes und ihre Auswirkungen, *Schweizer Archiv fur Neurologie, Neurochirurgie und Psychiatrie* 60:145–176.

Johnson, M. H. 1964. Social and psychological effects of vasectomy. *American Journal of Psychiatry* 121:482–486.

Laidlaw, R. W. and Bass, M. S. 1964. Voluntary sterilization as it relates to mental health. *American Journal of Psychiatry* 120:1176–1180.

Landis, J. F. and Poffenberger, F. 1965. The marital and sexual adjustment of 330 couples who chose vasectomy as a form of birth control. *Journal of Marriage and the Family* 27:57–58.

Lee, H. Y. 1966. Studies on vasectomy. III. Clinical studies on the influences of vasectomy. *Korean Journal of Urology* 7:11–29.

Marshall, D. S. 1971. Too much in Mangaia. *Psychology Today* 4:43–44, 70, 74–75.

Masters, W. H. and Johnson, V. E. 1966. *Human Sexual Response*. Boston: Little, Brown.

Melody, G. F. 1962. Depressive reactions following hysterectomy. *American Journal of Obstetrics and Gynecology* 83:410–413.

Phadke, G. M. 1964. Sterilization as a method of family limitation. *Maharashtra Medical Journal* 11:237–244.

Phadke, G. M. and Padukone, K. 1964. Presence and significance of autoantibodies against spermatozoa in the blood of men with obstructed vas deferens. *Journal of Reproduction and Fertility* 7:162–170.

Poffenberger, T. and Poffenberger, Shirley B. 1963. Vasectomy as a preferred method of birth control: a preliminary investigation. *Marriage and Family Living* 25:326–330.

Popenoe, P. 1929. Effect of vasectomy on the sexual life. *Journal of Social and Abnormal Psychology* 24:251–268.

Presser, H. B. 1970. Voluntary sterilization: a world view. *Reports on Population/Family Planning*, no. 5. New York: The Population Council.

Rodgers, D. A. and Ziegler, F. J. 1967. Cognitive process and conversion reactions. *Journal of Nervous and Mental Disease* 144:155–170.

———. 1968. Changes in sexual behavior consequent to use of noncoital procedures of contraception. *Psychosomatic Medicine* 30:495–505.

Rodgers, D. A.; Ziegler, F. J.; Altrocchi, J.; and Levy, N. 1965. A longitudinal study of the psycho-social effects of vasectomy. *Journal of Marriage and the Family* 27:59–64.

Rodgers, D. A.; Ziegler, F. J.; and Levy, N. 1967. Prevailing cultural attitudes about vasectomy: a possible explanation of postoperative psychological response. *Psychosomatic Medicine* 29:367–375.

Rodgers, D. A.; Ziegler, F. J.; Rohr, P.; and Prentiss, R. J. 1963. Socio-psychological characteristics of patients obtaining vasectomies from urologists. *Marriage and Family Living* 25:331–335.

Rümke, P. and Hellinga, G. 1959. Autoantibodies against spermatozoa in sterile men. *American Journal of Clinical Pathology* 32:357–363.

Sacks, S. and LaCroix, G. 1962. Gynecologic sequelae of postpartum tubal ligation. *Obstetrics and Gynecology* 19:22–27.

Schmidt, S. S. 1969. Vas anastomosis. Paper presented at the Conference on Human Sterilization, Cherry Hill, New Jersey, October 28–31, 1969. Cited by H. B. Presser, Voluntary sterilization: a world view. *Reports on Population/Family Planning*, no. 5. New York: The Population Council.

Simon Population Trust. 1969. *Vasectomy: Follow-up of a thousand cases*. Cambridge: Simon Population Trust.

Tietze, C. 1960. The current status of fertility control. *Law and Contemporary Problems* 25:426–444.

Wolfers, H. 1970. Psychological aspects of vasectomy. *British Medical Journal* 4:297–300.

Ziegler, F. J. and Rodgers, D. A. 1968. Vasectomy, ovulation suppressors, and sexual behavior. *Journal of Sex Research* 4:169–193.

Ziegler, F. J.; Rodgers, D. A.; and Kriegsman, S. A. 1966. Effect of vasectomy on psychological functioning. *Psychosomatic Medicine* 28:50–63.

Ziegler, F. J.; Rodgers, D. A.; and Prentiss, R. J. 1969. Psychosocial response to vasectomy. *Archives of General Psychiatry* 21:46–54.

PART V

Some Measurement Issues in Fertility

[12]

PERSONALITY ASSESSMENT
IN THE STUDY OF
POPULATION

HARRISON G. GOUGH

Even a cursory glance at past and current work on birth planning and population policy will reveal that psychologists and others interested in assessing personality factors, drives, and motives have not been conspicuously successful in relating these factors to criteria in the field of population. The deficiencies within this realm of analysis have been noted by many leading scholars. Stycos (1963), for example, remarked that until the last few years scientific study of motivational aspects of population problems has been virtually nonexistent. Davis (1967) used the phrase "the neglect of motivation" in his critique of current programs of population control, and Freedman (1962) observed that little has as yet come from the search for social-psychological and psychological factors capable of accounting for variations in fertility and other indices of reproductive behavior.

Psychologists themselves have been ready to acknowledge these shortcomings. Pohlman (1966) called it "ironic" to find psychologists almost totally unrepresented in the bibliographies on birth planning and population control, and in his book on birth planning (1969) he could list scarcely a handful of psychologists who had contributed to the field prior to the 1960s. Fawcett (1970) viewed one of the key functions of his book as that of stimulating more research by psychologists, and David (1970b) in a transnational conference called for work on psychological measurement as a major goal.

Lest the impression be given that population research is a simple puzzle waiting to be solved by the magic of psychological analysis, it should be stated at once that the problems in the field are complex and difficult, in fact too refractory to permit of anything other than step-by-step progress. Individual actions affecting fertility will invariably derive from a constellation of factors, some of which will be in opposition to others (cf. Flapan, 1969), and few of which are readily measurable at the present time (Bogue, 1966). Relevant variables must be distinguished from irrelevant ones, and problems of levels of awareness will be encountered (cf. Westoff, Potter, Sagi, and Mishler, 1961). What the assessment psychologist needs to do in this field, as in most others, is to look at what has already been done and try to discern leads and paths along which exploration of his particular kind might profitably be undertaken. With this admonition in mind let us turn to some prior work that can help set guidelines.

Prior Analyses

One of the pioneering inquiries in this domain is the Indianapolis study of social and psychological factors affecting fertility (Whelpton and Kiser, 1946–1958). Two concerns prompted this study—worry over the generally low urban birth rate in the 1930s and lack of understanding of the social and psychological factors underlying this phenomenon (cf. Whelpton and Kiser, 1959). Although a great deal of interesting demographic information was generated in this project, the yield in the psychological domain was discouraging. The project was carefully reviewed and criticized and shortcomings acknowledged (cf. Kiser, 1962). In the psychological realm a key deficiency was the brevity and relative inadequacy of the measures employed. In the 1950s another major project was initiated on the growth of American families (Freedman, Whelpton, and Campbell, 1959; Whelpton, Campbell, and Patterson, 1966). Over 5,000 subjects were studied in the two phases of the project. More than 90 percent of the wives reported at least some acceptance of family planning, although of course, opinions differed on preferred and legitimate methods. The findings in this investigation, however, were mostly demographic and socioeconomic and did not shed a great deal of light on motivational and psychological processes. The so-called Princeton study of family growth (Westoff et al., 1961; Westoff, Potter, and Sagi, 1963), also initiated in the 1950s, attempted to use psychological measurement and did include indices of ability and personality; the relationships between personality indicators and fertility were, however, disappointingly low. The prediction of family size, i.e., fertility, from psychological measures on individuals, is clearly an unsolved problem at the present time.

A certain degree of success has been achieved with indices of alienation (cf. Rainwater, 1960, 1965; Groat and Neal, 1967), but relationships are still modest. Although better measures may be available today than at the time the Indianapolis and Princeton studies were being planned, it is unlikely that the failure to attain impressive findings rests entirely on this one element. A more probable explanation is that the criterion itself—family size—is a resultant of too many factors, including accidental factors, to permit accurate forecasting from just the psychological perspective. The implied message in this comment is to look for more discrete and delimited targets for analysis.

Some Examples of Measurement

One such target might be termed "motivation for parenthood." Rabin (1965) employed the incomplete sentences method in a study of college students in New York and Michigan. Respondents were asked to complete thirty stubs beginning with phrases such as "men want children because . . ." and "women want children because. . . ." Questionnaire data on the 194 respondents in this study indicated that all but two expected to have children, and that the median number of wanted children was three; this figure is quite close to the mean of 3.02 for ideal size found by Gustavus and Nam (1970) in their survey of students in the southern United States and is also similar to findings of Blake (1966) in her twenty-fifth-year survey of white Americans.

Responses to the incomplete sentences were evaluated by two interpreters and classified under various categories of motivation such as altruistic and narcissistic. Almost half of the protocols were judged to indicate that the male's motivations for parenthood are primarily narcissistic—involving self-aggrandizement, perpetuation of self, and proof of vigor and virility. Only 9 percent of the protocols mentioned "proof of femininity" as a factor in women's motivation for having children. However, more than half of the protocols identified a sense of destiny or fulfillment as a major motive for childbearing in women.

This study using the incomplete sentences method was followed up in 1968 (Rabin and Greene, 1968) with an eighteen-item Child Study Inventory constructed to assess the four major categories of motivation found in the earlier work: altruistic, fatalistic, narcissistic, and instrumental. For each stub four completions were given, each expressing one category of motivation; the respondent was then asked to rank these completions in order of preference. Scoring was achieved by adding the ranks assigned to each type of motivation.

Adequate reliability for the four scales was claimed, and several applications of the Inventory were presented. For example, students with low scores on the altruistic motivation tended to see their own mothers and fathers as rejecting, and those scoring high on narcissistic motivation viewed their mothers as unloving. In a contrast between normal and schizophrenic respondents the schizophrenics were found to place greater stress on instrumental motivations (seeing the child as having utilitarian values to the parent) and less stress on altruistic ones. The Child Study Inventory would appear to be a useful research tool for the study of parental motivations, particularly if its findings are interpreted in conjunction with case-study analyses (cf. Flapan, 1969), factors of social change (Hoffman and Wyatt, 1960), and the "new femininism" (Carter, 1970).

The decision to use birth-control methods is another target to which measurement has been directed. Although contraceptive practices are as old as man (Tietze, 1965), relatively safe and effective methods (other than abstinence and withdrawal) have not been available for much more than the last 100 years. Oral ovulation suppressors, as is well known, did not become available until the late 1950s, and the intrauterine device or IUD, although described in the early years of the century, did not gain much attention until the late 1950s and early 1960s. The newest approach, the abortifacient prostaglandins, is only now coming into visibility.

Current estimates are that from 90 to 97 percent of American women ages eighteen to thirty-nine have used or expect to use some form of contraceptive practice (Westoff and Ryder, 1969). With figures this high, why suggest psychological study of those who do and do not decide on such usage? One answer to this is that usage varies between continuous and discontinuous, and another is that even though the percentage of nonusers is low the diagnostic problem is important.

A relatively new measuring device in psychology is the scale for "locus of control" introduced by Rotter (1966). The purpose of this measure is to assess the degree to which the respondent visualizes control over his behavior as being internal and self-governed or external and under the regulation of forces outside of the self. MacDonald (1970), using this scale, hypothesized that subjects with external orientation, lacking belief in the efficacy of personal control, might be less likely to attempt to control pregnancy, whereas subjects with internal orientation would be more likely to seek prevention of impregnation.

To check on this hypothesis 508 undergraduate students were given the Rotter scale, and subsamples were selected of 101 women with very low scores (internal orientation) versus 111 with high scores (external orientation). Data were analyzed separately for married and unmarried women. Among the unmarried thirty-nine "internals" and forty-five "externals" reported coital experience; 64 percent of the internals and 37 percent of the externals reported use of birth-control methods, a significant difference in line with expectations. The percentages for married students were in the same direction, eighty-seven versus sixty-three, but because of small N's the difference was not significant.

Attitudinal consistency is another psychological factor that has been found to differentiate between users and nonusers (Insko, Blake, Cialdini, and Mulaik, 1970). Consistency was evaluated by means of concordance between lists of forty-seven beliefs and attitudes. For example, the numerical endorsement of the notion that a wife should be able to work outside the home was multiplied by the degree of agreement with the statement that use of birth-control methods will give the wife more time for such work. An attitude x belief score was derived in this way for a sample of 263 females. The correlation between this index of consistency and the reported frequency of birth-control usage was .25 (p < .05). As a practical method for differentiating between potential users and nonusers this technique would be cumbersome, but as a way of demonstrating the role of individual attitudinal structures it is quite revealing.

"Fear of pregnancy" is one of the factors investigated in the Indianapolis study (Schachter and Kiser, 1953), the hypothesis being that the greater the fear of pregnancy, the greater the likelihood that the couple would employ contraceptive methods. Various indices of fear were used, including statements by husband and wife on the amount of risk in childbirth and the degree to which the couple had been discouraged from having children. About 8.5 percent of the 1,444 wives reporting indicated moderately high to quite high fears of pregnancy. In general, however, relationships between fear of pregnancy and criterion measures were modest and of little practical importance.

Recently (Kutner and Duffy, 1970) the "fear of pregnancy" variable has been reintroduced into birth-planning studies by way of the Kutner Fear of Pregnancy Test. In this test ten possible fears are listed, and the respondent is asked to assign personal ranks; the rank given to becoming pregnant is taken as the score on the test. Reliabilities of .83 (retest) and .89 (alternate form) were obtained for this brief assessment device. In a pilot study of women beginning to use oral contraceptives, the incidence of side effects was positively associated with greater fear of pregnancy as measured by the test.

Kapor-Stanulovic (1970) also investigated the incidence of unpleasant side effects in use of the pill. She worked with 184 women being seen at the Oakland, California, Planned Parenthood Clinic. In addition to interviews and the gathering of biographical information two psychological tests were administered. The first was the Franck Drawing Completion Test (Franck and Rosen, 1949), scored for feminine identification. This scoring is quite reliable and produces a variable often interpreted as an index of sex-role identification or even as a measure of "unconscious" femininity. The second was the Fe (femininity) scale (Gough, 1966) from the California Psychological Inventory (CPI) (Gough, 1957). The Fe scale is a thirty-eight-item measure previously shown to differentiate reliably between male and female samples in the United States and other countries (e.g., Korea, Norway, Venezuela, and Turkey) and is often interpreted as an index of sex-role preference or even of "conscious" femininity.

By selecting extreme cases on both variables Kapor-Stanulovic was able to define three special groups for study: high Franck + high Fe, high Franck + low Fe, and low Franck + high Fe. There were eleven subjects in each of these clusters. A fourth cluster of eleven subjects was composed, including women with average scores on both measures. Age, education, ethnic background, and occupational ratings did not differ significantly among the four groups, but variables pertaining to side effects and complaints did differ. The group with the lowest incidence of side effects was the high Franck + low Fe with a mean rate of 1.0 per subject, and the group with the highest incidence was the high-high with a mean rate of 3.0. The "psychology" of the high-low cluster is that of strong feminine identity with minimal sex-role preference. For the high-high cluster the résumé would stress strongly feminine dispositions in both feeling and behavior. The pattern for complaints concerning the effects of the contraceptive agents followed this same hierarchy.

Another difference noted in the clusters was the greater tendency to experiment with different methods of contraception among the high-low subjects. On the contrary the low-high cluster of women revealed an almost exclusive preference for the pill. When asked whether they would ever seek to become pregnant (or to become pregnant again), four of the women in the low-high cluster said no, whereas no more than one in any of the other three clusters gave this reply.

Kapor-Stanulovic interpreted her findings in the following way: for the high-low cluster initiative, freedom, and personal expression are important, and birth control is a welcome aid in the seeking of personal identity; for the low-high cluster contraception is a protection against an unwelcome possibility, one that therefore must be used consistently in spite of unpleasant effects; for the high-high cluster conflict is minimal if the life situation is compatible with the postponement or avoidance of pregnancy, but otherwise severe.

There are obviously factors other than fear of pregnancy influencing family-planning practices. In an intensive study of ten couples using family-planning methods versus ten not using any, Keller, Sims, Henry, and Crawford (1970) were able to identify a number of differentiating factors. For example, feelings of efficacy as inferred from Thematic Apperception Test (TAT) stories were significantly higher among users than nonusers. The tendency to plan ahead, as estimated from incomplete sentence protocols, was also more prominent among users. On the other hand, negative qualities attributed to members of the opposite sex in the TAT protocols were more prominent in the stories of nonusers. Classification of the twenty couples according to their standing on all of the variables analyzed showed ten out of ten users to have a preponderance of positive scores and seven out of ten nonusers to have a preponderance of negative scores; a simple 2 x 2 classification table based on these variables would therefore yield an 85 percent "hit rate." Because of the small samples in this study and the lack of cross-validation, the specific signs and variables utilized must be interpreted with caution; the method of combining discrete signs into a total index, however, is one that warrants further application.

Choice of contraceptive method is another target that might be approached by way of measurement. Oral contraceptives appear to be preferred by American women (Westoff and Ryder, 1967), whereas in the Taiwan study (Berelson and Freedman, 1964) 78 percent of the women chose the IUD; it should be noted, however, that the IUD was recommended by field personnel in the Taiwan program. Kutner and Duffy (1970) suggest that among American women the IUD may be preferred by women who wish to shift responsibility for avoiding pregnancy to an outside agent (i.e., the physician), whereas the pill may be preferred by women who wish to take on this responsibility for themselves.

Choice of the pill versus the IUD should not be seen as an all-or-none matter. Murawski (1969) in a five-year follow-up of patients from the Peter Bent Brigham Hospital in Boston found 29 percent of the women to be still using the same ovulation suppressor (Enovid), 35 percent to be using a different oral contraceptive, and 36 percent to be using an IUD. One of the factors leading to termination of the pill was its suppression of "femininity," i.e., its interference with normal duration and intensity of menstrual functioning. It should be noted that Moos (1968) found about 80 percent of the women in his study to show a moderate reduction in menstrual discomfort while on an antiovulation regimen. Murawski cites a case example of a woman who switched from the pill to an IUD and who was "delighted" with the return of cramps, backache, and menstrual discomfort.

The role of the husband in the choice of contraceptive method must be kept in mind in this discussion, certainly with respect to so obvious an example as vasectomy, but also with respect to choices among the options open to the wife. Ziegler, Rodgers, Kriegsman, and Martin (1968) make the following observation:

> Most women apparently find the pills to be somewhat inconvenient to take and often to involve some disagreeable side effects. They apparently are willing to tolerate these annoyances if they do not perceive their husbands as being excessively sexually demanding, feel generally responsible for managing family matters, and enjoy sexuality. Conversely, they apparently are unwilling to endure the inconveniences and discomforts of contraceptive pills if they feel that sexuality is primarily for the benefit of the husband rather than themselves, and if they generally regard their husbands as willing or likely to assume primary responsibilities in the marriage. [P. 853]

There is also the possibility that use of the IUD may arouse anxiety reactions in the husband (cf. Murawski, 1969). A possible hypothesis is that anxiety-prone males would oppose the wife's use of the IUD.

As already suggested, continuous versus discontinuous use of a contraceptive method is a criterion that might be predictable from psychological measures. Bakker and Dightman (1964) studied seventy-two women using

Enovid, asking them and also their husbands to take the Edwards Personal Preference Schedule (EPPS) (Edwards, 1953), the Minnesota Multiphasic Personality Inventory (MMPI) (Hathaway and McKinley, 1943), and the Sixteen Personality Factor Questionnaire (16PF) (Cattell and Stice, 1957). Criterion classifications in this study related to the occurrence of pill forgetting and the presence and type of major somatic complaints.

With respect to erratic or discontinuous use of the pill women who forgot tended to score higher on the psychopathic deviate scale of the MMPI and on the surgency scale of the 16PF; they also tended to score lower on the emotional maturity scale of the 16PF. There were no significant differences on the EPPS. Women who are less mature, more impulsive, less constrained, and more inclined toward action than contemplation seem to be more likely to experience lapses in use of the pill.

A similar contrast between those who complained or did not complain of side effects showed no significant differences on the three inventories. However, when husbands' profiles were taken into account an interesting phenomenon was observed: the more highly correlated the two profiles, the more likely was the woman to be classified as a complainer, whereas the more different the two profiles, the more likely was the wife to be a forgetter in use of the pill. These findings must be viewed as heuristic only, it should be stated, because of the small size of the samples and because of the lack of cross-validational evidence.

Rodgers and Ziegler (1968) also reported on continuous versus discontinuous users of the pill. They established a subsample of fifteen continuous couples who had revealed regular usage of oral contraceptives throughout a four-year period. Contrasting samples were formed of nine couples in which the wife stopped usage of the oral contraceptive, but without the intention of conceiving, and eleven couples in which usage was terminated in order to attempt impregnation. "Continuous" wives were significantly differentiated from "discontinuous" wives on five of the personality scales surveyed: the continuous users scored higher on the CPI scales for social presence, self-acceptance, and achievement via independence, lower on the MMPI scale for masculinity, and higher on the MMPI scale for hypomania. Husbands of wives who were continuous users scored higher than other husbands on the MMPI psychopathic deviate scale, and lower on the CPI scales for good impression, achievement via conformance, and socialization. The general pattern here is for the wife in a continuous-usage couple to be self-assured, expressive, versatile, and to have a wide range of interests, and for the husband to be somewhat impulsive, counteractive, and impatient with rules and other forms of social constraint.

Another method of analysis of the personality and demographic variables (see Ziegler et al., 1968) called for a combination of husband's and wife's scores on the CPI scales for dominance, capacity for status, and responsibility, plus age, preferred frequency of intercourse, and previous kind of contraception. By setting a cutting score on each of these six factors an index was established with possible variation between —6 and +6; actual scores for the twenty-four copies varied from —5 to +5. Seven of the eight couples with scores of +1 and above were discontinuous users, and fourteen of the sixteen couples with scores of zero and below were continuous users; the "hit rate" for this cutting point on the composite was therefore 87.5 percent. Chance in this dichotomy would be best represented by calling all couples continuous and would give a hit rate of 62.6 percent, so the empirical index exceeds the chance rate by a substantial amount. As with the Bakker and Dightman analysis these findings can be accepted as heuristic only because of the small N's and the lack of cross-validation.

Vasectomy is still another target that might be looked at from the standpoint of measurement. Rodgers, Ziegler, Altrocchi, and Levy (1965) reported on thirty-five men tested with the MMPI prior to vasectomy and then retested one year after the operation. Nearly all of these men expressed satisfaction with the results of the operation, but on the MMPI their scores showed significant increases on the scales for hypochondriasis, depression, hysteria, psychopathy, femininity, psychasthenia, and schizophrenia. Psychiatric diagnoses obviously should not be attached to these increments, but there seems little reason to doubt that the general level of maladjustment as measured did increase as an aftermath of the operation.

A new study of the effects of vasectomy on psychological functioning was then initiated (Ziegler, Rodgers, and Kriegsman, 1966), involving forty-two respondents. A control sample in which the wife was using an oral contraceptive was also tested with the battery of personality measures used in this study. Retest changes on the CPI and MMPI in the vasectomy group were compared for magnitude with those occurring in the control sample. Four significant differences were observed among the husbands: the vasectomy subjects had relatively greater drops on the CPI scales for socialization and femininity, and relatively greater increases on the CPI scale for social presence and the MMPI scale for psychopathy. The net effect appeared to be a movement toward great self-assertion, diminished control of impulse, and less willingness to endure social constraint or inhibition. For wives two changes were significantly different; the wives of the vasectomized husbands showed greater increments on the MMPI scales for psychasthenia and schizophrenia. The implication here is for an increase in anxiety, self-doubt, and emotional turbulence. With the exception of heightened emphasis on male masculinity (drop on the CPI Fe scale), the shifts are in the direction of greater friction with the environment and others and a higher incidence of personal discomfort. In spite of the directionality in these measured changes, the personal reports of couples in the vasectomy sample continued to reflect positive affect and even enthusiasm.

In a subsequent study (Rodgers, Ziegler, and Levy, 1967) the team of investigators found prevailing attitudes concerning vasectomy to be negative. The strongly favorable attitudes expressed postoperatively by vasectomized males could thus be seen in part as defensive assertions against these cultural norms. The conclusion was reached (Ziegler, Rodgers, and Prentiss, 1969) that vasectomy is reacted to by most men and by their wives as having a "demasculinizing potential," with a resulting increase in psychological upset or compensatory stereotypic masculine behavior or both. These effects are usually minimal to moderate and are outweighed by positive outcomes particularly where the husband is little affected by hypochondriacal concerns and is relatively confident of his own masculinity prior to the operation.

A final topic to be mentioned is that of abortion. Two national conferences on abortion in recent years have stressed the need for increased research on this problem (Beck, Newman, and Lewit, 1969; Newman, Beck, and Lewit, 1970). Questions were raised such as what are the psychological and other characteristics of the woman who seeks abortion, what is the effect on mother and child if abortion is denied, and what is the effect of repeated abortion-seeking? With laws governing abortion being liberalized both in the United States and elsewhere (cf. David, 1970a; Tietze and Lewit, 1969), more knowledge is needed concerning psychiatric indications and contraindications for abortion and the effects of denial.

Although laws are changing, public opinion in the United States has not yet advanced to the stage of endorsing elective abortion (Blake, 1971). Whereas 87 percent of white American adults would not disapprove of abortion in case of a threat to the mother's health, approximately 80 percent would disapprove if the reason was simply a wish not to have the child. Gallup Poll data indicate that support for legalized abortion is strongest among non-Catholic, well-educated, and economically advantaged persons.

Earlier psychiatric writing suggested that pathological outcomes could be expected following abortion because of excessive guilt and other untoward reactions. However, a careful review of psychiatric writing from 1935 to 1964 by Simon and Senturia (1966) revealed that many of these "studies" were highly biased, poorly controlled, merely retrospective, and based on small numbers of case vignettes.

More recent work has indicated that fears of psychiatrically negative sequelae have been overstressed. Peck and Marcus (1966) observed fifty women before and after abortion and found forty-six to be either unchanged or improved in psychiatric status; furthermore, in hindsight forty-nine of these women would repeat the abortion if they had it to do again. Simon, Senturia, and Rothman (1967) followed forty-six women at the Jewish Hospital in St. Louis. Women whose psychiatric status was normal prior to abortion tended to respond with self-limiting, transient, mild depression; those who manifested personality disturbances prior to abortion tended to hold their own or even improve after termination. Patt, Rappaport, and Barglow (1969) followed thirty-five women at Michael Reese Hospital in Chicago who were aborted on the basis of psychiatric recommendation. After termination twenty-six were judged improved, four unchanged, and five to be in poorer psychiatric condition. Sloane (1969) reported similar findings in his review of current work, and Simon (1970) noted that approximately 75 percent of women denied abortion could be expected to show subsequent disturbances of the mother-child relationship.

The only one of these studies using formal psychological measurement was that of Simon et al. (1967), in which several testing devices were employed. One of the most interesting findings was on the MMPI, where almost half of the patients had psychopathic deviate standard scores twenty or more points greater than their scores on masculinity. This pattern of high impulse expression plus "excessive" femininity is often referred to in MMPI lore as a sign of masochistic and self-rejecting dispositions. Even these patients, however, appeared to respond to the abortion without serious psychiatric disturbance.

The studies reviewed above do not, of course, include all that could have been mentioned. An attempt has been made to comment on most of those using personality-assessment methods and to stress questions in each of the target areas that might be amenable to analysis by means of assessment methodology. The role of measurement in any such inquiry is to provide tools by which significant and relevant variables may be brought into the conceptual domain. In other words measurement can furnish reliable information. The value of this information will be determined by the uses to which it is put by the scholar and the scientist.

Most of the assessment devices in widespread use in personality evaluation today are multivariate instruments taking from forty minutes to an hour to complete. The tests used by Bakker and Dightman (1964)—the EPPS, MMPI, and 16PF—are all in this category, and the CPI used by Rodgers and Ziegler (1968) is also of this type. In settings where intensive study of individual respondents is possible and where this much time can be given to a single instrument, use of tests such as those just mentioned is to be recommended. In many situations, however, only ten to fifteen minutes can be devoted to personality evaluation, and the tool of appraisal must be self-administering and capable of being applied in a waiting room or even in a field interview. Furthermore, if the results of one study are to be linked to those of another, the assessment device must be adapted to cross-cultural and transnational usage, and non-English language editions should be available.

The Personal Values Abstract

In reviewing the theory and research evidence on the California Psychological Inventory (Gough, 1957, 1968) with these considerations in mind, the perspective that seemed most compelling was that stressing normative behavior. Interpersonal behavior that is governed by social conventions and sanctions may be termed normative; these sanctions will include specifics as to time, place, manner, and permissible object. Sexual behavior, being subject to these sanctions, can be conceptualized from the normative standpoint.

With regard to measurement the task then becomes one of finding some small set of reliable indices capable of assessing fundamental parameters within the normative domain. Inasmuch as the CPI is intended to measure "folk concepts," universal dispositions emerging from and entering into social behavior, it would seem likely that at least certain of its scales would be relevant to this formulation of objectives. An additional criterion is that any scales selected for inclusion in a minimal kit should be relevant to what is known or hypothesized about birth planning.

This kind of thinking led to the conclusion that a minimal kit should include measures of norm-setting, norm-observing, and norm-changing dispositions. Given these specifications, the task becomes one of selecting the three scales best suited to the assessment of the three dispositions. In the sexual sphere the norm-setting component would seem to be adequately represented by a measure of masculinity-femininity. Research findings such as those of Kapor-Stanulovic (1970) confirm the relevance of this index, and there is also a more or less common-sense logic in including a masculinity-femininity scale in a minimal kit. The Fe (femininity) scale of the CPI was therefore selected as one of those to be included.

In the full inventory the Fe scale is composed of thirty-eight items, and in this version it has been validated in American studies and in work in France, Italy, Korea, Norway, Venezuela, and Turkey (Gough, 1966; Gough, Chun, and Chung, 1968). The underlying continuum of measurement is addressed to initiation (masculine mode) versus conservation (feminine mode); in symbolic terms the references are to man the protector and warrior and to woman the restorer and preserver, i.e., Zeus and Demeter, Jupiter and Ceres. Four items from the Fe scale whose functioning had been erratic in cross-cultural applications were dropped, leaving a thirty-four-item scale (called Fy) for the kit being assembled.

Adherence to norms is the second focus of measurement, and for this parameter the CPI So (socialization) scale was chosen (Gough, 1960, 1965a, 1965b). This scale has been validated in more than ten cross-cultural applications, including work in India, Japan, and Taiwan as well as in Europe and South America. The underlying dimension of measurement is addressed to the internalization of norms and the degree to which behavior is spontaneously guided by normative sanctions. The full version of the So scale contains fifty-four items; for the kit being assembled a thirty-two-item extract (called Sn) was defined by selecting those items with most significant differentiations in the original validation.

The third variable identified for measurement is that concerned with norm-changing and norm-improving. No single scale on the CPI is directly focused on this parameter, but the first cluster of scales seeks to assess different facets of social initiative and personal independence. Item-cluster analyses were therefore carried out to identify the thirty-two items having highest correlations with this first factor on the inventory. The thematic principle in norm-innovating and norm-changing dispositions is conceptualized as that of modernity, and for this reason the thirty-two-item index is designated My for "modernity."

Modernity has been frequently mentioned as a key concept in analyses of social change and receptiveness to birth-planning practices. Berelson (1964), for example, stressed the need to adapt recommendations for birth-planning methods ("hard" versus "easy") to the degree of modernity of the society in which work was being done. Various writers on social change and social structure (cf. Kimmel and Perlman, 1970; Peshkin and Cohen, 1967) have emphasized this concept, and attitudinal scales for "modernity" have been proposed by a number of investigators (cf. Doob, 1967; Kahl, 1968; Smith and Inkeles, 1966). Fawcett (1970) urged that more attention should be paid to the relationship between individual or psychological modernity and fertility.

These three scales—My (modernity), Sn (socialization), and Fy (femininity)—were therefore assembled into a new, brief assessment device that would cover three basic facets of normative and family-planning behavior and that could still be administered in ten- to fifteen-minute periods under conditions of minimal supervision. The scales contain thirty-two, thirty-two, and thirty-four items, but because of one overlap item between Sn and Fy the total length of the questionnaire is ninety-seven items. The device is called the *Personal Values Abstract*, reflecting its origin in the California Psychological Inventory, and copies for research use may be obtained from the publisher of the CPI.[1]

Psychometric Information

To gather basic psychometric information on the three scales of the *Personal Values Abstract* (PVA), a random selection of CPI protocols from the author's files was scored, including 529 males and 431 females. The means, standard deviations, and intercorrelations among the scales are given in Table 12–1.

Sex differences on the Fy (femininity) scale are highly significant, as would be expected. Males are slightly higher on My (modernity) although the difference is not significant. Females score higher on Sn (Socialization), and this difference is statistically significant ($p < .05$). The intercorrelation matrices are worth noting, as all values are insignificantly different from zero save the .22 between My and Fy for males. This relative independence among the three scales is an attractive property for the kind of typological analysis that a three-variable system like this invites.

[1] The Consulting Psychologists Press, 577 College Avenue, Palo Alto, Calif. 94306.

TABLE 12-1

Descriptive Information on the Modernity, Socialization,
and Femininity Scales of the Personal Values Abstract

Scale	Correlations[a]			Males[b]		Females[c]	
	My	Sn	Fy	M	SD	M	SD
My	—	.01	−.06	19.07	4.15	18.62	4.30
Sn	−.04	—	.06	23.99	3.60	25.78	3.40
Fy	−.22	.10	—	14.11	3.19	21.11	3.21

[a]Coefficients above diagonal, males; below diagonal, females.
[b]N = 529.
[c]N = 431.

The next step in the documentation of the PVA deals with the immediate psychological meaning to be attached to each variable. To develop information pertinent to this need the three scales were scored on samples of male and female college students for whom adjectival descriptions by peers were available. Each student in these samples had been described by three acquaintances, using the Gough Adjective Check List (Gough and Heilbrun, 1965) as the report form. The number of tallies for each adjective in the 300-item list is taken as the score of the student on that attribute, and the tallies are then correlated with the scale or index being evaluated.

For a sample of 192 women the descriptions correlating most highly with the My scale were these: aggressive, spontaneous, versatile, dominant, pleasure-seeking, outspoken, outgoing, show-off, ingenious, and witty. The descriptions with largest negative correlations were cautious, reserved, shy, timid, withdrawn, retiring, mild, silent, simple, and conventional.

For 194 male students the two clusters of correlations included these descriptions: positive coefficients—sharp-witted, self-confident, witty, outgoing, sociable, optimistic, talkative, pleasure-seeking, intelligent, and interests wide; negative coefficients—silent, shy, timid, meek, commonplace, quiet, mild, dull, awkward, and cautious.

No single person will be characterized by all of these words, of course. The task for conceptual analysis of the scale is to bring these nomothetic findings together into a psychological formulation that will be generally valid and informative in making interpretations of the scale. From this standpoint the following interpretational summary is offered: the My scale seeks to measure the kind of self-confidence, spontaneity, and personal verve one finds in individuals interested in new experience and variation in routine. High scorers are often seen as self-assured, outgoing, and pleasure-seeking, whereas low scorers are seen as diffident, conventional in outlook, and lacking in social grace and poise.

For the Sn scale key positive correlations for females included conservative, responsible, reliable, self-controlled, patient, peaceable, trusting, kind, cooperative, and obliging; key negative correlations included unconventional, disorderly, reckless, impulsive, rebellious, sarcastic, cynical, careless, coarse, and headstrong. For males the two clusters were as follows: positive —reliable, reasonable, steady, honest, sincere, wholesome, responsible, stable, organized, and modest; and negative—undependable, irresponsible, careless, reckless, thankless, impulsive, hard-hearted, rebellious, distrustful, and argumentative.

The Sn scale, in an inductive résumé, attempts to reflect the degree to which one has internalized societal values concerning self-discipline, the management of impulse, and the acceptance of order. High scorers tend to be seen as responsible, organized, and self-controlled, whereas low scorers are described as rebellious, undependable, and headstrong.

For Fy the positively correlated descriptions among women included feminine, discreet, gentle, tactful, submissive, warm, modest, reflective, quiet, and sympathetic, and the negatively correlated descriptions included argumentative, fickle, robust, restless, lazy, tough, loud, boastful, daring, and opinionated. The positive cluster for males included weak, nervous, worrying, self-pitying, whiny, dependent, reflective, prudish, complaining, and quitting, and the negative cluster daring, masculine, adventurous, clear thinking, forceful, aggressive, robust, outspoken, strong, and independent.

As before, these descriptions are starting points for inferences concerning the implied meanings of the scale, not end points. The formulation of Fy derived from these and other data stresses its focus on patterns of interest and preference indicative of nurturance and the conservation of human relationships on the one hand, versus enterprise and potency on the other. High-scoring women will tend to be seen as feminine, gentle, and sympathetic, low-scoring as restless, self-assertive, and dissatisfied. High-scoring men will tend to be seen as dependent, irresolute, and sensitive, low-scoring as masculine, forceful, and self-reliant.

Pilot Analysis of Birth-Planning Behavior

To permit a pilot analysis of the utility of the PVA in the study of birth-planning behavior, Rodgers and Ziegler were kind enough to score seventy-three of their couples on the My, Sn, and Fy scales and to make these data available to the author.[2] Thirty-eight of the couples were from the vasectomy sample, and thirty-five were couples in which the wife had used oral contraceptives. Within the group of thirty-five, fifteen were continuous users, nine discontinuous, and eleven had made voluntary decisions to cease use of the pill in order to attempt conception. Each of these categories can be treated as a criterion classification for purposes of analysis.

[2] The writer wishes to thank Dr. David Rodgers of the Cleveland Clinic and Dr. Frederick Ziegler of the Carmel, California Community Hospital for their kindness in providing these data.

Table 12-2 gives descriptive data on the contrast between those choosing the two different forms of contraception. The males selecting vasectomy as a birth-preventing method score lower on modernity and higher on socialization and femininity, although none of these differences is significant. The wives in the vasectomy subgroup score higher on modernity and lower on socialization and femininity, but again the differences are not significant.

TABLE 12-2

Comparison of Husbands and Wives in Couples Using Different Methods of Contraception

Scale	Husbands					Wives				
	Vasectomy[a]		Pill[b]			Vasectomy[a]		Pill[b]		
	M	SD	M	SD	t	M	SD	M	SD	t
My	18.24	4.59	19.09	4.75	−0.78	16.63	4.25	16.34	4.47	0.28
Sn	23.45	3.41	21.86	3.77	1.89	24.34	3.96	25.57	3.02	−1.48
Fy	14.05	3.01	13.26	2.56	1.21	21.55	3.13	22.23	2.87	−0.96

[a] N = 38.
[b] N = 35.

Although these differences are not statistically discriminating for either husbands or wives, considered separately, one wonders if a score for couples could be developed that would distinguish between the two subgroups. This method, it will be recalled, was used to advantage by Keller et al. (1970) and by Ziegler et al. (1968). Accordingly an index was set up in which the husband's contribution was defined as 50 — My + Sn + Fy and the wife's contribution as 50 + My — Sn — Fy. The two constants of fifty are used so as to avoid any negative numbers in the pretotals, and the weights are simple derivatives of the directions of difference identified in Table 12-2. The score that is evolved pertains to the *couple*, and seventy-three such scores were computed.

The mean value of this linear index turned out to be 87.40, with a standard deviation of 8.69. If couples with an index score of eighty-eight or above are classified as vasectomy users, thirty-eight of the seventy-three couples are so identified; of these thirty-eight, twenty-five were in fact in the vasectomy subgroup. Thirty-five of the couples had scores of eighty-seven or below, and of these twenty-two were in fact in the oral contraceptive subgroup. The 2 x 2 table incorporating these figures gives a chi-square of 5.83, which with one degree of freedom is significant beyond the .01 level, and the level of accuracy in classifying individual cases is 64.4 percent. Chance in this particular example would be best indicated by putting all couples in the vasectomy subgroup, in which case the hit rate would be 52 percent (thirty-eight hits out of seventy-three calls).

Obviously this simple three-scale index for husbands and wives is not proposed as a diagnostic method for recommending method of contraception. However, the fact that the two subgroups from the Rodgers and

Ziegler studies could be significantly differentiated suggests that the variables chosen for measurement are at least relevant to the important topic of contraceptive choice.

If we look only at the scores for husbands, regression analysis may be used to develop a three-scale equation to identify those choosing vasectomy. This equation takes the form $44.43 - .10My + .23Sn + .14Fy$. The multiplying weights are for use with raw scores on the three scales, and the constant of 44.43 is selected so that the array of a new set of scores computed on the equation will tend toward a mean of fifty. Computed scores of greater than fifty, it follows, will be indicative of choice of vasectomy, and scores of less than fifty will be contraindicative.

Any empirically derived equation, such as that just given, must be confirmed in cross-validation before credence can be given to it. The equation should be seen as an inductive hypothesis, based on seventy-three cases, concerning the way in which the three variables in the PVA relate to the likelihood that a male subject will opt for vasectomy as a mode of contraception. The psychological implications of the three-scale equation are for self-control, reserve, and moderateness at the higher end, versus surgency, assertiveness, and impatience at the lower end.

The next criterion chosen for study is that of continuous versus discontinuous use of the pill. There were fifteen couples in the former category and nine in the latter. Table 12–3 furnishes the descriptive data for the husbands and wives in these two classifications.

TABLE 12-3

Comparison of Husbands and Wives in Couples Manifesting Consistent versus Erratic Use of Oral Contraceptives

| | Husbands | | | | | Wives | | | | |
| | Continuous[a] | | Discontinuous[b] | | | Continuous[a] | | Discontinuous[b] | | |
Scale	M	SD	M	SD	t	M	SD	M	SD	t
My	20.20	5.78	18.89	4.23	0.58	19.00	4.91	14.78	2.49	2.39[c]
Sn	21.07	2.69	24.11	3.48	−2.41[c]	26.00	2.54	25.67	3.97	0.25
Fy	12.80	2.40	13.67	2.60	−0.83	22.13	2.75	20.89	2.15	1.16

[a]N = 15.
[b]N = 9.
[c]p < .05.

The husbands of wives who make continuous use of the pill score significantly lower ($p < .05$) on the Sn scale than do husbands of discontinuous users. Among wives there is also one significant difference—continuous users are higher on the modernity scale.

If attention is paid only to the wife in regard to continuous versus erratic or discontinuous use of the pill, a weighted combination of the three scales can be derived to forecast continuous usage. Since it is based on only twenty-four subjects such a venture must be viewed as highly speculative and in compelling need of cross-validation. Nonetheless, the forecast is of such great intrinsic interest that even a speculative probe of this kind is worth noting.

The multiple-regression analysis of the three-variable system yielded the equation $37.6 + .47My - .12Sn + .32Fy$. The multiplying weights are for use with raw scores on the three scales, and the constant of 37.6 is chosen so that an array of computed scores on a cross-sectional sample of women will approximate fifty. Computed scores above fifty would therefore be suggestive of more reliable use of the oral contraceptive, and scores of less than fifty of more erratic usage. The psychological implications of this mode of weighting the three scales are for self-confidence, progressive social attitudes, and independence at the higher end, versus a slower interpersonal style, conservatism, and emotional constraint at the lower end.

To develop a simple index to forecast continuous use by a couple, attention must be paid to the regression analysis just summarized, as it indicates that the weighting of the Sn scale for wives should be negative, not positive as would be suggested by the direction of difference in Table 12–3. With this proviso the husband's contribution to the continuous usage index becomes $50 + My - Sn - Fy$, and the wife's becomes $50 + My - Sn + Fy$. As before, the constants of fifty are employed so as to avoid any negative numbers in either component.

For the full sample of seventy-three couples the mean score on this index was 95.59, standard deviation 8.77. A cutting score of ninety-seven and above would identify fifteen of the twenty-four couples for whom usage is to be forecast; of these fifteen, twelve were in fact continuous users. Nine of the twenty-four couples in the continuous versus discontinuous use subsample had scores of ninety-six or below on the index, and of these six were in fact discontinuous users. The chi-square value for the 2 x 2 table of prediction versus outcome is 5.23, $p < .01$ with one degree of freedom. The hit rate of the psychometric index is eighteen out of twenty-four, or 75 percent. Chance would be best estimated by calling all twenty-four couples continuous and would be correct 62.5 percent of the time (fifteen out of twenty-four cases).

The 75 percent hit rate of the three scales in differentiating between the fifteen continuous and nine discontinuous couples should be compared with the 87.5 percent figure computed for the index proposed by Ziegler et al., (1968). These authors used six variables for their index, including three scales of the CPI, age in years, preferred frequency of intercourse, and kind of contraception previously used. Continuous usage was associated with the wife being of the same age as her husband, or older, the wife preferring intercourse more frequently than her husband, and previous method of contraception being primarily "feminine" (e.g., diaphragm or IUD). It seems quite likely that the My, Sn, and Fy scales of the PVA could be substituted for the three scales in the six-variable index of Ziegler et al. without loss of differentiating power.

The remaining criterion selected for analysis is the differentiation between the twenty-four couples continuing to use oral contraception (whether persistently or erratically) and the eleven couples deciding to terminate usage in order to conceive. Table 12-4 gives the statistical data on the three scales for husbands and wives in these samples.

TABLE 12-4

*Comparison of Husbands and Wives in Couples
Who Continue or Terminate Oral Contraception*

| | Husbands | | | | | Wives | | | | |
| | Continue[a] | | Terminate[b] | | | Continue[a] | | Terminate[b] | | |
Scale	M	SD	M	SD	t	M	SD	M	SD	t
My	19.71	5.14	17.73	3.20	1.14	17.42	4.51	14.00	3.22	2.20[c]
Sn	22.21	3.23	21.09	4.74	0.79	25.88	3.00	24.91	2.95	0.87
Fy	13.12	2.40	13.55	2.88	−0.45	21.67	2.51	23.45	3.24	−1.72

[a] N = 24.
[b] N = 11.
[c] $p < .05$.

The differences in Table 12-4 are small and, except for that between the two subsamples of wives on the My scale, are not significant. The directionality for both sexes, however, is congruent with those who terminate scoring lower on My and Sn and higher on Fy.

An index for couples set up to identify those who cease use of the oral contraceptive in order to conceive employs this combination for both husbands and wives: $50 - My - Sn + Fy$. Computation of this index on the seventy-three couples in the complete sample produced an array with a mean of 52.96 and standard deviation of 10.09. It was not possible to set a cutting score on this index that would reproduce exactly the eleven versus twenty-four split in the criterion. The closest approximation that could be made was to call couples with scores of fifty-nine and above terminators; of the thirteen couples in this category eight did in fact terminate.

Of the twenty-two couples with scores of fifty-eight and below nineteen were in fact either continuous or discontinuous users of the contraceptive. The chi-square value for the 2 x 2 table was 8.70, which with one degree of freedom is significant beyond the .01 level of probability. Twenty-seven of the thirty-five couples were correctly classified by the index, a hit rate of 77.1 percent. The phi correlation—another way of expressing the relationship between index and criterion—computed on these same data gives a coefficient of .50.

It should be repeated once more that the intention in the above analyses of the three scales from the PVA is not to set up practical methods of forecasting outcome, nor to claim a particular degree of relationship between scales and criteria. New validation on different samples is necessary before confidence can be placed in these relationships. The purpose of the analyses is heuristic only, to suggest that variables such as modernity, socialization, and femininity can be measured in a way that will prove fruitful when the scales are applied to criteria in the realm of birth planning and population policy.

Thinking need not be confined to empirically evolved combinations. Take, for example, the criterion of age of first heterosexual experience for males. Men vary in the age at which first sexual experience occurs, and most observers would expect motivational and other personality factors to play a part in determining age of onset. How might the three scales in the PVA be related to this criterion? Higher scores on socialization and on femininity ought to be predictive of later initiation because of inhibition and constraint in the former and reduced drive in the latter. Modernity might have either a facilitating or a delaying impact—facilitating because of greater self-confidence and verve, but delaying because of heightened interest in cognitive and intellectual issues.

Inasmuch as the example is speculative, let us resolve the matter by assigning all three variables positive weights, with socialization considered the most important element. An a priori forecaster of the form $.3My + .7Sn + .2Fy — 6$ could then be sketched. The weights reflect the tentative judgment of the experimenter concerning the role of each variable in the additive model, and the constant of six is included so that the mean age of onset for a random sample of adult males would be postdicted to be about eighteen years, with a range of from eight or nine to twenty-seven or twenty-eight. A score computed on the index would thus be equivalent to the hypothesized age in years when the first heterosexual experience occurred.

To conclude this sketch of illustrative applications and findings, a final empirical study should be mentioned. Jaccard (1971), in a senior honors thesis,[3] administered the PVA to seventy-eight female and sixty-five male married students at a California State college; protocols from both husband and wife were obtained for fifty-eight couples. One of the questions asked the respondents was "If you could afford as many children as you desire, how many children would you choose to have in your completed family?" The mean number for females was 2.78 and for males 2.34.

A trichotomy of the female sample into those wanting zero or one, two or three, and four or more children yielded corresponding means on the modernity scale of 23.3, 21.4, and 17.7, a highly significant progression (chi-square $= 8.08$, $p < .01$). This finding is in accord with the intended implications of the scale.

The socialization scale was not significantly related to this index of ideal family size, but the femininity scale related positively ($p < .05$); i.e.,

[3] Professor Thomas Crawford was the adviser for this thesis. The writer thanks Mr. Jaccard and Professor Crawford for permission to cite findings from the study.

higher-scoring women indicated a desire for larger families. Although the socialization scale did not relate to ideal family size among women, it did relate ($p < .05$) to favorability of attitudes toward use of oral contraceptives.

The three scales for husbands did not relate to the index of ideal family size nor to attitudes toward oral contraceptives. However, combinations of scores for husband and wife did show some interesting relationships to the nontest criteria. For example, the conjoint scoring of spouses on modernity revealed that for couples in which both partners scored low on modernity the wife wanted an average of 4.1 children in the completed family, as opposed to means of 2.4, 2.8, and 2.2 for pairings on modernity of husband high-wife high, husband high-wife low, and husband low-wife high. A similar comparison on femininity gave a mean number of desired children of 3.7 for wives in the couples in which husband scored low and wife high, as contrasted with means of 2.3, 2.2, and 2.3 for the high-high, high-low, and low-low pairings.

These data are based on young couples (mean ages of 24.0 for males and 22.6 for females) from one region of the country only and must therefore be viewed with restraint. Such caution, however, would not seem to preclude the inference that the three scales possess at least minimal relevance to problems in which researchers on family planning and fertility are vitally interested. Jaccard's findings also confirm the value of looking at husband-wife combinations as well as at scores for individuals.

Discussion and Summary

Although past research on the relationships between personality factors and population has not produced any very compelling findings, there are current leads that appear to offer promise of better results in the future. Comments on the form and direction of possible new study is therefore justified.

One inference from current work is that multivariate approaches are superior to univariate ones. Where time permits, personality inventories covering a range of factors are preferable to an approach limited to a single variable; similarly a battery of tests touching on different domains of functioning is better than one instrument used alone. Single-score tests might well be included in such a battery, but they should be supplemented by additional measures that can broaden and diversify the scope of assessment. Part of the appeal in these admonitions is to the common-sense notion of scanning: when the location of an object or relationship is unknown it is wise to survey as many possibilities as one can. Another important basis for the appeal is logical: the key concepts in the personality realm may well turn out to rest on patterns or combinations of variables, rather than on the positioning of a single measure without regard to such interaction.

With hundreds of available testing devices (see Buros, 1970) selection is necessary even for the most ambitious project. Barring new evidence from frankly empirical exploration, the most promising results to date appear to be coming from devices having at least some degree of theoretical relevance to the issues in birth planning. Variables such as motivation for parenthood, locus of control, fear of pregnancy, modernity, socialization, and femininity may be mentioned as among those for which current findings are encouraging.

During this period of exploratory analysis of techniques of measurement, speculative as well as algorithmic methodologies should be investigated. An example of an algorithmic method would be the fitting of a regression equation to a multivariate set of personality measures in order to forecast an outcome such as inconsistent use of the pill. An example of such an equation based on the My, Sn, and Fy scales was given above (p. 346).

An example of a speculative approach would be the specification of a priori patterns of interaction within a set of variables and then a follow-up to see if any particular patterns were characterized by interesting departures from modal behavior in the psychosexual sphere. More concretely one might take the same three scales—My, Sn, and Fy—and establish interaction typologies based on median splits within each measure. This would give a type having high scores on all three scales, a type having the combination high-high-low, down to an eighth type with the combination low-low-low. One would hypothesize quite different reactions to birth-control practices for men in the high-low-high and low-high-low categories.

Studies of personality factors cannot, of course, be carried on in a vacuum without reference to the larger goals of research on fertility. In addition practical issues such as the acceptability of the instruments to respondents, the ease and rapidity with which they can be completed, and the degree to which they are adaptable to transnational and cross-cultural application are important. In the not too distant future it should be a common practice for studies in different parts of the world all to be using the same basic kit of personality-assessment devices. Psychological measurement today is able to furnish tools possessing this kind of general applicability, and researchers who want to use testing methods in their studies of population questions should be satisfied with nothing less.

It is recognized that before these techniques of assessment will be employed there must be a recovery of optimism concerning their utility. Skepticism concerning the value of personality assessment is certainly justified on the basis of past evidence. At the same time there are clear signs that things are improving, and there are now several promising new devices that population researchers would do well to try out. Advances in measurement as in all other scientific disciplines come from the identification and correction of error. The new tools of today have profited from the correction of mistakes found in yesterday's methods. Now these new tools must themselves be used and evaluated, so that revised and even better techniques will become available to the researchers of tomorrow.

REFERENCES

Bakker, C. B. and Dightman, C. R. 1964. Psychological factors in fertility control. *Fertility and Sterility* 15:559–567.

Beck, M. B.; Newman, S. H.; and Lewit, S. 1969. Abortion: a national public and mental health problem—past, present, and proposed research. *American Journal of Public Health* 59:2131–2143.

Berelson, B. 1964. On family planning communication. *Demography* 1:94–105.

Berelson, B. and Freedman, R. A. 1964. A study in fertility control. *Scientific American* 210:29–37.

Blake, J. 1966. Ideal family size among white Americans: a quarter of a century's evidence. *Demography* 3:154–173.

————. 1971. Abortion and public opinion: the 1960–1970 decade. *Science* 171:540–549.

Bogue, D. J. 1966. Family planning research: an outline of the field. In B. Berelson, R. K. Anderson, O. Harkavy, J. Maier, W. P. Mauldin, and S. J. Segal, eds., *Family planning and population programs: a review of world developments*. Chicago: University of Chicago Press. Pp. 721–735.

Buros, O. K., ed. 1970. *Personality tests and reviews: including an index to the mental measurements yearbooks*. Highland Park, N.J.: Gryphon Press.

Carter, L. J. 1970. New femininism: potent force in birth-control policy. *Science* 167: 1234–1236.

Cattell, R. B. and Stice, G. F. 1957. *Handbook for the Sixteen Personality Factor Questionnaire*. Champaign, Ill.: Institute for Personality and Ability Testing.

David, H. P. 1970a. *Family planning and abortion in the socialist countries of Central and Eastern Europe*. New York: The Population Council.

————. 1970b. Psychosocial factors in transnational family planning research. In H. P. David and N. Bernheim, eds., *Proceedings of the Conference on Psychological Factors in Transnational Family Planning Research*. Washington, D.C.: American Institutes for Research. Pp. 8–15.

Davis, K. 1967. Population policy: will current programs succeed? *Science* 158:730–739.

Doob, L. W. 1967. Scales for assaying psychological modernization in Africa. *Public Opinion Quarterly* 31:414–421.

Edwards, A. L. 1953. *Edwards personal preference schedule*. New York: The Psychological Corporation.

Fawcett, J. T. 1970. *Psychology and population*. New York: The Population Council.

Flapan, M. 1969. A paradigm for the analysis of childbearing motivations of married women prior to birth of the first child. *American Journal of Orthopsychiatry* 39: 402–417.

Franck, K. and Rosen, E. 1949. A projective test of masculinity-femininity. *Journal of Consulting Psychology* 13:247–256.

Freedman, R. 1962. American studies of family planning and fertility: a review of major trends and issues. In C. V. Kiser, ed., *Research in family planning*. Princeton: Princeton University Press. Pp. 211–227.

Freedman, R.; Whelpton, P. K.; and Campbell, A. A. 1959. *Family planning, sterility, and population growth*. New York: McGraw-Hill.

Gough, H. G. 1957. *Manual for the California Psychological Inventory*. Palo Alto, Calif.: Consulting Psychologists Press.

————. 1960. Theory and measurement of socialization. *Journal of Consulting Psychology* 24:23–30.

————. 1965a. Conceptual analysis of psychological test scores and other diagnostic variables. *Journal of Abnormal Psychology* 70:294–302.

————. 1965b. Cross-cultural validation of a measure of asocial behavior. *Psychological Reports* 17:379–387.

————. 1966. A cross-cultural analysis of the CPI femininity scale. *Journal of Consulting Psychology* 30:136–141.

————. 1968. An interpreter's syllabus for the CPI. In P. McReynolds, ed., *Advances in psychological assessment*. Palo Alto, Calif.: Science and Behavior Books 1:55–79.

Gough, H. G.; Chun, K.; and Chung, Y-E. 1968. Validation of the CPI femininity scale in Korea. *Psychological Reports* 22:155–160.

Gough, H. G. and Heilbrun, A. B., Jr. 1965. *The adjective check list manual*. Palo Alto, Calif.: Consulting Psychologists Press.

Groat, H. T. and Neal, A. G. 1967. Social psychological correlates of urban fertility. *American Sociological Review* 32:845–959.

Gustavus, S. O. and Nam, C. B. 1970. The formation and stability of ideal family size among young people. *Demography* 70:43–51.

Hathaway, S. R. and McKinley, J. C. 1943. *Manual for the Minnesota Multiphasic Personality Inventory*. Minneapolis: University of Minnesota Press.

Hoffman, L. and Wyatt, F. 1960. Social change and motivation for having larger families: some theoretical considerations. *Merrill-Palmer Quarterly* 6:235–244.

Insko, C. A.; Blake, R. R.; Cialdini, R. B.; and Mulaik, S. A. 1970. Attitude toward birth control and cognitive consistency: theoretical and practical implications of survey data. *Journal of Personality and Social Psychology* 16:228–237.

Jaccard, J. 1971. Beliefs and personality in fertility research. Unpublished senior honor's thesis, University of California, Berkeley.

Kahl, J. A. 1968. *The measurement of modernism: a study of values in Brazil and Mexico*. Austin: University of Texas Press.

Kapor-Stanulovic, P. 1970. Sex-role identification and family planning. Unpublished master's thesis, University of California, Davis.

Keller, A. B.; Sims, J. H.; Henry, W. E.; and Crawford, T. J. 1970. Psychological sources of "resistance" to family planning. *Merrill-Palmer Quarterly of Behavior and Development* 16:286–302.

Kimmel, P. R. and Perlman, D. 1970. Psychosocial modernity and the initial accommodation of foreigners visiting the United States. *Journal of Social Psychology* 81:121–123.

Kiser, C. V. 1962. The Indianapolis study of social and psychological factors affecting fertility. In C. V. Kiser, ed., *Research in family planning*. Princeton: Princeton University Press. Pp. 149–166.

Kutner, S. J. and Duffy, T. J. 1970. A psychological analysis of oral contraceptives and the intrauterine device. *Contraception* 2:289–296.

MacDonald, A. P., Jr. 1970. Internal-external locus of control and the practice of birth control. *Psychological Reports* 27:206.

Moos, R. H. 1968. Psychological aspects of oral contraceptives. *Archives of General Psychiatry* 19:87–94.

Murawski, B. J. 1969. Psychological considerations for the evaluation of long-term use of oral contraceptives. *Journal of Reproductive Medicine* 3:151–155.

Newman, S. H.; Beck, M. B.; and Lewit, S. 1970. Abortion, obtained and denied: research approaches. *Studies in Family Planning* 53:1–8.

Patt, S. L.; Rappaport, R. G.; and Barglow, P. 1969. Follow-up of therapeutic abortion. *Archives of General Psychiatry* 20:408–414.

Peck, A. and Marcus, H. 1966. Psychiatric sequelae of therapeutic interruption of pregnancy. *Journal of Nervous and Mental Disease* 143:417–425.

Peshkin, A. and Cohen, R. 1967. The values of modernization. *Journal of Developing Areas* 2:7–22.

Pohlman, E. 1966. Birth control: independent and dependent variable for psychological research. *American Psychologist* 21:967–970.

————. 1969. *The psychology of birth planning*. Cambridge, Mass.: Schenkman.

Rabin, A. I. 1965. Motivation for parenthood. *Journal of Projective Techniques and Personality Assessment* 29:405–411.

Rabin, A. I. and Greene, R. J. 1968. Assessing motivation for parenthood. *Journal of Psychology* 69:39–46.

Rainwater, L. 1960. *And the poor get children.* Chicago: Quadrangle Books.

———. 1965. *Family design: marital sexuality, family size, and contraception.* Chicago: Aldine.

Rodgers, D. A. and Ziegler, F. J. 1968. Social role theory, the marital relationship, and the use of ovulation suppressors. *Journal of Marriage and the Family* 30:584–591.

Rodgers, D. A.; Ziegler, F. J.; Altrocchi, J. C.; and Levy, N. 1965. A longitudinal study of the psycho-social effects of vasectomy. *Journal of Marriage and the Family* 27:59–64.

Rodgers, D. A.; Ziegler, F. J.; and Levy, N. 1967. Prevailing cultural attitudes about vasectomy: a possible explanation of postoperative psychological response. *Psychosomatic Medicine* 29:367–375.

Rotter, J. B. 1966. Generalized expectancies for internal versus external control of reinforcement. *Psychological Monographs*, Vol. 80, no. 1 (whole no. 609).

Schachter, N. and Kiser, C. V. 1953. Social and psychological factors affecting fertility: XIX. Fear of pregnancy and childbirth in relation to fertility-planning status and fertility. *Milbank Memorial Fund Quarterly* 31:835–884.

Simon, N. M. 1970. Psychological and emotional indications for therapeutic abortion. *Seminars in Psychiatry* 2:283–301.

Simon, N. M. and Senturia, A. G. 1966. Psychiatric sequelae of abortion. *Archives of General Psychiatry* 15:378–389.

Simon, N. M.; Senturia, A. G.; and Rothman, D. 1967. Psychiatric illness following therapeutic abortion. *American Journal of Psychiatry* 124:65–97.

Sloane, R. B. 1969. The unwanted pregnancy. *New England Journal of Medicine* 280:1206–1213.

Smith, D. H. and Inkeles, A. 1966. The OM scale: a comparative socio-psychological measure of individual modernity. *Sociometry* 29:353–377.

Stycos, J. M. 1963. Obstacles to programs of population control—facts and fancies. *Marriage and Family Living* 25:5–13.

Tietze, C. 1965. History of contraceptive methods. *Journal of Sex Research* 1:69–85.

Tietze, C. and Lewit, S. 1969. Abortion. *Scientific American* 220:21–27.

Westoff, C. F.; Potter, R. G., Jr.; and Sagi, P. C. 1963. *The third child.* Princeton: Princeton University Press.

Westoff, C. F.; Potter, R. G., Jr.; Sagi, P. C.; and Mishler, E. G. 1961. *Family growth in metropolitan America.* Princeton: Princeton University Press.

Westoff, C. F. and Ryder, N. B. 1967. United States methods of fertility control, 1955, 1960, and 1965. In W. T. Liu, ed., *Family and fertility.* South Bend, Ind.: University of Notre Dame Press. Pp. 157–169.

———. 1969. Recent trends in attitudes toward fertility control and in the practice of contraception in the United States. In S. J. Behrman, L. Corsa, Jr., and R. Freedman, eds., *Fertility and family planning: a world view.* Ann Arbor: University of Michigan Press. Pp. 388–412.

Whelpton, P.; Campbell, A. A.; and Patterson, J. E. 1966. *Fertility and family planning in the United States.* Princeton: Princeton University Press.

Whelpton, P. K. and Kiser, C. V., eds. 1946–1958. *Social and psychological factors affecting fertility.* New York: Milbank Memorial Fund. 5 vols.

———. 1959. Social and psychological factors affecting fertility. *Eugenics Review* 51:35–42.

Ziegler, F. J.; Rodgers, D. A.; and Kriegsman, S. A. 1966. Effect of vasectomy on psychological functioning. *Psychosomatic Medicine* 28:50–63.

Ziegler, F. J.; Rodgers, D. A.; Kriegsman, S. A.; and Martin, P. L. 1968. Ovulation suppressors, psychological functioning, and marital adjustment. *Journal of the American Medical Association* 204:849–853.

Ziegler, F. J.; Rodgers, D. A.; and Prentiss, R. J. 1969. Psychosocial response to vasectomy. *Archives of General Psychiatry* 21:46–54.

[13]

RESEARCH ON MEASUREMENT
OF FAMILY-SIZE NORMS

E. I. GEORGE

A social norm can be described as a set of ideas regarding acceptable behavior under given circumstances. A social norm can also mean the ideal patterns of behavior in a community or group. These ideal patterns are used as criteria in judging the conduct of individuals, provided such conduct or behavior is controllable by the individual. The concept of family-size norms implies the standards held by a given population concerning the number of children a couple should ideally have and also the attitudes toward deviations from the ideal. From the point of view of measurement the concept of family-size norms has two aspects:

1. Family-size ideals. This refers mainly to the number of children considered to be ideal by the members of the population, including the extent of deviations that could be permitted considering, of course, such factors as economic affluence, physical health, the desire to have at least one son or one daughter, and so on.
2. Attitudes toward a small family. An attitude may be defined as a disposition a person has to favor or not to favor a type of social object or social action (Guilford, 1959). As part of the family-size norm, this refers to the position of a given group of people on an attitude continuum representing extreme favorableness toward a small family at one end and extreme unfavorableness toward a small family at the other end, with a neutral position in between. (The same can be regarded as a continuum representing attitude toward a large family with the extremes reversed.)

NOTE: The author wishes to acknowledge the help rendered by Dr. V. George Mathew and Mr. B. Dharmangadan, his colleagues in the Department of Psychology at Kerala University, and Dr. A. George of the Department of Statistics, in the program of research on family-size norms sponsored by the Ministry of Health and Family Planning, Government of India.

Measurement of Family-Size Norms: General Considerations

Measurement of family-size norms is important in launching programs of population control. It is important to know what number of children the people consider to be ideal and also whether they favor large families or small families. Any family-planning program is likely to be successful if initially a wide gap exists between the ideal family size and a larger actual number of children born to an average couple by the end of the reproductive period. If, on the other hand, it is found that people favor medium or large families, the first step will be to bring about a change in the family-size norm. By suitable interview techniques the reasons for the large family ideal should be investigated, and propaganda should be initiated pertaining to the advantages of a small family. Special techniques of persuasion also may be used in changing the beliefs and attitudes. The success of the program can be assessed periodically through instruments capable of detecting changes in the family-size norm.

Do Crystallized Norms Exist?

The first problem is whether the population concerned has any crystallized norms whatsoever regarding family size. There is no point in attempting to measure something that does not exist. It is sometimes argued that people, when directly questioned, may start thinking and then give a suitable answer, though prior to the questioning they had no concept of an ideal family size. It is therefore necessary to find out whether there is a norm relating to family size.

Method of Measurement

The obvious method is the use of single direct questions such as "What is the ideal number of children in a family?" or "Do you favor a small family or a large family?" Such questions are generally used as part of the KAP studies and fertility surveys. Many criticisms have been leveled against this method. The respondents may resent the direct question as an unwanted invasion of privacy. It is said that respondents can easily avoid revealing their true attitude when questioned directly. The unsophisticated villager may not be able to make an objective assessment of his own position and state it precisely in a few words. Another important question concerns the reliability of responses. To what extent are the responses to different questions in a survey consistent? Is it likely that the same responses will be elicited on a subsequent interview? Many investigators say that the single direct questions do not tap the real attitudes and ideals. Often failure to find significant relationships is attributed to inadequacies of the measures of family-size norms.

Many of the traditional psychometric techniques and techniques of attitude scale construction can be applied to the field of family-size norms. It remains to be seen how the single-question method fares in comparison with the more sophisticated methods of measurements. The reliability of the measures of family-size norms can be estimated using the retest, split-half, or parallel form techniques. Validity can be estimated by intercorrelations between different measures of the same attitude or ideal and of similar attitudes or ideals and by correlations with criteria like fertility, acceptance of family planning, attitude toward family planning, ratings by self, investigator, or others, and so on.

Family-Size Norms and Attitude toward Family Planning

It is important to differentiate between attitude toward family size and attitude toward family planning. There are instances where test constructors have included both indiscriminately in the same measuring instrument to derive a single total score. Theoretically it appears that both can be to some extent independent. An individual may favor a small family, but can be opposed to artificially limiting family size. Moreover, an individual may favor limiting family size but may oppose the present family-planning methods because no easy, one-time, reversible contraceptive is available. For instance, there are many Gandhians in India who advocate limiting family size through continence but who oppose the governmental family-planning program that popularizes other methods of birth control. Conversely one may consider a large family to be an ideal one, but may resort to family planning to obtain desired spacing or because of some purely health or economic considerations. There may be some justification for including questions on family-size norms in a scale measuring the attitude toward family planning, but it may not be proper to include questions on family planning when measuring attitude toward family size.

Studies are required to find out to what extent the two attitudes vary together.

Measurement of Family-Size Ideals

In KAP studies different questions have been used to measure family-size ideals. The most typical question concerns the number of children that a couple should ideally have. This is often referred to as the ideal family size, though the measure is the number of children. Mauldin, Watson, and

Noe (1970) report twenty-six major variations of this question. It is likely that the wording has some influence on the responses. Responses to question variations like "If you were to live your life all over again, how many children would you like to have?" may be influenced by the number of children the respondent has at present and therefore may not truly reflect the ideal. Most people do not like to admit that they are dissatisfied with their own present performance. The personal reference in the question "What is the ideal number of children for a couple like you?" may arouse suspicion and put the respondent on the defensive. Asking the ideal number of children "for an average couple" puts a restriction on the respondent that may not be of any use. It appears that the simple form of the question is the best. In our study the question used was "In your opinion what is the ideal number of children in a family?" The part "in your opinion" was included to indicate that we were not asking the respondent to guess the number that is considered ideal by people in general.

If the Model Questionnaire for KAP studies is widely used (The Population Council, 1970) it may make results obtained from different countries comparable, though when translated into different languages slight differences in meaning may be unavoidable.

Supplementary questions on family-size ideals would include questions on the ideal number of male and female children, the minimum number of children that there should be in a family, the maximum number, the number an economically affluent couple should have, and so on.

Ryder and Westoff (1969) measured ideal, desired, expected, and intended family size in connection with the 1965 National Fertility Survey of the United States. On the basis of the results obtained they found that expected and intended are virtually indistinguishable. It is possible that the distinction between desired and expected also is partly artificial because the two questions would have had a suggestive effect on the respondents, forcing them to give different replies to the two questions. The results show that the three concepts fall on an ideal-actual dimension with the ideal showing maximum overlap with desired, desired with intended, and intended with current.

The suspicion that people may not reveal their true family-size preferences when directly questioned (assuming they have definite preferences) has made some researchers use more complex measuring devices. It is expected that some of these tests may help in measurement when the degree of crystallization is low and may provide a more reliable measure than is yielded by direct questions. Sastry (1966) devised a Pictorial Choice Test, consisting of realistic pictures of eight families with number of children varying from one to eight with an equal number of boys and girls (in pictures with an odd number of children one was a baby with sex not distinguishable). The pictures were arranged in random order. The respondent had to indicate which family he liked most. Sastry also tried stick figures, which eliminate the effect of irrelevant features of the different pictures and make the test culture-free, but discarded the method because the stick figures did not give "a sense of reality."

The traditional scaling techniques of pair comparison and rank order (Guilford, 1954) can be applied to scale preferences for different family sizes. Myers and Roberts (1968) have attempted to scale, by the pair comparison method, preferences (considered ideal) for various combinations of boys and girls, each varying from zero to six. There would be forty-nine possible combinations of boys and girls. Each combination was then paired with every other, and thus there would be 1,176 pair comparisons. In each pair the respondent has to express a choice between the two combinations on a ratio scale (of the type 1:9, 2:8, 3:7, 4:6, 5:5, 6:4, 7:3, 8:2, 9:1). The preference scores were derived by the constant sum method of Torgerson (1958). The preference scores for any combination would be the geometric mean of the ratio judgments in the corresponding column of the matrix (one-half of the matrix containing the ratio judgments and the other half their reciprocals, with unity in diagonals). A contrast measure was derived that indicates the intensity or strength of preference for a given combination over other combinations. To get this the ratio judgment or its reciprocal, whichever is greater, is entered in the cells of the matrix, and the geometric mean in the corresponding column is determined. The time and labor involved in administration and computation would be enormous, and the authors had only eighteen Puerto Rican women subjects, who were paid for acting as subjects for the study.

The results obtained show the importance of sex balance in family-size ideals. Considering total number of children alone, the preferred numbers are two, four, three, and five, in that order. But when the different combinations were considered separately the most preferred combination was two girls and two boys, followed by one girl and one boy, and two girls and one boy. The alternatives of three girls and one boy, one girl and three boys, four girls and no boys, and no girls and four boys have low scores, bringing down the total preference for the family size of four children.

Measurement of Attitude toward Family Size

When the single-question method is used, often the questions on family-size ideals are considered to reflect the attitude toward a small family, or no attempt is made to measure the attitude. An additional question can be included, asking the respondent to state whether he is in favor of a small family or a large family. A neutral category also may be provided. A larger percentage of individuals expressing a favorable attitude toward a small family would mean a greater number of people not favoring families growing larger and would indicate a greater proportion of potential acceptors of contraceptives. However, there is the likelihood that the number of children considered "small" in one culture is "large" for another culture. Therefore, the fact that a larger percentage of individuals say that they prefer a small family does not necessarily mean that their ideal family size is smaller than that of another country. The attitude score indicates favorableness toward the growth of family size; it need not have a one-to-one correspondence with the absolute number of children considered to be ideal.

Instead of asking the respondent to choose one of the two or three response categories provided, a more elaborate rating scale of five or more points can be thought of. Ratings made by the interviewers on the basis of the whole interview also may be of some value. When the single-question method is used to measure attitude, the final estimate for the population usually will be in terms of the proportion of respondents favoring a small family.

The different techniques of attitude scale construction (Edwards, 1957; Fishbein, 1967) have been used to measure attitude toward family size. In the Thurstone procedure (Thurstone and Chave, 1929) a large number of simple, direct, unambiguous statements of opinion expressing different attitudes toward family size is prepared, and about 100 educated judges are asked to arrange them into eleven (sometimes five, seven, or nine) piles on a continuum having as the two extremes a maximum pro and maximum anti attitude toward a small family. The items about whose scale position there is high agreement among the judges are selected. The final scale is made up of a limited number of items (twenty-two or less) such that the scale values spread evenly over all parts of the continuum. The items should also satisfy the criterion of irrelevance. This is to ensure that an item is endorsed only by persons near the scale position represented by the item on the scale and not by those whose attitude level is different from the attitude level of the item. Unlike other attitude scales the Thurstone scale has a "neutral interval" though its midpoint cannot be regarded as a true zero point. It also has the equal-appearing-interval property, though this does not ensure equality of scale units. The main disadvantage is that the criterion of irrelevance is difficult to apply and many items do not satisfy this criterion. The Thurstone scale may lack unidimensionality also. Several scales of the Thurstone type have been developed in India to measure the attitude toward a small family (Govindachari, 1966; Warti, Pandit, and Amin, 1969; Sengupta, 1965).

In the development of the Likert scale a large number of propositions are administered to a group of individuals (preferably 400), and each of them has to indicate whether he strongly approves, approves, is undecided, disapproves, or strongly disapproves with respect to each of the items. Each item is scored by giving the weights five, four, three, two, and one to the above categories, and each person gets a total score for all the items. Then the score of each item is correlated with the total score, and items having high correlations (internal consistency) are retained for the final form. Likert scales usually have high unidimensionality.

Among the many attitude scales of this type developed in India the one by Mohanty (1966) deserves special mention. This instrument yields different kinds of information. It can indicate a person's (1) ideals of reproduction, (2) attitude toward family size, (3) desired family size, (4) values attached to children, and (5) attitude toward family planning. The instrument also indicates what the respondent thinks is the position of "other people" in each of these areas. The summed scores give the attitude of the testee toward a small family (personal dimension) as well as an estimate of what he thinks is the attitude of other people toward a small family (normative dimension). The personal and normative scores correlate 0.67. The reliabilities of the two scores are not reported. If the reliabilities of the two scales are not much higher than the above correlation, the possibility of using the normative dimension to estimate the personal scores as a projective technique can be considered. The main drawback of the scale is that it is too long; there are forty-eight questions given as twelve items, each having four parts.

In the Guttman technique of attitude scale construction the criterion for item selection is the consistency that endorsement of a given item is accompanied by sanction of all other items that are less extreme. The scale has good unidimensionality, but often all the items selected finally are variations or rephrasings of a single theme. Ahmed (1965) has developed a Guttman scale to measure the attitude toward family planning.

Eysenck and Crown (1949) proposed the scale-product method of scoring Thurstone scales, which combines the Thurstone scale values and Likert weights in the form of products, and showed that it gives higher reliability than the Thurstone or Likert methods. Panda and Kanungo (1964) developed a scale to measure the attitude toward family planning and found the scale-product method to have higher reliability than the simpler methods. Sastry (1966) developed the "Thematic Reaction Test" in which a story is told and questions based on the story are put to the respondent, eliciting his family-size ideals and attitudes.

In our study (George, Mathew and Dharmangadan, 1971) an attempt was made to measure family-size norms using different methods so that their relative merits could be compared.

From the same initial pool of 100 statements of opinion, three attitude scales were developed: Form T of the Thurstone type, Form L of the Likert type, and Form TL_1 and TL_2, parallel forms that can be scored either by the scale-product method or the Likert method. Item-total point-biserial correlations were used as indices of item validity. They were given some consideration in item selection for the Thurstone scale also as this can partly replace the criterion of irrelevance and increase unidimensionality (Edwards and Kilpatrick, 1948). Most of the statements favoring a small family were endorsed by large proportions of the respondents and so were less useful for the final forms of the tests than were items favoring a large family. This would make the final form of the tests look like propaganda for a large family, so a few of the best among the available items favoring a small family were also included. The Eysenck-Crown scale-product method was tried in the case of Form T and the parallel forms, but it did not prove to be more reliable than the simpler Thurstone and Likert procedures.

Examples of statements included in the attitude scales are, "More contentment and happiness are seen in the members of a small family," "Whether a family is small or large does not matter very much," and "Children are the joy of life; it is good to have a large number of them." For each statement the respondent has to choose one from five alternate responses: "strongly agree, agree, undecided, disagree, and strongly disagree."

A Story Response Test, following the model of Sastry's Thematic Reaction Test, was also prepared. A story about a recently married couple, the husband and wife (with two female children) having different family-size ideals and attitudes, is read to the respondent and seven questions about the story are asked. Each question has three alternative answers, "yes," "don't know," and "no." An additive attitude score is obtained, a high score indicating a favorable attitude toward a large family.

We also used the Picture Response Test in which six pictures are shown to the respondent with multiple-choice answers following each picture. The pictures depict a poor rural family with five children, a family with five female children, a rich couple with three children, a rural family with five children working in the fields, an old couple with nobody to look after them, and a family with five male children. Here also a summed attitude score is derived. In addition eight small pictures of families with the number of children varying from one to eight (following Sastry's Pictorial Choice Test) were included as an appendix to measure ideal parity.

Percentile norms were prepared for all the tests. In addition family-size ideals were measured by the single questions (ideal, minimum, maximum, and ideal for the rich). A total additive score also was derived. The sum of the four estimates of boys divided by the total scores on family-size ideals gave the sex-preference ratio.

Crystallization of Family-Size Norms

Ease and efficiency of measurement increase if what is measured is highly crystallized. One can expect to measure an attitude by means of a single question only if there is a high degree of crystallization. In such a case the single-question responses will have a reasonably high reliability, and only a few questions are needed to form a test.

In our study most of the 100 statements used in the trial form had high correlations with the total score. The median correlation was 0.46 with only three correlations below 0.15 and four correlations above 0.60. This is in spite of the fact that most of the p values (proportions marking the keyed answer) were extreme, a condition that brings down point-biserial correlations. This indicates that people respond in a consistent manner to different statements of opinion regarding family size. With only fifteen items the Likert scale has an odd-even reliability of 0.91. In the Ryder and Westoff study ideal parity was found to have smaller variance in relation to desired parity and intended parity. This also indicates that in the population there is general agreement about the ideal number of children. In the study by Myers on preferential family size, average contrast scores were highest for the most popular combination of two girls and two boys, and the next highest was for the next most popular combination of one girl and one boy. This also indicates that there is high agreement among people about the ideal combination. There is a consistent preference for male children in India, while in certain countries there is a consistent preference for females, e.g., Puerto Rico (Stycos, 1955; Myers and Roberts, 1968). In our study women, rural, older, and less educated people belonging to the lower-middle-income group, and men working as unskilled laborers were found to be more large-family oriented. However, no attempt was made to keep constant or partial out the effect of education while studying the relationship of other variables to the attitude. Such meaningful relationships also reflect the crystallization of norms in the population at large.

In our study husband-wife agreement was found to be low (the attitude score correlates only 0.19). This could be a result of poor husband-wife communication in such matters and not due to the lack of crystallization of the attitude. In contrast, in metropolitan America husband-wife agreement in family-size ideals has been found to vary from 0.39 to 0.76 for various religious groups (Westoff, Potter, Sagi, and Mishler, 1961). The correlation of the attitude scale score to attitude toward family planning (whether favorable or not) was also small (point-biserial correlation of 0.30, proportion favoring family planning being 0.92), indicating that the two attitudes do not have high covariation.

In a study by Stycos (1961) in Haiti a highly unstructured type of interview was used to measure family-size norms. To the question "What do you think is the best number of children for a person in your circumstances?" 70 percent replied that it is a matter entirely up to God. But those who did state a preference named a small family, the median number of children being 2.4. This result would appear to support the belief that responses given to direct questions in KAP studies are artificial or superficial and that crystallized norms do not exist. Stycos comes to the conclusion that the norm is an avoidance of mentioning a number or fatalism. In our opinion the number of children in a family is one of the most salient things in the psychological world of a villager, and he would be quite conscious of the economic and other consequences of different family sizes. Specific meanings and implications are likely to be associated with different boy-girl combinations also. What we experience in an interview situation is not the absence of a norm but a reluctance to state it. To the ordinary villager it might appear to be bad manners to state preferences for the number of children. It is significant that among those who stated a number as ideal in the above study there was high agreement. To mention a number as ideal (which is usually small) would imply disapproving the later arrivals, and it would not be proper to value those human beings less. It would also place parents who have many children in a bad light for no fault of theirs. The number of children one already has or the number of siblings he has may be larger or simply different from his ideal, making it slightly embarrassing for him to state it. However, when directly questioned or when the interviewer persists the norm may be revealed. In fact it is possible that an impersonal, quick, businesslike research attitude is better than an informal personal relationship. Stycos presented photographs of a large family (six children) and a small family (three children) and asked the respondents how the two families differed. About 22 percent did not see any difference, and among those who saw a difference just over a third mentioned size. Stycos does not hesitate to conclude that family size is a matter of low salience. On the contrary it is possible that family size was not mentioned as a factor because it is too evident and obvious. The ordinary respondent might not think that the interviewer is expecting him to make such a silly differentiation. It is unlikely that if a photograph of a man and another of a woman were presented simultaneously many respondents would mention sex as one of the important differences between the two photographs, but from this one should not conclude that sex is a matter of low salience!

In conclusion it may be stated that people have a well-defined concept of ideal family size and also well-defined attitudes toward family size. Therefore, it can be supposed that people have definite attitudes toward deviations from the ideal family size also. Until they know that family size is not beyond human control, they are likely to be reluctant to express the norm. Till then there may be no attempt to look down upon or criticize persons who diviate from the norm. It may be noted in this connection that birth control was not totally unknown in many primitive societies, though the indigenous methods used were difficult, dangerous, or ineffective. Traditionally people were shy of sex, and birth control was associated with infanticide. The very existence of such methods is proof that a norm exists, and a desire to limit family size, though subliminal, is present.

Family-Size Norms and Fertility

The family-size ideal and attitude toward family size of an individual can affect his fertility performance to the extent to which he is able and willing to plan the size of his family. In underdeveloped countries where the idea of family planning has not gained currency and people are fatalistic and do not plan their future to any considerable extent, we can expect the correlation to be low. In our study the correlation between the attitude score of Form L and fertility, after partialing out the effect of age, was only 0.05 (the sample consisting of 448 ever married women).

A positive association has been found between ideal family size and number of births in the United States (Whelpton, Campbell, and Patterson, 1966). Desired family size has moderate negative correlations with birth intervals (Westoff et al., 1961).

It is difficult to disentangle cause-effect relations in fertility performance and family-size norms. There is some evidence that current family-size preferences are consequences rather than causes of family size (Hill, Stycos, and Back, 1959). Studies relating fertility desires at the time of marriage to actual completed fertility later on are required to find out how far initial attitudes influence fertility performance. In one study fertility preferences of engaged couples were correlated with the number of births twenty years later. The correlation was 0.26 for husbands and 0.27 for wives. In another study husbands and wives were asked to state from memory their desired family size at the time of marriage twelve to fifteen years ago. The correlations with number of children were 0.30 and 0.32 for husbands and wives respectively (Westoff et al., 1961).

The Single-Question Method: An Evaluation

While we do not expect the single-question method to have a reliability and validity as high as those of sophisticated tests, the reliability and validity may be high enough to justify its use in many situations. The factors of time taken for administration and of economy have to be taken into account. Usually a wide variety of data are collected in surveys, and it is difficult to keep the respondent cooperative for a long time. Moreover, sophisticated tests require special tryouts and statistical treatment in the process of development and are therefore costly. So it is necessary to know in which situations we can manage with single questions and when we have to resort to specially devised tests. Ordinarily we need measuring devices with reliabilities above 0.9 when we want to predict the behavior of an individual. For research purposes where we are concerned with the group as a whole, instruments with reliabilities as low as 0.5 can often reveal relationships among variables and can be used to prepare norms.

A test ordinarily will not have a validity coefficient larger than its reliability. Under no circumstances can validity exceed the square root of reliability. Therefore, if a high validity coefficient can be obtained, then reliability is taken care of.

The reliability of a single question can be determined by reinterviewing a subsample of at least 100 respondents. A reestimation of the proportion may not give a true picture because individual errors may be mutually compensatory and get canceled out. The proportion giving the *same* answer in both interviews is a good measure of reliability. The reliability thus estimated is likely to be an underestimate as even slight deviations from the original response make the second response different from the first. Ryder and Westoff (1969) recommend the reliability ratio. The proportion giving the same response is corrected for the extent to which such responses would be expected by chance, given the configuration of the marginal distributions in the first and second interviews. Specifically the reliability ratio is defined as the ratio (O-E) / (N-E), where O is the number of cases observed in the equality diagonal, E is the number of cases expected on the equality diagonal under the assumption of randomness, and N is the total number of cases. Ryder and Westoff report reliability ratios of 0.65 for ideal number of children, 0.63 for desired number of children, and 0.86 for intended number of children.

With regard to validity it is often believed that "courtesy bias" (tendency to give a response that the respondent thinks will be pleasing to the interviewer) and superficiality of responses will be greater with single questions. On the other hand, response sets and biases like that of acquiescence (Guilford, 1954) have been found to operate in tests as well. Tests can also make the respondent suspicious, and the respondent may misunderstand what is being measured and give irrelevant answers.

In our study the odd-even reliabilities of the different attitude scores were as follows—Form L: 0.91; Picture Response Test: 0.90; Parallel Forms: 0.85; Form T: 0.84; and Story Response Test: 0.77. There were fifteen items in Form L and Parallel Forms and fourteen in Form T. The results are in agreement with the general finding that Likert scales often have high reliability. Discrimination among those favoring a small family is very poor for the Picture Response Test and to some extent for the Story Response Test and the Thurstone scale. Discrimination of these tests can be improved by trying out new items and selecting items discriminating individuals at this part of the scale. Ratings made by the investigators on a seven-point scale correlated 0.64 with the attitude score of Form L.

Attitude scores often are not normally distributed. It is therefore necessary to take recourse to nonparametric statistical tools unless we find the scores to be normal. The scores of Form L were found to be normally distributed in the case of men, but not in the case of women, when the chi-square test of normality was applied.

The single questions on family-size ideals had high correlations with the attitude scores on Form L. The number of children considered ideal correlated 0.79, minimum number of children (opinion) correlated 0.72, maximum permissible number of children correlated 0.75, and the number of children a rich couple should ideally have correlated 0.68. The total score on family-size ideals had a split-half reliability of 0.87 and correlated 0.81 with the attitude score of Form L and 0.79 with the rating made by interviewers. Some of the above correlations come close to the reliability of some of the attitude scale scores; considering the fact that family-size ideals can be to some extent independent of attitude, the single-question method appears to have sufficiently high reliability and validity to justify its use in the measurement of family-size norms. In this study the section on family-size ideals always followed the administration of some other test. Therefore, it may be argued that the same reliability and validity would not have been obtained if the family-size ideals questions were given first. The high reliability and validity of the sum of the responses to the four questions on family-size ideals indicate the possibility of combining the responses to different questions in KAP studies to obtain a more reliable and valid measure of attitude than is yielded by a single question. A comparison of results obtained in our study using different methods of measurement is shown in Table 13–1.

TABLE 13-1

Reliabilities and Validities of Different Measures of Family-Size Norms Obtained in the Present Study

Measure	Number of Items	Reliability	Validity[a]	Discrimination among Respondents
Attitude scales				
Form L	15	0.91	0.57 to 0.81	Very high
Form T	14	0.84	0.56 to 0.74	High
Parallel forms	15	0.85	0.65 to 0.72	Very high
Picture Response Test	6	0.90	0.54 to 0.72	Very low
Story Response Test	7	0.77	0.57 to 0.70	Low
Single-question method	1	—	0.68 to 0.79	—
Total score derived from single questions on family-size ideals	4	0.87	0.54 to 0.81	Low

[a]Correlations with other measures of family-size norms.

More than 400 KAP studies have been conducted all over the world (nearly sixty in India). The general finding is that contrary to expectation people do not want large families. In our study the mean ideal number of children was 3.1, while the average current number of children was 3.6. In view of the fact that most of the respondents (ever or currently married) had not reached the end of the reproductive period, this indicates a wide gap between the ideal and the performance. In fact our respondents reported having an average of 6.1 siblings, giving the impression that typical completed fertility is more than six. Mohanty's (1969) data indicate that even the number of children to guarantee at least one son was only 4.6 and at least one daughter 4.0, the ideal being 3.5. Moreover, ideal family sizes are often an overestimate as people hesitate to mention a number less than what they have at the moment.

Many people argue that villagers really want large families and that when questioned directly in countries where there is a government-sponsored family-planning program, people give small numbers as ideal because of fear or the "courtesy bias." If this is so, when sophisticated measuring devices or depth interview techniques are used, different results should be obtained. However, irrespective of the technique of data collection employed, the ideal family size is usually obtained as three or four children. Often when depth interview techniques are used the number is smaller. In the study by Stycos (1961) Haitian people were chosen as the study population since they were representative of relatively primitive populations who had never heard of family planning. With the highly unstructured interview technique it was found that the median ideal of those who stated an ideal was 2.4. It is very important to note that the characteristic statement of the villager is not that "I wish God would give me many children," but "Whatever number God gives me, I will accept." Therefore, the norm is certainly not in favor of a large family.

In our study the ideal number of children measured using the single-question method was compared to the ideal number of children obtained from a smaller but comparable sample using the eight pictures forming the second part of the Picture Response Test. The pictures were found useful in arousing the interest of the respondents and in eliciting their cooperation. If the courtesy bias operates more in the case of the question and if it will be minimized because of the interest aroused by the pictures, we may expect the pictures to give a higher mean ideal family size. However, the means are more or less the same for both methods. The mean for men was actually slightly lower with the pictures. The responses to the pictures showed more variability.

In the study by Myers and Roberts of the preferential family size using the pair-comparison method, respondents were independently asked to state their ideal family size and composition. A high correspondence was found between the most valued composition obtained by the scaling approach and the responses to the question regarding the ideal. It appears that investigators often distrust results obtained in KAP studies because of the stereotyped belief that traditionally people favor a very large number of children. This is not the case in most places, at least under the present socioeconomic conditions.

Eysenck and Crown (1949) suggest that the single-question method can also be made use of for the measurement of attitude. The fact that in our study some statements had correlations above 0.6 with the total score indicates the possibility of a single statement yielding a reliable measure of attitude in the area of measurement of family-size norms. Statements or questions should be selected after a proper tryout. Statements that are endorsed by about 50 percent of the respondents offer maximum discrimination. Statements having different stereotypy values (proportions) should be selected depending upon the cutoff point desired. If there are many statements to start with, their scale values can be determined by the Thurstone method, which would give a better understanding of the results obtained using the selected single statement. Two statements having the same scale value and stereotypy values can be used in the "split-ballot" technique to check the comparability of results.

When to Use Tests?

Sophisticated tests and methods of measurement will certainly have a place in research on small samples. In large-scale surveys the single-question methods can be used, but their reliability and validity should be determined objectively. Test scores can provide sensitive measures of family-size norms in many situations. For instance, in comparing the effectiveness of different methods of communication, sensitive measures of change in family-size norms may be required. A change in mean test scores will be a more sensitive measure than a change in the proportion of people favoring a small family. The Thurstone scale with the equal-appearing-interval property will be useful in comparing the amounts of change in two subsamples who occupied two different initial positions on the scale. Parallel forms will be useful where the attitude level of the same sample is to be measured twice with a relatively short time interval. Tests like the Picture Response Test will be useful where there is the problem of arousing the interest and eliciting the cooperation of the respondents and helping them to visualize different situations. Other things being equal, the Likert scale is to be preferred because of higher reliability and unidimensionality.

Diagnosis of individual cases and prediction of individual behavior (as contrasted with prediction of the behavior of the group as a whole) require sophisticated tests. When we want to locate individuals who are most favorable or most unfavorable tests will also be useful. Again, if we require an estimate of the range of attitude in any given subpopulation as compared with the general population, test scores are required. In general test construction is worth the effort only if the tests will be used by many investigators for a variety of purposes.

Summary

By family-size norms we refer to the standards held by a given population concerning the number of children a couple should ideally have and the attitudes toward a small family.

The high intercorrelation of statements of opinion regarding family size, agreement among people as to the ideal family size, and meaningful and consistent differences in family-size norms held by different subsections of the population indicate that family-size norms are generally highly crystallized. However, it is found that there is a reluctance on the part of respondents to express their ideals and attitudes because their own number of children may be different from the ideal and the number of children is often considered to be beyond human control.

The reliability of single questions should be objectively determined by reinterviewing, and their validity should be tested by correlating with suitable criteria. In the area of measurement of family-size norms the single-question method has been found to have sufficient reliability and validity to justify its use. It is possible to combine responses to different questions in KAP surveys to get more reliable estimates of the attitude.

Many investigators distrust the results of the single-question method because of their preconception that people have large-family ideals while the results obtained indicate that norms favor a small family. The ideal parity obtained using single questions is comparable to results obtained with depth interviews, a Pictorial Choice Test, and the pair-comparison scaling method.

Single direct questions can be used to measure attitude as well. When a single statement of opinion is to be used for the measurement of attitude, it should be selected after a proper tryout. Test construction will be useful in cases where it is necessary to get sensitive measures of family-size norms on small samples for several research investigations. Attitude scales of the Thurstone and Likert types and other tests like the Picture Response Test will be useful in different situations.

REFERENCES

Ahmed, S. F. 1965. *Attitude scale to measure attitude towards family planning.* New Delhi: Lady Hardinge Medical College.

Edwards, A. L. 1957. *Techniques of attitude scale construction.* New York: Appleton-Century-Crofts.

Edwards, A. L. and Kilpatrick, F. P. 1948. A technique for the construction of attitude scales. *Journal of Applied Psychology* 32:374–384.

Eysenck, H. H. and Crown, S. 1949. An experimental study in opinion attitude scales. *International Journal of Opinion and Attitude Research* 3:47–86.

Fishbein, M., ed. 1967. *Readings in attitude theory and measurement*. New York: Wiley.

George, E. I.; Mathew, V. George; and Dharmangadan, B. 1971. *Family size norms in Kerala*. (In press).

Govindachari, A. 1966. In K. R. Sastry and A. Govindachari, *Action Research Monographs No. III*. Gandhigram, Madurai: Institute of Rural Health and Family Planning.

Guilford, J. P. 1954. *Psychometric methods*. New York: McGraw-Hill.

———. 1959. *Personality*. New York: McGraw-Hill.

Hill, R.; Stycos, J. M.; and Back, K. W. 1959. *The family and population control*. Chapel Hill: University of North Carolina Press.

Mauldin, W. P.; Watson, W. B.; and Noe, L. F. 1970. *KAP surveys and evaluations of family planning programmes*. New York: The Population Council (mimeo).

Mohanthy, S. P. 1959. Attempts at measuring family planning attitudes in India: an assessment of traditional and emerging techniques. Chembur, Bombay: All India Seminar on Models in Demographic Analysis. Demographic Training and Research Centre.

———. 1966. *Family size attitude inventory*. Chembur, Bombay: Demographic Training and Research Centre.

Myers, G. C. and Roberts, J. M. 1968. A technique for measuring preferential family size and composition. *Eugenics Quarterly* 15:164–172.

Panda, K. C. and Kanungo, R. 1964. A scale of measurements of attitude towards family planning. *Indian Journal of Social Work* 25:125–130.

The Population Council. 1970. *A manual for surveys of fertility and family planning: knowledge, attitudes and practice*. New York: The Population Council.

Ryder, N. B. and Westoff, C. F. 1969. Relationships among intended, expected, desired and ideal family size: United States 1965. *Population Research*, March 1969.

Sastry, K. R. 1966. In K. R. Sastry and A. Govindachari, *Action Research Monographs No. III*. Gandhigram, Madurai: Institute of Rural Health and Family Planning.

Sengupta, A. 1965. Constructing a scale for measuring attitude towards family planning: an experiment with Thurstone. *Technical Paper No. 5*. Calcutta: Family Planning Research Unit, Indian Statistical Institute.

Stycos, J. M. 1955. *Family and fertility in Puerto Rico*. New York: Columbia University Press.

———. 1961. Haitian attitudes toward family size. *Human Organisation* 23:42–47.

Thurstone, L. L. and Chave, E. J. 1929. *The measurement of attitude*. Chicago: University of Chicago Press.

Torgerson, W. S. 1958. *Theory and methods of scaling*. New York: Wiley.

Warti, M. S.; Pandit, P.; and Amin, D. 1969. *Measurement of family size norm*. Department of Psychology, Baroda University.

Westoff, C. F.; Potter, J. R.; Sagi, P. C.; and Mishler, E. G. 1961. *Family growth in metropolitan America*. Princeton: Princeton University Press.

Whelpton, P. K.; Campbell, A. A.; and Patterson, J. E. 1966. *Fertility and family planning in the United States*. Princeton: Princeton University Press.

[14]

A NEW HUMAN LIFE
AND ABORTION: BELIEFS, IDEAL
VALUES, AND VALUE JUDGMENTS

ANDIE L. KNUTSON

Beliefs about human life are centered within the philosophical and religious perspectives of culture. So, too, are assessments of the relative ideal value of the lives of men versus women, young versus old, the educated versus the uneducated, and so forth, and value judgments about the treatment of human life under various conditions of our changing society. Relatively little attention has been given in research to the patterning of such beliefs and ideal values and to their relation to value judgments about abortion.

Perhaps one can best understand how such beliefs and values function by determining their meanings within the cognitive structures of individuals and by seeing how they relate to each other and to activities of significance to these persons. Several beliefs about life, together with assessments about the ideal value of a human life at given ages during development, have been examined in terms of their functional relationship to value judgments about abortion and other practices that involve decisions about continuing or ending a life.

This preliminary report is primarily based on a sample of U.S. public health professionals who returned to school for further graduate training. Since this sample varies little in terms of age, education, intelligence, orien-

NOTE: This research was supported in part by Public Health Service General Research Support Grant Number FR–05441 (School of Public Health), Research Career Program Award Number K–3 MH 20976 (School of Public Health and Institute of Human Development), a small grant Number MH–19217 and an award from the Russell Sage Foundation (Institute of Human Development), and a travel award from The Population Council. During this research David Day served as my assistant. A discussion of theory and methodology will be included in a monograph in preparation for the Russell Sage Foundation.

tation toward health and the care of human life, one would expect that relationships found in this sample will be present to a greater degree in the general public. More limited data are presented for smaller samples of health professionals in Taiwan and advanced medical students in Thailand. The analysis of the data from these and other overseas samples is still to be completed.

Rationale

Two general hypotheses have guided this research: (1) value judgments about abortion are more closely associated with religious orientations than with age, sex, profession, or other demographic and sociological variables; and (2) value judgments about abortion are closely associated with beliefs about a human life and the ideal value assigned a human life during development.

The beliefs, ideal value assessments by age, and value judgments studied in this research were identified and formulated on the basis of intensive interviews with prior samples of U.S. and other health professionals similar to those whose responses are reported here. Subjects were queried at length about the practices under study to determine how they viewed each behavior and the situation to which it is related, the beliefs they held of concern to that behavior and how they formulated these beliefs, and the value judgments they made regarding the behavior. The items used in measures of beliefs and value judgments developed for this research are therefore formulated in terminology consonant with the cognitive patterns of these health professionals.

Predictions about actual behavior cannot be made with confidence on the basis of the present data, however, since what one ought to do or should do is not always consonant with what one does.

The Sample

The primary sample for this report is 290 U.S. public health professionals, who returned to the School of Public Health at Berkeley for further graduate training, and includes about two-thirds of these graduate students during each of four academic years, 1965–1968. All were volunteers.

Professional identifications held prior to entering the School of Public Health included physicians (33 percent), nurses (12.5 percent), health educators, nutritionists or home economists, teachers, hospital administrators, sanitarians, social workers, biostatisticians, epidemiologists, radiologists, engineers, behavioral scientists, other specialists, and advanced students of various disciplines. Males outnumber females (60 percent to 40 percent). Fifty-nine percent of the subjects are married, 11 percent are divorced or widowed, and 30 percent have never been married. The median age is about thirty-five with 31 percent in their twenties, 35 percent in their thirties, 25 percent in their forties, and 10 percent over fifty years of age. Fourteen percent have completed only college or its equivalent (sixteen years of education), 42 percent have completed from one to three years of graduate education, and 44 percent have completed four or more years of graduate education. No valid measure of socioeconomic status is available. Twenty-six specific religions are represented.

The Taiwan sample, obtained in 1967, includes fifty members of health departments in Taichung and Taipei and a few public health students. The professional distribution is not greatly different from the U.S. sample, with physicians (34 percent), nurses (22 percent), health educators (15 percent), and other professionals (29 percent). About two-thirds are men, 66 percent are married, 4 percent widowed, and 30 percent single. The educational level is somewhat lower than the U.S. sample, with 16 percent not having completed college, 32 percent being college graduates, 40 percent having one to three years of graduate education, and 12 percent having four or more years of graduate education. Thirty percent identified themselves as Buddhist, 6 percent as Confucian, 32 percent as having no organized religion, and the remaining 32 percent vary widely in religion.

The Thailand sample, obtained in 1967, includes sixty-four graduate students, interns, and physicians in a Bangkok medical school. Twenty-seven percent are physicians and 70 percent are students. They are young (98 percent under thirty), primarily male (81 percent), unmarried (97 percent), and Buddhist (92 percent). Twenty-three percent have sixteen years or less of education, 64 percent have from one to three years of graduate education, and 8 percent have four or more years of graduate education.

Beliefs and Their Distributions—U.S. Health Professionals

The Definition of a New Human Life

Two beliefs about a new human life have particular relevance to abortion. These beliefs concern: (1) when in the course of development a new life is believed to exist as a new human life; and (2) the primary criterion whereby one judges a new life to be a human life.

When a Human Life Begins. Beliefs regarding the time a new human life begins were obtained by asking each subject to check from an age-ordered series of eight statements "the one statement with which you personally most agree in answering the question: at what point in development would you say *this* is a new human life?" While public health professionals must adhere to legal definitions, their personal beliefs about when a new life begins vary widely. Only a small proportion of the subjects hold personal beliefs fully consistent with the professional and legal definition of about twenty weeks that is followed in most states (Knutson, 1967a, 1967b).

For the purposes of comparative analysis U.S. health professionals were grouped into three categories: those who believe a new human life begins at conception or during the first trimester (47 percent), those who believe it begins during the second or third trimester or at birth (31 percent), and those who believe it begins at viable birth or later (22 percent).

The Primary Criterion of a Human Life. In the exploratory study subjects discussed the characteristics they considered most significant in differentiating between a prehuman life and a human life and between human life in general and a specific new human life. Subjects participating in the major study were presented these criteria as a series of alternatives ranging from those relating to God-given or spiritual characteristics to those concerning sociocultural and personality characteristics. They were asked to indicate "the statement that best describes your point of view." U.S. health professionals have been ordered into five groups in terms of their beliefs about the primary criterion of a human life:

1. Spiritual criterion (22 percent): when the soul or spirit enters or infuses the body.
2. Biogenetic criterion (30 percent): the fact that it has the biological potential for being a human being, and this fact alone, makes it a human being.
3. Demographic-physiological criterion (14 percent): when it can be perceived and recognized.
4. Psychophysiological criterion (17 percent): when it is physiologically self-sufficient and functioning on its own.
5. Psychosocial criterion (17 percent): when it is alert and recognizes environment, begins to interact with others, or begins to become socialized and to have a personality.

The Human Soul

In recent years relatively little attention has been given by social scientists to beliefs about the presence and nature of a human soul. Nor has much attention been given to the significance of these beliefs as dynamic variables of concern to health-related behavior. Depth interviews with members of the health professions yielded information that beliefs about the concept of a human soul and the time of its infusion into the new life have significant implications for value judgments about abortion.

The Concept of a Human Soul. Beliefs about who has a human soul and when a soul is present in a human life hinge upon whether a person believes in the concept of a soul and, if so, how he defines this concept. At the heart of this issue is a belief in or rejection of the concept of God. About 45 percent of the U.S. health professionals say they believe in a God-given soul, and most of these also believe the soul to be eternal. Twenty-eight percent believe the soul to be a useful humanistic construct representing awareness, conscience, and the like; 19 percent question the value of the concept; and 8 percent reject the concept. For purposes of comparative analysis the latter two groups were combined, totaling 27 percent.

When the Soul Infuses. In the inquiry on beliefs about the time the soul infuses a new life, alternatives were provided for those who reject the concept of a soul or question whether the soul is a meaningful concept. For the purpose of comparative analysis U.S. subjects were ordered into three belief positions: (1) 42 percent believe the soul is present at conception or before birth; (2) 26 percent believe the soul enters or develops at birth or after birth; and (3) 32 percent question or reject the concept of the soul.

Locus of Control over a Human Life

Beliefs about the right of control over a human life include beliefs about the right to decide whether a new human life should be born, about whom a new human life belongs to, about the right to decide whether to continue or end a mature human life. From responses to questions on these issues a general locus of control index was developed.

Right of Decision over a New Life. Decisions about whether a new life should be born include decisions about the practices of sterilization, contraception, abortion, infanticide, and artificial insemination. Such decisions are made before the new life is capable of making decisions for itself and, indeed, before the new life may exist or may be defined as a human life. The neonate is not yet defined as a human life by one-third of the sample; many judge it to be a part of the mother rather than an independent individual.

About one-fourth of the U.S. health professionals believe that only God or no one has this right of decision over a new life; two-thirds believe that the mother or parents have this right; and the remainder believe that other members of society have this right of control. Evidence from other analyses indicates that many who assign to the mother or parents this right of control over a new life believe that the individual himself has this right once he is mature.

Ownership of a New Human Life. The question "To whom does a new human life belong?" specifically identifies a concern with a new *human* life. Since subjects vary in belief about when a new human life begins, responses need to be viewed with a recognition that they are in disagreement about the minimum age of this new human life. Therefore, responses have greater meaning when related to beliefs about the beginning of a new human life.

About 29 percent of the U.S. health professionals believe a new human life belongs to God, about 21 percent to its parents, 5 percent to "society," and 45 percent believe a new human life is "inherently independent and belongs to no one." Subjects choosing this latter alternative tend to divide between those who assign control to the individual himself on maturity and those who assign control to no one once the individual has matured.

Decisions about Continuing or Ending a Mature Life. "Who has a right to make decisions about continuing or ending a human life after it has grown up?" deals with a belief of primary concern to the prolongation of life. However, this, like other beliefs about the locus of control over a human life, appears to tap basic orientations toward control. Thus even though questions are specific to a particular period, responses have general relevance.

About 26 percent of the U.S. health professionals assigned this right of decision over a mature life to "only God," 25 percent to no one, 9 percent to society or its members, and the remaining 40 percent only to the individual himself.

The Goseso Index of the Locus of Control (God, Self, or Society). A belief index of the locus of control over human life was empirically developed through a contingency analysis of beliefs about the right of control over birth, the ownership of a new human life, and the right to continue or end a mature human life. In constructing this index responses obtained during the first two years of the study were employed, but no significant differences are found between these first two years and subsequent years. By this measure subjects are grouped in terms of their primary beliefs about the locus of control over a human life, whether this control belongs to no one, God, the individual himself, or society.

Ideal Value of a Human Life

Many problems arise in attempting to develop measures of the ideal value of life since direct questions about terminal values are hazardous. One cannot be certain that a respondent clearly distinguishes between his judgments about what is, what is desired, and what should be. Accordingly terminal values can perhaps best be inferred from indirect measures, some of which have been employed in the current research. However, one direct attempt was also made to obtain assessments of the ideal value of a human life by age. Subjects were asked to respond to a series of items regarding the relative worth that *should* be assigned an individual at various stages of development. Responses to this question yielded a nearly perfect Guttman scale, the index of reproducibility being .99. The scale has a good step distribution beginning with conception and continuing on into maturity. Subjects varied widely in their responses to this task. Some assigned full ideal value to new life at conception; others assigned ideal value by degrees with increments of age; and for others the shift from little or no value to high value was abrupt at a particular point in development.

Value Judgment Scales

Two types of value judgment scales were developed and given a rigorous preliminary test on a pilot sample prior to use in this research in order to assure the testing of hypotheses with minimal *post hoc* effects. An empirical scale with seventeen items is used to determine the strength of associations and to facilitate multivariate analysis. Nonparametric Guttman-type scales employing the same items permit the comparison of value judgments in an ordered sequence. While major attention is given here to selected findings using the empirical scale, comparisons using nonparametric scales are also presented.

Scale items were randomly imbedded within a list of 164 items to limit structured responses. In responding to the questionnaire subjects were asked to: "(1) assume there are no legal issues involved; (2) assume that any action will be carried out under good medical care and social services; (3) assume you are in position to make the decision and have the time to decide what should be done." For each item subjects were asked to indicate "What you personally feel that one *should do* or *should not do*" by responding in terms of five alternatives ranging from "should do; always good" to "should not do; always bad."

Nonparametric Value Judgment Scales

The nonparametric scales were developed by dichotomizing the five-point range of alternatives, with the "usually bad" and "always bad" responses serving as a primary scale matrix. The dichotomy was made at this point since a person who responds "neither good nor bad" was assumed to hold a value position that was not actively in opposition to the action being judged.

The method of scaling has features of the Guttman cumulative scale in that the scales satisfied the criterion of unidimensionality and items are ranked in a cumulative manner from bad to good. It deviates from the usual cumulative scale, however, in that the items were developed and the scales constructed prior to use in the study. The method of scoring differs in that the first two steps are scored like a summated scale, permitting greater use of the data. "Neither good nor bad" responses imbedded in the "should not do" matrix are scored as one-half errors, whereas those within the "should do" matrix are not scored as errors.

A comparison of the three samples on a general scale of value judgments about abortion is presented in Table 14–1. This scale may be viewed as a ladder with the value positions ordered from zero to seven. Step 7, at the bottom of the ladder, represents a position disapproved by 8 percent of the U.S., 14 percent of the Taiwanese, and 17 percent of the Thai subjects. Persons in step 7 judge all the actions of the scale as bad to do. The next step in the scale, step 6, is opposed by 12 percent of the U.S. sample. These are persons who pass the seventh step of the scale but not the other six.

TABLE 14-1

General Scale of Value Judgments about Abortion,
Comparative Positions on Cumulative Scale—
U.S. and Taiwanese Public Health Professionals, and Thai Medical Students and Physicians

Scale Steps		Scale Step Distribution			Cumulated Distribution		
		U.S. (N = 290)	Taiwan (N = 50)	Thailand (N = 64)	U.S. (N = 290)	Taiwan (N = 50)	Thailand (N = 64)
0	All acts are good to do.	13%	0%	0%	100%		
1	No act is bad to do: Some acts are good to do; others are all right.	15	20	2	87	100%	100%
2	Step 2 only is bad to do: An unmarried woman having an abortion because having a child will bring dishonor upon her family.	10	2	0	72	80	98
3	Steps 2, 3 only are bad to do: A married woman having an abortion because she wants one—no other reason given.	10	2	6	62	78	98
4	Steps 2, 3, 4 only are bad to do: A married woman having an abortion because she does not want any children at all.	12	36	20	52	76	92
5	Steps 2, 3, 4, 5 only are bad to do: An unmarried woman having an abortion because she does not feel she can adequately provide for the child.	20	12	39	40	40	72
6	Steps 2, 3, 4, 5, 6 only are bad to do: Obtaining an abortion when the child would be likely to suffer from physical or mental abnormality.	12	14	16	20	28	33
7	Steps 2, 3, 4, 5, 6, 7 all are bad to do: A married woman with children having an abortion to protect her own life.	8	14	17	8	14	17
		100%	100%	100%			

Guttman Rep   .93 (N = 150) Does not include subjects who give "neither good nor bad" responses.
K Rep   .96 (N = 290) (½ error scored for "neither good nor bad" responses when imbedded in "bad" matrix).

The scale thus yields an ordered comparison of the various value positions in terms of their acceptability. Most acceptable is the practice of a married woman having an abortion to protect her own life (8 percent of the U.S. professionals judge this as bad). An additional 12 percent oppose obtaining an abortion when the child would be likely to suffer from physical or mental abnormality, and an additional 20 percent oppose an unmarried woman having an abortion because she cannot adequately provide for the child. Thus of the U.S. professionals 40 percent oppose this latter position (step 5).

By this scale the U.S. health professionals are least opposed to abortion;

Taiwanese health professionals are next; and Thai medical students and physicians are most opposed to abortion. Note that 52 percent of the U.S., 76 percent of the Taiwanese, and 92 percent of the Thai samples oppose step 4 of the scale (a married woman having an abortion because she does not want any children at all), whereas 28 percent of the U.S., 20 percent of the Taiwanese, and 2 percent of the Thai samples judge all the acts as good to do or all right to do.

Two of the nonparametric scales permit a comparison of value judgments about abortion involving unmarried and married women (Tables 14–2 and 14–3). For all three samples opposition to a married woman having an abortion tends to be stronger than opposition to an unmarried woman hav-

TABLE 14-2

Scale of Value Judgments about Abortion for Married Women—
U.S. and Taiwanese Public Health Professionals, Thai Medical Students and Physicians

Scale Steps		Scale Step Distribution			Cumulated Distribution		
		U.S. (N = 290)	Taiwan (N = 50)	Thailand (N = 64)	U.S. (N = 290)	Taiwan (N = 50)	Thailand (N = 64)
0	All acts are good to do.	19%	0%	0%	100%		
1	No act is bad to do: Some acts are good to do; others are all right.	14	14	0	81	100%	
2	Step 2 only is bad to do: A married woman having an abortion because she wants one—no other reason given.	10	2	3	67	86	100%
3	Steps 2, 3 only are bad to do: A married woman having an abortion because she does not want any children at all.	11	28	13	57	84	97
4	Steps 2, 3, 4 only are bad to do: A married woman having an abortion because she does not feel she can adequately provide for the child.	35	30	61	46	56	84
5	Steps 2, 3, 4, 5 all are bad to do: A married woman who has no children having an abortion to protect her own life.	11	26	23	11	26	23
		100%	100%	100%			

Guttman Rep .93(N = 188) .88(N = 28) .99(N = 42).
K Rep .95(N = 290) .94(N = 50) .97(N = 64).

TABLE 14-3

Scale of Value Judgments about Abortion for Unmarried Women—
U.S. and Taiwanese Public Health Professionals, Thai Medical Students and Physicians

Scale Steps		Scale Step Distribution			Cumulated Distribution		
		U.S. (N = 290)	Taiwan (N = 50)	Thailand (N = 64)	U.S. (N = 290)	Taiwan (N = 50)	Thailand (N = 64)
0	All acts are good to do.	30%	14%	2%	100%	100%	100%
1	No act is bad to do: Some acts are good to do; others are all right.	15	16	6	70	86	98
2	Step 2 only is bad to do: An unmarried woman having an abortion because she wants one—no other reason given.	9	12	13	55	70	93
3	Steps 2, 3 only are bad to do: An unmarried woman having an abortion because she does not want to have a child.	6	22	6	46	58	80
4	Steps 2, 3, 4 only are bad to do: An unmarried woman having an abortion because she does not feel she can adequately provide for the child.	30	26	47	40	36	74
5	Steps 2, 3, 4, 5 all are bad to do: An unmarried woman having an abortion to protect her own life.	10	10	27	10	10	27
		100%	100%	100%			

Guttman Rep .97(N = 202) .90(N = 30) .91(N = 41).
K Rep .98(N = 290) .94(N = 50) .93(N = 64).

ing an abortion. The relative positions with respect to abortion for the three samples are quite similar to that found for the general value judgment scale. These differences between the samples are significant both for value judgments concerning married women (Kruskal-Wallis H = 3.60; p < .0001) and unmarried women (Kruskal-Wallis H = 38.5; p < .0001).

The Empirical Scale

The empirical scale was developed by assigning weights to the responses on each of seventeen scale items, with "always good" scored as one and "always bad" scored as five (Likert, 1932). Thus the scale can have values ranging from a score of seventeen to a score of eighty-five, with a high score on the Likert scale reflecting a value position opposed to abortion and a low score reflecting a value position more favorable to abortion. The reliability coefficients for this scale are high for the U.S. sample (r = .95) and good also for the Taiwanese (r = .81) and Thai (r = .81) samples as computed by the Kuder-Richardson formula 20 (Guilford, 1954, pp. 383–385; Winer, 1962, pp. 124–132).

The three samples differ significantly in their value judgments about abortion (F = 16.45; p < .001 with 2 and 400 d.f.), with the U.S. sample being the least opposed (mean = 46.5), the Taiwanese sample next (mean = 48.4), and the Thai sample being the most opposed (mean = 58.5). In addition the distribution of scores of U.S. public health professionals appears to be more variable than the distributions of the Taiwan and Bangkok samples, reflecting the greater heterogeneity of this sample on various relevant characteristics, especially religious affiliation.

Research Findings—U.S. Sample

Demographic Variables

Value judgments of U.S. health professionals about abortion are found to have some statistically significant but no important associations with the demographic or sociological variables other than those concerned with religion. No significant differences are found by sex, age, or marital-parental status. Professional identification accounts for only 3 percent of the variance of scores on the scale, with physicians tending to be slightly more opposed in their value judgments than nurses and other health professionals (p < .05). The grouping of a large number of specific occupations in this third category may mask more important relationships. No difference is found between the four samples of health professionals responding in successive years, assuring that the pooling of these four samples is appropriate.

Health professionals who have had courses in family planning or population control tend to be more favorable in value judgments about abortion in comparison with those who had attended lectures or had not been involved. The difference, however, accounts for only 4 percent of the scale variance ($p < .01$).

Although neither sex nor marital-parental status have any direct effect on the abortion scale, they combine to yield a significant interaction ($F = 5.69$; $p < .005$, with 2 and 280 d.f.).[1] Single women and married men with children tend to be very opposed to abortion, and single men and married women with children tend to be very favorable to abortion. Married men and women without children tend to hold intermediate value positions and appear to be in close agreement on their value judgments about abortion.

Religion. It was hypothesized that the most important factors in value judgments about abortion are those related to religion. Therefore, subjects were asked about the dominant religion in their home during childhood, their current religious affiliation, and the relative strength of their religious convictions. In addition an attempt was made to assess the effect of the subjects' changes of religion from childhood to adulthood.

To test these hypotheses with minimal *post hoc* influence, religions were precoded and preordered (with only minor changes) into eight religious categories along a conservative-humanistic-secular dimension. Some errors in precoding are reflected in the distributions. Primary among these is an error in grouping Congregational and United Church of Canada religions with Unitarians in the liberal category.

Religious identification is found to account for about 39 percent of the variance of the scale of value judgments about abortion by the U.S. sample; parental religion of childhood accounts for 25 percent. Subjects who rate themselves as more religious tend to be more opposed to abortion, this variable accounting for 18 percent of the scale variance. Few religious conservatives classify themselves as being not very religious or not religious at all, and few liberals or secularists classify themselves as being somewhat or very religious. The religious commitment variable therefore does not have equal application to all religious categories. Subjects who have changed their religious identification to a more liberal religion tend to be more favorable to abortion than those who have not changed or who have changed to a more conservative group, with this variable accounting for 7 percent of the scale variance. All associations with these religious variables are significant ($p < .0001$).

Religious identification together with parental religion (the dominant

[1] The percentages of variance accounted for that are reported in this chapter were estimated through the use of multiple regression and dummy variable coding (Cohen, 1968). The effects for the two-way analysis of variance were estimated in accordance with the Method 1 summarized by Overall and Spiegel (1969), which controls for both the covariance between main effects and the covariances between main effects and interaction effects.

religion of childhood) is found to account for 42 percent of the variance in value judgments about abortion (F = 13.65; p < .001 with 14 and 264 d.f.). Adding information about a subject's current religion to that of his dominant religion of childhood therefore increases the proportion of variance in the abortion scale accounted for by 17 percent (F = 7.72; p < .001 with 7 and 264 d.f.).

For this group of health professionals Catholics, Jews, minority sects, and fundamentalist groups appear to have lost membership from one generation to the next. Nearly half of those raised as fundamentalists (Lutheran, Baptist, Methodist) have changed in religious identification, primarily in the liberal direction. On the other hand, the moderate, no-organized-religion, liberal, and secularist groups have all gained members, with the greatest proportional gains being in the liberal (Unitarian) and secularist (agnostics and atheists) groups. The dominant religious and philosophical orientation of childhood was secular for only about one-fifth of those who now identify themselves as secularists. More than half of the members of this group have conservative religious backgrounds.

There is a general tendency for subjects who have changed to a more liberal religion than the religion of childhood to be more liberal in value judgments about abortion, but some tend to retain the position of the more conservative group. Greater variation is noted within those religious categories that include members of several specific religions or members whose parents were of another religion. Subjects who were raised as Catholic and changed religion tend to among those most opposed to abortion within each of the religious groups to which they have become affiliated. Even in the secular group (agnostics and atheists) the order of position on value judgments is closely related to the conservative-secular positions of parental religion, with those raised as Catholics or fundamentalists being more opposed to abortion than those raised as liberals or secularists.

Belief Variables

Belief variables as compared with demographic and sociological variables other than religion are found to be of considerably greater importance in their association to value judgments about abortion. Included here are beliefs about the criterion whereby one judges a life to be human, the time a human life begins, the presence and nature of a human soul, and the locus of ownership and control of a human life. It was hypothesized that persons holding traditional or spiritual beliefs about these issues would tend to have value judgments more opposed to abortion. This hypothesis is strongly supported for each of the several measures of belief, with confidence levels all exceeding p < .0001.

The specific beliefs about a human life are found to account for from 25 percent to 31 percent of the variance of the scale of value judgments about abortion. The Goseso Index of the Locus of Control over a human life is found to account for 38 percent of the scale variance. These beliefs appear to be part of a common belief system, with overlapping effects relative to the value judgments. In no instance, however, is this overlap of effect complete for this group of beliefs.

Beliefs about the concept of a human soul and when a soul infuses, for example, are rather closely associated ($\emptyset^1 = .56$; $X^2 = 178$ with 4 d.f.; $p < .01$) (Hayes, 1963, p. 606). Together these two belief orientations account for 37 percent of the scale variance ($F = 41$; $p < .001$ with 4 and 277 d.f.), while alone they account for 31 percent of the scale variance. While there is overlap in variance accounted for, the two-way least-squares analysis of variance (Figure 14–1) shows that the time of infusion of a

Figure 14–1. Value Judgments about Abortion, as Related to the Concept of a Human Soul and the Time the Soul Infuses—U.S. Public Health Professionals.

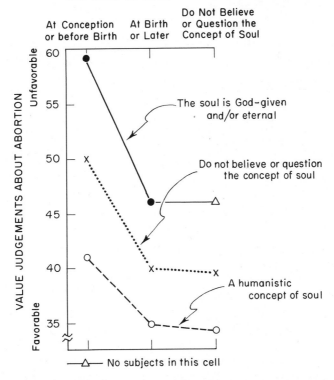

human soul has a significant main effect over and above the effects of the concept of a human soul and the interaction term. Most opposed in value judgments about abortion are those who believe both that there is a God-given soul and that it infuses before birth. Least opposed are those who define the soul in humanistic ways as conscience, awareness, and so forth and believe it infuses at birth or later. In an intermediate value position are those who reject the concept of the soul but believe the soul infuses at birth or later (two conflicting beliefs) or who question or reject the concept of the soul in response to both belief questions. The tendency of those who reject the soul to be more conservative than those who redefine the soul is of interest. When conflicts are present in responses to questions about the soul, these conflicts are represented in intermediate value judgment positions about abortion.

Beliefs about when a human life begins together with beliefs about the locus of control over a human life, as measured by the Goseso Index, are found to account for about half of the variance in value judgments about abortion ($F = 14.8$; $p < .001$ with 17 and 263 d.f.) (Figure 14–2). Here

Figure 14–2. Value Judgments about Abortion, as Related to When a Human Life Begins and the Locus of Control over a Human Life—U.S. Public Health Professionals.

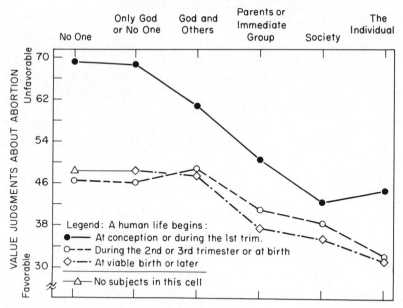

THE RIGHT OF DECISION BELONGS TO:

the two-way analysis of variance shows both main effects as significant, but the interaction effect is not. Most opposed to abortion are health professionals who believe that a human life begins at conception or during the first trimester and that God or no one has the right to make life/death decisions. Most favorable to abortion are those who believe a human life begins at birth or later and that the parents, "society," or the individual have this right of decision. Included in the most favorable group also are those who believe that a human life begins during the second and third trimester and that the individual has this right of control. The pattern of association to abortion is thus strong along the God-society individual continuum.

Religious identification together with beliefs about the beginning of a human life is found to account for 53 percent of the variance in the scale of value judgments about abortion (F = 12.5; p < .001 with 23 and 258 d.f.) (Figure 14–3). An important group of health professionals in each religious

Figure 14–3. Value Judgments about Abortion, as Related to the Religious Identification of Subject and Beliefs about When a Human Life Begins—U.S. Public Health Professionals.

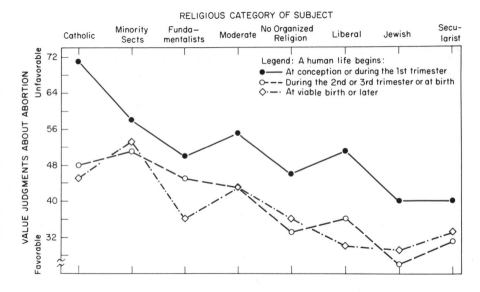

category believes that a human life begins at conception or during the first trimester, and within each category this group tends to be considerably more opposed to abortion. The association is present even for those health professionals who identify themselves as secularists (agnostics or atheists). About half the secularists have parents who were conservative in religion, and this group tends to be among those secularists somewhat more opposed to abortion. Further analysis is needed to determine if these are the secularists who believe a human life begins at conception.

Ideal Value of a Human Life

The assessment of the ideal value of a human life at different ages during development is found to account for about 21 percent of the variance in value judgments about abortion for this group of U.S. health professionals (p < .001). Those subjects who assign average or higher relative ideal value before conception, at conception,. or immediately afterward (N = 99) tend to be considerably more opposed to abortion than those who do not assign average or higher ideal value until the second trimester or later.

Assessments of ideal value during development are significantly associated with religion and with each of the several belief variables. The degree of these associations is not high, the closest association being with beliefs about the beginning of a human life ($\emptyset^1 = .35$; $X^2 = 70$; $p < .001$ with 4 d.f.), and the lowest association being with beliefs about the concept of a soul ($\emptyset^1 = .18$; $p < .001$; $X^2 = 18$ with 4 d.f.). Accordingly ideal value during development contributes effectively when used together with these belief variables in association with value judgments about abortion.

Beliefs about the primary criterion of a human life together with the assessment of ideal value during development are found to account for about 45 percent of the variance in value judgments about abortion (F = 15.6; $p < .001$ with 14 and 270 d.f.) (Figure 14–4). Health professionals who assign average or higher ideal value at conception or immediately afterward tend to be most opposed to abortion if the primary criterion of a human life they employ is spiritual, biogenetic, or demographic-physiological. Those who assess the new life as attaining average or higher value

Figure 14–4. Value Judgments about Abortion, as Related to the Primary Criterion of a Human Life and the Ideal Value by Age during Development— U.S. Public Health Professionals.

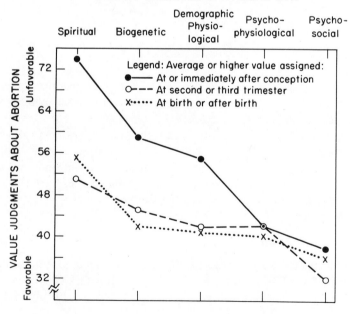

PRIMARY CRITERION OF A HUMAN LIFE

after the second trimester do not differ in their value judgments about abortion. Within each ideal value category those who employ the spiritual criterion of a human life tend to be most opposed to abortion, and those who employ the psychosocial criterion tend to be most favorable to abortion.

Therapeutic Abortion and Legislation

It was not possible to measure the behavior of health professionals regarding abortion. However, subjects were asked how they would respond if a legislative body in their state or country were exploring the possibility of legislation to permit qualified professionals greater freedom of action regarding therapeutic abortions. In response to this question the U.S. health professionals indicate they would probably: actively support (speak for), 65 percent; passively support, 25 percent; be indifferent, 1 percent; passively oppose, 4 percent; and actively oppose, 5 percent. Eighty-one percent of the Taiwanese and 71 percent of the Thai health professionals would actively or passively support such legislation.

The finding that 9 percent of the U.S. sample would passively or actively oppose legislation permitting greater freedom for therapeutic abortions is consonant with the finding that 8 percent judge therapeutic abortion to be bad, those found to be opposed to step 7 of the abortion value judgment scale (Table 14–1). Of special interest, however, is the finding that twenty-one of the twenty-seven U.S. professionals who say they would passively or actively oppose this legislation are Catholics. Among the forty-one Catholics 27 percent would actively support, 17 percent passively support, 5 percent be indifferent to, 24 percent passively oppose, and 27 percent actively oppose legislation for greater freedom of therapeutic abortion.

Summary and Discussion

The findings presented in this preliminary report have been selected to draw particular attention to the importance of religion, beliefs, and ideal values in relation to value judgments about abortion within a fairly homogeneous U.S. public health sample. Presented are findings that employ two types of value judgment scales. The empirical (Likert) scales prove to be reliable and efficient for comparative and multivariant analysis. The nonparametric cumulative scales serve to pinpoint issues of agreement or disagreement in value judgment. Through their use one can identify specific points of conflict between groups in value judgments about abortion, and one may be able to relate the issues on which there is disagreement to specific beliefs, ideal values, or other factors. Such information should be useful in both research and program planning.

Primary attention has been given to the beliefs and ideal values of U.S. public health professionals as they relate to value judgments about abortion. Preliminary comparisons of the United States, Taiwanese, and Thai samples, in terms of beliefs and ideal values as related to value judgments about abortion, yield interesting and significant interactions. Some beliefs and ideal values contribute to the variance in value judgments of the overseas samples in ways different from that found for the U.S. sample. Additional analysis will be necessary to identify the factors associated with these interactions in order that such findings can be presented with an identification of contributing factors.

U.S. public health professionals are found to vary widely in their beliefs about a human life, in their assessments of the ideal value of a new life, and in their value judgments about abortion. When the U.S. health professionals are compared with smaller samples of health professionals in Taiwan and medical students and physicians in Thailand, the U.S. and Taiwanese health professionals tend to be most favorable and the Thai medical students and physicians most opposed to abortion. All three groups are somewhat more favorable to abortions for unmarried than for married women.

For this research religions were precoded into religious categories, and these categories were preordered along a conservative-secular continuum to minimize *post hoc* effects. This precoding was based on best estimates in 1965 based on pretest and pilot data, opinion data, and the like. Inadequacies and errors, even when noted, have not been corrected. The Jewish category, while primarily reform Jews, includes several orthodox members who tend to be more conservative than reform Jews on many issues. The liberal category includes Unitarian, Congregationalist, and the United Church of Canada. Various analyses indicate that the Congregationalist and United Church of Canada should be included in the moderate religious category.

Value judgments about abortion are found to be associated to an important degree with the religious identification of subjects, the dominant parental religion of childhood, and the degree of religious commitment. Religion of subject together with dominant religion of childhood is found to account for a large proportion of the variance of the value judgment scale. Other demographic variables, such as age, sex, profession, and marital-parental status, or training in family planning, are found to be insignificant or to have very little association to value judgments about abortion. Single women and married men with children are found to be relatively opposed to abortion, but single men and married women with children tend to be relatively favorable to abortion. Married men and women without children tend to have intermediate value positions and do not differ greatly.

Value judgments about abortion are closely associated with beliefs about a human life. Among the beliefs that contribute in important ways to variance in value judgments are the primary criterion of a human life, the time a human life begins, the concept of a human soul and the time the soul infuses, and beliefs about the locus of control over a human life. These beliefs, when paired in the analysis or employed together with religious identification, account for as much as half the variance of value judgments about abortion.

Assessments of the ideal value of a new human life by age are found to have an important association to value judgments about abortion. This association is highly important when ideal value assessments together with religion or beliefs about a human life are related to value judgments about abortion.

It is significant that physicians and nurses who have had more training and experience dealing with pregnancy, abortion, and delivery do not as groups differ greatly from other health professionals in value judgments about abortion. Nor does training related to family planning appear to be as significant a factor as might be expected. Instead, religious identification, childhood religion, and those beliefs and ideal values relating to a human life that appear to be transmitted from generation to generation as part of religious and philosophical socialization are of greatest importance to these value judgments. This finding would appear to have important implications for those responsible for formulating policies and programs related to family planning and population control. The findings do not include measures of field behavior. Value judgments regarding therapeutic abortion are, however, consonant with responses of subjects about their expected actions regarding legislation favoring therapeutic abortions. Primary opposition to this legislation for the U.S. public health sample is found to be within the Catholic group.

Findings reported are based upon a preliminary analysis of a sample of health professionals who are relatively homogeneous in age, education, income, intelligence, and general orientation toward health and the care of human life. One would expect an equal or greater degree of association to religious orientation, beliefs, and values within the general population.

The samples employed in this analysis were "bunch" samples that are not representative of major professional parameters. Accordingly distributions in beliefs, values, and value judgments cannot be assumed to be representative. The U.S. sample is judged adequate, however, for testing the hypotheses under study.

REFERENCES

Cohen, J. 1968. Multiple regression as a general data-analytic system. *Psychological Bulletin* 70:426–443.

Edwards, A. L. 1957. *Techniques of attitude scale construction.* New York: Appleton-Century-Crofts.

Guilford, J. P. 1954. *Psychometric methods.* 2nd ed. New York: McGraw-Hill. Pp. 383, 385.

Hays, W. L. 1963. *Statistics for psychologists.* New York: Holt, Rinehart & Winston.

Knutson, A. L. 1967*a*. The definition and value of a new human life. *Social Science and Medicine* 1:7–29.

———. 1967*b*. When does a human life begin? Viewpoints of public health professionals. *American Journal of Public Health* 57:2163–2177.

Likert, R. A. 1932. A technique for the measurement of attitudes. *Archives of Psychology,* no. 140.

Overall, J. E. and Spiegel, D. K. 1969. Concerning least squares analysis of experimental data. *Psychological Bulletin* 72:311–322.

Winer, B. J. 1962. *Statistical principles in experimental design.* New York: McGraw-Hill. Pp. 124–132.

PART VI

Research Related to Social Action Programs

[15]

POPULATION AND YOUTH

NANCY F. RUSSO
AND YVONNE BRACKBILL

Approximately 40 percent of the U.S. population is less than twenty-one years of age. Half the female population marries before age twenty-one, and over one-third of first births in 1968 were to women under twenty. One-fourth of the females between the ages of fifteen to nineteen have at least one child.

Such stark considerations dictate that today's youth receive high priority in action programs that seek to alleviate population pressures. Marriage at an early age not only increases the number of years a woman is exposed to pregnancy but also reduces the time span between generations if the first child is born soon after marriage. The significance of younger age groups should also be reflected in research priorities. Unfortunately individuals under twenty years of age have been relatively ignored by fertility researchers.[1] However, several investigators have recently begun to study the attitudes of young people toward family size and other population-related variables, and the rising interest in population education has contributed to the initiation of research in this area.

Obviously no single program (nor chapter!) could address itself to all the factors concerning youth that need to be considered for such a comprehensive perspective. However, it is important at least to identify the multiple factors involved before priorities can be assigned and objectives selected. This chapter attempts to provide a reference work that will be useful to

NOTE: The authors would like to thank Nöel-David Burleson, James T. Fawcett, Barry McCarthy, Martha Mednick, Thomas Poffenberger, Thomas A. Russo, Michael L. Stadter, and Raymond Yang for their comments and criticisms on this chapter. The authors are also grateful to Henry P. David and the staffs of the American Institutes for Research and American University for their assistance in the preparation of this chapter. This work was supported in part by Grant MH 5925 from The National Institute of Mental Health to Yvonne Brackbill.

[1] Though there are notable exceptions, cf. Westoff and Potvin, 1966.

population programmers in two ways. First, it presents data obtained in studies of U.S. youth that may be of use to population educators and action programmers, delineating some of the implications of the existing research findings for population education and action programs. Second, it explores ways in which psychologists may contribute toward the goal of effective population education and action programs.

Research on Youth

Fertility is the result of a series of life events and decisions. Factors affecting the probability of a young person's exposure to intercourse, conception, and gestation (the "intermediate variables" of Davis and Blake, 1956) are numerous, and the data on the diverse kinds of variables that have implications for action programs are fragmented and not easily organized. Some areas, such as correlates of early marriage, have been investigated for some time, while others, such as population awareness, have yet to be widely studied. Psychologists and other social scientists have a major task in filling gaps in existing data, monitoring the tremendous changes taking place, and opening new areas not yet explored. The research on youth relevant to action programmers has been divided into four major topical areas for this summary: (1) marriage, career, and family; (2) sexual behavior, pregnancy, and fertility; (3) contraception, abortion, and sterilization; and (4) population awareness. It should be kept in mind that the topics do overlap to some extent.

Marriage, Career, and Family

Marriage

Early marriage, here considered as marriage with the bride under twenty-one years of age, has received much attention because it tends to be followed by familial poverty, divorce, and other marital problems (Burchinal, 1959b, 1959c: Gingles and Voss, 1965; Glick, 1957; Herrmann, 1965; Inselberg, 1962; Lowrie, 1965; Monahan, 1953–1954; Muller, 1970; Rele, 1965). In addition women who marry younger also have a higher total number of children, even when duration of marriage is controlled (Rele, 1965).[2]

---

[2] In order to interpret changes over time in rates of early marriage, one must consider the age/sex structure of the population. For example, the downward trend in mean age

What antecedent variables are associated with early marriage? If one analyzed the correlates of marital age, premarital conception stands out as the predominant factor. Approximately one-third to one-half of all high school brides are premaritally pregnant (Christensen, 1963; Lowrie, 1965). In general the younger the bride, the more likely that she is pregnant (Lowrie, 1965). Note that errors in such statistics are likely to be in the direction of underestimation. Variables associated with premarital pregnancy will be discussed later.

Other antecedent variables that have been associated with early marriage are socioeconomic status, race, regional differences, and early dating (Bartz and Nye, 1970). Both racial and regional differences in early marriage have been evident in the past, but the relationship between these variables and early marriage has declined sharply in recent years (Moss, 1965). Studies relating early dating and going steady to early marriage have been carried out by Burchinal (1959a, 1959d), Inselberg (1962), and Moss and Gingles (1959). In interpreting these relationships the reader is cautioned against inferring a simple causal relationship. On the surface it would appear that early dating leads to early marriage. But in reality it may be that orientation toward marriage leads to early dating (Broderick, 1966).

Early marriage has also been found, though with some inconsistency, to be related to difficulties in adolescents' personal adjustment and parental relations and to their unrealistic perception of the advantages of getting married (Burchinal, 1965; Havighurst et al., 1962; Herrmann, 1965; Lowrie, 1965; Martinson, 1955, 1959; Moss and Gingles, 1959).

Another group of variables associated with early marriage involves education and career orientations of both males and females. Early marriage is inversely related to interest in obtaining higher education (DeLissovoy and Hitchcock, 1965; Moss and Gingles, 1959) and higher parental education and occupational status (Almquist and Angrist, 1970; Burchinal, 1959d; Burchinal and Chancellor, 1963; Glick, 1957; Havighurst et al., 1962; Perrucci, 1968; Rele, 1965). These interests are developed early in life, and research related to their development will be discussed later.

Many findings in the literature on early marriage have been organized by Bartz and Nye (1970). These authors categorize the adolescents who marry early into two groups: those who are "forced" into marriage because of premarital conception and those who voluntarily choose to enter married status because they view it as yielding more rewards than staying single.

If one can assume that most premarital pregnancies are unintended by-products of sexual behavior, then the implications for the action programmer are clear: widespread sex education and contraception information and ac-

---

of marriage has diminished of late. However, in the past there has been an age gap between bride and groom of approximately 2.5 years. At present the ratio of marriageable men to women is decreasing. Therefore, unless the age gap at the time of marriage decreases, there may be an increase in the number of unmarried females or an increase in the average age at which females marry (Park and Glick, 1967).

cessibility should receive top priority for this group. To design programs for those who voluntarily seek marriage at an early age, it is necessary to delve further into the research literature. The question of why some individuals hold educational and career aspirations that affect marriage and childbearing patterns is especially important.

Career

Higher education and career achievement have been shown to be associated with preference for delay in marriage and childbearing for both males and females (Almquist and Angrist, 1971; Burchinal, 1965; Perrucci, 1968; Rele, 1965). Fertility has sometimes been found to be inversely associated with the female's education and employment status (Rele, 1965), though the relationship is complex, interacting with religion and educational institution (Westoff and Potvin, 1966). It is difficult to draw causal inferences from correlational data. However, female career-oriented graduate students do say they desire smaller families than noncareer-oriented female graduate students (Farley, 1970). This indicates that desire for smaller families is in some cases antecedent to employment experience. High-school and college dating occurs with the same frequency for career-oriented and noncareer-oriented women, but the pattern differs. Career-oriented college women are less likely to be going steady, engaged, or married before their senior year (Almquist and Angrist, 1971).

Although career-oriented women are thus potentially different from non-career-oriented women in ways that are relevant to population planners, career women still do maintain many characteristics of their more traditional counterparts. In fact the vast majority of career-oriented women do not seek a career *instead of* a husband and family, *but in addition to* a husband and family (Almquist and Angrist, 1970; Angrist, 1970; Empey, 1958; McMillin, Cerra, and Mehaffey, 1971; Oppenheimer, 1968; Poloma, 1970; Poloma and Garland, 1970; Turner, 1964).

Although there is evidence that traditional sex roles have been changing (McKee and Sherriffs, 1959), acceptance by both males and females of the woman's role in the home is still pervasive in our society (Epstein, 1970). Acceptance of the traditional limitations of the feminine role by many young people is reflected in the findings of a recent study of more than 180,000 entering college freshmen by the American Council on Education (ACE, 1970). According to these norms over half the freshmen men and 9 percent of the women did not agree that women should receive the same salary and opportunities for advancement as men in comparable positions. Despite lack of reliability data for the survey instrument, these percentages may be substantial enough to indicate that traditionalism is not confined to the older generation.

A recent study of 530 graduate women that focused on differences between career-oriented women and noncareer-oriented women also underscores the persistence of traditional attitudes (Farley, 1970). It demonstrated that career-oriented women are more likely than noncareer-oriented women to have a desire for fewer children, to plan to work full time even with preschool children, to believe the husband should have equal responsibility for housework, and to be reluctant to yield priority to a husband's career automatically. Nevertheless, when considering the career-oriented group only 36 percent still desired three or more children, 73 percent did not plan to work when they had preschool children, 48 percent did not believe that the husband should have equal responsibility for housework, and 57 percent would still automatically yield priority to a husband's career.

The conflict between career and family priorities for women has been widely discussed (e.g., Epstein, 1970; Kammeyer, 1964; Komarovsky, 1946, 1953; Matthews and Tiedeman, 1964; Turner, 1964; Wallin, 1950). Some writers have noted that those professional women who do give family needs priority over career needs are sometimes considered neither dedicated nor emancipated (Almquist and Angrist, 1971; Poloma and Garland, 1970, 1971). Ironically little is said about the number of men who place their family needs above career goals, and this cultural bias is reflected in the research literature by the lack of studies on such conflict for males.

Despite the fact that many career-salient women do have family values similar to those of their more traditionally oriented peers, we have seen that as a group their life styles do differ and their desired family size may be lower. In fact career-salient attitudes affect decisions on life options even in the early teenage years, since career-oriented females are more likely to select a demanding college preparatory curriculum than other types of programs in high school (Matthews and Tiedeman, 1964).

The great personal ambivalence caused by conflict between achievement needs, which may be satisfied by career and educational attainments, and the fear that success will bring peer rejection is still with today's female college student (Horner, 1969). The female's perception of what the male peer believes is desirable behavior on her part, especially with regard to intellectual accomplishment, is particularly important (French and Lesser, 1964; Horner, 1969; Komarovsky, 1946, 1953; Matthews and Tiedeman, 1964; Wallin, 1950). The contribution of the male attitude is also demonstrated by the finding that influence of male peers plays more of a role in the formulation of goals for career-salient women than for noncareer-salient women (Almquist and Angrist, 1971).

Traditionally achievement has been seen even by college students as a characteristic limited to the male sex role (Veroff, Wilcox, and Atkinson, 1953). Many females still see rejection of the woman's role as necessary for intellectual attainment (French and Lesser, 1964) and regard intelligence as grounds for social rejection (Horner, 1969; Matthews and Tiedeman, 1964). Research on the effects of the post-Sputnik governmental campaign to stimulate achievement in science and mathematics found that the campaign was successful in motivating males, but not females, to succeed in these traditionally male areas (Poffenberger and Norton, 1963). This evidence implies that males and females respond to differing cultural cues and that if population education is to have major behavioral effects, the cues that affect each sex must be identified. If women define achievement and success in terms of marriage and children, population awareness is likely to have little effect; the priority goal would first be to redefine what is regarded as achievement for women. The evidence cited in this section consistently indicates that current patterns of sex-role socializaton propel females toward accepting marriage and childbearing roles and toward rejecting other sources of self-fulfillment as improper. These studies overwhelmingly underscore the need for change in sex-role socialization as a necessary condition to voluntary control of population growth in this society.

There is some evidence that the traditional perception of male attitudes of what is appropriate behavior for a woman may not be completely accurate. As early as 1959 it was reported that college men appear to have a less restrictive stereotype about what is appropriate for females than women believe them to have (McKee and Sherriffs, 1959). Some males in fact reject the homemaker as a "dull" companion (Poloma and Garland, 1971), and a recent study of college students found that two out of five college men sampled prefer to have a wife who has a career (McMillin et al., 1971).

Despite their potential for contributing to the widening of women's sources of self-fulfillment, young males, especially black males, generally have continued to have a less egalitarian orientation toward marriage than do females (ACE, 1970; Kalish, Maloney, and Arkoff, 1966; McMillin et al., 1971; Payne, 1956). In view of the adverse effects that the husband's negative attitude toward the wife's working has traditionally had on the frequency of her employment (Weil, 1961) and on marital happiness (Gianopulos and Mitchell, 1957), the effects of current male attitudes toward the woman's role in career and marriage merit investigation. A recent study of the attitudes of over 2,800 college students by McMillin et al. (1971) indicates that this cultural lag in egalitarianism by males is persistent. Those authors found that 72 percent of the college females sampled said they wished to work after marriage, quitting only while the children were young and going back to work after they were in school. In contrast only 40 percent of the males sampled preferred this arrangement for their wives, 38 percent did not want their wives to work unless it was essential, and 12 percent did not want their wives to work at all. These data suggest that changes in sex-role conceptualization are occurring more quickly for females than for males.

Religious variables also influence the conception of woman's role. For example, according to ACE norms freshmen at Catholic colleges for men are more likely than freshmen at nonsectarian colleges for men to agree that the activities of married women are best confined to home and family.

Percentages of agreement are 56 and 48, respectively. Corresponding percentages for female freshmen at Catholic and nonsectarian schools are 38 and 24. It seems likely that parochial institutions only reinforce such restrictive attitudes. A survey of 104 presidents of Catholic colleges that admit women revealed that the majority of them believe that the average college woman should be guided into a field of study and work that represents "typically feminine interests and abilities" (Smith, 1962).

Racial differences in attitudes toward the woman's role indicate that caution must be exercised in generalizing to black populations from studies using white subjects. In the ACE study mentioned earlier 58 percent of the freshmen at predominantly black colleges agree that the activities of married women are best confined to home and family, while only 43 percent of the freshmen at nonblack, nonsectarian colleges hold this opinion. Nevertheless, other data provide substantial evidence that college blacks, especially black females, hold a stronger career orientation than their white peers (ACE, 1970; Hedegard and Brown, 1969). For example, 78 percent of the freshmen at predominantly black colleges feel that it is very important for them to become authorities in their field, while only 65 percent of freshmen at nonblack, nonsectarian colleges agreed to this statement. Considering the females only, 76 percent attending black colleges and 60 percent attending nonsectarian colleges feel that becoming authorities in their chosen field is very important (ACE, 1970). In a study of high school sophomores Kuvlesky and Obordo (1969) found that black females both desired marriage at a later date and more often expected to work after having children than did their white counterparts.

The development of career orientation has been associated with a variety of familial variables. Early evidence indicates that females from families of higher socioeconomic status show less restriction in their range of occupational choices (Boynton and Woolwine, 1942). Recent studies with females have demonstrated that maternal employment and parental encouragement, especially paternal encouragement, are important variables in influencing career aspirations (Almquist and Angrist, 1970, 1971; Astin, 1967; Poloma and Garland, 1971; Siegel and Curtis, 1963; White, 1967).

Educational and occupational experience may provide reinforcement that can encourage or discourage a career-salient orientation. The number and variety of jobs a college girl holds is directly associated with her career salience (Almquist and Angrist, 1971). Career-salient college women are more likely than noncareer-salient women to name professors and work models as important influences on their occupational choice (Almquist and Angrist, 1971; Simpson and Simpson, 1961), which indicates the great potential that work models and college faculty have in influencing the goals of young women. Unfortunately, however, there is evidence that the status of women in the world of work is declining (Knudsen, 1969). In academe many faculty members still feel that women would (and should) "just get married and have babies" (Graham, 1970) and discriminate against female students and faculty accordingly. This discrimination not only limits the role models available to young females but legitimizes blocking of their aspirations, contributing to a self-fulfilling prophecy and perpetuating a cycle of earlier marriage, childbearing, and population growth. The action programmer certainly is confronted by a multifaceted task, and the concerned psychologist could begin in his own departmental backyard.

Family

Despite the differences in sex-role conceptions of varying groups of males and females in the United States, there is still a near universal consensus for males and females on the desirability of getting married and having children (Goldsen, Rosenberg, Williams, and Suchman, 1960; Landis and Landis, 1963; Rabin, 1965). Of a random sample of the 1970 incoming freshman class at American University, Washington, D.C., all of the sixty-five females and seventy-five of the seventy-six males intended to marry (Russo and Stadter, 1971). Not only is having a family seen as desirable by the current younger generation, it also receives a high priority in terms of sources of life satisfaction. The 1970 ACE norms indicate that 62 percent of incoming freshman men and 71 percent of the females feel raising a family to be essential or very important to their life objectives, and as we have seen even the dedicated career-salient graduate woman of the 1970s desires a career in addition to a husband and family (Farley, 1970).

Recent research on the details of proposed family formulation, size, and structure among young people is still scanty, but some conclusions are possible. Although the majority of young people agree that it is desirable to limit family size (Eisner, van Tienhoven, and Rosenblatt, 1970; van Tienhoven, Eisner, and Rosenblatt, 1971), young people, like their parents, generally agree on the desirability of having from two to four children (Darney, 1970; Eisner et al., 1970; Gustavus and Nam, 1970; Hendershot, 1967, 1969; Kuvlesky and Obordo, 1969; Purdue Opinion Poll, 1970; Russo and Stadter, 1971; Wanderer, Seaver, and Wagner, 1970). Note that the mean desired family size is higher than that needed for population replacement, and unintended pregnancies are not even considered.

Young people are like their parents in their wish to avoid both childlessness and an only child (Eisner et al., 1970; Gustavus and Nam, 1970; Hendershot, 1969; Poffenberger, Bachman, and Weiss, 1970; Purdue Opinion Poll, 1970; Russo and Stadter, 1971; van Tienhoven et al., 1971). Also evident is the traditional preference for having at least one child of each sex and a preference for male children (Freedman, Freedman, and Whelpton, 1960; Markle and Nam, 1970; Pohlman, 1967).

Young people, especially young girls, start thinking about how many children they would like to have as early as elementary school (Gustavus and Nam, 1970), which suggests that family size and composition are appropriate concepts for the action programmer to include in his approach to this young age group.

Because of methodological differences between studies, reported differences in desired family size are difficult to interpret. Confidence in the validity of such differences increases, however, when they are replicated in a number of studies. One of the most widely found differences is that females prefer a larger family size than males (American Institute of Public Opinion, 1961; Markle and Nam, 1970; Nobbe, 1968; Purdue Opinion Poll, 1970; Wanderer et al., 1970), which is consistent with the direction of socialization of the female role. In general a large proportion of young people, especially males, are undecided as to how many children they expect to have (Purdue Opinion Poll, 1970).

Differences in family-size preference have shown a sometime relationship to a number of variables, including age (American Institute of Public Opinion, 1961; Eisner et al., 1970; Purdue Opinion Poll, 1970; van Tienhoven et al., 1971), parental education (Purdue Opinion Poll, 1970), region of the country (Purdue Opinion Poll, 1970), marital status (Eisner et al., 1970; Markle and Nam, 1970), experience with parenthood (Eisner et al., 1970), and race (Buckhout, 1971; Gustavus and Mommsen, 1969; Gustavus and Nam, 1970; Kuvlesky and Obordo, 1969; Nobbe, 1968).

Size of family of origin appears to be related to desired family size for both males and females (Gustavus and Nam, 1970; Hendershot, 1969). The relationship, not a strong one, is larger for females who are first borns or who feel closer to their families (Hendershot, 1967).

Religion is a powerful variable in many attitudes toward the family, even in the "modern" generation. Markle and Nam (1970) studied 283 college students' attitudes toward sex predetermination, i.e., the ability to choose the sex of one's child before birth. They found that 40 percent were opposed to the idea, that Catholics were most opposed, and that Protestants and those with no religion were least opposed. Like their parents Catholic youth of high-school and college age report a larger preferred family size than Protestants, Jews, or atheists (American Institute of Public Opinion, 1961; Gustavus and Nam, 1970; Nobbe, 1968; Wanderer et al., 1970; Westoff and Potvin, 1966). Students in Catholic schools desire larger families than students in non-Catholic schools (Westoff and Potvin, 1967). The relationship between desired family size, religion, and sectarian education is complex. Westoff and Potvin (1966) concluded that the self-selection process operating in the religious student's choice to attend a Catholic school was the basis for the higher desired family size associated with such institutions. Nobbe (1968), however, found that this relationship held for males, with religiosity of parents predicting their fertility preferences. For females extent of Catholic schooling was the better predictor of fertility values.

Although it has been established that nearly all young people want to have children, there is little research on why they want to have children.

Rabin and his colleagues have explored this question (Rabin and Greene, 1968) and have developed a scale to measure motivation for parenthood. They found that the reasons college students give for having children can be grouped into four categories: altruistic, fatalistic, narcissistic, and instrumental (Rabin and Greene, 1968). The scale, called the Child Study Inventory, is still experimental and has not been widely used, but there is evidence that there may be sex differences in the perception of the functions of children. Females rank fatalistic reasons for having children (e.g., having children is a natural instinct) higher than do males, while instrumental reasons (e.g., children are needed to enhance social status) are ranked higher by males than by females (Major, 1967).

The population programmer has a long way to go in order to have an impact on population growth. Early socialization, especially with respect to sex-role conception and religious values, appears to play a major role in the development of family-size preferences. Studies of how such socialization affects motivation for parenthood and perceived functions of children are logically of high priority for the action programmer.

Sexual Behavior, Pregnancy, Fertility

Sexual Behavior

As night follows day, so does pregnancy follow sexual activity among highly fecund young persons who do not consistently use contraception. That this simple fact of life goes unrecognized by the young (and those responsible for their education and guidance) is evident in the predominant role premarital conception plays in early marriage. Further evidence comes in the large number of illegitimate births to girls under twenty years of age (165,700 reported in 1968). How many pregnancies are kept secret or result in abortions can only be estimated, but they are probably numerous (Kinsey, 1966; Steinhoff, Smith, and Diamond, 1970). Knowledge of the variables involved in sexual practices, premarital conception, and resulting fertility is another necessary facet of a comprehensive attack on population growth.

There has been a controversy whether the well-publicized sexual revolution in attitudes has actually been accompanied by a rise in premarital sexual intercourse (Blaine, 1967; Christensen and Gregg, 1970; Guttmacher, 1969; Hacker, 1965; Kaats and Davis, 1970; Reiss, 1966b). Because of sampling differences and the problems of obtaining reliable and valid data on this personal subject, it is difficult to make comparisons among current studies, much less comparisons between generations when retrospective data are involved. Since sexual behavior has been found to be correlated with personal attitudes and social norms in both Denmark and the United States (Christensen, 1966; Reiss, 1964), it would be surprising if some behavioral change did not follow the verbal revolution. Recent evidence suggests that there has been a striking rise in premarital coitus for middle-class females (Bell and Chaskes, 1970; Christensen and Gregg, 1970; Kaats and Davis, 1970).

The major earlier research findings in the United States on sexual attitudes and behavior of young persons have been summarized in several places (Bell, 1966b; Ehrmann, 1959, 1964; McCary, 1967; Reiss, 1966b, 1967; Schofield, 1965), and a comprehensive review will not be attempted here. Race, sex, class, and education have generally been found to be influential variables. Results of more recent studies affirm many of the earlier findings. There is a relatively high incidence of premarital sexual behavior: the most recent estimates for college students range around 30 to 45 percent for females and 60 percent for males (Bell and Chaskes, 1970; Christensen and Gregg, 1970; Kaats and Davis, 1970). Males continue to be more permissive in both sexual attitudes and behavior than females (Christensen, 1966; Christensen and Gregg, 1970; Ehrmann, 1959; Kaats and Davis, 1970; Katz, 1968; Miller and Wilson, 1968; Reiss, 1966b). Despite the evidence that suggests that the female's position is becoming more liberal (Christensen and Gregg, 1970), the sex difference is still a persistent one and affects many aspects of behavior. Males have more positive attitudes toward sex (Russo and Stadter, 1971) and give greater approval toward premarital coitus (Christensen and Gregg, 1970). They are younger when they engage in first intercourse than are females (Lowry, 1969), and compared to females, their first partner is less likely to be a steady or fiancée (Christensen and Gregg, 1970). Most girls confine their sexual behavior to one boy (or at least one boy at a time), and promiscuity is a relatively rare phenomenon (Furstenburg, Gordis, and Markowitz, 1969; Hacker, 1965; Lowry, 1969; Reiss, 1966b; Von Den Ahe, 1969), though intercourse without a strong commitment appears to be increasing (Christensen and Gregg, 1970). The male's willingness to have more sexual experience on the first date and thereafter (Miller and Wilson, 1968) probably underlies the finding that females remain more concerned with "how far they should go" than with contraceptive information (Angrist, 1966; Poffenberger, 1961).

The increased sexual permissiveness of the younger generation does not mean that the traditional double standard no longer exists, however. Kaats and Davis (1970) reported that the majority of both the males and females of their college sample held a double standard of sexual behavior and noted that "in this sample where barely more than half of the females were still virgins, 45 percent of the men wanted to marry a virgin" (p. 395).

The double standard is especially strong when applied to sexual intercourse between individuals who share little affection (Kaats and Davis, 1970). This finding underscores the necessity of studying complex interpersonal relationships if premarital sexual intercourse is to be understood (Kirkendall and Libby, 1966). Sex and affection are reported as strongly linked by a larger proportion of college females than males (Katz, 1968), and when asked why they engage in premarital intercourse, girls more often give reasons related to love and maintaining a close relationship, while males reveal exploitative, self-indulgent, esteem-related attitudes (Hacker, 1965; Reiss, 1964; Von Den Ahe, 1969). Girls are seen as conquests, especially in some subcultures in the lower classes (Blood, 1962; Ehrmann, 1959; Grant, 1957; Green, 1960; Rosenburg and Bensman, 1968). There is evidence that sexual morality of college students is based on the concept of a mutual interpersonal relationship (Kirkendall, 1961). Serious involvement for both sexes is a factor in sexual permissiveness for a couple (Bell and Chaskes, 1970; Blood, 1962; Ehrmann, 1959; Kaats and Davis, 1970; Miller and Wilson, 1968; Zelnick and Kantner, 1970), and the nature of the relationship is central to the understanding of premarital intercourse (Kirkendall, 1961; Kirkendall and Libby, 1966). Nevertheless, the situation for most young individuals, both black and white, is still aptly described by Lowry: "In every social class, girls look for love and boys look for sex" (Lowry, 1969, p. 95).

The effect of contraceptive accessibility and information on premarital sexual behavior has traditionally been a matter of concern, and recently questions about the effect on sexual activity of accessibility to abortion have also been raised (Reiss, 1966a). Although research on contraception, abortion, and sterilization will be discussed later, it should be noted at this point that whatever contribution contraceptive information may make toward sexual permissiveness is minor compared with the roles of basic cultural and personal values (Christensen, 1966; Reiss, 1966b, 1967), social pressure and coercion (Christensen, 1966), and whether or not the female is "in love" (Reiss, 1966a, 1967). The frequency of premarital pregnancy, illegitimacy, forced marriage, and abortion among the young obviously demonstrates that a significant amount of sexual activity goes on in the absence of contraception. Therefore, concern that sexual behavior of the young may increase if sex education and contraceptive information are implemented or if abortion is accessible seems misplaced.

Two conclusions can be drawn from the current findings on the sexual behavior of the young in America: (1) attitudes toward premarital sex have become more liberal, and (2) a sizable proportion of both males and females under twenty-one engage in premarital intercourse, with, as we have noted, a concomitant high incidence of premarital pregnancy, illegitimate birth, abortion, forced early marriage, and unwanted and neglected children (Blaine, 1967; Cutright, 1971; Kinsey, 1966; Lacognata, 1967; Martz, 1963; Miller and Wilson, 1968; Reiss, 1966a, 1967; Smith et al., 1971). These conclusions underscore the importance of sex and contraceptive education. Indeed, many younger persons, black and white, feel that their education on sexual and contraceptive matters is deficient (Burchinal, 1960;

Ehrmann, 1959; Furstenberg, 1970; Lacognata, 1967; Poffenberger, 1959, 1960). If their knowledge is tested objectively the data concur with this self-perception (Burchinal, 1960; Gottschalk et al., 1964; Stone, 1960; Von Den Ahe, 1969). Adolescents perceive their parents as disapproving of sexual activity (Kaats and Davis, 1970) and do not discuss their sexual behavior with their parents (Miller and Wilson, 1968), which cuts off their access to an important information source. In general young people learn about sex from their mothers, peers, siblings, or books (Angrist, 1966; Angelino, Edmonds, and Mech, 1958; Gottschalk et al., 1964; Grinder and Schmitt, 1966). A significant proportion of young persons recognize their informational inadequacies and express desire for information from authoritative sources (Angrist, 1966). Few report that sex education should not be taught in the schools (Poffenberger et al., 1970).

One of the problems in implementing sex education is that parents fail to recognize that there may be a problem with their own children until confronted with pregnancy (Bell, 1966a). An important task in this area is to mobilize those forces in the community who are now permitting a minority to determine the education of the majority of children. Teachers, clergymen, and mental health professionals are among those who need to be mobilized, but who may be themselves lacking in knowledge (Signell, 1969). Psychologists could play a useful role in designing informational and motivational programs and working out curricula and projects acceptable to diverse groups. Although adequate sex education of both young and old is not a sufficient condition for population control, it is certainly an important one, and given the personal tragedy of the pregnant teenager, in addition to societal concern with the effects of population growth, the sooner the action the better.

Pregnancy

When pregnant and nonpregnant teenage girls are compared two types of differences emerge, biological and socioenvironmental. Using age of menarche as an indicator of physical maturity, it appears that pregnant girls are more likely to have matured sexually earlier than nonpregnant girls of the same chronological age (Gottschalk et al., 1964; Rosen, Campbell, and Arima, 1961).

Notwithstanding biological differences, socioenvironmental factors contributing to pregnancy are numerous and important. When pregnant and nonpregnant black and white unmarried teenage girls are compared on a variety of social factors, avoidance of pregnancy is associated with less permissiveness by parents, church attendance, less dating, and more sources of information on dating, marriage, and sex (Gottschalk et al., 1964).

When teenage brides are considered the chance of the bride's being pregnant is inversely associated with her age (Christensen, 1963; Lowrie, 1965). In addition the pregnant bride appears to come from a family with

lower educational attainment than that of the groom (Lowrie, 1965).
Lowrie (1965) has indicated that in adolescent marriages pregnancy—
whether obviously premarital or within the first seven to nine months after
marriage—is inversely related to the female's educational level and also to
the educational level of the male's parents. Religious preferences are not
closely related to pregnancy in brides, although Catholics marry earlier
after conception than non-Catholics, and there is no consistent relationship
between the age of the first date and the probability of pregnancy (Lowrie,
1965).

Much has been written about the unwed pregnant teenager in which
psychological factors and class differences are the major focuses of research
interest. Summaries of the literature are available (Cutright, 1971; Roberts,
1966; Semmens and Lamers, 1968; Vincent, 1961, 1966). Some writers have
suggested that such pregnancy is a result of the girl's unconscious desire
to become pregnant (Blaine, 1967; Giel and Kidd, 1965; Young, 1966),
while others feel that it is an unintended by-product of her sexual behavior
(Fürstenberg, 1970; Fürstenberg, Gordis, and Markowitz, 1969; Vincent,
1961). In either event some maintain that the role of unconscious desire is
minimal compared with the role of lack of sexual knowledge and accessibility of means of birth limitation (Fürstenberg et al., 1969).

Although premarital pregnancy is generally viewed as undesirable,
social reaction to it differs with race and class (Fürstenberg et al., 1969;
Zelnick and Kantner, 1970). Rejection or fatalistic acceptance of the
occurrence of pregnancy are common responses, but a minority (who
generally hope to marry soon) report that they are happy about it
(Fürstenberg et al., 1969; Greenburg, Loesch, and Lakin, 1959; Von Den
Ahe, 1969). Unwed mothers can and do make adjustments to their situation
(Hill and Jaffe, 1966; Kogan, Boe, and Valentine, 1965; Zelnick and
Kantner, 1970). However, that does not mean that they did not wish to
avoid the situation in the first place.

Despite the fact that lower-class unwed teenage mothers report that they
are anxious to avoid a second illegitimate pregnancy, they do often become
pregnant again within a few years. In 1967 Sarrel reported that 95 percent
of his sample of 100 unwed adolescent mothers had a repeat pregnancy
within five years. In the five-year span of the study these 100 teenagers
had 340 babies and nine known abortions (Sarrel, 1967). That such pregnancies are not desired and are not inevitable is domonstrated by the effectiveness of the special clinic for the teenage unwed mother instituted after
this study (Sarrel, 1967, 1969). Unfortunately such clinics are scarce, and
private physicians hesitate to provide preventive services to minors without
their parents' consent, partially because of the fear of legal sanction (Pilpel
and Wechsler, 1969). Although the physicians' fear is not completely supported by the legal facts, and no case of criminal prosecution against a
physician for supplying contraceptives to a minor is known (Pilpel and
Wechsler, 1969), the legal situation still is not clearly favorable for the

physician in all states. A high-priority task of the population planner is still to initiate changes in the legal structure so that contraception can be made available to all without fear of legal penalties as long as sound medical judgment is practiced.

Fertility

Young persons begin their family building early in marriage, intentionally or unintentionally. In 1968 there were 496.5 births for every 1,000 married women in the fifteen to nineteen age group. This was the highest birth rate for married women of any age group, with mothers of twenty to twenty-four years of age second highest, having 255.2 births for every 1,000 married women in that age bracket. In addition to the fertility of married women in this age group, one must also consider the fertility of unmarried women. In 1968 there were approximately 19.8 births per thousand unmarried women in the fifteen to nineteen bracket, which contributed approximately 158,800 additional births to the total fertility of the fifteen to nineteen year olds.[3] Of the total number of babies born to married and unmarried teenagers under fifteen in 1968, 97.1 percent were first births, 2.8 percent were second births, and 0.1 percent were third births. Of the babies born to fifteen to nineteen year olds, 77 percent were first births, 18.7 percent were second births, 3.5 percent were third births, and 0.7 percent were fourth and fifth births. Most of these multipara are nonwhite. The impact of having one or two children, let alone three or more, on the economic, social, educational, and physical well-being of these teenagers is devastating (Campbell, 1968; Muller, 1970), and compensatory resources such as counseling services or special educational programs are inadequate or nonexistent.

Since the number of females in the fifteen to nineteen age group will probably increase by approximately a million persons in the next five years, an upswing in the number of babies born to this group is to be expected, whether or not the birth rate remains stable. The inadequate services now supplied to these young mothers—both wed and unwed—will be in even stronger demand.

The undesirable personal and social outcomes of early marriage have already been noted. The high financial, social, and psychological costs of children (Pohlman, 1969) probably play a major factor in shaping such outcomes, especially when the high rate of premarital conception is considered (Bartz and Nye, 1970).

Illegitimacy has long been considered a social problem, and much has been made of the racial differences in such births, but the inadequacies of

---

[3] It should also be noted that illegitimate births are not restricted to fifteen to nineteen year olds; on the contrary three-fifths of unwed mothers are past their teens (Vincent, 1966). However, the focus of this chapter is on youth, defined as twenty-one years of age or younger, and the discussion is focused on their fertility.

statistical reporting and the differential access to contraception, abortion, and travel to states that do not record such births as illegitimate make racial comparisons difficult (Hill and Jaffe, 1966; Vincent, 1966). Analysis of some of the problems in interpreting the statistics on racial differentials in illegitimacy can demonstrate how difficult it is to infer underlying causation without a broad knowledge of the dynamics of the situation. For example, differences in the number of out-of-wedlock births between the races cannot be used to infer differences in the number of women involved, since blacks are more likely to have repeat illegitimate pregnancies than whites. When this factor is taken into account the racial difference is reduced (Pratt, 1965). Also, out-of-wedlock conceptions are more likely to result in early marriage before the birth when the mother is white; marriage often comes after the birth with nonwhites, but the child is still labeled "illegitimate." The impact of this technicality on interpretation of statistics is considerable. The white-nonwhite ratio of illegitimate births in general is 1:8; for out-of-wedlock conceptions it is 1:3; when repeaters are considered the proportion of women involved drops to 1:2 (Hill and Jaffe, 1966).

The population programmer has two tasks—to discourage voluntary fertility and help to eliminate involuntary fertility. The research on marriage and career identifies factors that will especially assist in the former task; the research on sex and pregnancy will be of partciular use in the latter. Given the value structure in our society that emphasizes individual choice, it is logical that priority has been assigned to the elimination of involuntary fertility. Indeed, the extent of involuntary fertility will delineate the scope of the action programmer's task, for it can be argued that unwanted fertility is the major contributor to the population problems in the United States (Bumpass and Westoff, 1970). Nevertheless, research on desired family size indicates that without considering both factors we will be unable to cope effectively with the problem of overpopulation. In order to avoid the necessity of instituting compulsory limitation of family size, programs dealing with both aspects must be implemented.

Contraception, Abortion, Sterilization

Contraception

One of the major tasks to be accomplished before involuntary fertility can be eliminated is to change public opinion toward greater acceptance and practice of effective means of birth limitation. Evidence suggests that young people are very much in favor of contraception, both for themselves and for others (ACE, 1970; Hacker, 1965; Markle and Nam, 1970). Most hold no moral, religious, or political objections to birth control in general (van Tienhoven et al., 1971). In fact the recent ACE 1970 college norms indicate that 73 percent of incoming college freshmen feel the federal government should be more involved in distributing birth-control information, pills, or devices to the general population (ACE, 1970), and 80 percent of a national probability sample of post-high-school-age males were in favor of having contraceptive information taught in the school (Poffenberger et al., 1970).

Nevertheless, young people are selective in considering who should receive such material. One poll of fifteen to nineteen year olds living at home indicated that the majority favored the distribution of birth-control information, but only a third felt that such information should be available to anyone who wanted it (Erskine, 1967). This discrepancy underscores the importance of the wording of the question when measuring attitudes toward contraception, and caution is warranted when comparing responses obtained by different instruments.

Young people do not appear to know much about most topics related to sex, but they do seem to be relatively knowledgeable about the existence of various methods of contraception (Angrist, 1966; Grinder and Schmitt, 1966; Kantner and Zelnick, 1969; Lacognata, 1967; McCreary-Juhasz, 1967). Although the depth of their knowledge is not great (Eisner et al., 1970; Kantner and Zelnick, 1969; Poffenberger et al., 1970; van Tienhoven et al., 1971; Von Den Ahe, 1969), it might be adequate enough to protect them from pregnancy if motivation to use contraception were present (Angrist, 1966).

College students are most familiar with the pill as a method of contraception. They also prefer it most, with the diaphragm, IUD, and condom also receiving favorable ratings (Russo and Stadter, 1971; van Tienhoven et al., 1971). Despite these preferences the condom was the method actually used by most young people; the pill was next, followed by withdrawal and the diaphragm (van Tienhoven et al., 1971). These results parallel the findings of Fürstenberg and his colleagues (1969) that lower-class females also report the use of the condom most frequently, although they possess knowledge of the pill and IUD. These investigators concluded that "girls tend to be most aware of forms of birth control to which they have the least access (pills, IUD) and over which they have the least control (condoms)" (p. 40).

Studies of contraceptive use among the young are fragmentary, with widely differing sampling methods and data-collection instruments, so that few firm conclusions can be drawn. In general, however, race and religion do stand out as influential variables. Racial differences have been obtained in widely different studies, with blacks having more restrictive attitudes than whites both toward their own and others' use of contraceptives (Kantner and Zelnick, 1969; Markle and Nam, 1970; Zelnick and Kantner, 1970). Fewer freshmen at predominantly black colleges than integrated colleges agree that the federal government should be more involved in distributing birth-control information, pills, or devices (ACE, 1970). Kantner and Zelnick (1969) suggest that such attitudes may reflect a "sense of biological inevitability" by blacks (p. 12).

Results with regard to religion are less consistent, perhaps because of the lower degree of religiosity of college students, but it does appear that today's young Catholics have shown greater resistance to contraceptive information than other religious groups (Garai, 1964). It is not unreasonable to infer that most freshmen who attend Catholic colleges and universities are individuals who have been more influenced by the Church, either directly or through parental behavior, and who may be considered as more religious. This inference is supported by the ACE finding that incoming freshmen of Catholic schools were more likely to have discussed religion or to have attended a religious service than freshmen who attend nonsectarian institutions. It is not surprising, therefore, to discover that these individuals are less likely to agree that the federal government should be more involved in programs distributing birth-control information, pills, or devices. What is surprising, however, is that even among this selective sample over half of the men and women do agree to more federal involvement (ACE, 1970).

A poll conducted in 1965 indicated that 47 percent of the teenagers sampled perceived the Roman Catholic Church as trying to prevent the distribution of birth control in the United States (Erskine, 1967). However, the recent publicity campaign initiated by the Vatican against birth and population control may drastically change the perceptions of youth with respect to the actions of the Catholic Church, so that generalizing from earlier studies is unwise. One study has demonstrated that the Ecumenical Council's consideration of the birth-control issue in 1965 was associated with a positive attitude change on the part of Catholic students toward birth control (Ward and Barrett, 1968). The authors concluded that the shifts in Catholic attitudes could be due to the Council's consideration of the pro-birth-control position, which gave birth control some legitimacy, and they also suggested that the anticipation of a pro-birth-control decision by the Council may have initiated the attitude change. Whether or not the Pope's public pronouncement (*Time*, 1971) will also have such a powerful effect in the opposite direction has yet to be seen. The ACE norms suggest that effecting such a reversal would not be an easy task.

Despite the positive attitudes toward birth control generally held by young people, it has been reported that over half of the girls who become pregnant have not been using contraception (Fürstenberg et al., 1969). That attitudes do not necessarily predict behavior is a truism in psychology. The important question is *Under what conditions* do attitudes generalize to behavior? A major task of the psychologist interested in population is to delineate the factors that contribute to the gap between contraceptive attitudes and contraceptive behavior. For example, if females do not accept the fact that they are having sexual intercourse (each time being considered the last time), then they may reject the "planning ahead" for sex that the use of contraception implies (Spicer, 1969; Zelnick and Kantner, 1970), even though they have favorable attitudes toward contraception in general.

One of the reasons for a discrepancy between contraceptive attitudes and behavior is the relative inaccessibility of effective contraception for the young. Doctors not only hesitate to advise minors without parental consent (Ortho-Panel, 1968; Pilpel and Wechsler, 1969), but pharmacists keep contraceptives, including condoms, behind the drug counter, making them psychologically unavailable to embarrassed teenagers (Wagner, Millard, and Pion, 1970). Increasing the accessibility of contraception is one of the easiest first steps to reduce the discrepancy between attitudes and behavior in this case.

Abortion

Although a substantial number of abortions are performed that involve youth, in general their attitudes toward abortion are less positive than their attitudes toward contraception (Eisner et al., 1970; Russo and Stadter, 1971). As with attitudes toward sex and contraception males' attitudes toward abortion tend to be more liberal than females' (ACE, 1970; Maxwell, 1970). However, 89 percent of incoming college freshmen do agree that "under some conditions abortions should be legalized" (ACE, 1970, p. 80).

Race and religion continue to be influential variables. A large proportion of both male and female incoming freshmen at predominantly black colleges and universities show restrictive attitudes toward abortion, with only 71 percent agreeing that abortions should be legalized under some conditions (ACE, 1970). This attitude parallels that found with lower-class black subjects, who expressed the belief that life must be preserved once begun (Kantner and Zelnick, 1969). As would be expected, freshmen attending Catholic colleges show more restrictive attitudes toward abortion than freshmen attending nonsectarian institutions. Seventy percent of Catholic college freshmen agree that abortion for some conditions should be legalized, whereas 85 percent of nonsectarian college freshmen hold this opinion (ACE, 1970).

There is evidence that favorable attitudes toward abortion are associated with more education, urban rather than rural residence, less participation in church activities, smaller families of origin, exposure to peers who have had an abortion experience, and positive attitudes toward premarital sex (Maxwell, 1970).

Further studies are needed on such variables, especially because they help in understanding the dynamics of racial and religious differences. It has only been recently that attitudes of youth toward abortion have become a research topic of interest to psychologists. The lack of data reflects earlier neglect. Considering the incidence of premarital pregnancies, illegitimate births, and abortions in young people, such neglect is unfortunate to say the least.

Sterilization

There is a wealth of data on abortions compared to that available on young people's attitudes about sterilization. The Cornell study, which included student attitudes toward sterilization, has been widely reported (Eisner et al., 1970; van Tienhoven et al., 1971). This was based on a highly selective sample of students and faculty at Cornell University. Despite the intelligence and supposedly superior quality of education received by this Ivy League population, there was considerable ignorance among both students and faculty with respect to the effects of sterilization. Even among the biology faculty 14 percent of the respondents said that they were certain that vasectomy would impair the ability to ejaculate, and 10 percent were certain that cutting the oviducts would affect menstruation. Poffenberger et al. (1970) found that only 19 percent of their sample knew what vasectomy was. Clearly youth's knowledge about sterilization is minimal. Perhaps such ignorance and misinformation partially underlies the negative attitudes toward sterilization exhibited by the 40 percent of Cornell students who stated that they would *never use* vasectomy or cutting the oviduct to limit family size even after attaining their desired number of children (van Tienhoven et al., 1971, p. 20).

Population Awareness

The social and cultural "press" in the United States has traditionally been toward childbearing. The basic premise in this country is that "people should have as many children as they can afford," and individuals who do less have been viewed negatively. The unwritten assumption has been that couples should demonstrate reasons for *not* having children (i.e., cannot educate them, clothe them, and so forth) or else be considered selfish, egocentric, and otherwise inadequate (Pohlman, 1969; Rainwater, 1960, 1965). The recent emphasis on the social and environmental problems caused by population pressures provides a potential counterforce to the traditional perspective on childbearing, i.e., that couples should now demonstrate reasons for *having* children. The foundation of this new perspective on childbearing is population education. Population education is a new field, and as yet there is dispute about its best definition and means of implementation. Most broadly defined it is the study of the causes and consequences of population growth, be they proximal or distal. Simmons

(1970) has divided the educational approaches in the field into four areas: sex education, family living, population awareness, and basic value orientation associated with sexual and family behavior. In general the focus of population-education programs has been on population awareness, or knowledge and understanding of population dynamics. Such awareness is a major factor in changing what childbearing means, although that is not to say that such knowledge will automatically yield reduced childbearing for all couples. However, the decision to have children is no longer a private matter when the number of persons born so profoundly affects the welfare of the other individuals in society.

Hence, population awareness becomes a crucial variable in providing motivation for control of population on the basis of enlightened self-interest. The question becomes not what families can afford but what society can afford. The more persons who realize that having an overabundance of children is maladaptive, the greater the likelihood that action programs will be instituted. Given the extreme importance of this variable, the lack of comprehensive research on the subject becomes distressing to the action programmer. Certain conclusions can be made, however.

Young people do consider population a serious problem (Darney, 1970; Dykstra, 1965; Poffenberger et al., 1970; Wanderer et al., 1970), although other issues such as the Vietnam war, race relations, and pollution are considered more important (Poffenberger et al., 1970). Nevertheless, their population *knowledge* is not great. A substantial proportion of youth is unfamiliar with basic population facts, such as the population of the United States (Dykstra, 1965; Poffenberger et al., 1970; Wanderer et al., 1970). Of course, lack of factual population knowledge does not necessarily mean underestimation of the problem. Poffenberger et al. (1970), for example, found that their subjects generally overestimated the U.S. population and also that 90 percent of the sample felt that the U.S. population should either not increase or should decline in number.

On the other hand, overestimating the problem does not mean that individuals will modify their fertility goals accordingly. Only 64 percent of the subjects questioned by Poffenberger and his associates (1970) agreed with the statement, "I feel strongly enough about preventing overpopulation that I would be willing to limit my family to two children," and the mean desired family size of this particular sample was 2.9. This apparent inconsistency in attitude was also reported by Wanderer et al. (1970), who found that although 91.3 percent of their sample agreed that reduction of population growth was desirable, mean ideal family size was 3.7 for Catholic school students and 2.4 for non-Catholic students.

The relationship between population awareness and individual attitudes and behavior has yet to be adequately studied. The research by Poffenberger and his colleagues (1970) indicates that the form of the question is highly important. For example, these investigators found that 43 percent of their subjects agreed that "a couple should have as many children as they want, without worrying about increasing population," while 70 percent agreed that "to prevent overpopulation, each couple has a responsibility to limit the number of children they have."

Disagreement as to the causes of the problem and the appropriate means for solution should affect the link between perception of overpopulation and the feeling that one should modify personal fertility goals. Darney (1970) found that 78 percent of his sample agreed that overpopulation was a problem in the United States, but only 4 percent said that this influenced their personal family-size decisions. The mean desired family size of his sample was 2.9. Over 30 percent of this group reported that the reason that overpopulation was a serious problem was "poor people have more children than they can support." Persons desiring four or more children were more likely to give this reason for problems of overpopulation than were those who desired smaller families (45 percent versus 25 percent). Persons desiring smaller families were more likely to mention the effects of environmental crowding as the reason that overpopulation was a problem in the United States (45 percent versus 17 percent). If middle-class individuals perceive the problems of overpopulation as being caused by the fertility of "the poor," then one can understand how they could consider population as a serious problem, yet still maintain relatively high personal fertility goals.

Little research has been done with respect to delineating the perceived effects of population growth. Darney asked his subjects "How do you think overpopulation might affect you or your children in the future?" and found that the three effects most often mentioned were increase of environmental crowding, greater competition for education and jobs, and decreased opportunity for recreation, in that order. Interestingly pollution was mentioned by only 8 percent of the sample. It is logical to assume that perceived effects as well as perceived causes of overpopulation may affect both personal fertility goals and recommended solutions, but data are lacking.

The effect of population awareness on individual action, therefore, requires much research effort. In general, attitudes toward birth control are apparently becoming more favorable, and motivation to acquire more information is being aroused as population increases. However, the extent of the change differs, depending on religion, with Catholics showing fewer effects of population awareness on attitudes toward birth control (Garai, 1964). Whether such attitude change becomes translated into behavioral change is unknown. A poll conducted in 1965 asked "What, if anything, should be done to control the increase in population?" (Erskine, 1967). Young people showed a lack of consensus on a solution. One-third of the teenage sample replied "don't know" or did not give an answer; 25 percent said "do nothing, it's up to the individual"; 23 percent mentioned use of birth control; and 13 percent mentioned education and advice on birth control (Erskine, 1967). More recent data in this form are not available.

The majority (74 percent) of incoming college freshmen do feel that the government should be more involved in "provision of birth-control information, pills, or devices to the general population," and 51 percent feel that there should be more government involvement in use of tax incentives to control the birth rate (ACE, 1970).

If reporting that the government should be more involved in the use of tax incentives to control the birth rate can be considered an index of concern about population, it is apparent that not all segments of the incoming freshman population are equally concerned. Once again, race and religion are influential variables. Fifty percent of the incoming freshmen at nonsectarian coeducational colleges feel the use of tax incentives to control the birth rate should be increased, as compared with 36 percent of those entering Catholic coeducational colleges and 38 percent of those entering predominantly black colleges (ACE, 1970).

A recent survey of 163 high school and college students underscores the racial differences in population awareness (Russo et al., 1971). Seventy-three percent of the white students as compared with 44 percent of the black students reported that the rate at which the U.S. population is growing is a very serious problem. Seventy-two percent of the whites as opposed to 38 percent of the blacks agreed that the U.S. government should have tax incentives for small families, but only 29 percent of the whites versus 22 percent of the blacks felt there should be government penalties for large families. Seventy-four percent of the whites versus 26 percent of the blacks said that population affected them personally.

Buckhout (1972) and his students have emphasized the contrast between the attitudes of white students and their black and chicano peers toward population-control policies. When compared to white students blacks and chicanos saw the population explosion as less serious and rated voluntary limitation of family size to two children as less favorable. The black subjects showed hostility and suspiciousness in their spontaneous comments when approached to be interviewed for the study. Many black students do impute genocidal motives to population-control advocates and respond accordingly.

Little is known about the sources of population awareness in young people. High school students reported in the early 1960s that overpopulation was usually referred to in school only briefly, if at all (Dykstra, 1965). With the recent efforts to organize the field of population education and implement population-education programs (Burleson, McArthur, and Taylor, 1969; Simmons, 1970; Viederman, 1970a, 1970b), the situation may change. Population awareness is a relatively new area. As population education becomes more widespread, the relationship between population awareness and individual fertility may increase. At present, however, it appears that until researchers identify the conditions that are necessary and sufficient for translation of population awareness into limitation of personal fertility the efficacy of population education will remain in the realm of speculation.

Role of the Psychologist in Action and
Research Relating to Population and Youth

The literature on youth demonstrates that there are many unanswered questions in the population field that are within the purview of psychology, but that have so far escaped the attention and concern of psychologists. Of the 36,000 members and associates of the American Psychological Association, only a handful are actively engaged in population research or action programs.

From the point of view of professional interest child psychologists, educational psychologists, and school psychologists—all of whom together account for about 16 percent of APA membership—have as a common bond a commitment to the welfare of children and youth. One natural outcome of such a commitment is (or should be) a realization that population overgrowth is antithetical to the optimum environmental quality necessary for rearing children properly.

In the past few years there have been many technological advances in contraception as well as considerable liberalization of abortion laws. Nevertheless, a large number of children are still being born to parents, some very young parents, who do not want them or who cannot care for them properly. The cry of "murder" is frequently raised by opponents of abortion. But to classify a child as "living" is a mere technicality if the "living" child is a victim of malnutrition, disease and improper medical care, social discrimination, inadequate intellectual stimulation, and inadequate or warped emotional ties to significant adults.

Aside from compelling moral reasons why psychologists should interest themselves in youth and population, there are also compelling professional reasons. By virtue of their particular training psychologists are well qualified to deal effectively with many aspects of population research and action programs. Besides the role of filling data gaps in the research literature, those aspects of population that are most akin to psychologists' training and experience relate to population education, the provision of counseling, clinical, and advocacy services, methodology in population research and its applications, and development of motivational theory appropriate to population issues.

Population Education

Within the field of population education one of the most obvious areas in which child psychologists, educational psychologists, and school psychologists may help is that of curriculum design. Population education is not limited to any one particular age, so that a correct analysis of age-appropriate methods and content is essential. Abstract discussions of fertility rates may be appropriate for college sophomores, but they are not appropriate for elementary schoolchildren. Additionally, when considering age-appropriateness from a cross-cultural frame of reference, it must be remembered that in the United States the majority of thirteen-year-olds can be reached in schoolrooms whereas the majority of thirteen-year-olds in many underdeveloped countries have left school forever, so that different routes of communication must be used to reach them (Poffenberger, 1971).

Another example of this type of help psychologists may give to curriculum design concerns the optimum size of chunks of population information for any population curriculum and the degree to which it is integrated with other material. Specifically the question is whether population information is best conveyed in a direct, concentrated curriculum—such as algebra or metal working—or whether it is best conveyed by "infusion," whereby bits of information are slipped into other standard curricula.[4]

The evaluation of the relative effectiveness of different curricula and modes of curriculum presentation is just as important as the design of the curriculum itself and equally requires the attention of education and school psychologist. If population information is presented for the first time to a group of eight-year-olds and a group of thirteen-year-olds, how much will each have retained at age fifteen? Is it possible that the first group of children, by virtue of subsequent sensitization to incidental sources of population education, will have the better informational grasp?

A third subarea of population education needing the assistance of psychologists concerns the motivational analysis necessary to maximize information input to the learner, information output on the part of the teacher, and acceptance of this dual process on the part of the community. Psychologists are particularly well equipped to identify and deal with attitudes that constitute sources of resistance to effective population education. To give an example, it is obvious that teaching about population problems involves an admission that there *are* population problems. But to what extent should the solutions to these problems remain tacit, be made explicit, or be made explicit *and* emphasized as the "only" proper mode of behavior for citizens with a social conscience? To what extent is the teacher of population seen as justified in presenting his own opinion on "proper" family size?

Counseling, Child Advocacy, and the Training of Counselors and Advocates

Counseling psychologists, clinical psychologists, and social psychologists number about 9,800 or 27 percent of the membership of the American Psy-

---

[4] For an example of population-education curriculum as a concentrated, demarcated entity at the secondary-school level, see Hertzberg, 1965. For a presentation of the advantages of the diffusion method, see Viederman, 1970a, 1970b.

chological Association. By way of research or clinical practice these psychologists deal with people's unrealistic attitudes and behaviors, with their fears and undue sensitivities, with problems in communication, with techniques of adjusting discrepancies between personal and social values, and with techniques of persuasion and behavior change.

Many of the problems in the area of youth and population call for skills and techniques of this sort. To list some examples, many parents oppose sex education, but oppose still more the involvement of their unmarried child in a pregnancy. Many also oppose population education because they confuse it with sex education. Many unmarried girls become pregnant because they are unwilling to admit either that they are having intercourse or that pregnancy is a probable outcome of intercourse. Many girls, upon finding themselves pregnant, are both terrified and uncertain about the course they should follow. Many young people are aware that a population problem exists, but see it as someone else's problem, preferring large families for themselves. All of these circumstances are at variance with reality and call for the expertise of clinical, counseling, and social psychologists.

Recently the Joint Commission on the Mental Health of Children proposed that the United States establish a child advocacy system for the youth of this country. A child advocate is a professional person whose main job is to protect the welfare of children. His loyalty and obligation is not to the child's family or to any institution but to the child himself. The child advocate is responsible for a group of children living within some geographical area. The group may consist of all the children within that area or a particular subgroup, e.g., children with physical disability or mental retardation.

Underlying the adoption of a child advocacy system are at least two basic assumptions that are highly relevant to the pursuit of quality of life for the nation's young people. The first assumption of a child advocacy system is that children are a valuable natural resource and as such must be cultivated with care. Second, a child advocacy system recognizes that children's needs are not always met by their parents or by societal institutions as those are now constituted. The fact that adults' and children's interests may not coincide can be illustrated by the very reasons that some adults give for conceiving and bearing children. These reasons, as documented, for example, by Pohlman (1969) or by Rabin and Greene (1968), center around reasons why adults want to become parents. They focus on the advantages of parenthood rather than looking at life's future prospects from the child's point of view. More than one disillusioned and apathetic teenager has said in desperation, "But I never asked to be born!" Literally he is right. Perhaps no one did consider the quality of his prospects before he was conceived. In all too many cases there is no one to consider them after he is born either. That is the role of the child advocate.

A limited child advocacy system is being used to great advantage in other countries such as Denmark. Whether American parents and American institutions would find it acceptable remains to be seen. On March 30, 1971 Senator Abraham Ribicoff introduced a bill (S.1414) to create a nation-wide child advocacy system in the United States. It is too early at the time of writing to determine the bill's legislative fate or public palatability.

Methodology in Population Research and Its Application

Within the behavioral and social sciences psychology has been a leader in research methodology, both in terms of experimental design and statistical analysis. In interdisciplinary settings psychologists are often turned to as methodologists, and it is precisely in this capacity that psychologists need to lend their assistance to population research and its applications. Some examples from the field of population research may help to illustrate the need for methodological improvement and to convince psychologists that their talents in this respect are called for. One such example involves the need to use smaller samples in many population settings. In terms of their training and experience sociologists and demographers are predisposed to use very large samples in their research, but in many cases the use of very large samples is dictated more by habit than by necessity. With the advances in precision and validity of small-sample designs and statistics made by both psychologists and mathematical statisticians, the uniform use of N's in the thousands is no longer necessary for accurate generalization to populations. Furthermore, large-scale sampling must be eyed carefully nowadays in terms of its consumption of time (a luxury in population research) and in terms of its consumption of money (a luxury in times of decreased financial support for grant research).

Another research area in need of the methodological help that psychologists could provide is that of assessing the accuracy or reliability of population measurements. Almost all of the research in the area of population has been carried out by means of questionnaires, surveys, or interviews. Nevertheless, relatively little of this research has attempted to assess the extent to which these questionnaires, surveys, or interviews are measuring accurately. As Cronbach has pointed out, "An inaccurate test cannot be a good predictor. The error portion of the test score will not correlate with any criterion; consequently, the greater the error variance the lower the validity coefficient" (1970, p. 171).

Most population research is concerned with prediction. A common problem, for example, involves prediction to the criterion of completed family size from prior statements of desired family size. If such statements were in fact valid predictors of this criterion, we would know automatically that the statements were reliable predictive measures. But there is no evidence in the literature that completed family size is being predicted accurately. Therefore, it is imperative to examine the predictive or measuring instruments with the goal of pinpointing sources of unreliability, i.e., error variance contributions to the prediction. When reliability of the *criterion* variable is also suspect, as in questions conveying the threat of negative social sanction (e.g., have you had an abortion?), then the need to assess reliability becomes all the more imperative.

The Development of
Motivational Theory Appropriate to Population Issues

When one gets right down to it the question that is basic to all of population research and all of population programming is why do people want children? Until the answer to this question is known there will be no sure way of controlling fertility through voluntary means. Fertility is not reduced by the development of new and better modes of contraception. It is reduced through the cooperation of people who actively seek not to become fertile, who align their motives for one reason or another with the goals of bearing fewer children with longer intervals between births. As documentation for these conclusions, consider that the birth rate during the Depression era of the 1930s, before significant advances in contraception had taken place, was far lower than it was subsequently during the 1950s and 1960s, the period during which the most effective contraceptives yet developed were introduced, namely, the pill and the IUD.

The question, therefore, of why people want children is central to all of population research and population programming aimed at voluntary control of fertility. By definition the question is a motivational one and calls for the skills of those who have been trained in motivational assessment and in affecting motivational changes.

Another crucial area for motivational management falls within the area of population education. As currently conceived by some population educators, population education rests on two psychologically untenable assumptions. The first is that knowledge transforms itself into action. The second is that knowledge will cause personal goals to change so that they accord with the needs and goals of society. But it is clear by now, unfortunately, that there are an increasing number of people who are aware that population problems exist but still desire three or more children.

If population knowledge remains cognitively compartmentalized, unincorporated into personal behavior and divergent from societal needs, population education will have little impact on population growth. In both its research and clinical training psychology emphasizes, more than any other discipline, that human beings do not behave logically and rationally, that verbal behavior is no sure predictor of nonverbal behavior, that cognitive dissonance and cognitive compartmentalization are common psychological characteristics, and that personal conscience and social conscience are discordant under many conditions. If population-aware people are to become population-oriented citizens, if population education is to generate population action, then psychology must join forces with other social sciences to effect those motivational changes that will aid in transforming population awareness into action.

REFERENCES

Almquist, E. M. and Angrist, S. S. 1970. Career salience and atypicality of occupational choice among college women. *Journal of Marriage and the Family* 32:242–249.

———. 1971. Role model influences on college women's career aspirations. *Merrill-Palmer Quarterly* 17:263–279.

American Council on Education (ACE). 1970. *National norms for entering college freshmen—fall 1970.* Washington, D.C.: ACE Research Reports, Vol. 5, no. 6.

American Institute of Public Opinion, 1961. Attitudes of young adults—college and high school students, #POS544.

Angelino, H.; Edmonds, E.; and Mech, E. 1958. Sex-expressed "first" sources of sex information. *Psychological Newsletter* 9:268–269.

Angrist, S. S. 1966. Communication about birth control: an exploratory study of freshman girls' information and attitudes. *Journal of Marriage and the Family* 28: 284–286.

———. 1970. Changes in women's work aspirations during college (or work does not equal career). Paper presented at the meeting of the Ohio Valley Sociological Society, Akron, Ohio, May 1970.

Astin, H. 1967. Factors associated with the participation of the woman doctorate in the labor force. *Personnel and Guidance Journal* 45:240–246.

Bartz, K. W. and Nye, F. I. 1970. Early marriage: a propositional formulation. *Journal of Marriage and the Family* 32:258–268.

Bell, R. R. 1966a. Parent-child conflict in sexual values. *The Journal of Social Issues* 22:34–44.

———. 1966b. *Premarital sex in a changing society.* Englewood Cliffs, N.J.: Prentice-Hall.

Bell, R. R. and Chaskes, J. B. 1970. Premarital sexual experience among coeds, 1958 and 1968. *Journal of Marriage and the Family* 32:81–84.

Blaine, G. B., Jr. 1967. The adolescent's crisis today: sex and the adolescent. *New York Journal of Medicine* 67:1967–1975.

Blood, R. O. 1962. *Marriage.* Glencoe, Ill.: The Free Press.

Boynton, P. L. and Woolwine, R. D. 1942. The relationship between the economic status of high school girls and their vocational wishes and expectations. *Journal of Applied Psychology* 26:399–415.

Broderick, C. B. 1966. Sexual behavior among pre-adolescents. *Journal of Social Issues* 22:6–21.

Buckhout, R. 1972. Toward a two-child norm: changing family planning attitudes. *American Psychologist* 27:16–26.

Bumpass, L. and Westoff, C. 1970. The "perfect contraceptive" population. *Science* 18:1177–1182.

Burchinal, L. G. 1958. What about school-age marriages? *Iowa Farm Science* 12:12–14.

———. 1959a. Does early dating lead to school-age marriage? *Iowa Farm Science* 13:11–12.

———. 1959b. How successful are school-age marriages? *Iowa Farm Science* 13:7–10.

———. 1959c. Comparison of factors related to adjustment in pregnancy-provoked and nonpregnancy-provoked youthful marriages. *Midwest Sociologist* 21:92–96.

———. 1959d. Adolescent role deprivation and high school age marriage. *Marriage and Family Living* 21:378–384.

———. 1960. Research on young marriages: implications for family life education. *The Family Life Coordinator* 9:6–24.

————. 1965. Trends and prospects for young marriages in the United States. *Journal of Marriage and the Family* 27:243–254.

Burchinal, L. G. and Chancellor, L. E. 1963. Social status, religious affiliations, and ages at marriage. *Marriage and Family Living* 25:219–221.

Burleson, N.-D.; McArthur, D.; and Taylor, D. 1969. The time is now: population education. Unpublished manuscript, Center for Population Research, University of North Carolina.

Campbell, A. A. 1968. The role of family planning in the reduction of poverty. *Journal of Marriage and the Family* 30:236–245.

Christensen, H. T. 1963. Child spacing analysis via record linkage. *Marriage and Family Living* 25:272–280.

————. 1966. Scandinavian and American sex norms: some comparisons with sociological implication. *Journal of Social Issues* 22:60–75.

Christensen, H. T. and Gregg, C. F. 1970. Changing sex norms in America and Scandinavia. *Journal of Marriage and the Family* 32:616–627.

Cronbach, L. J. 1970. *Essentials of psychological testing.* 3rd ed. New York: Harper & Row.

Cutright, P. 1971. Special feature: illegitimacy: myths, causes and cures. *Family Planning Perspectives* 3:25–48.

Darney, P. D. 1970. Attitudes of married college students on overpopulation and family planning. *Public Health Reports* 85:412–418.

Davis, K. and Blake, J. 1956. Social structure and fertility: an analytic framework. *Economic Development and Cultural Change* 4:211–235.

DeLissovoy, V. and Hitchcock, M. 1965. High school marriages in Pennsylvania. *Journal of Marriage and the Family* 27:263–265.

Dykstra, J. W. 1965. The population explosion: a neglected topic. *Social Studies* 56: 190–193.

Ehrmann, W. H. 1959. *Premarital dating behavior.* New York: Holt, Rinehart & Winston.

————. 1964. Marital and nonmarital sexual behavior. In H. T. Christensen, ed., *Handbook of marriage and the family.* Chicago: Rand McNally. Pp. 585–622.

Eisner, T.; van Tienhoven, A.; and Rosenblatt, F. 1970. Population control, sterilization and ignorance. *Science* 167:337.

Empey, L. T. 1958. Role expectations of young women regarding marriage and career. *Marriage and Family Living* 20:152–155.

Epstein, C. F. 1970. *A woman's place: options and limits in professional careers.* Berkeley: University of California Press.

Erskine, H. G. 1967. The polls: more on the population explosion and birth control. *Public Opinion Quarterly* 31:303–311.

Farley, J. 1970. Graduate women: career aspirations and desired family size. *American Psychologist* 25:1099–1100.

Freedman, D. S.; Freedman, R.; and Whelpton, P. K. 1960. Size of family and preference for children of each sex. *American Journal of Sociology* 66:141–146.

French, E. G. and Lesser, G. S. 1964. Some characteristics of the achievement motive in women. *Journal of Abnormal and Social Psychology* 68:119–128.

Fürstenberg, F. F., Jr. 1970. Premarital pregnancy among black teenagers. *Trans-Action* 7:52–55.

Fürstenberg, F. F., Jr.; Gordis, L.; and Markowitz, M. 1969. Birth control knowledge and attitudes among unmarried pregnant adolescents: a preliminary report. *Journal of Marriage and the Family* 31:34–42.

Garai, J. E. 1964. The effects of information on students' knowledge of population problems and their attitudes toward population control. *Psychology: A Journal of Human Behavior* 1:16–21.

Gianopulos, A. and Mitchell, H. E. 1957. Marital disagreement in working wife marriages as a function of husband's attitude toward wife's employment. *Marriage and Family Living* 19:373–378.

Giel, R. and Kidd, C. 1965. Some observations on pregnancy in the unmarried students. *British Journal of Psychiatry* 111:591–594.

Gingles, R. and Voss, J. 1965. Young couples look at teenage marriage. *Nebraska Experiment Station Quarterly* 12:12–13.

Glick, P. C. 1957. *American families.* New York: Wiley.

Goldsen, R. K.; Rosenberg, M.; Williams, R. M.; and Suchman, E. A. 1960. *What college students think.* Princeton: Van Nostrand.

Gottschalk, L. A.; Titchner, J. L.; Piker, H. N.; and Stewart, S. S. 1964. Psychosocial factors associated with pregnancy in adolescent girls. *Journal of Nervous and Mental Disease* 138:524–534.

Graham, P. A. Women in academe. 1970. *Science* 169:1284–1290.

Grant, V. M. 1957. *The psychology of sexual emotions: the basis of sexual attraction.* London: Longmans, Green & Co.

Green, A. W. 1960. The "cult of personality" and sexual relations. In N. W. Bell and E. F. Vogel, eds., *A modern introduction to the family.* Glencoe, Ill.: The Free Press. Pp. 608–615.

Greenberg, N. H.; Loesch, J. G.; and Lakin, M. 1959. Life situations associated with the onset of pregnancy. *Psychosomatic Medicine* 21:296–310.

Grinder, R. E. and Schmitt, S. S. 1966. Coeds and contraceptive information. *Journal of Marriage and the Family* 28:471–479.

Gustavus, S. O. and Mommsen, K. G. 1969. Negro-white differentials in the formation of ideal family size among young people. Paper presented at the annual meeting of the Southern Sociological Society, New Orleans, Louisana, April 1969.

Gustavus, S. O. and Nam, C. B. 1970. The formation and stability of ideal family size among young people. *Demography* 7:43–51.

Guttmacher, A. F. 1969. How can we best combat illegitimacy? *Medical Aspects of Human Sexuality* 3:49–61.

Hacker, A. 1965. The pill and morality. *New York Times Magazine*, 32:128–129.

Havighurst, R. J.; Bowman, P. H.; Liddle, G. P.; Matthews, C. V.; and Pierce, J. V. 1962. *Growing up in River City.* New York: Wiley.

Hedegard, J. M. and Brown, D. R. 1969. Encounters of some Negro and white freshmen with a public multiversity. *Journal of Social Issues* 25:131–144.

Hendershot, G. E. 1967. Fertility values in two generations. Paper presented at the annual meeting of the Population Association of America, Cincinnati, Ohio, April 1967.
———. 1969. Family satisfaction, birth order, and fertility values. *Journal of Marriage and the Family* 31:27–33.

Herrmann, R. O. 1965. Expectations and attitudes as a source of financial problems in teenage marriages. *Journal of Marriage and the Family* 27:89–91.

Hertzberg, H. W. 1965. *Teaching population dynamics: an instructional unit for secondary school students.* New York: Teachers College.

Hill, A. C. and Jaffe, F. S. 1966. Negro fertility and family size preferences: implications for programming of health and social services. In *The Negro American.* Boston: Houghton-Mifflin Co. Pp. 205–224.

Horner, M. 1969. Why bright women fail. *Psychology Today* 3:36ff.

Inselberg, R. M. 1962. Marital problems and satisfaction in high school marriages. *Marriage and Family Living* 24:74–77.

Kaats, G. R. and Davis, K. E. 1970. The dynamics of sexual behavior of college students. *Journal of Marriage and the Family* 32:390–399.

Kalish, R. A.; Maloney, M.; and Arkoff, A. 1966. Cross-cultural comparisons of college student marital-role preferences. *Journal of Social Psychology* 68:41–47.

Kammeyer, K. 1964. The feminine role: an analysis of attitude consistency. *Journal of Marriage and the Family* 26:295–305.

Kantner, J. F. and Zelnick, M. 1969. United States: exploratory studies of Negro family formation—common conceptions about birth control. *Studies in Family Planning* 43:10–13.

Katz, J. 1968. Four years of growth, conflict, and compliance. In J. Katz, ed., *No time for youth.* San Francisco: Jossey-Bass.

Kinsey, A. C. 1966. Illegal abortion in the United States. In R. W. Roberts, ed., *The unwed mother.* New York: Harper & Row. Pp. 191–200.

Kirkendall, L. A. 1961. *Premarital intercourse and interpersonal relationships.* New York: Julian Press.

Kirkendall, L. A. and Libby, R. W. 1966. Interpersonal relationships—crux of the sexual renaissance. *Journal of Social Issues* 22:45–59.

Knudsen, D. D. 1969. The declining status of women: popular myths and the failure of functionalist thought. *Social Forces* 48:183–193.

Kogan, W. S.; Boe, E. E.; and Valentine, B. L. 1965. Changes in the self-concept of unwed mothers. *Journal of Psychology* 59:3–10.

Komarovsky, M. 1946. Cultural contradictions and sex roles. *American Journal of Sociology* 12:184–190.

———. 1953. *Women in the modern world.* Boston: Little, Brown.

Kuvlesky, W. P. and Obordo, S. A. 1969. Racial differences in teenage girls' orientations toward marriage: a study of youth living in an economically depressed area of the South. Paper presented at the meeting of the Southern Sociological Association, New Orleans, Louisiana, April 1969.

Lacognata, A. A. 1967. Birth control information and practices among college students. *National Association of Women Deans and Counselors Journal* 30:180–181.

Landis, J. T. and Landis, M. G. 1963. *Building a successful marriage.* 4th ed. Englewood Cliffs, N.J.: Prentice-Hall.

Lowrie, S. H. 1965. Early marriage: premarital pregnancy and associated factors. *Journal of Marriage and the Family* 27:48–56.

Lowry, T. 1969. First coitus. *Medical Aspect of Human Sexuality* 3:91–97.

McCary, J. L. 1967. *Human sexuality.* New York: Van Nostrand Co.

McCreary-Juhasz, A. 1967. How accurate are student evaluations of the extent of their knowledge of human sexuality? *Journal of School Health* 37:409–412.

McKee, J. P. and Sherriffs, A. C. 1959. Men's and women's beliefs, ideals and self-concepts. *American Journal of Sociology* 64:356–363.

McMillin, M. R.; Cerra, P. F.; and Mehaffey, T. D. 1971. Opinions on career involvement of married women. *Journal of the National Association of Women Deans and Counselors* 34:121–124.

Major, M. A. 1967. Assessment of motivation for parenthood in parents of disturbed and normal children. Unpublished Ph.D. diss., Michigan State University.

Markle, G. E. and Nam, C. B. 1970. The impact of sex predetermination on fertility. Paper presented at the annual meeting of The Population Association of America, Washington, D.C., April.

Martinson, F. M. 1955. Ego deficiency as a factor in marriage. *American Sociological Review* 20:161–164.

———. 1959. Ego deficiency as a factor in marriage—a male sample. *Marriage and Family Living* 21:48–52.

Martz, H. E. 1963. Illegitimacy and dependency. *Health, Education and Welfare Indicators,* September 1963, pp. 15–30.

Matthews, E. and Tiedeman, D. V. 1964. Attitudes toward career and marriage and the development of life style in young women. *Journal of Counseling Psychology* 11: 375–384.

Maxwell, J. W. 1970. College students' attitudes toward abortion. *The Family Coordinator* 19:247–252.

Miller, H. and Wilson, W. 1968. Relation of sexual behaviors, values, and conflict to avowed happiness and personal adjustment. *Psychological Reports* 23:1075–1086.

Monahan, T. P. 1953–1954. Does age of marriage matter in divorce? *Social Forces* 32:81–87.

Moss, J. J. 1965. Teenage marriage: cross-national trends and sociological factors in the decision of when to marry. *Journal of Marriage and the Family* 27:230–242.

Moss, J. J. and Gingles, R. 1959. The relationship of personality to the incidence of early marriage. *Marriage and Family Living* 21:372–377.

Muller, C. 1970. Socioeconomic outcomes of present abortion regulations and practices. *Studies in Family Planning* 53:8.

Nobbe, C. E. 1968. Correlates of desired family size among college-educated Catholics. Unpublished Ph.D. diss., University of Washington.

Oppenheimer, V. K. 1968. The sex-labeling of jobs. *Industrial Relations* 7:219–234.

Ortho-Panel. 1968. Teen-age and premarital sexual counseling. In *Ortho panel 3: report and commentary on current problems in medical practice.* Ortho Pharmaceutical Corp.

Parke, R., Jr., and Glick, P. G. 1967. Perspective changes in marriage and the family. *Journal of Marriage and the Family* 29:249–256.

Payne, R. 1956. Adolescents' attitudes toward the working wife. *Marriage and Family Living* 18:345–348.

Perrucci, C. C. 1968. Mobility, marriage and child spacing among college graduates. *Journal of Marriage and the Family* 30:273–282.

Pilpel, H. and Wechsler, N. 1969. Birth control, teenagers and the law. *Family Planning Perspectives* 1:29–36.

Poffenberger, T. 1959. Family life education in this scientific age. *Marriage and Family Living* 21:150–154.

———. 1960. Responses of eighth grade girls to a talk on sex. *Journal of Marriage and the Family* 22:38–44.

———. 1961. Sex-courting concerns of a class of twelfth grade girls. *The Family Life Coordinator* 10:75–81.

———. 1971. Population learning and out-of-school youth in India. Unpublished manuscript, Center for Population Planning, University of Michigan.

Poffenberger, T.; Bachman, J. G.; and Weiss, E. 1970. Survey of population knowledge and attitudes of post high school age boys in the United States. Paper presented at the meeting on student knowledge of and attitudes toward population matters, Population Council, New York, December 1970.

Poffenberger, T. and Norton, D. 1963. Sex differences in achievement motive in mathematics as related to cultural change. *Journal of Genetic Psychology* 103:341–350.

Pohlman, E. 1967. Some effects of being able to control sex of offspring. *Eugenics Quarterly* 14:274–281.

Pohlman, E., with the assistance of Pohlman, J. M. 1969. *The psychology of birth planning.* Cambridge, Mass.: Schenkman.

Poloma, M. M. 1970. The myth of the egalitarian family: familial roles and the professionally employed wife. Paper presented at the meeting of the American Sociological Association, Washington, D.C., September 1970.

Poloma, M. M. and Garland, T. N. 1970. Role conflict and the married professional women. Paper presented at the meeting of the Ohio Valley Sociological Society, Akron, Ohio, April 30–May 2, 1970.

———. 1971. Jobs or careers? The case of the professionally employed married woman. In A. Michel, ed., *Family issues of employed women in Europe and America.* Leiden, Netherlands: E. J. Brill.

Pratt, W. F. 1965. Premarital pregnancy in a metropolitan community. Paper presented at the meeting of the Population Association of America, Chicago, Ill., April 1965.

Purdue Opinion Poll. 1970. People problems: population, pollution, prejudice, poverty, peace. Lafayette, Ind.: Purdue University, Measurement and Research Center.

Rabin, A. I. 1965. Motivation for parenthood. *Journal of Projective Techniques* 29: 405–411.

Rabin, A. I. and Greene, R. J. 1968. Assessing motivation for parenthood. *Journal of Psychology* 69:39–46.

Rainwater, L. 1960. *And the poor get children.* Chicago: Quadrangle Books.

———. 1965. *Family design: marital sexuality, family size, and contraception.* Chicago: Aldine.

Reiss, I. L. 1964. Premarital sexual permissiveness among Negroes and whites. *American Sociological Review* 29:688–698.

———. 1966a. Contraceptive information and sexual morality. *Journal of Sexual Research* 2:51–57.

———, ed. 1966b. The sexual renaissance: a summary and analysis. *The Journal of Social Issues* 22:123–137.

———. 1967. *The social context of premarital sexual permissiveness.* New York: Holt, Rinehart & Winston.

Rele, J. R. 1965. Some correlates of the age at marriage in the United States. *Eugenics Quarterly* 12:1–6.

Roberts, R. W., ed. 1966. *The unwed mother.* New York: Harper & Row.

Rosen, E. J.; Campbell, C.; and Arima, L. A. 1961. A psychiatric, social, and psychological study of illegitimate pregnancy in girls under the age of sixteen years. *Psychiatric Neurology* 142:44–60.

Rosenburg, B. and Bensman, J. 1968. Sexual patterns in three ethnic subcultures of an American underclass. *Annals of the American Academy of Political and Social Science* 376:61–75.

Russo, N. F.; Cohen, G.; Blasi, C.; Marber, D.; Reed, J.; and Wholey, A. 1971. A survey of population and environmental awareness among youth. Unpublished manuscript, American University.

Russo, N. F. and Stadter, M. 1971. Sex and religion: college students and family planning. Paper presented at the meeting of the American Psychological Association, Washington, D.C., September 1971.

Sarrel, P. M. 1967. The university hospital and the teenage unwed mother. *The American Journal of Public Health* 57:1308–1313.

————. 1969. Teenage pregnancy. *Pediatric Clinics of North America* 16:347–354.

Schofield, M. 1965. *The sexual behavior of young people*. Boston: Little, Brown.

Semmens, J. P. and Lamers, W. M. 1968. *Teenage pregnancy*. Springfield, Ill.: Charles C Thomas.

Siegel, A. E. and Curtis, E. A. 1963. Familial correlates of orientation toward future employment among college women. *Journal of Educational Psychology* 44:33–37.

Signell, K. A. 1969. Prevention of teenage illegitimate pregnancy: a consultation approach to sex education. *The Family Coordinator* 18:222–225.

Simmons, O. G. 1970. Population education: a review of the field. *Studies in Family Planning* 52:1–5.

Simpson, R. L. and Simpson, I. H. 1961. Occupational choice among career-oriented college women. *Marriage and Family Living* 23:377–390.

Smith, Sr. M. L. 1962. Catholic viewpoints about the psychology, social role, and higher education of women. *Journal of Home Economics* 54:228.

Smith, R. G.; Steinhoff, P. G.; Diamond, M.; and Brown, N. 1971. Abortion in Hawaii: the first 124 days. Unpublished manuscript, School of Public Health, University of Hawaii.

Spicer, F. 1969. Adolescents—family planning. *Journal of the Royal College of General Practitioners* 17 (monograph supplement 2): 17–22.

Steinhoff, P. G.; Smith, R. G.; and Diamond, M. 1970. The characteristics and motivations of women receiving abortions. Unpublished manuscript, School of Public Health, University of Hawaii.

Stone, W. L. 1960. Sex ignorance of college students. *Family Life* 20:1–3.

Time. 1971. The rhythm lobby. *Time* 19:54.

Turner, R. H. 1964. Some aspects of woman's ambitions. *American Journal of Sociology* 7:271–285.

van Tienhoven, A.; Eisner, T.; and Rosenblatt, R. 1971. Education and the population explosion. *Bio Science* 21:16–21.

Veroff, J.; Wilcox, S.; and Atkinson, J. W. 1953. The achievement motive in high school and college age women. *Journal of Abnormal and Social Psychology* 48:108–119.

Viederman, S. 1970a. Developing education programs for population awareness. Paper presented at the Conference on Education and the Environment in the Americas jointly sponsored by the Organization of the American States and the American Association for Colleges of Teacher Education, Washington, D.C., October 1970.

————. 1970b. *Population education: a world-wide review of programs in process and planned*. Unpublished manuscript, Population Council.

Vincent, C. 1961. *Unmarried mothers*. Glencoe, Ill.: The Free Press.

————. 1966. Teenage unwed mothers in American society. *Journal of Social Issues* 22:22–23.

Von Den Ahe, C. V. 1969. The unwed teenage mother. *American Journal of Obstetrics and Gynecology* 104:279–287.

Wagner, N. N.; Millard, P. R.; and Pion, R. J. 1970. The role of the pharmacist in family planning. *Journal of the American Pharmaceutical Association* NS10:258–261.

Wallin, P. 1950. Cultural contradictions and sex roles: a repeat study. *American Sociological Review* 15:288–293.

Wanderer, M.; Seaver, R. M.; and Wagner, N. N. 1970. Preliminary reports on population education research. Unpublished manuscript, University of Washington School of Medicine, Division of Family Planning Education.

Ward, C. D. and Barrett, J. E. 1968. The ecumenical council and attitude change among Catholic, Protestant, and Jewish college students. *Journal of Social Psychology* 74: 91–96.

Weil, M. W. 1961. An analysis of the factors influencing married women's actual or planned work participation. *American Sociological Review* 26:91–96.

Westoff, C. F. and Potvin, R. H. 1966. *College women and fertility values.* Princeton: Princeton University Press.

White, K. 1967. Social background variables related to career commitment of women teachers. *Personnel and Guidance Journal* 45:48–52.

Young, L. 1966. Personality patterns in unmarried mothers. In R. W. Roberts, ed., *The unwed mother.* New York: Harper & Row.

Zelnick, M. and Kantner, J. F. 1970. United States exploratory studies of Negro family formation—factors relating to illegitimacy. *Studies in Family Planning* 60:5–9.

[16]

SOME PRACTICAL APPLICATIONS
OF SOCIAL PSYCHOLOGY TO
FAMILY-PLANNING PROGRAMS

GEORGE P. CERNADA
AND THOMAS J. CRAWFORD

Introduction

In this chapter we will discuss what we believe to be some practical uses of social psychology in a family-planning communications program in a field setting. A good deal of our emphasis is on attitude theory and measurement. The chapter grew out of a series of conversations between the two authors first inside and later outside the classroom. One of us looks at the problems we will discuss from the vantage point of experience in family-planning action research programs abroad, and the other approaches these problems from the perspective of a continuing interest in attitude theory and research. Since much of the chapter represents a continuing dialogue it may be less systematic than other chapters in this volume. Certainly we have not attempted to be comprehensive in our coverage. At best we will provide some descriptions of program situations and problems that arise in field settings and sketch out some possible practical applications of social-psychological concepts and techniques to these problems. The topics, explored with varying degrees of intensity, include: measurement problems in the knowledge, attitude, and practices (KAP) surveys; organizational and personnel training problems; and family planning communication program strategies. The ordering of topics is loosely chronological, reflecting the usual development from initial fact-finding about the need and demand for a birth-planning program through development of an organization to implement the program and consideration of the kinds of communication approaches to be used to reach the population.

Survey Measures of Family-Planning Knowledge, Attitudes, and Practices

Family-planning programs provide birth-control information and services, usually on a voluntary basis. The programs are directed toward a target population, mostly women, in order to lower fertility and enhance family and societal welfare. The major contraceptive methods offered have been the intrauterine contraceptive device—the Lippes loop—and more recently the oral contraceptive. In some countries sterilization, primarily vasectomy for males, has been offered. The major program approach has been systematic home visiting by family-planning field workers.

Before most family-planning communication and persuasion programs are carried out, there usually is an assessment of preprogram levels of family-planning knowledge, attitudes, and behaviors in the population in which the program is to be undertaken. The nature of the audience to be reached in most family-planning communication programs is often assessed by standardized KAP, or knowledge, attitude, and practice surveys. These are large-scale representative sample surveys, of which more than 400 have been carried out in "virtually all of the world's major geographic and cultural areas" (Fawcett, 1970, p. 38). They attempt to assess *knowledge* about reproduction and contraception, *attitudes* about size of family, pregnancy, fertility, and use of contraception, and birth-control *practice*. While the strategic value of survey results for indicating public interest in family planning to political leaders is generally acknowledged, there appears to be an increasing sense of dissatisfaction with the use of KAP surveys as instruments for assessing attitudes toward, and readiness to adopt, contraceptive methods. Part of this disillusionment may be due to the evidence of unreliable and invalid responses to questions about contraceptive practices and family-size ideals (Mauldin, Watson, and Noe, 1970).

It seems clear, as Hauser (1962, 1967), Stephan (1962), and others have pointed out, that the usefulness of KAP surveys could be increased if more attention were given to careful measurement procedures. For example, Caldwell found that although 62 percent of the women interviewed in a KAP survey of Ghana said that they would use a contraceptive recommended by a physician, only 25 percent queried afterward said that they would use it if it were complicated and difficult to use (Mauldin et al., 1970). Unfortunately many KAP surveys do not probe beyond the surface level represented by the initial 62 percent positive response. The inadequacies of attitude measurement in KAP surveys are summarized by Fawcett (1970):

> In KAP and fertility surveys the aspect of attitudes that is usually measured is direction; occasionally, there is measurement of intensity; almost never is attention given to different components of attitudes (cognitive, affective, behavioral), or to the functional bases of attitudes, or to the salience of an attitude in a particular context. Measuring instruments are designed mainly on the basis of face validity. Response sets, such as acquiescence and effects of the interviewer-respondent relationship are seldom assessed [pp. 75–76].

Since attitudes and beliefs cannot be measured directly but must be inferred from verbal report or other behaviors, the possibility of measurement error cannot be completely eliminated. Nevertheless, a variety of techniques could be employed to reduce some of the more obvious sources of error. Attitude questions that indicate *degree* of approval or disapproval, multiple-item unidimensional scales in place of single-item measures, wording of questions to minimize yea-saying, social desirability and other response sets, and checks on interviewer effects should help to reduce bias in KAP surveys. A "funnel-sequence" procedure (Kahn and Cannell, 1957), which begins with general open-ended questions and then proceeds to specific fixed-alternative questions, may reveal more about the existence, salience, dimensions, and importance of family-planning-related concepts than an approach that relies entirely on direct, fixed-alternative questions. This technique would help to determine whether individuals even have an attitude toward a specific family-planning topic, or whether the answers given to certain items in surveys are merely "efforts at politeness to meaningless inquiries or forced responses to questions to which the respondent really has no answer" (Hauser, 1967). Salience and importance might also be assessed by asking respondents to select or rank concepts from an array that includes non-family-planning-related as well as family-planning-related terms, especially if the selection or ranking is done early in an interview that has not yet obviously focused upon family planning. A useful set of guidelines for the construction of KAP questionnaires is contained in the *Manual for Surveys of Fertility and Family Planning: Knowledge, Attitudes, and Practice* (The Population Council, 1970).

Part of the so-called unreliability problem in KAP surveys may result not from measurement error but from real instability and fluctuation in family-planning attitudes. Information about the stability and resistance to change of such attitudes might be obtained by a field "persuasion experiment" in which an interviewer would read a message advocating a different ideal family size or a different opinion about contraceptives from that expressed by the interviewee. A great deal of change by the interviewee in the direction advocated might indicate either an unstable, noninvolving attitude or a desire to please the interviewer. In either case our confidence in the verbal report measures of attitude would be reduced.

In common with the usual emphasis in attitude research, the KAP surveys have concentrated more upon the affective or evaluative component of attitudes than upon the cognitive and behavioral components. Research by Crawford, Stocker, and Heredia (1968), by Insko, Blake, Cialdini, and Mulaik (1970), and by Jaccard (1971) suggests that studies of the cognitive or belief component of family-planning attitudes may have important practical and theoretical implications. These studies of cognitive structure indicate that the perceived relationships between birth control and other positively or negatively valued concepts (e.g., minor discomforts, smaller families, poverty, good health, and so forth) are related both to evaluation of birth control and to use of birth-control methods.

Of perhaps even more practical significance are two recent doctoral dissertation studies of the behavioral component of family-planning attitudes. Laing (1969) and Kothandapani (1971) found that behavioral intentions with regard to family planning were more closely related to family-planning behaviors than were feelings or beliefs about family planning. In his methodologically sophisticated study Kothandapani developed measures of the affective, cognitive, and behavioral components of birth-control attitudes. Four measures of each of the three attitudinal components were constructed, using the techniques of Thurstone equal-appearing intervals, Likert summated ratings, Guttman scalogram analysis, and Guilford self-rating. The twelve scales developed by Kothandapani to measure birth-control feelings, beliefs, and intentions to act should be useful in organized family-planning programs.

In addition to the concern over reliability and validity, another source of dissatisfaction with KAP surveys is the frequently observed discrepancy between verbal report of attitudes toward family planning and family-planning behavior. Even if we had perfectly valid and reliable measures of family-planning attitudes and beliefs, we would not expect such measures to bear a perfect one-to-one correspondence to family-planning behavior. The social-psychological literature is replete with studies that demonstrate the inadequacies of verbal reports of attitude for predicting overt behavior. Several critics of verbal measures of attitudes have cited the apparent inconsistency between measured attitudes and behavior as grounds for entirely abandoning verbal-report attitude-measurement techniques. More sophisticated analyses of the attitude-behavior relationship, however, recognize that *situational* constraints as well as attitudes are operating to influence behavior (Campbell, 1963; Smith, 1969). When both variations in the intensity of the individual's attitude and variations in the intensity of counterattitudinal situational constraints are jointly considered, it becomes clear that many of the studies of the verbal report-overt behavior relationship are describing a pseudo-inconsistency (Campbell, 1963). Similarly this conceptualization of behavior as a function of both attitudes and situations suggests that much of the debate between sociologists and psychologists as to whether attitudes or situations determine behavior is a pseudo-controversy (Smith, 1969).

With the best imaginable attitude-measurement procedures we may obtain an approximation of the individual's overall evaluation of some class of objects or events, such as "small families" or "birth control." This evaluation may be taken directly from perceived membership and reference-group norms, or it may reflect the externalization of perhaps unconscious conflicts, as Smith, Bruner, and White (1956) point out. In addition this overall evaluation is supported by, and is to some extent a function of, all the beliefs the individual has concerning the attitude object, including its perceived consequences for obtaining or blocking other objects and events valued by the individual. But not all of the beliefs the individual has about an attitude object are operating to influence his behavior at a particular time and in a particular situation. This might be illustrated in a family-planning context by the following example. If matched groups of users and nonusers of condoms were asked to list the various advantages and disadvantages of the method (as is sometimes done in follow-up surveys of contraceptive acceptors), both groups might list roughly equivalent evaluations of the effectiveness of the method, the relative cost, and so on. But in actual practice those who fail to use condoms might not use them because they felt that they diminish sexual pleasure or make lovemaking mechanical and impersonal. Given the actual circumstance of use with a partner, those beliefs relating to effectiveness and cost might not be engaged in terms of a decision to use or not use a condom. The beliefs relevant to this action when the action is taken may only concern the sexual pleasure of self and partner. When situational constraints, involving, for example, the accessibility and convenience of contraceptives, are taken into account and weighed against the intensity of the individual's attitudes and the nature of his beliefs, more precise behavioral predictions will result.

More generally it is important to distinguish between the overall attitude toward an activity or object and the "engaged" attitudes and beliefs (Smith, 1969), which are only those beliefs about the object that are perceived by the individual as relevant to the pursuit of his currently salient goals. It is the situationally engaged beliefs and attitudes, and not the overall attitude or the total system of beliefs, that relate to behavior. Attitude-measurement procedures that generate tangible, quantifiable responses may be responsible for the tendency of attitude researchers to reify attitudes and beliefs and to think of them as frozen, semipermanent structures that operate to influence all behaviors relevant to the attitude object. It may be more fruitful to think of the mind as a response-selecting process whose function is to choose an appropriate behavioral means for attaining currently salient goals (Sperry, 1952). Depending upon the nature of these currently salient goals and upon the present situational cues and constraints, certain beliefs about a concept such as birth control may be seen as relevant to goal-striving behavior, but in all likelihood most of the beliefs the individual has about the concept will remain "unengaged" in "storage" or memory and therefore irrelevant to his present actions.

There are several practical implications of this conception of the mind as a goal-striving process, apart from the obvious implication that an inventory of the individual's family-planning beliefs and attitudes will not, by itself, provide an adequate basis for predicting his family-planning behavior. One line of research suggested by this perspective is the study of those beliefs or perceived relationships that differentiate those who report favorable attitudes and practice family planning from those who report favorable attitudes but do *not* practice family planning. The belief measures developed by Insko et al. (1970) and by Crawford et al. (1968) and based upon Rosenberg's (1956) procedures may be useful for this purpose. Another implication of this analysis, and one that is consistent with the Laing (1969) and Kothandapani (1970) studies, is that predictions of family-planning behaviors based upon expressed behavioral intentions will be more accurate than behavioral predictions based upon beliefs and attitudes. In expressing a behavioral intention the individual not only takes into consideration his own attitudes and beliefs, but he also anticipates to some extent the situation in which he will enact behavior relevant to the attitude object. Consequently as Laing and Kothandapani found, behavioral intentions are more closely related to family-planning behavior than either family-planning attitudes or family-planning beliefs. The predictive utility of reported behavioral intentions has also been demonstrated in family-planning programs. In Taiwan the contraceptive acceptance rate was 44 percent among those who had earlier said that they intended to accept soon, but only 15 percent among those who said that they intended to accept "eventually" (Freedman and Takeshita, 1969).

Family-Planning Organizations

Organizational Problems

Once an assessment of the knowledge, attitudes, and practices of the population to be served has been made, an organization is formed to provide contraceptive services, education, and information to a target group. As with any agency organizational problems often abound. The focus of this section is on intra-agency communication and on the selection and training of family-planning field workers.

The effectiveness of the flow of communication from a program to an audience is largely determined by the flow of communication *within* the program organization itself. As Schramm points out, ". . . it must be recognized that public communication is merely the part of family-planning communication that floats above the water; it rests upon a large amount of communication of which the public may never be aware" (1971, p. 2).

Schramm illustrates this point with examples from development extension services in India (Pelz, 1966) and the use of communication in support of development, also in India (Childers, 1966). These examples indicate the variety of internal communication paths and the need for two-way communication. Schramm (1971) cites Kanagaratnam, who previously directed Singapore's extensive family-planning program:

> Before the general public can be effectively informed . . . information and training must be given to trainers, technical administrators, medical and paramedical staff in hospitals and clinics, operating personnel (including health educators), peripheral field workers (health assistants, nurse-midwives, etc.), personnel of communication units in the family planning program, mass media specialists . . . , legislators and administrators, staff of related departments, voluntary agencies, and key members of organizational groups. [P. 2]

That internal communications play a vital role in the implementation of any family-planning program is obvious. In practice, however, relatively little attention is given to intra-agency communication. A simple mapping out in diagram form of the flow of communications within an agency at headquarters level and its diffusion to the field staff would probably contain surprising information for most staff members. In studying intra-agency communication the methods of organizational and industrial psychology may be of some benefit.

One particular problem area in many family-planning programs is communication between the research and evaluation units and other units such as program planning, education and information, training, supervision, supplies, and so forth. Some carefully managed group discussion with related staff might delineate the existence and extent of the mistrust other program staff feel toward evaluation personnel and programs. A large part of intra-agency hostility may relate to the threat of evaluation of staff activities. This threat would be increased by any tendency of the evaluation staff to project images of themselves as more well trained, academic, and scientific than other staff members. This phenomenon is probably intensified in developing countries where education is a more unique status indicator. Another source of difficulty is the fact that by the time data for program evaluation are collected and analyzed, they are frequently obsolete except as history. In many cases data are not collected in close coordination with field supervisory and operational units, and hence these latter staff members, who should be able to implement the findings, have little or no commitment to them or are openly skeptical about how much the academically oriented study staff knows of the field situation. In some areas such as Taiwan there have been attempts to abstract the major findings of studies with action-program implications and to translate these into simple language, with clear statements of possible recommendations for program action. With these capsulized summaries busy administrators are better able to integrate evaluative findings into their program decision-making.

Training Problems

The extension-education component of most family-planning programs is centered on group meetings and systematic home visiting by family-planning field workers. In many countries these field workers are considered to be the most valuable component of the informational and educational approach. The Korean and Taiwan programs center on such home-visiting and meeting-organizing techniques.

In Taiwan selection of the house-to-house visiting field workers assumes high program priority. The type of worker sought is one who is reasonably similar in her beliefs and attitudes to the women in her geographical area. The selection guidelines spelled out in this program include the following characteristics:

1. *Emotionally Mature.*
2. *Over 30, up to 40.* Program experience suggests that emotional maturity is correlated with age. Also of significance is that the median age of marriage for females in Taiwan (twenty-two years) is higher than most Asian countries. In other areas a lower age might be acceptable.
3. *Being Married.* Helps her talk at an equal level with the potential acceptor. Also lessens the likelihood of her leaving her job to marry one of the local health personnel.
4. *With Children.* Having children seems to help since there is an endless source of experience to relate to the economic values of planning family size. She should have, however, someone to take care of the children. And if she is breast feeding, remember she may not be available when desired.
5. *Using a Contraceptive Method.* All the better if she herself is spacing or has had as many children as she wants and is satisfactorily using a method to plan her family size. Most desirable is that she is using one of the effective methods the program is promoting, i.e., IUD or pill. She also is not likely to become pregnant and add to the vacancy rate.
6. *Indigenous.* She should be living in the community in which she works. This means she will not be looked on as an "outsider," and she will speak the local dialect.
7. *At Ease in Discussions.* She should be able to talk and be at ease with wives she visits. One factor that helps is experience in meeting people, particularly a job in which she dealt with women on a face-to-face basis.
8. *Education.* In Taiwan this requirement has been lowered from twelve to nine years minimum. In other places qualifications would be acceptable if they correspond to the level of schooling in the area in which she will work. Tests should not place too much weight on written answers; otherwise one may reject the wives who are able in discussion but weak at writing. Keep the examination weighted heavily on oral response. (Taiwan began to observe this in 1966.) After all, the job in the field depends almost entirely on oral communication. [Cernada and Huang, 1968, pp. 2–3]

In selecting workers there has been less standardization of the selection procedures than is desirable and virtually no use of personality assessment tools as screening devices. The workers, however, are often selected with practical, simple tests administered orally by several earthy midwives with relatively advanced education and extensive experience. The problems posed for candidates are the following types:

> You are a family-planning worker. I am a local village leader. I am opposed to your work. We are having tea together at my house. What would you say to me to convince me of the value of your bringing family-planning information to my village?

or

> How many children do you think most wives in your village have by the time they reach forty? Do you think most want more or less? What number is the one most would like to have had? Do you think younger women these days want fewer children? Do you think you want less or more than others? Why are you different? [Cernada and Huang, 1968, p. 3]

Training is probably the most neglected area in family-planning programming. Yet the training of field workers provides many opportunities for applying practical principles of social psychology and learning theory. Examples abound. Unnecessary lectures often predominate in training sessions. These formal educational approaches suppress active exchange of ideas between teacher and student, and continuing feedback is minimal. Lecturers seldom know whether they are talking over the heads of their audience. Where possible, lectures should be replaced with educational approaches that more actively involve those who are to be trained; for example, the main points of the usual fifty-minute talk could be summarized in fifteen minutes, a mimeographed outline of the main points passed out, and the rest of the time devoted to group discussion so that the trainer knows that the trainees understand the important points he wants to make.

Improvised role-playing needs further use in both the selection and in the training of field workers, since both experimental and field studies suggest that individuals who actively play the communicator role are more likely to be influenced than are those who are passively exposed to lectures. In terms of continuing in-service education role-playing may also produce change with respect to evaluation of previously disliked tasks.

Group discussions could also be used more effectively in training programs, and the potential use of this technique has been stressed in the Taiwan program:

> If you tell a worker that only two to three of 100 women using the loop for one year become pregnant, it does not mean that she believes you. Trainees need to be encouraged to express their doubts openly so that these doubts can be answered and discussed. Tape recordings of satisfied users should be heard. If possible, satisfied acceptors should be brought in to talk with workers; all the better if the satisfied users are regular field workers or the new trainees [Cernada and Huang, 1968, p. 5].

With the exception of East Pakistan there seems to have been virtually no attempt to determine the family-planning attitudes and program expectations of field workers. Little is usually done beyond establishing a baseline of knowledge about physiology and contraception, and even this step is sometimes omitted. The need for more assessment of field workers' attitudes is suggested by a recent study in Taiwan that indicates that family-planning workers have considerable ambivalence about birth-control pills, and many believe the pills are very likely to produce serious side effects, including cancer. To what extent do these negative or mixed feelings of workers affect the acceptance or continuance of contraceptive use? The University of Michigan is conducting an interesting study using path analysis to determine the sociological characteristics of effective field workers in Taiwan. The possibility of complementing this effort with a study of the personality and attitudinal correlates of field workers' effectiveness, as suggested by Fawcett (1970), is intriguing:

> The psychological correlates of field worker effectiveness is another topic that might appropriately be investigated by industrial psychologists. . . . Research in Taiwan and Korea has revealed some demographic factors associated with field worker effectiveness and has identified some productive field work techniques but a thorough study of the attitudes, personality variables or modes of performance associated with field worker effectiveness has yet to be done. While there are some obvious problems in attempting to implement a study of this kind, particularly in an alien cultural setting, the difficulties do not seem insurmountable [pp. 103–104].

Communication

Principles of Communication and Persuasion

Most current family-planning programs are composed of a provision of services, personal contact by field staff, and public education and information provided through media and community organizations. In this section we will be concerned with the flow of information from family-planning organizations to the general public.

Bogue (1965) was one of the earliest family-planning researchers to develop fully the idea that theory and research on communication and attitude change could be an important source of family-planning action-program hypotheses and recommendations. The communication and persuasion literature suggests a number of studies that not only should add to our understanding of the psychology of family planning, but also should furnish important positive and negative feedback for theories of attitude organization and change. The latter consideration seems especially important since, as Hovland (1959) pointed out, many of these theories have been developed primarily on the basis of data gathered in an artificial laboratory situation, using topics and issues that are relatively trivial and noninvolving.

Once a would-be change agent has clearly formulated the goals of an action program, perhaps the most fundamental psychological question he should try to answer is: what needs or functions are currently being served by the attitudes and behaviors that the agency will attempt to change? The answer to this question should then influence the strategy and approach of a communication and information campaign. Katz (1960) has argued that unless we know the psychological needs that are served by an attitude or a behavior pattern, we are in a poor position to design a program to change the attitude or behavior. The attitude functions suggested by Smith et al. (1956) may provide a useful framework for understanding the functional bases of family-planning beliefs and attitudes. These authors propose three needs that may be served by attitudes:

Object Appraisal. In a general sense attitudes help the individual to appraise reality and thus prepare for the benefits and harms it holds in store for him. Presented with an object or event, the individual is able to categorize it in some class of objects and events for which a predisposition to action and experience already exists.
Social Adjustment. This function serves the individual in his adjustments to the groups in which he participates and gives him a badge of identity with his significant reference groups.
Externalization. Externalization occurs when an individual, often responding unconsciously, senses an analogy between a perceived environmental event and some unresolved inner problem. He adopts an attitude toward the event in question that is a transformed version of his way of dealing with his inner difficulty. [Adapted from Smith et al., 1956]

To the extent that family-planning attitudes serve an "object appraisal" or knowledge function, they should be susceptible to modification through persuasive communications that present rational arguments. For example, if preference for large families or opposition to a particular method of contraception stems from beliefs about the positive and negative consequences of large families or contraceptives, a rationally argued information campaign that presents evidence to alter negative beliefs and to reinforce existing positive beliefs or introduce new positive beliefs should meet with some success. The literature from experimental studies of attitude change is relevant to this rational-argument mode of social influence.

One of the most important sets of findings in social psychology has emerged from the experimental study of communication and persuasion. McGuire (1969) has provided a comprehensive and critical review of this literature, and the practical principles of persuasion that can be derived from these studies have been ably summarized by Zimbardo and Ebbesen (1969) and by Karlins and Abelson (1970). In Table 16–1 the Zimbardo and Ebbesen summary of principles of persuasion (which was in turn derived largely from Abelson's earlier [1959] summary) is presented.

While well-designed and clearly reasoned messages from highly credible sources should have an impact upon attitudes that serve a knowledge

TABLE 16-1

Summary of Social-Psychological Findings Regarding Communication and Persuasion[a]

A. The Persuader

1. There will be more opinion change in the desired direction if the communicator has high credibility than if he has low credibility. Credibility is:
    a. Expertise (ability to know correct stand on issue).
    b. Trustworthiness (motivation to communicate knowledge without bias).
2. The credibility of the persuader is less of a factor in opinion change later on than it is immediately after exposure.
3. A communicator's effectiveness is increased if he initially expresses some views that are also held by his audience.
4. What an audience thinks of a persuader may be directly influenced by what they think of his message.
5. The more extreme the opinion change that the communicator asks for, the more actual change he is likely to get.
    a. The greater the discrepancy (between communication and recipient's initial position), the greater the attitude change, up to extremely discrepant points.
    b. With extreme discrepancy and with low-credibility sources there is a falling off in attitude change.
6. Communicator characteristics irrelevant to the topic of his message can influence acceptance of its conclusion.

B. How to Present the Issues

1. Present one side of the argument when the audience is generally friendly, or when your position is the only one that will be presented, or when you want immediate, though temporary, opinion change.
2. Present both sides of the argument when the audience starts out disagreeing with you, or when it is probable that the audience will hear the other side from someone else.
3. When opposite views are presented one after another, the one presented last will probably be more effective. Primacy effect is more predominant when the second side immediately follows the first, while recency effect is more predominant when the opinion measure comes immediately after the second side.
4. There will probably be more opinion change in the direction you want if you explicitly state your conclusions than if you let the audience draw their own, except when they are rather intelligent. Then implicit conclusion drawing is better.
5. Sometimes emotional appeals are more influential, sometimes factual ones. It all depends on the kind of audience.
6. Fear appeals: the findings generally show a positive relationship between intensity of fear arousal and amount of attitude change if recommendations for action are explicit and possible, but a negative reaction otherwise.
7. The fewer the extrinsic justifications provided in the communication for engaging in counternorm behavior, the greater the attitude change after actual compliance.
8. No final conclusion can be drawn about whether the opening or closing parts of the communication should contain the more important material.
9. Cues that forewarn the audience of the manipulative intent of the communication increase resistance to it, while the presence of distractors simultaneously presented with the message decreases resistance.

C. The Audience as Individuals

1. The people you may want most in your audience are often least likely to be there. There is evidence for selective seeking and exposure to information consonant with one's position, but not for selective avoidance of information dissonant with one's position.
2. The level of intelligence of an audience determines the effectiveness of some kinds of appeals.
3. Successful persuasion takes into account the reasons underlying attitudes as well as the attitudes themselves. That is, the techniques used must be tailored to the basis for developing the attitude.

TABLE 16-1 (continued)

Summary of Social-Psychological Findings Regarding Communication and Persuasion[a]

4. The individual's personality traits affect his susceptibility to persuasion; he is more easily influenced when his self-esteem is low.

5. There are individuals who are highly persuasible and who will be easily changed by any influence attempt, but who are then equally influenceable when faced with countercommunications.

6. Ego involvement with the content of the communication (its relation to ideological values of the audience) decreases the acceptance of its conclusion. Involvement with the consequences of one's response increases the probability of change and does so more when source-audience discrepancy is greater.

7. Actively role-playing a previously unacceptable position increases its acceptability.

D. The Influence of Groups

1. A person's opinions and attitudes are strongly influenced by groups to which he belongs and wants to belong.

2. A person is rewarded for conforming to the standards of the group and punished for deviating from them.

3. People who are most attached to the group are probably least influenced by communications that conflict with group norms.

4. Opinions that people make known to others are harder to change than opinions that people hold privately.

5. Audience participation (group discussion and decision-making) helps to overcome resistance.

6. Resistance to a counternorm communication increases with salience of one's group identification.

7. The support of even one other person weakens the powerful effect of a majority opinion of an individual.

8. A minority of two people can influence the majority if they are consistent in their deviant responses.

E. The Persistence of Opinion Change

1. In time the effects of a persuasive communication tend to wear off.

    a. A communication from a positive source leads to more rapid decay of attitude change over time than one from a negative source.

    b. A complex or subtle message produces slower decay of attitude change.

    c. Attitude change is more persistent over time if the receiver actively participates in, rather than passively receives, the communication.

2. Repeating a communication tends to prolong its influence.

3. More of the desired opinion change may be found some time after exposure to the communication than right after exposure (sleeper effect).

[a]From Philip Zimbardo and Ebbe B. Ebbesen, *Influencing attitudes and changing behavior* (Reading, Mass.: Addison-Wesley, 1969), pp. 20-23. Reprinted by permission of the publisher.

function, such messages may have little or no influence upon attitudes that serve either to externalize unconscious inner conflicts or to facilitate the individual's social relationships with important others. It seems plausible to us that deeper lying sexual needs and fears, and unconscious impulses and characteristic modes of dealing with these impulses, play some role in influencing family-planning attitudes and behavior. To the extent that such forces do operate, attitudes and behaviors will be relatively immune to attack through reasoned evidence in persuasive messages. Relatively little is known about this source of "hard-core resistance" to family planning, though some suggestive leads are provided by Wyatt (1967) and by Keller, Sims, Henry, and Crawford (1970).

Without minimizing the importance of clinical research on resistance to family planning or the role of unconscious motivation in determining family-planning attitudes, we would suggest that social adjustment needs play an even more critical part in determining family-planning attitudes. By gaining social approval for the individual his expressed attitudes may facilitate his adjustment to the groups to which he belongs. A related social adjustment function of attitudes is that of identification with positive reference groups. The individual may bolster his self-esteem by adopting attitudes and beliefs that are similar to those he believes are held by groups and individuals he respects. A mass-communication campaign that ignores the social context in which family-planning attitudes, beliefs, and behaviors are embedded stands an excellent chance of failure or even of producing boomerang effects. On the other hand, a campaign that takes advantage of the existing natural group structure by utilizing respected reference persons, indigenous opinion leaders, and group meetings may greatly increase its effectiveness.

Mass Communications

Most family-planning programs, particularly those supported by an official government policy, use the mass media to some extent. Researchers seem to "have accepted the position of most practitioners that media and personal channels belong together and doubtless interact in whatever they accomplish" (Schramm, 1971, p. 32). There have been a large number of field studies and several experimental studies of both formal and informal communication in family-planning programs (see summary reviews by Schramm, 1971, and by Fawcett, 1970). Schramm (1971), in summarizing the state of the art of family-planning communications, reports that people learn about contraception from the mass media, but that the "evidence is not so clear as to how much the mass media can do by themselves to motivate acceptors" (p. 32). The report also raises a variety of questions that might be posed regarding the messages and channels of communications. Schramm concludes that there is little hard evidence to support the kind of messages that are presently widely used in family-planning programs, despite their appeal to the common sense of program personnel (Schramm, 1971, p. 37). We really do not know, for example, how much to stress economic appeals vis-à-vis health appeals, or in what circumstances programs can effectively appeal to the general public to act for the national good.

Because of this lack of reliable information on the effects of variations in message content, the potential use of mass media in the preparation of special communications aimed at particular groups in family-planning information campaigns has not as yet been sufficiently explored. Research identifying the social and psychological characteristics of opinion leaders and the development of communications with particular appeal to them is needed. However, it should be remembered that the opinion leaders on matters of family planning may not be opinion leaders on other subjects. For example, a male Muslim village chief, who owns the only transistor radio, may well be a source of political news and opinions, but he seldom may be referred to by the wives of the village for consultation on pregnancy or contraception.

To provide an illustration of a mass-communication question with both theoretical and practical implications, let us consider the question of the ideal number of children, ignoring for a moment the problems involved in measuring this ideal in KAP surveys. Assuming that the ideal number of children in a given population is four or five, or more, what optimum number of children should a family-planning message advocate? More generally what is the relationship between communication distance and opinion change? A great deal of attitude-change theory and research has been addressed to this problem of how the amount of induced opinion change varies as a function of the size of the gap between the message receiver's initial opinion and the position taken in a discrepant communication. While there is still some unresolved controversy surrounding this question, in general it appears that the more opinion change the communicator requests, the more opinion change he will obtain, *provided that*: (1) the communicator is seen as a trustworthy expert by the audience, and (2) the topic of the communication is not particularly important or ego involving to the audience. In other words the highly credible communicator discussing an uninvolving topic can "get by" with more extreme arguments and for strategic reasons probably should take an extreme stand—i.e., one that is widely discrepant from the opinions of the message receivers. When the communicator has less credibility, or when the topic is more ego involving to the audience, the communicator should take a less extreme position if he wishes to induce the maximum amount of possible opinion change.

After many years of study in one Asian country it was concluded that most couples were having about five children but actually thought that four was "ideal" (according to KAP findings). From a demographic viewpoint, however, a net reproductive rate of one (i.e., two children) to achieve a zero-growth rate of population by the year 2030 has been considered advisable. After an official population policy was announced in 1969 personnel from the family-planning program and officials of government education and communication agencies met to plan a campaign to influence couples to think more in terms of two children as the ideal number. The focus of attention at the time was the planned issue of a postage stamp depicting the ideal family size. A great deal of discussion centered on whether to have one, two, or three children on the stamp. Demographers argued that population growth would never be curbed unless couples thought in terms of two children as the ideal family size. Those espousing one were considered too radical. The more practical minded contended that three was closer to the real present ideal and hence more likely to be acceptable, considering the ego involvement of parents. The debate raged, with the whole litany of communication and persuasion experiments being invoked. Finally through compromise and negotiation the local ministry and department-level officials decided upon depicting two children (one boy and one girl) with their mother and father.

When the stamp was issued some nine months later, however, three children and their parents were depicted. It was alleged that legislators had screened the stamp design and had decided that three was a better size. Apparently these legislators were older individuals who themselves had large families. Thus despite the considerable concern from the viewpoint of communication theory, the final word was said by those whose authority was greater than that of the program technicians. This example may serve not only to point out that there is room for more attitude-change theory in the field, but also to point out the practical limitations of applying these findings in field situations. Perhaps part of the solution lies in more emphasis on getting the appropriate information to the people who make the final decisions. Had concrete evidence from a family-planning-oriented, communication-distance study been available, the argument for a two-child stamp would have been strengthened.

Messages: Pretesting

An economical method of evaluating the kinds of appeals integrated into program approaches is pretesting. While most family planners acknowledge the value of pretesting in theory, all too often this potentially valuable step is omitted from an action program. An illustration of what may well be common occurred in an Asian country with a long history of extended family life, where the message on thousands of colorful outdoor posters read "A small family is a happy family." Field workers were asked "Is it not a good thing that we have our father and mother living with us?"

International agencies might play a significant role in promoting pretesting by simply including with program funding a contractual requirement for pretesting, and by drawing up a methodological guideline or "cookbook" for the pretesting of materials in the groups for which the materials are intended. Few approaches provide a better cost-effectiveness return on the dollar invested in international family-planning programs than pretesting.

Motivation and Postpartum Period

An example that may concretely illustrate the complexity of the problem of communication effectiveness and its relationship to the functions of attitudes is that of the postpartum approach. At present considerable attention is being given by national and international agencies to postpartum approaches—that is, reaching a mother with contraceptive information and services just after she has had a child. The obvious advantage of this approach is the logistical accessibility of women in a hospital setting who have clearly proven that they are part of the fertile target group. Family planners are currently providing information and services during this period in numerous urban hospitals throughout the world as part of an international study (Taylor and Berelson, 1971; Zatuchni, 1970). There is considerable interest in expansion of the postpartum approach to rural areas, and a feasibility study has been completed (Taylor and Berelson, 1971) to assess the problems and costs involved in setting up maternal and child health centers in rural areas, where contraceptive services on a postpartum basis could be provided. From the humanitarian viewpoint of providing health care to rural populations and from the political viewpoint of lessening the impact of cries of genocide by Western providers of contraceptive services, the stratagem is probably sound. A question that arises, however, relates to the psychological state of readiness to adopt contraception of a woman who has just given birth to a child (Taylor and Berelson, 1971). Recent literature on the subject (Berelson, 1970) tends to assume that the postpartum period is one of very high motivation for family-planning service. Unfortunately little supporting evidence beyond acceptance rates (which vary considerably among the various postpartum programs) has been introduced to support this assumption.

Indeed, an argument could be made to support the opposite contention —that is, the postpartum period is a time when women are less likely to be willing to accept contraception. The results of several studies of post-abortion reactions, reported primarily in psychiatric and medical journals (e.g., Fleck [1970], Kummer [1963], and Peck and Marcus [1966]), may be partially applicable to the postpartum period. The results of intensive postabortion follow-up interviews show that these women have surprisingly few negative reactions. Some investigators have interpreted these results in terms of cognitive dissonance theory. Dissonance theory suggests than an individual will attempt to justify to himself a voluntary behavioral action that cannot be undone. This justification may take the form of selective overemphasis of positive consequences and selective underemphasis of negative consequences of the voluntary action, whether it be childbirth or having an abortion. The key factor operating here appears to be defense of self-esteem against the implication of having made a wrong decision. Interestingly enough this evidence seems not to be considered in terms of its applicability to a postpartum-oriented program, where it might suggest resistance to family planning. For example, since becoming pregnant normally involves voluntary behavior, a woman may justify her pregnancy by selectively emphasizing to herself all the positive aspects of having a child. On the other hand, a woman who has given birth to a child may regret her pregnancy and still maintain her self-esteem if she places the blame for the pregnancy upon her husband, thus eliminating the "voluntary commitment" element that is presumably critical for dissonance arousal. These and other questions remain to be answered by research.

Some obvious research questions to be asked are: is the postpartum period really a time of high motivation for family planning? Is the reason for a high rate of postpartum contraceptive acceptance due entirely to women being easily identified as fertile and as a captive audience in a hospital setting, or are women also more ready psychologically to stop having children at this time? One problem with determining the motivational intensity of the postpartum period is the absence of a good "control group." Perhaps a postabortion period could be considered comparable in certain respects to a postpartum period. A study providing equivalent contraceptive-oriented education to both postpartum and postabortion women and matching them for other characteristics in selection, such as parity, marital status, and so forth, might provide useful information about motivation for family planning.

These questions assume great importance in terms of the tentative plans to expand postpartum approaches from urban to rural areas. Certain considerations seem to argue against the notion that the postpartum period is one of high motivation to adopt contraception. For example, in Taiwan, where women have a rest period of thirty days after childbirth, they are then a focal point of attention, often in the home of their husband's parents. Would wives be likely to be even more motivated *after* their postpartum rest period is over, when they must themselves begin caring for the child and resume the household drudgery? Should we also ask to what extent the postpartum approach is a projection by Westerners of their common value orientations about childbirth to an Asian society where women's liberationists are few and childbirth is not recognized as an economic and social disaster for individuals? More research is necessary here, particularly in light of the enormity of the costs of such programs.

Discontinuation of Contraceptive Use

One problem in most family-planning programs abroad has been the low continuation rates after initial adoption of contraceptive methods. Even in a relatively sophisticated Asian setting such as Singapore, only about half of the women who begin use of the oral contraceptive pill are still using it after eighteen months (Kanagaratnam and Kim, 1969). In Taiwan only half of those who began use of the IUD still have it after two years (Taiwan Institute of Family Planning, 1969). To increase continuation rates has become a high-priority goal in most family-planning programs, but little research has been devoted to this topic. Most approaches have involved standardized interviews or follow-ups of contraceptive acceptors, with primary emphasis on creating a demographic profile of the IUD dropouts.

An attitude-change principle that appears to be relevant here is the experimental finding that presenting both sides of the argument will be more effective when it is likely that the audience will be hearing the other side elsewhere or initially disagrees with the communicator. In addition two-sided arguments have the advantage of "inoculating" the message receiver against subsequent counterpropaganda (McGuire, 1964). In the practical, day-to-day field operation in most countries there may be a trend toward providing data on "both sides of the argument," since in areas such as Taiwan and Korea field workers contend that most women have already heard rumors about side effects of the IUD. Thus house-to-house visiting field workers in Taiwan are trained to use the analogy of wearing the IUD to wearing a new pair of shoes—at first the body has to adjust to this foreign object, and there may be some pain for a while, *but* you usually do not throw the shoes away, do you? So, too, with the loop. The information on the extent to which either program-policy or field-worker practice consciously puts the two-sided argument strategy into effect (and, assuming it is practiced, its effectiveness vis-à-vis a one-sided argument approach) is sketchy. Research in field settings on the effectiveness of one-sided versus two-sided arguments in producing attitude and behavior change and inoculation against subsequent counterarguments could have some value here in substantiating and justifying the apparent preference for two-sided arguments. Control-group experiments, even in less representative clinic settings, also could be of value and might be less subject to the confounding variables in field situations.

An important determinant of the efficacy of persuasive appeals is the perceived social acceptability of the induced behavior. Field-worker training in Taiwan includes a two-hour block of classes on the use of satisfied acceptors, not only as an approach to recruit clients, but as a kind of social support device at the local level, based on the hypothesis that potential clients want to know what other people are doing, how widespread a practice is, and so forth (Cernada, 1968). Another approach to providing social support for contraceptives and one that is geared to sustaining continuation of their use, as well as increasing initial acceptance, is the use of mothers' clubs in Korea. These are organized women's groups meeting on a quarterly basis and subsidized by the family-planning program (Ross, Finnigan, Keeny, and Cernada, 1969). Their effectiveness is currently being evaluated.

Areas of concern relevant to continuation as well as initial adoption that may be amenable to the methodologies of social psychology include the whole spectrum of communication networks, from communicator, through channel and message, to opinion leaders, and finally to grass-roots audience. From field and clinic studies of family-planning communication we might learn the answers to important questions, such as:

What do Mrs. Chen and Mrs. Kim, who are visited, perceive as the vested interests of the home-visiting field workers?

To what extent do incentive and target systems cause home visitors to "hard sell" the contraceptive methods they offer and to fail to warn clients about possible side effects? To what extent does the "hard sell" affect initial acceptance and continuing use of a contraceptive method?

To what extent do other women, neighbors, and relatives who have had side effects or have heard rumors about them influence whether a woman tries the contraceptive method and whether she continues with it? Perhaps valuable information could be obtained from a study that exposes matching groups of women to such rumors in field settings. What kinds of fears about side effects need to be allayed with what kinds of women or men?

In what ways can potential acceptors be told about side effects in order to provide them with reassurance and enable them to keep loops in longer? When is it best to provide information about side effects—before insertion by the worker? just before insertion by the physician? by the physician after insertion? Should the discussion be with both husband and wife? What are the barriers to effective communication between physicians and their patients in terms of differing frames of reference? [cf. selections from Roberts, 1970.]

The Neglected Husband

One relatively neglected topic in many family-planning programs is the role of the husband in decision-making with regard to acceptance and discontinuation of contraceptive methods. The husband's role takes on particular importance in Asia, Africa, and South America, where the position of the female is generally more subordinate to the male in many areas of decision-making than in the United States and Europe. In programs such as those in Taiwan and Korea, which are female-method oriented and employ only female home visitors who visit only wives, the importance of the male may be underestimated. Studies of couple concurrence and empathy (Yaukey, Griffiths, and Roberts, 1967) and of familial structure (Hill, Stycos, and Back, 1959) should be replicated and extended. Questions worthy of further exploration include:

What kinds of educational approaches are most likely to appeal to males?

Are males more likely to be interested in the economic implications of larger families than in matters of maternal health?

To what extent do pamphlets provided by female workers to wives only, and mildly flavored with a "women's liberation from childbirth" appeal, later elicit unfavorable reaction from husbands?

Would a two-pamphlet approach, as once advocated in Taiwan (Cernada, 1968), be beneficial if the pamphlet for the wife stresses female interests and the one for the husband stresses the economic values of having fewer children?

Conclusion

It seems to us that the burden of proof that social psychology has an important role to play in family-planning programs is on the shoulders of social psychologists. It is to be hoped that some of the illustrations we have presented will suggest possibilities of applying social psychology's theory and methods to the problems of family-planning programs. As we noted with regard to the question of communication distance and ideal family size, however, there are practical obstacles to the implementation of social-psychological hypotheses in family-planning field programs. Nevertheless, it is our belief that the concepts and methods of social psychology are of great potential usefulness in action programs, and that the application of these concepts and methods will benefit social-psychological theory at least as much as it benefits family-planning programs.

REFERENCES

Abelson, H. I. 1959. *Persuasion, how opinions and attitudes are changed.* 1st ed. New York: Springer.
Berelson, B. 1970. The present state of family planning programs. *Studies in Family Planning* 57:1–11.
Bogue, D. J. 1965. *Inventory, explanation and evaluation by interview of family planning motives-attitudes-knowledge-behavior.* Chicago: University of Chicago Community and Family Study Center.
Campbell, D. T. 1963. Social attitudes and other acquired behavioral dispositions. In S. Koch, ed., *Psychology: a study of a science.* New York: McGraw-Hill. 6:94–172.
Cernada, G. P. 1968. Family planning communication in Taiwan, Republic of China. In *Communications in family planning: report of a working group.* Bangkok: United Nations Economic Commission for Asia and the Far East (ECAFE). Pp. 8off.
Cernada, G. and Huang, T. 1968. Taiwan: training for family planning. *Studies in Family Planning* 36:1–6.
Childers, E. 1966. *Outline specification for an Indonesia development support communication service.* Bangkok: Development Support Communication Service.
Crawford, T. J.; Stocker, E.; and Heredia, R. 1968. Family planning attitudes and behavior as a function of the perceived consequences of family planning. Paper presented at the meeting of the Population Association of America, Boston, April 1968.
Fawcett, J. T. 1970. *Psychology and population.* New York: The Population Council.
Fawcett, J. T. and Somboonsuk, A. 1969. Using family planning acceptors to recruit new cases. *Studies in Family Planning* 39:1–4.
Fleck, S. 1970. Some psychiatric aspects of abortion. *Journal of Nervous and Mental Disease* 151:42–50.
Freedman, R. and Takeshita, J. 1969. *Family planning in Taiwan.* Princeton: Princeton University Press.
Hauser, P. M. 1962. On design for experiment and research in fertility control. In C. V. Kiser, ed., *Research in family planning.* Princeton: Princeton University Press. Pp. 463–474.
———. 1967. Family planning and population programs. *Demography* 4:397–414.
Hill, R.; Stycos, J. M.; and Back, K. 1959. *The family and population control.* Chapel Hill: University of North Carolina Press.
Hovland, C. I. 1959. Reconciling conflicting results derived from experimental and survey studies of attitude change. *American Psychologist* 14:8–17.
Insko, C. A.; Blake, R. R.; Cialdini, R. B.; and Mulaik, S. A. 1970. Attitude toward birth control and cognitive consistency: theoretical and practical implications of survey data. *Journal of Personality and Social Psychology* 16:228–237.
Jaccard, J. 1971. Beliefs and personality in fertility research. Unpublished senior honors thesis, Department of Psychology, University of California, Berkeley, June 1971.
Kahn, R. L. and Cannell, C. F. 1957. *The dynamics of interviewing.* New York: Wiley.
Kanagaratnam, I. and Kim, K. C. 1969. Singapore: the use of oral contraceptives in the national program. *Studies in Family Planning* 48:1–9.

Karlins, M. and Abelson, H. I. 1970. *Persuasion, how opinions and attitudes are changed.* 2nd ed. New York: Springer.

Katz, D. 1960. The functional approach to the study of attitude. *Public Opinion Quarterly* 24:163–204.

Keller, A. B.; Sims, J. H.; Henry, W. E.; and Crawford, T. A. 1970. Psychological sources of "resistance" to family planning. *Merrill-Palmer Quarterly* 16:287–302.

Kothandapani, V. 1971. A psychological approach to the prediction of contraceptive behavior. University of North Carolina: Carolina Population Center Monograph no. 15.

Kummer, J. H. 1963. Post-abortion psychiatric illness—a myth? *American Journal of Psychiatry* 119:980–983.

Laing, J. E. 1969. The relationship between attitudes and behavior: the case of family planning. Unpublished Ph.D. diss., University of Chicago.

McGuire, W. J. 1964. Inducing resistance to persuasion: some contemporary approaches. In L. Berkowitz, ed., *Advances in experimental social psychology.* New York: Academic Press. Vol. 1.

———. 1969. The nature of attitudes and attitude change. In G. Lindzey and E. Aronson, eds., *Handbook of social psychology.* Reading, Mass.: Addison-Wesley. 3:136–314.

Mauldin, W. P.; Watson, W. B.; and Noe, L. F. 1970. KAP surveys and evaluation of family planning programs. New York: The Population Council (mimeo).

Peck, A. and Marcus, H. 1966. Psychiatric sequelae of interruption of pregnancy. *Journal of Nervous and Mental Disease* 143:417–425.

Pelz, D. C. 1966. *Co-ordination, communication, and initiative in agricultural development.* New Delhi: Indian Institute of Public Administration.

Pohlman, E. 1969. *The psychology of birth planning.* Cambridge, Mass.: Schenkman.

The Population Council. 1970. *A manual for surveys of fertility and family planning: knowledge, attitudes, and practice.* New York: The Population Council.

Roberts, B. J. 1970. Research in educational aspects of health programmes. *International Journal of Health Education,* Supplement to 13:1–33.

Rosenberg, M. J. 1956. Cognitive structure and attitudinal affect. *Journal of Abnormal and Social Psychology* 53:367–372.

Ross, J.; Finnigan, O. D.; Keeny, S. M.; and Cernada, G. 1969. Korea and Taiwan: review of progress in 1968. *Studies in Family Planning* 41:1–11.

Schramm, W. 1971. Communication in family planning. *Reports on Population/Family Planning* 7:1–43.

Smith, M. B. 1969. *Social psychology and human values.* Chicago: Aldine.

Smith, M. B.; Bruner, J. S.; and White, R. W. 1956. *Opinions and personality.* New York: Wiley.

Sperry, R. W. 1952. Neurology and the mind-brain problem. *American Scientist* 40: 291–312.

Stephan, F. 1962. Possibilities and pitfalls in the measurement of attitudes and opinions on family planning. In C. V. Kiser, ed., *Research in family planning.* Princeton: Princeton University Press. Pp. 423–431.

Taiwan Institute of Family Planning. 1969. *Taiwan family planning in charts.* 3rd ed. Taichung, Taiwan.

Taylor, H. C. and Berelson, B. 1971. Comprehensive family planning based on maternal/child health services. A feasibility study for a world program. *Studies in Family Planning* 2:1–54.

Wyatt, F. 1967. Clinical notes on the motives of reproduction. *Journal of Social Issues* 23:29–56.

Yaukey, D.; Griffiths, W.; and Roberts, B. 1967. Couple concurrence and empathy on birth control motivation in Dacca, East Pakistan. *American Sociological Review* 32: 716–726.

Zatuchni, E. I., ed., 1970. *Postpartum family planning: a report on the international program.* New York: McGraw-Hill.

Zatuchni, G. 1967. International postpartum family planning program: report on the first year. *Studies in Family Planning* 22:1–23.

Zimbardo, P. and Ebbesen, E. B. 1969. *Influencing attitudes and changing behavior.* Reading, Mass.: Addison-Wesley.

[17]

BIRTH-PLANNING INCENTIVES: PSYCHOLOGICAL RESEARCH

EDWARD POHLMAN

Recent writings about population policy show sharp disagreement as to whether it will ever be desirable or necessary to influence people to want fewer children (e.g., Berelson, 1969; Callahan, 1971; Davis, 1967; Enke, 1966; Kangas, 1970; Leibenstein, 1969; Pohlman, 1971a; Ridker, 1969a; Simon, 1969). Material incentives represent one way of seeking to change family-size desires; incentives may also be used to encourage or facilitate the adoption of birth-planning methods.

There have been a number of specific proposals for research and programs involving fairly large incentives. Such proposals have been drawn up for Pakistan (Sirageldin and Hopkins, 1969), for Mauritius (Titmuss and Abel-Smith, 1968), for the United States (Leasure, 1967; Loubert, 1970; Pohlman, 1970b), and particularly for India (Balfour, 1962; Enke, 1960; Mueller, 1967; Pisharoti, 1968; Pohlman, 1967; Ravenholt, 1967; Ridker, 1969b, 1971; Simmons, 1969; Simon, 1967, 1968). General discussions of incentives are provided by Gillespie (1968), the International Planned Parenthood Federation (1969), and Pohlman (1971a). (The present chapter is derived in part from material in the monograph cited last.)

Most of those who have advocated antinatalist incentives are economists, who portray incentives as an investment for developing countries to prevent population growth from continuing to offset the nation's economic advancement. A number of economists, such as Enke (1966) and Simon (1967, 1968), have tried to estimate the value to a nation of the average "avoided birth." Benefits occurring to the society in future years from a current "nonbirth" are discounted back to the present, much as one would figure interest, but in reverse. Estimates of the "discounted value of an avoided birth" in a developing country at the time of its prevention have ranged to twice the annual per capita income in that country or even more. (For India estimates have ranged from Rs. 540 to Rs. 21,000.)

Such estimates are greatly affected by intricate economic assumptions; the approach of estimating discounted values for avoided births has been challenged by Leibenstein (1969). Simon (1970), who seems to have revised his thinking about the urgency of population problems and the need for incentives, adds other criticisms.

Some advocates of incentives (e.g., Enke, 1966) claim that incentives are merely transfer payments using up no real resources. A government taxes some to give incentives to others, but nothing is really consumed or lost. If so the estimated value of an avoided birth does not provide any limit on the amount that might logically be spent on incentives to avoid a birth. Schemes that would pay rather large incentives on a nationwide basis are not extremely expensive when compared with total national budgets, defense spending, or space exploration costs. But taxation or international aid each has its problems as a way of paying for incentives, such as inflationary tendencies in the case of aid. There have been discussions of (1) the size of incentives required to get people to act; (2) the total cost of such schemes; (3) the source of funds for these programs; and (4) the economic effects of such large-scale incentive programs (see Pohlman, 1971a, chap. 10). Conclusions in these discussions are primarily educated guesses.

The Carolina Population Center held a major conference on incentives in June 1971, attended by many of the economists who have written about incentives, by representatives of funding organizations, and by others. Few new ideas emerged, and the major function of the conference was to facilitate exchange of information and views. The gap between the huge number of schemes proposed and the almost total lack of research to test the schemes was noted. Among new developments described at the conference was the decision of Taiwan to test an educational incentive amounting to approximately twenty-five dollars toward a child's higher school work, provided total family size was not too large.

Incentives are often in a precarious situation politically, and one major reason is the belief that they are unethical. Callahan (1971) and Pohlman (1971a, chap. 12) give extensive attention to the ethics of incentives. Both agree that under certain circumstances they would be ethically justifiable, and under others they would not. There is, however, disagreement on other specific issues between these two authors.

Psychologists and Family-Size Desires

Current population programs are geared almost completely to assisting people to have the number of children they want. But if parents continue to want "too many" children for population stabilization, then even the most perfect contraception, sterilization, and abortion techniques alone will not stop population growth. Partly because of their potential for guiding policy, projections of the average number of children people in various countries will want in coming decades are extremely important. Psychologists can contribute to the research on which such projections are made. Data available to date are based primarily on surveys with unsophisticated instruments. A summary of such data (Mauldin, 1965) shows that people in most developing countries seem to want far too many children for population stabilization. Pohlman (1971a, chap. 13) reviewed factors that might be expected to make people in coming decades actually have fewer children than these surveys suggest, and factors that might have the opposite results. This review suggested the distinct possibility that parents in most developing countries will have even more children on the average than the "too many" that surveys suggest they want.

There is little more than speculation about why people do or do not want an additional child's birth, but it seems clear that "wanting" or "not wanting" a child is often a precarious decision, growing out of complex ambivalence and subject to change (Pohlman, 1965, 1968, 1969, chaps. 4–8; 1971b). Psychologists should provide research to further understanding of why children are wanted and to predict possible broad cultural shifts in family-size desires, especially in developing countries. Direct efforts to influence people to want fewer children may soon be viewed as necessary, and psychologists (along with other social scientists) may become involved in designing those efforts (Pohlman, 1970a). Sizable material incentives represent one possibility and seem to lie somewhere intermediate between the present laissez-faire emphasis on free parental choice in family size and the opposite extreme of limits governed by coercion.

The case for incentives need not rest entirely on the assumption that parents want "too many" children. Even if they do not some parents may continue to have unwanted children, especially because birth-control methods are less than perfect. If so this "excess" might need to be balanced by other people having fewer children than they would ordinarily want. Incentives might achieve this, might encourage the hesitant or indifferent to take contraceptive steps (such as sterilization) they would otherwise delay, and in other ways might speed up population limitation.

Currently there is sharp controversy about the urgency of population control and the advisability of various strategies (including incentives) for particular countries; an edited collection brings together many of these conflicting statements (Pohlman, 1972). Much of the controversy springs from differing predictions about the success of completely voluntary or laissez-faire approaches; incentives represent one alternative. For example, Davis (1967) is extremely pessimistic about the current family-planning focus. Berelson (1969) is not; in "Beyond Family Planning" he reviews numerous alternative population-limitation programs, including compulsion. Berelson's evaluation of incentives given to clients of family-planning programs is that they are of uncertain value for ethical, political, administrative, and financial reasons. I believe that this negative verdict (which was tentatively stated) should not be accepted without much more study and empirical evidence.

Psychologists may contribute to knowledge and evaluation of incentives, especially through research. Scarcely any controlled research has been done on incentives.

Definition and Conceptualization of Incentives

English and English (1958) give three definitions of *incentive*:

1. An object or external condition, perceived as capable of satisfying an aroused motive, that tends to elicit action to attain the object or condition . . .
2. A supplementary goal object that elicits behavior tending toward attainment of the main goal; anything that increases the apparent satisfyingness of a goal: e.g., offering a child a prize for conscientious study . . .
3. Any manipulatable aspect of the environment that can be used to energize and direct . . . behavior . . .

I will use a definition consistent with these but more specific: an *incentive* is something of financial value, given by an organization to an individual, couple, or group to induce some birth-planning behavior. Birth-planning behavior may include not only that of potential parents, but also the behavior of medical or paramedical personnel or helpers to induce their clients to avoid births. However, incentives to these personnel include only per-act or per-case payments, not salaries. This chapter will give attention primarily to incentives paid to potential parents.

The terms "disincentive" and "negative incentive" will be used interchangeably for something negative (e.g. taxes) imposed or something withheld in view of a birth-planning failure or the failure to produce a desired birth-planning behavior. Pronatalist incentives are those that aim to produce more babies; unless otherwise indicated *incentives* refers to antinatalist incentives. These usages are consonant with custom in family-planning and population-control discussions.

What Incentives Do

There is disagreement whether incentives influence people to want fewer children or merely prod people into taking a contraceptive step (notably sterilization) they would otherwise avoid or defer until after unwanted babies are accidentally born. The nature of the influence probably varies with individuals and subgroups and may often be a combination of the two.

We might subdivide the factors leading men to want a vasectomy into (1) factors making them want to avoid fathering more children, (2) other factors making them want to achieve the sterile state, and (3) factors making them want the operation—including incentive offers. Similarly factors leading men to want to avoid vasectomy include (4) factors making them want to father more children, (5) other factors making them want to avoid the sterile state, and (6) factors making them want to avoid the operation itself. If (3) is sufficiently strengthened it may outweigh (4). Many combinations of factors and kinds and degrees of ambivalence are thus possible. Where ambivalence is extreme and absence of formalized decisions widespread, incentives might easily push parents toward a preference for smaller families, perhaps without their realizing this, and with the "it-makes-the-bitter-method-sweeter" reasoning adopted as their rationalization.

The government of India (1968) has staunchly maintained that the small payments (typically under four dollars) to men having vasectomies are not incentives but compensations for time off from work and for travel and other expenses. This implies that men neither make nor lose money by the transaction. But of 297 Indians asked their primary motivation for vasectomy, 43 percent cited money and 38 percent a desire to limit family size (Srinivasan and Kachirayan, 1968).

The term "compensation" has public relations value, however, and it may be accurate in a much broader sense. Sons are often perceived as the key to old-age security in developing countries with no bureaucratic social security, pension, or retirement programs for rural citizens. Curtailing family size may mean the loss of vastly larger sums than the small amounts typically given men in India after vasectomies, so that even much larger incentives might be no more than partial compensation.

Incentives and Psychological Theory

Additional conceptual work relating birth-planning incentives to psychological theory and to ongoing theory-oriented empirical work is needed. Incentives for using pills, condoms, or coitus interruptus might be conceptualized as positive reinforcements strengthening the likelihood of maintaining a recurring behavior pattern. Yet in practical programs it is difficult or impossible to use incentives in relation to these acts. Sterilization incentives cannot easily be viewed as reinforcements since sterilization typically occurs only once. Incentives paid after months or years of nonpregnancy may provide reinforcement for the acts that avoided pregnancy. But at least with sterilization incentives and possibly with all birth-planning incentives, the most productive conceptualization may be in terms of cognitive factors such as perceptions and expectations. The three definitions quoted above from English and English imply such orientations.

Of particular interest to population programs is the warning of cognitive dissonance theorists that an inducement perceived as large may "produce behavioral, but not attitudinal, shifts" (Festinger, 1957). At first glance this might seem to be no obstacle in a vasectomy program; but if all men with three or more children in a hypothetical village had vasectomies but maintained a negative attitude toward incentives, this might have undesirable effects on younger men and even the next generation. A large incentive, in Festinger's view, may produce little dissonance and little attitude change, because a person can justify his change in behavior as a way of getting the attractive reward. A smaller incentive may produce more attitude change. Elms (1967) summarizes cognitive dissonance theory on this point and competing theory, notably the conveniently labeled "incentive theory" of Hovland, Janis, and Kelley (1953).

Elms reviews relevant research, some supporting cognitive dissonance theory and some showing differences in the opposite direction. In the classic Festinger and Carlsmith (1959) study Elms claims that subjects learned that the investigator told lies and were asked to help him deceive another student. Suspicion, guilt, resentment over being forced, desire to show the investigator that the subject could not be "bribed," desire to wreck carefully laid plans, and anxiety about being evaluated might have been present in studies showing large incentives less effective; all these reactions might be expected to increase with the size of incentives offered. Elms and Janis (1965) found high incentives more effective in attitude change when recipients perceived funds as coming from a "good" source (the U.S. government) and low ones more effective with a "bad" source (the Russian embassy). Factors implied in the last two paragraphs have parallels in population-control incentive programs, although it does not take psychological theory to advise administrators that suspicion or anger toward the program may block effectiveness.

As usual, research is hardly conclusive. We must be cautioned, however, against either assuming that higher incentives always produce better results or assuming from the writings of dissonance theorists that lower incentives always produce better results. Dissonance theory is best suited to a situation where there is more than one opportunity for expressions of attitude change, but sterilization does not fit this model well. Research opportunities to test cognitive dissonance theory vis-à-vis sterilization in field settings might be devised.

Past Studies and Experience

Antinatalist Incentives

There is scarcely any controlled research on incentives in population-control programs, so that in a strictly scientific sense it is difficult to prove that they have any effect or to know whether larger incentives are more or less effective than smaller ones. A few studies that approach scientific rigor deserve mention. Madras State in India seems to have been the first place in the world to introduce sterilization incentives, in May 1958. In November 1959 the scheme was extended to the whole state, the amount of the incentive was raised, and a payment to canvassers was initiated. Sterilizations in the state (mostly vasectomies) showed the following trend during selected twelve-month periods: 1956, 8,000; 1962, 50,000; 1964, 32,000; 1965, 117,000; 1966–1967, 248,000; 1967–1968, 128,000.

Canvasser incentives were abolished in 1963 because of criticisms, producing an abrupt slump, and restored in full force in late 1964, producing a sharp increase. Repetto (1968) reviews this material. In informal discussions some have implied that these data show canvasser incentives to be more important than acceptor incentives. This conclusion is not testable by the data since canvasser incentives were never used without acceptor incentives. Incentives for potential parents were in effect throughout this period.

Repetto (1967) attempted statistical analyses through regression equations, with the annual number of vasectomies regressed on (1) the amount of incentives to promoters that year, (2) a linear time trend to allow for "historical" changes, and (3) a "dummy variable." Overall results suggested that the incentive program had had a substantial impact. In the period subsequent to Repetto's research the number of vasectomies slumped in Madras, starting in early 1967. This may be explained by a "depletion of supply" theory (Pohlman, 1971a, chap. 6); if so the slump is no discredit to the success of incentives in inducing men to have vasectomies relatively early in childbearing.

May (1967) plotted sterilizations per capita and per-case incentives to doctors and promoters for each Indian state as of late 1966 and got a very high correlation between the two. But his procedure failed to control for acceptor payments and other variables, and the product-moment procedure relied heavily on Madras—high on both variables in 1966, though somewhat changed in relative position since. Also causal trends are unknown; possibly the more progressive states were most open to incentives and also to vasectomy.

Pai (1968) has claimed that Bombay had 4,000 sterilizations from 1957 to 1967 and 100,000 between July 1, 1967 and December 31, 1968, and that Bombay's registered birth rate dropped from thirty-one per 1,000 for 1967 to twenty-eight per 1,000 for 1968. It seems likely that an increase in vasectomies was caused in part by a shift from emphasizing salaries to emphasizing incentives to physicians, "helpers," and potential parents. But several other variables were not controlled, including the simultaneous introduction of sterilization procedures in railroad stations and the driving enthusiasm of Pai and his team.

A study in Seoul in which health educators recruited agents (housewives, midwives, beauty operators, kinship leaders, and the like) is reported by Kwon (1967). Agents got a small per-case incentive for IUD cases, and so did the health educators who supervised them. Monthly average acceptances per agent climbed for agents who stayed with the task. The report does not attempt to show that successes were greater than they would have been without the program. Successes were reportedly so great that funds began to run out. Between January and mid-September 1967 the program was responsible for 28 percent of IUD acceptors in Seoul.

In urban Accra gift coupons were added to the usual referral slips during the first, third, and fifth weeks of an experiment (Perkin, 1970). These could be redeemed for a tin of dry milk by coming for family-planning help. These experimental weeks proved superior to the second and fourth (control) weeks in number of referrals, proportion of referrals accepting family planning, and alacrity of acceptance. The five-week block produced more new patients than earlier or later five-week blocks. In the fifth week milk was offered to workers also, as competitive prizes for referrals; the fifth week showed best results, though this might reflect the spread of effects started earlier. Milk was chosen as something of known monetary value with obvious relevance to health.

Pronatalistic Incentives

In a small experiment Flanagan (1942) offered couples a college scholarship for any additional child who would be born in 1940. Couples had significantly more children than expected, and others reported trying unsuccessfully. Possibly these "extra" births would merely have occurred later.

Have child allowances, whether intended to boost birth rates or not, done so? Canada instituted family allowances in 1945, and birth rates rose sharply thereafter. But they fell again after about 1959 without any decrease in allowances, and the United States had a closely parallel curve without allowances. France paid relatively higher allowances than Canada and aimed to increase birth rates; there is disagreement how much and whether these allowances influenced birth rates. Italy and Sweden used allowances but birth rates continued their downward trends. A 1964 suggestion to the Permanent Committee on Family Allowances for the International Social Security Association that it study effects on birth rates was rejected: data were thought insufficient for responsible interpretation (Schorr, 1965).

The dubious effects of pronatalist incentives cannot be used to predict ineffectiveness for antinatalist incentives. In strictly economic terms pronatalist incentives are offset by the additional costs of a child (one minus one equals zero), whereas antinatalist incentives are added to the savings achieved by avoiding births (one plus one equals two). Also pronatalist incentives have typically been relatively small; many advocate much larger antinatalist incentives.

Incentives in Industry and Agriculture

In industry research on incentives is often inconclusive since incentives are introduced in combination with other innovations (Marriott, 1968). There has been little tightly controlled research to show with scientific certainty that industrial incentives do what they were intended to do. There has also been some strong opposition to incentives from workers; laying a careful groundwork of labor-management acceptance seems important. Incentive schemes seem to work well under some conditions and not under others. These points may have parallels in population incentives. Unionized, urbanized, sophisticated Western groups may tell us little, however, about Indian peasants (for example), and once-only vasectomy is very different from daily industrial production.

The Food and Agriculture Organization (1967) of the United Nations reported extensive use of agricultural incentives in many developing countries. Prices have often been supported to mold behavior toward an overall policy. Historically when laissez-faire approaches were abandoned compulsion was substituted—but has seldom proved effective. Even in communal farms planned to permit compulsion it has been necessary to augment "compulsion" with incentives. Farms are widely scattered and are in small units (in contrast to mining or manufacture), making administration difficult. Birth planning may be like agriculture; incentives may not only be more politically acceptable but also more administratively feasible than compulsion. The FAO report reviewed evidence suggesting that incentives will work even with poor and supposedly nonmaterialistic, unambitious peasants.

Independent and Dependent Variables

Independent Variables

One class of independent variables deals with what is offered as the incentive. Possibilities include cash and material goods, savings bonds or retirement bonds of various kinds, pensions, food, clothing, housing and housing materials, education benefits, agricultural supplies and equipment, radios or television, health care, employment opportunities, wedding costs or dowries, lottery-type chances on a huge prize, various government-controlled favors and priorities in such matters as government housing, education, court waiting lists, and so forth. Negative incentives primarily involve taxes. Incentives may be given to individuals, couples, extended families, castes or other subgroups, villages, residential areas, or even whole nations in the case of international aid (Kangas, 1970).

Questions about what is given as incentives include not only the form (commodity or item) but also the amount (how much cash, how many years of free schooling). In trials and initial stages of a program would it be better to start with larger incentives and then if necessary shift to smaller ones, or vice versa? Should the amount given as a vasectomy incentive be tied to family size so that, for example, the man having the operation after two children gets more than the one operated on after four?

Two programs will differ substantially if one offers incentives for female sterilization, and the other for delaying marriage. Since it is within the program's administrative control to decide what act or acts an incentive program will focus on, the type of incentive program (classed as vasectomy incentive program, child-spacing incentive program, etc.) may be considered among the independent variables to be systematically varied. (Of course, in another sense the behavioral responses for which the programs are christened are dependent variables.) The desired achievements for which incentives may be given include temporary methods such as condoms or pills, IUD's, sterilization, contraceptive implants or long-term injections, undiscovered methods, remaining unmarried or childless, older age at marriage, delaying first birth after marriage or later births, smaller total family size, education or employment of women (presumed to affect fertility indirectly), and so forth. These divide into methods and results. Ideally, controlled experiments might compare the relative merits of these approaches; in practice this is probably impossible, and the best vehicles for incentives must be chosen on the basis of experience and armchair perspectives. In view of many criteria for judging "candidates" there appear to be currently two promising prospects for large incentive schemes: sterilization, and postponement or nonpregnancy at periodic inspections

(Pohlman, 1971a, chap. 2). Long-lasting implants or injections also seem promising, but the techniques must be perfected first. IUD's can be too easily removed; some Indian women have accepted an IUD for the incentive, had it removed at a cost lower than the incentive, and then repeated the process.

What are the relative merits of offering incentives to physicians, paramedical personnel including midwives, "helpers," or agents, community leaders, administrators, potential parents or grandparents, or various combinations of these? What are the relative merits of money spent on incentives, of traditional "supplies and services" approaches, of mass-communications efforts, of better administration, or of various combinations of these? What are the value of incentives to individuals for individual achievement, to groups for group quotas in population control, to individuals for group achievements, or combinations of these? Should salaries or incentives be given to medical and other population-control helpers? Should positive or negative incentives be used? Should alternative rationales be publicized to explain why incentives were being offered? Under what circumstances, if at all, can various incentive schemes work administratively? Can fraud, bribery, and corruption be kept within ranges that are administratively, politically, and financially tolerable? What administrative and other steps may be taken to reduce these unsavory elements?

Tables 17-1 and 17-2 present schematic research designs for the most promising current "candidates" for incentives: vasectomy and nonpregnancy

TABLE 17-1

Schematic Research Design for Vasectomy Incentives[a]

	I			II			III		
	Cash			Bonds			Other forms of payment		
1. Same amount to each eligible man (no gradation by family size; no group quotas)	A	B	C[b]	A	B	C	A	B	C
2. Gradations by family size; no group quotas	A	B	C	A	B	C	A	B	C
3. Group quotas; no gradation by family size	A	B	C	A	B	C	A	B	C

[a] Each cell (for example, A of I-1) should involve several villages to neutralize idiosyncrasies of any one particular village.

[b] A, B, C: different magnitudes of incentives, large, medium, small, and so forth.

at inspection. Although Table 17-1 involves vasectomy incentives and Table 17-2 nonpregnancy incentives, the two might be interchanged with modifications. In Table 17-1 the columns compare *forms* of payment; subcells A, B, and C compare large, medium, and small *amounts*. Rows check on the possible advantages of higher incentives offered if vasectomy comes after smaller families and if higher proportions of eligible men participate. Ideally each cell should be replicated. Fragments of the table could be studied: one row, one column, one magnitude; magnitudes A, B, and C for one cell only, and so forth.

TABLE 17-2

Schematic Research Design for Non-Pregnancy Incentives[a]

Group	Incentive	Special Contraceptive Help?
Experimental 1	large	yes
Experimental 2	small	yes
Experimental 3	large	no
Control 1	none	yes
Control 2	none	no

[a]Each group should involve several villages to neutralize idiosyncrasies of any one particular village.

Dependent Variables

Dependent variables of special interest to psychologists involve the changes in attitudes and other psychological characteristics as a result of incentive schemes. In addition to simple pretest and post-test comparisons repeated sequential measurements may permit fine-grained analyses of reactions. Psychologists interested in testing cognitive dissonance theory or other theories can fit the measurement of dependent variables to these interests. Measuring changes in family-size norms and values is crucial; especially if psychologists can develop more sophisticated ways to tap such variables, they will find family-size-related attitudes of keen interest.

Other more pragmatic dependent variables are implied by these questions: Did people do what incentives aimed to get them to do, and if so in what proportions did particular subgroups respond? In schemes promoting some achievement other than contraception, what were the effects on sales, distribution, knowledge about or reported use of methods? What are the attitudes among those who accepted and refused the offer toward the offer, the method advocated (if any), and birth planning in general? What are the reactions of influential political, professional, and community leaders and of the general public? What is the extent of fraud, bribery, and corruption? What are the changes in birth rates and associated demographic indices?

Some Illustrative Hypotheses

These hypotheses serve as examples of what might be tested in research designs. Tables 17–1 and 17–2 imply some of the hypotheses: larger incentive amounts will produce more vasectomies than smaller ones within some limits; incentives tied to family size will tend to produce vasectomies after smaller families, but will be more difficult to handle administratively and will produce more political objections; incentives made larger if specified quotas join together in vasectomy will produce higher proportions having the operation; incentives are more effective than control schemes using no incentives.

It is hypothesized that as the size of incentives increases, people become motivated proportionately more by incentives and proportionately less by intrinsic desire to avoid pregnancy; hence there is more fraud and corruption and, in the case of sterilization, more regrets. The size of incentives, it is hypothesized, produces a curvilinear relationship with the effects because extremely large incentives produce more suspicion and hostility. Cash or material goods with clear cash value are predicted to be more effective than bonds, but bonds are more acceptable politically, more easily financed since payment is deferred, and less inflationary. Cash labeled as providing opportunities for existing children, it is hypothesized, will be more politically acceptable than cash simply labeled as such.

Positive incentives are likely to have more favorable public-relations effects and more overall effectiveness with low-income families. But among affluent middle and upper classes positive incentives should have relatively less appeal, and negative incentives may have greater effectiveness in avoiding births. In a given community incentives are likely to have greater impact on those with less income. Incentives made available only to the poorest groups in areas where the poorest are largely of a different race, religion, caste, or other such grouping will be criticized as prejudicial.

It is hypothesized that incentive schemes will be more effective and more politically acceptable if they arouse less suspicion and less guilt, and if they are perceived as being sponsored by a source that is viewed favorably. In developing countries, which have poor birth records, incentives for sterilization will be more administratively manageable and will probably produce less corruption and more avoided births (per money invested) than incentives for small families or nonpregnancy. In developed countries with better records incentives for nonpregnancy will be more manageable and successful than in developing countries. If sterilization becomes more reversible, sterilization incentives will reach more acceptors and reach them after fewer children than otherwise.

Eventually research should compare programs of contraceptive services and supplies, incentives with no contraceptive supplies (but perhaps contraceptive information) provided, a combination of both these programs, and controls. We hypothesize that all three of the experimental programs will be superior to the controls and that the combination will be superior to either program alone.

Since a newly introduced birth-planning program can count on a backlog of people eager to stop having children, services and information to them are crucial. Hence incentives to physicians and "helpers" are relatively more effective in the early stages of a program; those to potential parents in later stages. For the same reason a new program that starts with small incentives and moves toward larger ones will be more effective than one that follows the reverse sequence.

Research on communities in one stage may tell us little about relative merits of incentives versus services and supplies for communities at another stage. Incentives research in one country should at best lead to hypotheses, not conclusions, concerning another dissimilar culture.

Rogers (1971) suggests a typology of incentives based on seven dimensions: (1) adoption-diffusion, (2) individual-group, (3) positive-negative, (4) monetary-nonmonetary, (5) immediate-delayed, (6) graduated-nongraduated, and (7) contraception-births prevented. These and other dimensions are elaborated in Pohlman (1971a). Most of these labels are self-explanatory; "adoption-diffusion" refers to a distinction between incentives to parents (or nonparents) and to physicians and other helping personnel. This terminology is unfortunately ambiguous since incentives to parents and to "helpers" alike involve both adoption and diffusion, but Rogers' attempt to embrace incentives within his descriptions of the diffusion of innovation is valuable.

Rogers also suggests five "propositions," though granting that the empirical foundation for them is not extremely strong: (1) incentives to parents (adopters) increase "rate of adoption of an innovation by emphasizing its perceived relative advantage"; and (2) "lead to adoption . . . by different individuals than would otherwise adopt"; but (3) the "quality of such innovation decisions may be relatively low," with resulting limitations; (4) incentives to helpers ("diffusion incentives") speed adoption "by encouraging interpersonal communication about the innovation with homophilous peers"; but (5) the "quality of such adoption decisions may be relatively low, leading to undesired consequences." On the second point Rogers notes some evidence that with incentives people of the lowest income and social status may adopt the innovation first, in contrast to patterns without incentives.

Research and Reality

Incentives are a politically volatile subject in many countries; administrators and politicians fear that citizens may regard incentives as immoral or as an attempt to reduce the proportional size of certain religious, ethnic, or racial groups. Practically it would seem best to start research with incentive schemes that have the greatest likelihood of success, rather than to compare systematically all possibilities. A comparison of the scale implied by Table 17–1 or Table 17–2 may be ideal but impossible in most countries. There are many knotty problems in translating research design ideals into practical field programs. For example, countries sufficiently interested in population programs to permit research on incentives will probably have many other relevant efforts going on simultaneously with the incentives. Untangling influences of the many independent variables therefore becomes complex.

Obviously there is a need for baseline studies of attitudes, birth rates, and other dependent variables before starting the incentive study, and for control villages. But it may be difficult to assure that while control areas or villages do not get the incentive offers, they do get the same "dose" as do the experimental area or villages of the other population efforts of the national program. Some national program administrators dislike experimental control studies or other complex designs because they seem to treat humans as guinea pigs. The logic of control groups—deliberately omitting some treatment—may seem a cruel neglect to some; if incentives are good they should be offered to all or at least to all as far as the funds permit— and not in a manipulated program that systematically helps only certain groups, neglecting others.

The literature shows an unfortunate preoccupation with designing new schemes and speculating about trying them out, instead of focusing on existing incentive programs. Despite the millions of incentive payments already made in India, for example, and the sizable proportion of India's family-planning budget spent in incentives, there is virtually no controlled research. At the Carolina Population Center conference on incentives mentioned earlier, representatives of some fund-granting agencies indicated that they had little interest in supporting strictly experimental controlled research on new incentive ideas, but would be much interested in supporting analyses of existing programs.

It should be possible for researchers tactfully to gain the ear of administrators so that the two groups could cooperatively design decisive studies on the effects of India's ongoing incentive and disincentive schemes. Since the size of incentives and other aspects of their use shift every now and then for administrative or political reasons, more "natural experiments" should be possible.

Surveys and attitude studies concerning incentives have a place, especially since experiments are hard to perform. People can be asked how they think they would react if an offer were made. But the crucial test of incentive schemes is field experimentation with built-in evaluative research. The psychologist who must confine his research to a university campus may be able to contribute less to the understanding of incentives than one who can participate in controlled field experiments.

REFERENCES

Balfour, M. C. 1962. *A scheme for rewarding successful family planners.* New York: The Population Council (mimeo).

Berelson, B. 1969. Beyond family planning. *Studies in Family Planning* 38:1–4.

Callahan, D. 1971. *Ethics and population limitation.* New York: The Population Council.

Davis, K. 1967. Population policy: will current programs succeed? *Science* 68:132–148.

Elms, A. C. 1967. Role playing, incentive, and dissonance. *Psychological Bulletin* 68: 132–148.

Elms, A. C. and Janis, I. L. 1965. Counter-norm attitudes induced by consonant versus dissonant conditions of role-playing. *Journal of Experimental Research in Personality* 1:50–60.

English, H. B. and English, A. C. 1958. *A comprehensive dictionary of psychological and psychoanalytical terms.* New York: McKay.

Enke, S. 1960. The gains to India from population control: some money measures and incentive schemes. *Review of Economics and Statistics* 42:175–181.

————. 1966. The economic aspects of slowing population growth. *Economics Journal* 76:44–56.

FAO. 1967. Incentives and disincentives for farmers in developing countries. In *The state of food and agriculture.* Rome: Food and Agriculture Organization. Pp. 75–117.

Festinger, L. 1957. *A theory of cognitive dissonance.* Stanford: Stanford University Press.

Festinger, L. and Carlsmith, J. M. 1959. Cognitive consequences of forced compliance. *Journal of Abnormal and Social Psychology* 58:203–210.

Flanagan, J. C. 1942. A study of factors determining family size in a selected professional group. *Genetic Psychology Monographs* 25:3–99.

Gillespie, R. W. 1968. *Economic incentives in family planning programs.* New York: The Population Council (mimeo).

Government of India. 1968. *Small family norm committee report.* New Delhi: Government of India.

Hovland, C. I.; Janis, I. L.; and Kelley, H. H. 1953. *Communication and persuasion.* New Haven: Yale University Press.

International Planned Parenthood Federation. 1969. *Incentive payments.* Working paper no. 4. London.

Kangas, L. W. 1970. Integrated incentives for fertility control. *Science* 169:1278–1283.

Kwon, E. H. 1967. *Use of the agent-system in Seoul.* New York: The Population Council (mimeo).

Leasure, J. W. 1967. Some economic benefits of birth prevention. *Milbank Memorial Fund Quarterly* 45:417–425.

Leibenstein, H. 1969. Pitfalls in benefit-cost analysis of birth prevention. *Population Studies* 23:161–170. See also 24:115–119.

Loubert, J. D. 1970. A national family support program (NFSP). Bethesda, Md.: Trans-Cultural Research Company (mimeo).

Marriott, R. 1968. *Incentives payment systems: a review of research and opinion.* 3rd ed. London: Staples Press.

Mauldin, W. P. 1965. Application of survey techniques to fertility studies. In M. C. Sheps and J. C. Ridley, eds., *Public health and population changes: current research issues.* Pittsburgh: University of Pittsburgh Press.

May, D. 1967. *Strategy for family planning in India.* Cambridge, Mass.: Harvard University Press.

Mueller, Eva. 1967. *Incentive payments for family planning.* New Delhi: AID (mimeo).

Pai, D. N. 1968. The great experiment. *Sukhi Sansar* 1:12–14.

Perkin, G. 1970. Non-monetary commodity incentives in family planning programs. *Studies in Family Planning,* no. 57:12–15.

Pisharoti, K. A. 1968. *Community incentives for population control in India: design and evaluation of a project.* A scheme proposed by the Institute of Rural Health and Family Planning, Gandhigram, India, in collaboration with the Carolina Population Center (mimeo).

Pohlman, E. 1965. "Wanted" and "unwanted": toward less ambiguous definition. *Eugenics Quarterly* 12:19–27.

———. 1967. *Incentives in population control: research in new directions in India* (mimeo).

———. 1968. Changes from rejection to acceptance of pregnancy. *Social Science and Medicine* 2:337–340.

———. 1969. *The psychology of birth planning.* Cambridge, Mass.: Schenkman.

———. 1970a. *Influencing people to want fewer children.* Paper presented at American Psychological Association convention, Miami, September 4, 1970.

———. 1970b. *Experiments and data on incentives: a project proposal.* Stockton, Calif.: University of the Pacific (mimeo).

———. 1971a. *Incentives and compensations in population programs.* Chapel Hill: Carolina Population Center Monograph Series, no. 11.

———. 1971b. Children born after denial of abortion requests. In S. H. Newman, M. B. Beck and S. Lewit eds., *Abortion obtained and denied: research approaches.* New York: The Population Council, 1971. Pp. 59–73.

———, ed. 1972. *Population: two sides.* New York: New American Library.

Pohlman, E. and Rao, S. 1967. Children, teachers and parents view birth planning. New Delhi: Central Family Planning Institute Monograph Series, no. 14.

Ravenholt, R. T. 1967. *Baltimore Sun,* May 2, 1967. Quoted as part of a speech by Senator Gruening, *Congressional Record-Senate,* S6215, May 2, 1967.

Repetto, R. 1967. *Temporal elements of Indian development.* Cambridge, Mass.: Harvard University, Ph.D. diss. Chap. 5.

———. 1968. A case study of the Madras vasectomy program. *Studies in Family Planning* 31:8–16. (Condensed from Repetto, 1967.)

Ridker, R. G. 1969a. *A proposal for a family planning bond.* New Delhi: AID. Portions later adapted as Ridker, 1969b.

———. 1969b. Desired family size and the efficacy of current family planning programmes. *Population Studies* 23:279–284.

———. 1971. Savings accounts for family planning. *Studies in Family Planning,* 2:150–152.

Rogers, E. M. 1971. Incentives in the diffusion of family planning innovations. *Studies in Family Planning* 2:241–248.

Schorr, A. 1965. Income maintenance and the birth rate. *Social Security Bulletin,* December 2–10, 1965.

Simmons, G. B. 1969. *The Indian investment in family planning.* Unpublished Ph.D. diss., University of California, Berkeley.

Simon, J. L. 1967. *Money incentives to reduce birth rates in low-income countries: a proposal to determine the effect experimentally.* Urbana: University of Illinois.

———. 1968. The role of bonuses and persuasive propaganda in the reduction of birth rates. *Economic Development and Cultural Change* 16:404–411.

———. 1969. The value of avoided births to underdeveloped countries. *Population Studies* 23:61.

————. 1970. *Should family size be regulated by law? Or, Science does not show that there is overpopulation.* Urbana: University of Illinois Press (mimeo).

Sirageldin, I. and Hopkins, S. 1969. *Proposal for a pilot project to test an economic approach to the promotion of family planning in developing nations.* Baltimore: Johns Hopkins University (mimeo).

Srinivasan, K. and Kachirayan, M. 1968. Vasectomy follow-up study: findings and implications. *Institute of Rural Health and Family Planning Bulletin* (Gandhigram) 3: 13–32.

Titmuss, R. M. and Abel-Smith, B. 1968. *Social policies and population growth in Maritius.* London: Frank Cass.

Part VII

Training for Psychological Aspects of Population

[18]

INTRODUCING POPULATION INTO A PSYCHOLOGY CURRICULUM: A CHALLENGE FOR PSYCHOLOGISTS

VAIDA THOMPSON,
MARK APPELBAUM,
AND JOHN HOLMES

The Noninvolvement Dilemma

Have you ever wanted to develop a course, a curriculum, or a research project relating to population, but felt reluctant to try? Why should such a venture be so different from all the others psychologists undertake? People have been known to embark on a new course or research project after hearing one good paper session at a convention or after reading a few conflicting research reports in the literature. Why then in the field of population is psychology the reluctant virgin?

Perhaps as approached in the past and as presented in the more generally accessible journals (such as *Science*), the population problem seems to belong to other disciplines: for example, to demography, economics, political science, or the biological sciences. The major references by members of other disciplines to psychological aspects of population tend to deal with seemingly dismal failures in earlier attempts to determine psychological correlates or predictors of reproductive behavior.

When scholars, our own among them, question psychological contributions those of us interested in population must decide whether to agree with them and stay out or to feel challenged and forge ahead. Let us suppose that one does choose to attack the problem, because of interest, of conviction, or of the challenge. We could begin by going back and examining the psychological contributions that have been deplored. If we do this we should be reassured by our observations that such studies have not really been psychological studies; the atheoretical approaches, the methodologies, the analyses, and even the interpretations that we observe in such studies do not strongly reflect a psychologist's *modus operandi*. However, even so assured, the potential difficulties in becoming involved in population are still numerous.

One inhibiting factor is no doubt the image of population derived from the accessible literature. Some psychologists indeed view population as a "problem"—but principally a matter demanding governmental policy and control. Others more clearly perceive it to be a problem deserving scientific consideration—but by disciplines other than psychology. In the same way that many psychologists assiduously avoid a scientific focus on other social problems, their recognition of the need for research relative to the population problem does not engender the awareness that psychologists possess unique skills, methodologies, and theoretical frameworks by means of which basic and crucial population questions could be considered. Such a misperception is no doubt abetted in part by the professional training of the psychologist.

Psychologists on the whole are highly trained specialists in rather discrete areas of psychology: operant conditioning with lower organisms, scaling techniques, small group research, and so on. In all such areas psychologists have developed their skills in rigorous programs geared predominantly toward highly controlled laboratory experiments. Neither the programs nor the majority of scholars produced are geared toward theoretical or experimental consideration of such vast real-world problems as population growth. This is not to deny that individual psychologists or groups of psychologists are not concerned with applying their knowledge and techniques to real-world problems; the entire Society for the Psychological Study of Social Issues, the recent text on *Psychology and the Problems of Society* (Korten, Cook, and Lacey, 1970), Abelson and Zimbardo's recent manual for peace canvassers (1970), and texts such as Evans and Rozelle's *Social Psychology in Life* (1970) or Baughman and Dahlstrom's award-winning contribution *Negro and White Children* (1968) are just a few examples that represent psychologists' interests in nonlaboratory problems. The major point is that programs in psychology are not often directed toward a major focus on such real-world considerations.

In a recent survey Driver[1] (personal communication) found that the majority of psychology departments he contacted did not have population programs as a major or a minor focus and did not see the relevance of such a focus in psychology. Given the understandable emphasis on the

[1] Edwin D. Driver, University of Massachusetts.

development of expertise in a chosen area of psychology and the existing lack of training in population (as in other real-world problem areas), it is not surprising that most graduates of psychology programs do not choose to explore or, if interested, do not have the means (from their perspective) of contributing to an analysis of population issues. It is equally understandable that many departments would no doubt be averse to incorporating population as a major focus of study; a program largely directed toward such a broad problem might realistically be seen as preventing the development of essential specialized disciplinary expertise. However, the development of psychological skills, even within a fairly narrow area of psychology, may ultimately be the most useful framework for approaching population problems. The population field may benefit more from engaging the interests of a large variety of trained specialists than it would from a vast corps of population generalists.

Even given the improbability that numerous psychologists would voluntarily become immersed in research or teaching in population, there are obviously many who are attracted to the problem and at least some who are deeply involved. Several interesting observations may be made about the way psychologists do become involved. The Director of the Carolina Population Center, for example, has noted that psychologists do not seem to pick up some theoretical or research problem in population as they would other problems they encounter in their field; rather, they tend almost to leave their disciplinary expertise behind and to become involved in massive educational or action programs requiring methodologies with which psychologists are less familiar. A similar observation could be made by an observer of gatherings of psychologists who are deeply committed to the need for psychological involvement in population. Some persons with obviously deep convictions that psychology should turn its attention to population seem more caught up with the immense overall problem, and with their convictions, than with reasoned suggestions about how psychologists with diverse interests might proceed toward meaningful contributions. Few of us would become emotionally involved, to the point of missionary zeal and mass proselytizing, with our usual research and teaching ventures; such involvement in fact might be deemed completely deleterious to objectivity. Nevertheless, one might wonder if this is not in fact what is happening with many who are interested and involved in population; they wish to charge madly at the entire beast, instead of selecting some part of its anatomy and exploring it patiently, thoroughly, and scientifically, as we would with our usual scientific ventures.

These then may be our most crucial problems: we are generally not trained to explore such vast real-world problems, and when we desire to become involved we fail to approach the issues as we would if we were exploring, say, interpersonal attraction, the measurement of personality variables, or the psychophysical responses of the elderly. It is within our own areas of expertise that we can competently and profitably explore population variables, rather than in attempts to invade and conquer the entire broad and strange territory of the population field.

Many who have become aware of the possibility of contributing in an area in which they feel competent may still have a great deal of reluctance on account of a lack of knowledge of the population literature, and concomitantly of an uneasy suspicion that much of the research or theory development that could be accomplished by psychologists must already exist. It is true that within the vast array of studies and speculative writings that exists relative to population, numerous "psychological" variables have been explored or touched upon, often by scholars who either are not aware that there exists psychological theory in the area they are exploring or who perceive the concepts as belonging strictly to their own disciplines. The psychological literature certainly contains a dearth of sophisticated material (actually of any material) related to population; the *Journal of Personality and Social Psychology,* for example, has only recently published its first article presenting a specific population-related study (Insko, Blake, Cialdini, and Mulaik, 1970). In perusing the *one* recent brief survey of psychological considerations of population (Fawcett, 1970) the novice population psychologists must bear in mind that what is summarized therein represents almost the total body of psychology and population. One must conclude that there is no aspect of the psychology of human fertility (be it correlates of family size; norms of family size; effects of human crowding; attitude assessment concerning birth control or population policy; means of effecting attitude and behavior change; or whatever the psychologist's area of interest) that has been thoroughly and adequately explored. Further there is almost no genuine psychological theory relating to fertility behavior. Therefore, a psychologist should be assured that a literature search in his area of concern might reveal a few useful research reports and perhaps a little more speculation, but that there is virtually no aspect of the problem to which he might not contribute, given carefully conceptualized research or carefully derived theoretical considerations.

Even believing this to be so, we would see the problem still in some lines from Tennyson's *Ulysses:*

> . . . yet all experience is an arch wherethrough
> gleams that untravelled world whose margin
> fades for ever and for ever when I move.

We certainly may possess the expertise, and the population field is there waiting for us to apply our skills, but as we approach it, our own ways of believing and doing within our field may block us from the application we envision. Even more true, perhaps, we may almost have an approach in our grasp only to lose it when we attempt to actualize it.

What we may have misperceived or failed to facilitate is the interest that students, graduates and undergraduates both, have in the problems of population. These students are learning that the aim of psychology is to explain, predict, and control behavior. Many are already eager to focus on behaviors related to family size and population growth. Perhaps we ourselves cannot quite shift to this new realm. However, in responding to student interests and demands we might yet produce a psychological focus on the problems by students whose skills as psychologists have been developed in a framework in which understanding and coping with real-world problems is a part of a program's goal. One might well ask, of course, how then if we can't shift our gears toward research in the population field, can we shift our teaching gears? The answer may lie in the readiness and even the demand of students to explore population from any angle—the survey course in population, the societal problems course, the measurements course, and so on. Because of their readiness we may easily develop courses in which we and our students can together learn and benefit from a psychological focus on population. Or if we examine the content of more traditional courses, and at the same time abandon our concern that we must cover the entire population field, we may find that we are much like Molière's gentleman; in our courses on early development, in our applications of social psychology, or whatever our focus, we may have been speaking about population all our academic lives.

For the remainder of this chapter let us look at some of the possibilities for teaching population in a psychology curriculum. It is not our intention that the reader seize upon one of our topics or suggested formats, nor do we propose to include an exhaustive list of possible courses. Rather, it is our hope that through our considerations those who have been eager to develop a course or a curriculum will perceive that they may already have the material at hand; better still, we would hope that each reader who desires to teach a course may find that he can develop a course or a curriculum that is superior to any we may have suggested.

From Zero to Less Than Zero Focus on
Population in the Psychology Curriculum

One-Shot Courses

Suppose someone interested in the population problem has sampled the population literature and is determined to take the first step toward introducing population into the psychology curriculum. As we see it, there are three possible one-course formats, two of which have more commonly been used. The first format is a general broad-based course that surveys the entire population field; the second, a course in which psychological theory structures the course content; and the third, a course in which a specific project structures both the theoretical considerations and the course content. Let us consider each of these in turn and then refer to examples of the various approaches.

The survey course in population offered by a psychologist would differ little in content or approach from one offered by a member of any other discipline. Essentially the focus would be the population field, and an attempt would be made to familiarize the student with diverse considerations of population and research approaches dealing with population. The flavor of the course would no doubt reflect a disciplinary interest; just as the anthropologist might focus on cultural aspects, the psychologist might focus more heavily on psychological approaches and issues in the population realm. Nevertheless, the intent of such a course would be to familiarize the student with the field of population, that is, to provide him with a general base of knowledge concerning what is going on in population.

In the theory-related content course there would be an initial (necessarily more cursory) consideration of population issues; then the course would become essentially cyclical though aiming toward a specific goal. The cyclical aspect would result from a repeated movement from (1) an introduction to psychological theory to (2) a consideration of its utility in application to or as characterization of population phenomena to (3) an introduction of other psychological theory. The ultimate goal of the course would be the generation of specific psychological theories of population or of reproductive behavior. Because a psychologist's *modus operandi* entails constant movement from basic theory relating to human behavior to research testing of the theory to expansion or modification of the model, the theory-originating, theory-generating approach would necessarily incorporate considerations of theory testing. However, the basic aim, in terms of student and instructor goals, would be principally to apply and develop theory, rather than to focus on methodological considerations and research development. Thus the final student product for such a course would most appropriately be a paper in which the student applied psychological theory to reproductive behaviors or population issues, rather than a research design per se. Nevertheless, one might well question one's success *if* students did not perceive the need and possibilities for research testing of the theory developed.

The third approach, that of a specific project dictating content and theory, would entail a movement from student effort (e.g., a proposal for a research project) to a provision by the instructor (or others) of necessary methodological and theoretical considerations to a final product—a behavioral outcome. Again, the typical approach in such a course would be an initial brief consideration of selected population issues followed by a charge to *produce* something. The product might be the same for the entire class, or it might be an individual or subgroup effort. Whatever the level of the student (freshman undergraduate through advanced graduate) the goals might conceivably vary from lab experiments to field experiments to community action programs geared toward social change.

Although we have presented the three possible courses in a specific order, we do *not* perceive the ordering in terms of appropriateness or desired outcomes. Rather, our ordering reflects more our view of the three as a hierarchy; given that one were planning a series of courses, we would see the need for moving from the survey course to the theory-generating course to the behavioral outcome course. However, given that one were able to provide *one* and *only one* course, we suggest the second alternative—the theory-generating course. Our reasoning is that from such a course the student could move backward toward the broad issues (perhaps under his own initiative) and forward toward research. It would probably be a more difficult and more frustrating experience for the student to attempt to move from the survey course to the theory and research level or from a behavioral outcome course to the more sophisticated theoretical level. Thus the survey course (particularly if very broad) may lead to a dead end in terms of channeling the student toward a psychological orientation, while the outcome-oriented course, standing alone, may not provide the theoretical depth essential for continued psychological exploration of population variables.

While we propose a hierarchy and conclude that a theory-generating course might be the most fruitful, we realize that the novice in population must begin wherever he sees the beginning to be. If we consider some "one-shot" efforts (our own included) we can see a diversity of approaches, each no doubt evolving both circumstantially and in accord with the instructor's perception of the best means to achieve his goal of introducing or integrating psychology and population.

If we can generalize from responses to a questionnaire distributed by the American Psychological Association Task Force on Population and from answers to requests for information placed by us, it would seem that a fairly common beginning is some broad survey or reading course in population. In such a course students sample readings of immeasurable diversity: population theory; economic considerations in population; political considerations; religious considerations—ad infinitum. Students then select topics, delve deeply, and produce oral and written reports.

Two things should be noted about such a broad-based course. First, if truly a population survey course the format does not demand that a psychologist be an instructor. Because the psychologist may not have the necessary background, it is thus open to question whether his greatest contribution *is* in the broad survey course. Second, there is an obvious danger in such a course. Students may become aroused zealots convinced that something must be done, but they may not even be close to tackling population as a psychological problem.

The psychologist who is aware of the problems inherent in a broad population survey course may attempt to avoid these by developing variants of the reading-discussion-report class that should both avoid the hazards of a blind alley and also lead the student toward psychological concerns. While our second alternative (theory suggests content) might well emerge as a possibility, it would seem that a population-problem orientation, rather than a psychological-theory orientation, has more frequently been adopted. That is, the course content appears to be a more narrow survey of population problems with a focus on issues that seem more salient to and more demanding of psychological consideration. For example, the focus may be on such things as: studies of attitudes toward family size, contraception, abortion, policy, and the like; nutritional problems; family-planning services; demographic factors that influence fertility; human crowding; correlates of family size; or contraception and abortion counseling. Indeed, such topics are legitimate concerns of psychologists. Further, a focus on such topics is no doubt preferable to the broader population survey course and more in the realm of psychologists. While such courses appear to be more survey than theoretical in nature, their adequacy depends on the degree to which they engender or expedite an explicit psychological orientation.

Although we do not know of an example of the type of course that we felt might be most productive (theory motivating content), we have seen several attempts to accomplish the third type of basic course (outcome determines theory and content). Perhaps the best example is that of Buckhout (see Sanford, 1970). The intent of the course appeared to be to guide students toward *doing* something related to population and psychology. To quote from the description of the course:

> The class (of eighteen students) focused on the population explosion as a societal issue which integrated the class efforts to learn how to do relevant psychological research. This time the goal of a published *article* was set, with all students sharing in the conception and execution of the research—and its authorship. A stratified sample survey of attitudes toward family planning, sterilization, and abortion was conducted on unmarried young people. In this case, undergraduates had to learn interviewing techniques, computer analysis, statistics, and the population literature from other students and faculty. The point was that in order to say something useful about the social problem—population—it was necessary to acquire rapidly the usual skills of social scientists. In addition, the students had to learn to communicate their topical findings in a way which would maximize their social utility—an elusive and somewhat unique skill for social scientists.

Because we have attempted similar courses we have some mixed feelings about the adequacy of such a course as a preliminary venture in psychology and population. Such a course is fun and stimulating but *hard* to supervise. Moreover, for students with no background in population and research one semester seems inadequate for such a course. As we noted earlier, it seems that some introduction to population issues and to research methods and theory may be essential before students can embark on a manageable research venture. Subsequently, though they may be guided at every stage of design and analysis, time may prohibit their doing other than a relatively simple and superficial project (unless the research pertains more specifically to a single aspect of the adviser's research, which then negates the student-origination goal). While students may enjoy the course they may perceive their somewhat simple and superficial approach as an adequate foundation and guide for pursuing research questions, yet they may not perceive their need for greater theoretical and research development.

We would like to stress that our conclusions concerning the most appropriate course (given that only one can be offered) or hierarchy of courses have evolved from our own experiences with courses in psychology and population on the graduate and undergraduate level. An undergraduate course, conducted by the senior author and an advanced graduate student, actually moved through all three levels of the hierarchy previously described. It began as a broad survey of population. Upon perceiving that we were drifting into stimulating and provocative discussions about the nature of the problem, we moved toward the second level, having students read theories concerning attitudes, norms, social comparison, bargaining, and so forth, and then attempting to apply these to reproductive behaviors. Finally, yielding principally to student interests in learning what students on campus "really thought" about family size, we continued the course for a second semester, during which the students were supervised in developing, administering, and analyzing a preliminary survey instrument and ultimately a Rosenberg-type instrument (similar to that used by Insko et al., 1970) focusing on attitudes and values associated with desired family size.

Immediately following the course, we felt very gratified with the students' involvement and with both their accomplishments and comprehension relative to one crucial aspect of population—family size and its determinants. However, our *post hoc* evaluations and our subsequent experiences suggest to us that the research accomplishments in themselves were not the major advantages. Research experiences did not provide the students with as much depth and breadth concerning psychological aspects of population as did the more theoretically derived considerations; it was the latter that appeared to provide the impetus for extended and in-depth consideration of population issues.

On the graduate level our first seminar (conducted by the senior author, a staff member in experimental psychology, and a visiting social psychologist from India) was intended principally as a theory-application, theory-generation course. Students were to focus on population issues from the standpoint of their own area of interest and expertise. At the students' request (because they did not feel well enough informed about the population field and the diverse approaches to it) much of the initial reading material for the course was a sampling of various aspects of the population field: population theory, demographic considerations, food and environment issues, economic considerations, and so on. The remainder of the readings were specifically oriented toward psychological issues and studies. For example, when studies of attitudes were discussed a wide range of approaches, from the traditional KAP studies to the more recent (and more sophisticated) psychological approaches of Crawford, Heredia, and Stocker (1968) and Insko et al. (1970), were included. In conjunction with readings about research in population theoretical and methodological papers from the psychological literature (e.g., by psychologists dealing with attitude theory and measurement) were included where useful. In dealing with field research, population studies in which social psychologists were involved were included. As the course progressed, it was suggested to students that they should be able to come up with a researchable group project or with individual or subgroup proposals.

In evaluating the course we found we certainly could not rate the course itself as A+ in all its aspects. Looking at the triadic approach we no doubt succeeded most in turning students' attention toward researchable population proposals. The more broad survey aspects were no doubt informative and useful; however, even with advanced graduate students, application of psychological theory or consideration of possible psychological interpretations of population issues did not spontaneously emerge. In fact we perceived anew the problems intrinsic in attempting to convey substantive background information concerning population; diffuse and opinionated responses were more likely to emerge than were counterchallenges and analyses couched in the theoretical or methodological frameworks of the participants. The theory that was applied emerged principally from the social-psychology realm; for example, viewing attitudes toward reproduction, the need to study these attitudes, and the perceived lack of focus on them from extant attitude and theoretical frameworks became a predominant focus of the course. As the social-psychology students began to move toward researchable ideas, they tended to propose research on attitudes as predictors of behavior and thus further enhanced the focus on attitude theories and methods of measurement. Again, we must note that psychological theoretical considerations and application of these considerations to population issues did not often spontaneously emerge, as we would have anticipated they would in this more sophisticated group. This suggests to us that in the somewhat foreign field of population, with its dearth of psychological concepts, the charge of the instructor is more appropriately that of directing a cyclical focus on psychological theory, then moving to the application of such theory to population issues, and then on to the development of psychological theory of reproductive behavior.

We should note that we were not disappointed with student-generated research on this level. We found that as the students oriented more toward researchable ideas, there was also a move toward operational understanding of the diffuse and speculative issues. In approaching their research designs students found themselves faced with the same problems many psychologists have encountered: they perceived the mammoth, threatening beast and were convinced that psychologists should become involved, but they found themselves flirting with massive educational programs rather than with manageable research problems. It was thus quite pleasing in the end to receive some highly sophisticated research proposals (e.g., in the measurement of family-size norms with a goal of predicting actual behavior, and in crowding research focusing on variables of concern to social psychologists) and some more general proposals for research or teaching within a given area (as dyadic decision-making as it relates to family size and spacing).

More Subtle Solutions: Substantive Courses with Population a Referent

So we offer that *one* basic course, and we get the demand (or see the need) for one more course focusing on population. Because of the typical orientation of most psychology departments, it is possible that we might be able to add just one course or a hodgepodge of unrelated courses. There is no reason at this point to deplore either alternative. A glance at many undergraduate and graduate psychology bulletins should convince us that many minor and even major programs are indeed made up of an apparent hodgepodge of courses seemingly derived as much from the interests of the staff as from a search for a well-ordered and comprehensive curriculum. If we have the interest most of us could no doubt add one more course, or one part to an extant course, concerning population. Such a contribution might seem small, particularly if we are eager for a comprehensive focus on population. However, we should consider that even one section of one course in social problems or contemporary trends or psycholinguistics, wherever we might fit it in, would be better than nothing at all; we should also consider just one course with a specific focus on some aspect of psychology and population as better than that. Again, however, if we are excitedly concerned with the overall "population problem" we may not see the means of producing courses, or parts of courses, that focus on one aspect of the problem. Even worse, whether true or not, we may feel that our particular program has no room for or would not condone a population course. Should this be the case, there are certainly very subtle ways of introducing population issues into our content courses.

One easy way that one of us (Appelbaum) has found to incorporate a focus on population into a course (in the absence of a basic course in psychology and population) is to treat population as a real-life problem to be considered as part of the basic general introductory course in psychology. Most basic courses have some room for picking a social problem to consider from the standpoint of the diverse concepts touched upon in the introductory course. The focus might be brief, and the student might not be advanced enough to apply thoroughly diverse concepts, but as a topic that will engage the interest of young students, our experiences have shown us that population is high on the list. True again, the focus may be more emotional than rational, and the students may approach the topic with the urgency for doing something, but with some maneuvering the instructor can nudge them toward more astute observations, particularly if they themselves have some concern with the issues involved.

Just as easily population could be incorporated in a "social problems" course subsequent to a basic course in social psychology. Since the basic course often has a more experimental laboratory approach, the social problems course can be used to apply the theories and experimental findings to diverse issues: ghetto problems, learning problems, campus unrest, racial issues, poverty—and population. Again, in such a course term papers that relate basic social-psychological theory to population might be a most fruitful goal.

Perhaps a less obvious, but potentially applicable, area for the inclusion of population topics as referent materials is in quantitative psychology, particularly in those courses dealing with game theory and mathematical models of human decisions. It must be remembered, however, that the usual objective of these courses is an understanding of the theory of rational interactive behaviors as formulated in mathematical models (the psychological variables contributing to decisions or the process of decision-making usually being in the domain of the social psychologist). Thus the inclusion of population topics would perhaps also require a limited extension of the usual scope of these courses, but this could be achieved without disturbing their basic focus or purpose.

While the current applications of games and decision theory in population per se are limited (Kahan, 1970), there are a number of works on the application of these areas to the more general area of social psychology, particularly research into interpersonal behavioral exchange (e.g., Gergen, 1969) and dyadic and N-person decision processes (e.g., Rapoport, 1970). These works should provide abundant materials for exploring population topics in terms of mathematical models, particularly if one is willing to conceive of reproductive behavior as a dyadic game or to approach population policy-making in terms of a large-scale Prisoner's Dilemma.

Perhaps the most subtle of all approaches (and one that, it would be our hunch, most of us already use) is that of making population our referent in residence. In developmental courses, for example, we may have a specific focus on such issues as density and the effects of early experiences, both of concern to populationists; but aren't there a diversity of topics (such as family size and sex composition and sex-role behaviors) that could be focused upon in such courses? Isn't comparative psychology replete with opportunities for considering population issues across species—including man? When we're dealing with the biological and physiological bases of human behavior, aren't there numerous fruitful focuses for considering issues that are relevant to population? And what about personality—can't one consider diverse theories (as has Wyatt, 1967) in terms of reproductive behaviors? Where, indeed, if we are dealing with human behavior, could we not introduce population issues as part of our core content or as a referent for extrapolation from our laboratory findings?

It would seem to be easiest and quite appropriate to introduce population considerations into courses in social psychology. When social psychology is taught by psychologists the research orientation generally defines his focus, so that the content tends to be experimental laboratory research. Despite the potential relevance and importance of the diverse concepts and the research directed at tests of these concepts, many students leave a typical undergraduate course in social psychology with the observation that the material is interesting but not "relevant." Even granted that many of our research findings cannot be generalized to real-life situations, given the demand for relevance and our desire to encourage a population focus, why not satisfy these dual needs by using population as a running referent, at least for classroom discussions?

Without attempting an exhaustive list of possibilities let's describe roughly how population might be a fitting referent. First, we could begin such a course as Zimbardo and Ebbesen (1969) begin their small book on attitudes. For example, we might ask as they do: "What if you . . . were hired to change people's attitudes toward birth control? . . . Let us assume that you are being hired to design a program for solving problems, such as promoting birth control. . . ." Such a beginning should prepare the student to be concerned with this and other real-life matters. Subsequently, as diverse and often complex theories are dealt with, a variant of the original question might aid the student in seeing that the theory is not just esoteric jargon but has meaning in terms of real-world topics. Obviously not all of the topics we focus on in social psychology readily lend themselves to a consideration of contraceptive or family-planning behavior. But what about such topics as: the development and maintenance of attitudes; methods of attitude measurement; approaches to attitude and behavior change, including communications; the importance of comparison and reference groups in developing and maintaining the diverse spectrum from attitudes to beliefs and emotions; concepts of social pressure and social influence; personal causation; motivation (as affiliation); small-group phenomena as they relate to persistence or change of attitudes; dyadic bargaining situations; norms? Ad infinitum, the skilled instructor who so desires could bring the students back to that common referent by asking: how would you look at and try to influence reproductive behavior from the standpoint of these concepts, these research findings, or this particular methodology? One of the writers has attempted this rather pervasive referent and has found that undergraduate students in particular understand such things as the attitude-change paradigms or models of attitudes better if they have been presented in such a format; they also seem better able to generalize such theories to other problems (such as drug usage or attitudes toward the Vietnam war) than if they are presented solely in terms of cold hard theory or research findings.

A Direct Attack: Make No Mistake, This Is a Course in . . .

But can you really develop courses that are presented as population *and* psychology courses—courses in which the student interested in population can learn how to look at or deal with the psychological aspects of the problem? Some of the broader courses cited above should meet this criterion. Surely other courses could be developed that would do this. Many persons now offer courses at the graduate level that focus on such things as human sexuality, the psychology of women, the psychology of reproductive behavior, and human crowding phenomena. While it seems most likely that such courses are offered subsequent to the basic course, an ingenious instructor might be able to develop courses in population that could serve as the basic course within a content area. We would like to offer a few examples of possible courses that might conceivably be a first or subsequent course. In offering examples, it should be noted, we are not attempting to be exhaustive, and we are obviously influenced by our own areas of interest. We are not in any case attempting to provide a complete listing of course material, since we feel that such extensive considerations would be useful only to someone interested in the specific kinds of courses we are describing. We realize that the content of a course must be determined by the individual instructor, and that such content is largely directed by professional interests and technical expertise gained in psychology and not in population. Thus we are providing general formats principally with the hope that they might aid in generating course ideas, rather than that they serve as models.

Social Psychology of Population

Because there are obviously many social-psychological phenomena that are applicable in considerations of reproductive behavior, an instructive approach would be to attempt to develop a course in the "social psychology of reproductive behavior." Since students in and out of psychology have shown strong interest in both relevancy and focus on real-world problems, such a course should serve as an exemplar for deriving courses in other more applied areas. It would indeed be quite a challenge to try to focus on the development of theory and research related to population and at the same time to really get across the important social-psychological concepts and research findings. In developing and conducting such a course one would not be able to cling tightly to traditional social-psychological approaches and yet one could not leave them far behind. While an experimental laboratory approach might receive less focus, an important goal would still be to convey salient and important theoretical concepts without distortion. Such a course would be a more specific example of the nature of our suggested "theory motivates content" approach in that it would be social-psychological theories that would be presented and from which population issues would be considered.

Again, all social-psychological theories and related research findings do not immediately lend themselves to application to population issues. One might include ill-fitting concepts anyway and wonder with the students why they are not applicable. If we are indeed trying to understand, predict, and control behavior, and we fall short, perhaps we need to examine our theories and research and not the target problem we are trying to consider.

In broad outline the format perhaps would be an overt version of the more subtle referent format focused on earlier. However, it should be perfectly clear that our underlying topic was population and that we were trying to see it from a social-psychological perspective. In the introductory section an approach such as that in Zimbardo and Ebbesen's (1969) first chapter might again be utilized to underscore the fact that we are establishing a set for the constant application of psychological concepts with the final goal of developing theory and research suggestions applicable to population.

We might follow this up with a focus on research methodology (field studies and experiments, laboratory experiments, and the like) presenting, where available, some examples of population-focused research utilizing the various approaches. Here, for example, the Hill, Stycos, and Back studies (cf., 1959), KAP surveys, and broad mass-communication experiments, such as the Udry and Blake[2] study on advertising effectiveness in influencing contraceptive behavior (in progress), could be introduced. The correlational, as opposed to the experimental, approach could be explored, with a stress on the importance of control, prediction, and causality in the experimental method. We could examine the many population studies that have used the correlational method (as the innumerable ones concerning family size and its correlates) and could question with our students the dearth of truly experimental or controlled studies.

As we moved into attitude-value theories and measurement, theories could be presented with contraception and family size as referents. The studies by Insko et al. (1970) and Crawford et al. (1968) could be reviewed as research examples of the Rosenberg (1956) model and as a demonstration of the utility of consistency models in examining population questions. In viewing attitude measurement Kothandapani's (1971) dissertation research, in which diverse measurement techniques (Semantic Differential, Likert, Thurstone, Guttman, and Guilford techniques) were used to focus upon the components of attitudes related to contraception, could provide both an excellent view of possible research approaches and at the same time a deeper understanding of the scaling methods *and* components of attitudes.

[2] J. R. Udry and R. R. Blake, An evaluation of the effect of a mass media program on fertility and fertility behavior, Department of Maternal and Child Health, School of Public Health, University of North Carolina, in progress.

In dealing with the development, maintenance, and change of attitudes, we could bring in population research that attempts to apply concepts of reference and comparison groups (e.g., Freedman, 1963), peer and other social influence, and social comparison processes as they relate to research on family-size norms. Conformity might also be an important process to consider in relation to family-size norms. Concerning actual attempts to change attitudes, we may find few adequate population-related examples; we could, however, attempt to generate research ideas on the basis of findings about the nature of the communicator and the communication, fear-arousal approaches, and behavioral change followed by attitude change in dissonance, self-persuasion, or other theoretical research paradigms.

Norms and normative behavior should occupy a certain prominent position in our approach; surely there is a plethora of population-related research in this area. As a basis for approaching norms, the bargaining and other dyadic and N-person games could be focused upon; here, of course, the "tragedy of the commons" (Hardin, 1968) can be comprehensibly integrated. Other aspects of dyadic and group behavior (e.g., responsibility diffusion, roles, leadership, and the group as a means of effecting attitude change) could also be incorporated and considered as they apply to population issues.

Individual phenomena should also be considered. For example, motivation would be an important focus; this might be considered in terms of Rosenberg's (1956, 1960) framework and also in terms of theory and research concerning such motives as affiliation and achievement as they relate to family size and birth order. One might also include intrapersonal processes such as attribution and person perception, individual characteristics such as internal-external control and dogmatism, and phenomena such as reactance.

Finally there is a very legitimate social-psychological population problem in human crowding and density, an area that is increasingly engaging the concern of social psychologists. This focus would provide a fitting denouement to a course in the "social psychology of population."

In suggesting the possibility for such a course we are aware that very little population-related research exists relevant to the suggested areas. Where available the research could be incorporated as examples of the application of social-psychological theory or methodology; where such research does not exist the course could focus on the need and suggestions for approaches.

If there is a question concerning the difference between the above total course and the more "subtle" approach cited previously, let us repeat: *there* the focus was on social psychology with population only a real-life referent; *here* the focus is on population with an attempt being made to apply social-psychological theory and research findings to population phenomena and to evolve a social-psychological theory for population.

What one might note from the above is that many of the topics cited could be the primary focus in a course specifically geared to population. Some of the possible courses described below are merely expansions of topics or areas.

Attitude Theories and Attitude Measurement: An Application to Population

The plethora of attitude studies reported concerning population-related variables should suggest the need for an understanding both of what attitudes are and how they can be measured. Given that the instructor has expertise in both attitude theory and attitude measurement, it is highly possible that the two might be integrated as one course or arranged as two sequential courses. However, as we noted earlier, the technical skills of the faculty involved might lead to a predominant focus on either attitude theories or the measurement of attitudes. If this were the case it would certainly be beneficial for the student to have an adequate comprehension of attitude theories prior to the predominantly measurement-oriented course or the opportunity to focus on attitude measurement subsequent to an attitude theory course. Even though prior considerations of attitudes in population research would not provide sufficient examples of the diverse attitude theories and measurement techniques, research suggestions could easily be derived from both the theories and the measurement techniques.

Attitude Theories. Space precludes an extensive consideration of the basic content or considerations in such a course. Principally one might wish to proceed from the views of attitudes as uni- or multidimensional concepts, in terms of the adequacy of the concepts for predicting behavior. A consideration of theoretical views of attitudes as incorporating affective, belief, and behavioral components, or some combination of these, would lead to a focus on theories such as those of Rosenberg (1956, 1960) and Fishbein (1963, 1965a, 1965b), both of which emphasize that one's attitude toward a given object is a function of an individual's belief that the object will in some way (positively or negatively) relate to diverse other positively or negatively evaluated attitude objects. Further extensions of either the Rosenberg model (e.g., Insko and Schopler, 1967) or the Fishbein model (1967), both of which include behavioral components (behavior or behavioral intention), would provide even broader frameworks from which to critically consider attitudes toward population variables (such as family size or population policy) and previous attempts to treat more unidimensional responses as predictors of reproductive behavior.

The use of multidimensional models provides a means not only for considering the interrelationships between the components but also for making predictions concerning consistency and the resolution of inconsistency. Such a focus would also lead to the incorporation of other consistency models, such as dissonance (Festinger, 1957), congruity (Osgood and Tannenbaum, 1955), and value consistency (Rokeach, 1968), which could then be applied to population questions such as behavior-attitude discrepancies, incentives, and the nature of communications. If one were to proceed to a consideration of attitude measurement (other than that intrinsic to the models cited), the Rosenberg and the Fishbein multidimensional models also serve as vehicles for considering diverse approaches.

There are other advantages to focusing extensively on multidimensional models. For example, they provide a means for considering a motivational basis for numerous reproductive behaviors and attitudes (e.g., contraceptive use or nonuse, various population policies, and so on). Further, some excellent population research has been done utilizing the Rosenberg method of attitude assessment (Crawford et al., 1968; Insko et al., 1970). These research reports could be used to clarify and enunciate the conceptual and methodological advantages of using more complex models of attitudes and to provide a means for elaborating motivational and attitude-change components inherent within the models.

There are other useful attitude models that have relevance for population. One might include learning-theory models (cf., Greenwald, Brock, and Ostrom, 1968), which focus on conditioning and reinforcement, and incentive theories, which deal with maximizing one's outcomes; functional considerations of attitudes (Katz, 1960) might also be included. One might also wish to incorporate frameworks that consider the development and maintenance of attitudes; useful references might include Kelman's (1958) conceptualization of compliance, identification, and internalization and the literature on reference and comparison groups (cf., Kelley, 1952) and on effect and information dependence (cf., Jones and Gerard, 1967).

Various other frameworks could also be considered. For example, assimilation and contrast (cf., Hovland, Harvey, and Sherif, 1957), models of fear arousal (cf., Janis, 1967; McGuire, 1967), hypotheses concerning selective exposure, cognitive models of resolution of inconsistency (cf., Abelson, 1959), reactance (Brehm, 1966), and communicator credibility could be focused upon. All of these perhaps have more narrow application, but they provide useful frameworks for considering attitude-change concepts as they relate to population variables.

Attitude Measurement. As noted above, theoretical models of attitudes both enable one to move from more specific theories to a consideration of population variables and provide a lead-in to a consideration of diverse methodological approaches to the measurement of attitudes. In turning to the methodological approaches we see again a more specific psychological focus (here theoretically derived measurement techniques) being used as a springboard to a consideration of *measurement* of population variables.

If we consider the multitude of attitude studies conducted by population researchers from diverse disciplines, we find that these studies predominantly utilize very simple, often dichotomous, response measures of one component of attitude, perhaps affective, but more frequently belief (or opinion). It would appear that such measurements are used principally because of the survey methodologies employed; one might assume that they may derive from either a less complex conceptualization of attitude structures or a conviction that the more complex measurement techniques cannot be employed in large-sample interview assessments. However, a recent dissertation by Kothandapani (1971) demonstrated both the multicomponent structure of attitudes toward birth control and the feasibility of measuring these components by multiple and more complex measurement techniques. This accomplishment with a low-income black population certainly suggests the utility of providing the opportunity for students interested in assessing population attitudes to learn such a variety of approaches to measurement.

In a course devoted principally to attitude measurement it would seem useful to aim toward comprehension of techniques and their research potential for considering attitudes toward relevant population variables. One would want to focus on complex attitude measurements (e.g., Thurstone equal-appearing intervals; Likert summated ratings; and Guttman scalogram techniques); these are delineated quite simply in Edwards' (1957) excellent book on scale construction. One would want also to elaborate on less complex techniques such as the Semantic Differential (Osgood, Suci, and Tannenbaum, 1957) and Guilford self-rating scales (Guilford, 1954).

In attempting to consider the utilization of such techniques in population-related research, we find the most useful and comprehensive application in Kothandapani (1971). Kothandapani has incorporated all of the methods cited above (i.e., Thurstone, Likert, Guttman, Guilford, and Semantic Differential techniques) in a multitrait-multimethod analysis (cf., Campbell and Fiske, 1959). A careful study of his research should clarify the relevance of these techniques for measurement of attitudes toward reproductive behaviors.

Such a course would also be an ideal locus for considering survey methodology, which is already widely used in population research. Although one would want to refer to and critically examine existing studies, the primary goal would be teaching about the methodology. A number of resources (cf., Cannell and Kahn, 1968) are available. However, because many psychologists are not as well grounded in survey methodology as are members of some other disciplines, student learning could be facilitated and the interdisciplinary nature of population issues could be explicated by planning a joint teaching (with perhaps a sociologist) of at least this aspect of the course.

We should note that a measurements course focusing on the techniques cited might not exist in many psychology programs; in the absence of such a course a field- and laboratory-oriented measurements course with a population focus might serve adequately as a core course in the psychology curriculum. That is, given that students can demonstrate their comprehension of and competence in such methods of measurement, a population focus should aid students in conceptualizing application of these methods.

Group Phenomena in Population Behavior

Group Crowding.[3] One might assume that this is a most appropriate course relating population and psychology since density is a recognized concern of both disciplines. Here, however, we would have only a minimal focus on animal research and population mechanisms (the more likely focus of the populationist); we would not ignore animal research concerning environmental stressors that contribute to pathological behavior or physiological changes, but would include it to the degree that it should pertain when one is focusing on humans.

We might emphasize environmental psychology (cf., Wohwill, 1966; Craik, 1970), and concomitantly research on behavioral settings (e.g., Barker, 1968) and on personal space (Sommer, 1969). We would have to incorporate certain cultural aspects, but our principal focus would no doubt be on intra- and interpersonal variables as precursors and consequences of crowding and density. The importance of psychological as well as physical space would be emphasized, and we would be concerned with both physical and psychological consequences. While there does exist a great deal of diverse research that has focused on the above aspects, the most important goal would be to apply extant psychological theory and to generate psychological theories concerning the variables that interrelate with or are affected by crowding.

As Stokols (1970) has pointed out, one would want to consider individual personal attributes and characteristics. For example, personal characteristics such as dogmatism, comparison levels, need achievement, and internal-external control; personal idiosyncratic skills such as IQ; characteristics of an individual derived from group membership such as roles, leadership, and the like; and clinical manifestations and etiologies of psychopathological behavior should be focused upon. All of the preceding may be affected by or may affect responses to overcrowding or undercrowding. We would want to explore perception of situations, relationships with others, and satisfaction with or need for interpersonal relationships as independent or dependent variables. Principally we would want to examine changes (adaptive or maladaptive) that evolve in the psychological make-up of the focal persons. We would not want to ignore the physical characteristics of crowding (such as spatial arrangements or noise) as they develop from or influence personal characteristics. However, the central focus would be the social or interpersonal characteristics that affect or are affected by crowd-

[3] In proposing the content of such a course, the writers are indebted to Dan Stokols, a graduate student at the University of North Carolina.

ing; for example, the relationship of persons in the situation (as friends or strangers), the task requirements of the situation, elements of competition (as for scarce resources), and aspects of group structure and activity such as cohesiveness and deindividuation. As noted above, we would not ignore the undercrowded situation, a potentially deleterious situation for persons with high affiliative or other needs.

Thus our social-psychological focus would be both sociological (the macroscopic focus of urban design and environmental behavioral sciences, concerned with factors such as suicide, crime, and disease) and psychological (behavioral, cognitive, or perceptual adaptation to stress as a result of the consistency or inconsistency with one's needs or expectations in the crowded situation). We would focus on norms of distance, individual styles and accustomed interactions, the nature of the setting, motivation, personality, and both situational and task variables. We would then look for the *consequences* of physical and psychological crowding in terms of their general effects and the interrelation of such moderating variables as sex, personality types, group organization, and attributional propensities.

The general goal would be to look constantly at causes, consequences, and problems of human density. However, the most important concern would be the reciprocal causal relationship between social-psychological variables and crowding. We would keep in mind the need to derive theory and to apply our accustomed research methodologies in testing our hypotheses, all derived from extant social-psychological theory relative to intra- or interpersonal characteristics. Milgram (1970) provides an excellent example of this approach.

Group Processes. The application of social-psychological theories of group behavior has been virtually ignored in the population literature. Yet the "true" family planners, the couple involved in the family-size decision-making processes, are immersed in an intricate web of interpersonal and intragroup affiliations that will almost certainly have a dramatic influence on their behavior. In addition the small-group processes that evolve within the *central* social unit itself, the couple that must in fact make the decisions, are of such vital consequence that the veritable absence of research in this area is incomprehensible.

Almost by definition the organizing principle of any course in this area of concern must be the outcome of these processes—the behavior decisions and attitudes related to family size. Within this context we could approach the course from two perspectives: (1) the external social system as the course of influence on the marital dyad; and (2) the reciprocal flow of influence patterns within the dyad as they affect the individual. It may be worthwhile to discuss each in turn.

1. The mosaic of external social influences is at first glance so complex that it would seem to defy analysis. Any attempts to treat group membership and identification without the supports of prevailing psychological theory would seem to be destined to spasmodic, short, and affect-laden

life spans. The basic concept of role theory (Biddle and Thomas, 1966; Sarbin and Allen, 1968) and reference-group theory (cf., Jones and Gerard, 1967) could provide the analytic tools for an entry into this area. The role expectations of women in our society, their relations to social class, education, and so on, require a careful and thorough discussion. The study of reference groups is absolutely crucial to any understanding of the dynamics of decision-making on family size. The distinction between comparative or informational influence and normative or effect dependence (cf., Kelley, 1952; Jones and Gerard, 1967) might lead to some differential hypotheses concerning the actual influence of distinct groups or agents upon behavior. Especially interesting are the effects of reference groups (including the media) with which people identify but in which they do not actually have membership. It may also be important to discuss general misperceptions and inaccuracies in people's judgment of the prevailing opinions of their referent groups; for instance, a culture lag of sorts may prevent the person from accurately construing the feelings of his group members on such things as birth control. The degrees of susceptibility to comparative influence could be described in terms of social comparison theory (cf., Collins and Raven, 1969), and different hypotheses might be generated from the diverse theoretical viewpoints (cf., Pettigrew, 1967). Related topics such as conformity (Allen, 1965) might be included with particular emphasis on the different bases of power involved (cf., Collins and Raven, 1969). In this regard a careful delineation of the potential agents of influence would seem warranted, particularly with respect to the degree of change predicted due to the various sources. For instance, the parents of the decision-makers (i.e., of the couple) may exert a strong influence through their informal reward or coercive power (e.g., approval or liking) but not through their comparative influence or identification processes. Further, one might consider the role of the negative referent groups and of public figures who attempt to effect change through prestige suggestion or "expert" knowledge.

Contemporary exchange theories, such as that of Thibaut and Kelley (1959), would provide a rather different approach to an analysis of the effects of group membership on the dyad. The effects of norms might also be examined within this framework. The concept of comparison level might be useful in specifying the perceived *outcomes* or satisfactions expected from small or large family sizes. These outcomes could be compared with those that are expected from the more general life style; for example, many young couples aspire to such amenities as yearly vacations, expensive cars, and an individual home, but the harsh realities of the expense and behavioral limitation connected with large families may not have been integrated into the general comparison level. The analytical approach of Thibaut and Kelley (1959) would also be an excellent technique for examining the social power of various other groups and individuals and perhaps even for integrating some of the influences of economic patterns (such as tax laws) on such decisions.

2. In terms of the second perspective the reciprocal flow of influence *between* the individuals in the marital relationship offers a great deal of potential for the innovative application of small-group theory. The Thibaut and Kelley (1959) theory includes many concepts that could be useful in this respect. Their theory of interpersonal power, including fate and behavior control, is especially relevant. The implications of value similarity or dissimilarity with regard to family size and its instrumental relationships could be considered. Further, some of the effects of correspondence or noncorrespondence of outcomes could be specified. If differential levels of decision-making power are evident, the consequences of the asymmetrical relation could be developed; for example, one might incorporate observations concerning dominance patterns in husband-wife relationships (Strodtbeck, 1951).

To be able to predict the influence patterns (in terms of reward-cost implications) that will occur in the marital dyad, one must have some knowledge of the degree to which each partner accurately perceives the values and preferences of the other in such matters as family size. A thorough study of the dyadic communication patterns is therefore necessary, and impediments to open, trusting communication must be examined. Patterns of communication within the marital dyad can be both analyzed and predicted in terms of "correspondence of outcomes" (cf., Kelley, 1966); for example, one might focus on certain ritualized norms in the dyad that may develop or impede the free flow of expression. The theories concerned with interpersonal inferences (cf., Jones and Davis, 1965; Kelley, 1967) would offer different bases for understanding the mechanisms through which attributions were developed and might provide clues to possible problem areas. A not infrequent condition in the dyad may be the case where the individuals are in reality in fairly complete accord in their choices (e.g., concerning family size) but where each has misperceived the preferences of the other. In general the literature related to decision-making in groups from a psychological perspective would also offer a wide variety of approaches not discussed here (cf., Collins and Guetzkow, 1964).

By means of either of the courses proposed in this section relating to group processes and crowding phenomena, our orientation is made even more explicit. Both courses incorporate highly sophisticated theoretical material that is extremely relevant to our understanding of intra- and interpersonal phenomena. However, despite its level the material is necessary if one is going to attempt to *understand* such behaviors as individual or dyadic decisions concerning family planning. Again, our intent should be quite clear: we do *not* perceive the utility in moving into research in this realm *until* the student has a firm basis in such important concepts. The population literature is replete with research that might have offered more clarification of population issues if it had been derived from a comprehensive *and* explicit understanding of important intra- and interpersonal phenomena.

Motivation for Parenthood

In a course concerning "motivation for parenthood" we find ourselves stretching further than our expertise. Every area of psychology has its motivational concepts, but apparently courses in motivation per se are rarely offered. Instead, motivation tends to be an integral component of diverse courses; physiological, instinctual, stimulus-response or social learning, and consistency theories of motivation are offered in accord with the framework of the instructor. In social psychology, motivation may be discussed in the context of several topics, such as social learning theory, affiliation and achievement, personality traits such as internal and external control, or perhaps more generally, consistency as an explanation of maintaining or changing interrelated attitudes, values, and behavior.

In attempting to conceptualize a course concerning motivation for parenthood, we find that we cannot think in terms of a single approach to motivation; that is, we cannot apply a purely social learning approach with a focus on the shaping of behavioral contingencies (a framework that seems implicit in many of the populationist views of motivation), nor can we move from a purely physiological approach in which fundamental drives and needs could be considered as the principal explanatory variables. Instead, we find ourselves considering and attempting to interrelate a variety of approaches to motivational questions. Again, we perceive that the most useful approach would be to consider a number of theories of motivation and to attempt to move from them to a consideration of reproductive behavior, with the final goal of delineating a motivational framework for reproduction for a first birth and subsequent ones. We believe that looking first at reproduction and then trying to intuit motivation through assessment of personality and attitude measures may not be as fruitful a goal as would be the development of a sound basis in motivational considerations. We must again note that the theories focused upon and the course format would largely depend on the orientation and expertise of the instructor.

Such a course might begin with a consideration such as that of Janis et al. (1969) of three broad categories of motivation: the learning-theory approach, psychodynamic theory (principally Freudian), and the cognitive approach. We might also incorporate a more fundamental "need" focus, dichotomizing and examining the more instinctual or physiological needs and the more socialized or socially conditioned needs or goals. In conjunction with traditional textbook considerations of such motivational considerations, we would be aided in our attempts to consider applications to reproductive behaviors by incorporating related population literature. For example, Wyatt (1967) has considered learning theory, psychodynamic theory, and physiological needs in his consideration of motivation for parenthood, and Pareek (1968) has considered the more socially conditioned needs in his paper on "Motivational patterns and planned social change."

As psychologists, we would perhaps focus predominantly on the socialized needs that reflect both overall cultural and subgroup or familial value systems. Perpetuation of socialized needs is of concern to psychologists from most areas; clinical, social, developmental, and personality theorists are all interested in some aspects of need socialization. Although we might spend much of a course focusing on a more restricted set of motives (e.g., affiliation, achievement, and extension), we might choose to look at diverse "secondary social motives" (cf., Cohen, 1970a, 1970b), which are thought to be derived and perpetuated for purposes of maintaining homeostasis or balance. Among the learned social motives that we might consider, as treated in Cohen's (1970b) small and comprehensive text, are: social stratification (caste and class); competition and cooperation (as normative behavior); societal norms (customs and fashions) and rules; and obedience to authority. Cohen also suggests a number of "innate social motives," which he perceives to be continuous over species but to have both innate and learned components in man. Examples of this class of motives that might be relevant in population considerations are: social facilitation, functional autonomy, competition and hierarchies (dominance-subordination, both generally and sexually), and social imitation. From our perspective these two types of social motives can be approached also from social-psychological concepts derived from observations of dyadic and small-group interactions.

In considering reproductive motivation there are also tailor-made considerations of social homeostatic mechanisms that may be pitted against the Malthusian and Darwinian theories. Although there are many sources for material concerning these controversies, Cohen's text (1970b) succinctly outlines these opposing views, presenting Malthusian and Darwinian theories and the "socioecology" hypothesis of Wynne-Edwards (1962). The latter, a more social-homeostatic theory, concerns animal and human individual and group selection and maintenance of behaviors such as social dominance and territoriality. While populationists may extrapolate from animal research concerning such behaviors, the importance of cognitive manipulation in humans provides a transition to intra- and interpersonal psychological considerations.

Incorporation of basic needs in such a course might be facilitated by utilizing texts such as Cohen's (1970a, 1970b) and a second text such as Maslow's (1970), which provides a more holistic approach to personality and motivation. For those not familiar with this text psychoanalytic and "instinctoid" concepts are incorporated. One chapter entitled "Is Destructiveness Instinctoid" provides not the content but perhaps the stimulus to ask this same question of reproduction. Maslow also focuses on instinctive needs that might be considered more socialized needs by others; such discrepant considerations are useful in demonstrating the breadth and complexity of motivational issues. In the same vein of encouraging diverse considerations one might wish to consider Maslow's need-hierarchy structure, which postulates that one must resolve conflicts and attain gratification at one level before one can move on to the next (and on to final self-actualization), and contrast it with the more Freudian consideration of fixations reflected in adult behavior and defense mechanisms or with need-gratification theories such as McClelland's (1961).

Aside from these approaches, however, one would not want to ignore more cognitive homeostatic mechanisms. For example, an application of Rosenberg's (1956, 1960) theory of attitude structure would reveal a motivational system based on the realization or interference with one's valued end states. Within such a framework the learned cultural and individual attitude systems could be productively explored. One would also want to refer to Rokeach's (1968) value-consistency model, which focuses on terminal and instrumental values; both this model and other consistency models (e.g., value-attitude, affect-belief, or behavioral-attitude consistency frameworks) certainly contain motivational implications. Personal perceptions of individual control or mastery of one's environment, as opposed to perceptions of fate or external control, are also salient considerations, particularly in terms of examining individual or cultural differences in family-planning behavior.

Finally one would not wish to omit the diverse motivational or value articles in the population literature. Many of these articles are quite speculative and tend to be derived as much from intuitive frameworks as from extant theoretical models. Still, they contain the crucial focus on specific questions of reproductive motivation. If we can move from theories toward constructive criticism and elaboration of hypothesized reproductive motivation, we should be more able to discern *both* the commonalities of reproductive and other motivations *and* motivational variables that may indeed be unique to reproductive behavior.

A Potpourri: The Family as a Unit

Many psychologists concerned with population have considered or developed courses that relate to reproduction (e.g., focusing on the psychology of human reproduction). However, we have discerned little emphasis on such topics as the characteristics and dynamics of families as units. Perhaps such considerations are perceived more as belonging to such disciplines as family sociology. It does seem to us that at least some aspects of the family are of intrinsic interest to psychologists, particularly to those psychologists who are interested in population. Further, if we are to achieve a more interdisciplinary focus it may be necessary for us to expand beyond the traditionally delineated boundaries of our disciplines. We perceive that there are at least three components of family characteristics or dynamics that might be focused upon by psychologists, dependent again upon explicit training and orientation. While each of these components might be the focus of an entire course, we would like merely to present them and discuss them generally. The three family aspects are: demographic characteristics, family size as it relates to individual characteristics and interpersonal relationships, and family interrelationships or dynamics. Again, one could focus on these separately or combine them in a course on the family as a unit.

If one were focusing specifically on demographic characteristics, the orientation might lean principally on variables that are generally considered within the domain of the sociologist. However, a developmental psychologist concerned with such variables as status, occupation, education, age of parents, residence (urban-rural, type of dwelling, and the like) would consider them more in terms of how such variables affect the mental and physical growth of the child, rather than as parental or background variables that are of more demographic concern. Such a course would also accommodate the myriad of questions and findings concerning family size and structure as they relate to developmental and maturational phenomena. Effects of ordinal position and of sex of child and of siblings might also be related to psychological development. Sex of a child and the behavioral concomitants could be dealt with more in terms of resultants of cultural and social learning than as demographic characteristics.

If one is concerned with family size and its correlates, there is certainly sufficient material to provide content for an entire course. In the literature we can find evidence that suggests that members of large families suffer from maternal deprivation, which in turn is thought to lead to physiological, psychological, and intellectual deficits (cf., Thompson, 1970; Thompson, 1960). We can also find evidence that density per se appears to lead to lethargy and later dependency (Waldrop and Bell, 1964, 1966). There is enough material concerning the consistently demonstrated negative correlation between family size and IQ to fill a course, or a major part of a course, in family size or IQ development. School and adjustment problems have also received a fair amount of attention, although correlations with family size are largely inconsistent. Ordinal data, particularly concerning first and only children versus later borns, is readily available. An examination of the numerous studies relating to family size reveals such inconsistent results that there should be a plethora of research questions that could be incorporated in developing a course. However, what is principally lacking is adequate theory concerning the causal sequences in correlational data relating family size to diverse intra- and interpersonal characteristics. Here again, numerous theories exist that have been given scant attention in the majority of research efforts. It would seem imperative that more attention be given to concepts derived from group research and from social learning theory in considerations of role behaviors, value transmission, and so on. As in our previous suggestions we again see the need for moving from theories to a consideration of existing research and finally on to more theoretically derived research by means of which causal sequences *can* be more clearly delineated.

If one is principally interested in the total family a more clinical focus might be in order. Marital relationships could be explored in terms of being precursors or consequences of large or small family size. One could also delve more deeply into individual member and family adjustment problems; family interaction patterns could be viewed in terms of models derived from family therapy (cf., Lowman, 1970). There does exist a fair amount of clinical research (e.g., Rainwater, 1960, 1965) concerning marital relationships and reproductive behavior; however, extant psychological theory concerning dyadic and group communications and relationships could again be used as a basis for examining the research that does exist and for generating further research to test explicitly salient theory.

We have again emphasized throughout the need for dealing with existing psychological theory first and then moving to an examination of the literature. In the area of the family such an approach should not only elucidate the findings but also provide a basis for further research. There are indeed some massive problems as yet unsolved, particularly concerning the causal sequence in family size and intra- or interpersonal correlations. If there is to be an appeal for reduced and altered family sizes and role behaviors, appeals should be accompanied by firmly substantiated facts concerning the precursors, correlates, and consequences of such family and role variations.

A Comment about Proposed Courses

All of the above courses are mere suggestions in terms of content and focus. As is quite obvious, the authors are principally concerned with social-psychological and measurement problems. Nevertheless, we believe that any psychologist truly interested in integrating population as a referent or in making population a direct focus of a course could meet the challenge. Given that the psychologist does not have space in his teaching for both a course, say, in motivation and one in motivational aspects of parenthood, quite obviously more subtle integration of population questions might be most feasible. However, should there be room for and interest in a more specific focus on population, our bent would be to look at population questions from the standpoint of extant theory and research findings and to gear the course toward the development of theory and research on population. Both theory and research concerning the psychology of reproductive behavior (and of other population-related behavior and attitudes) are urgently needed. We already have enough discussions or speculations about the nature of the population problem and the bleak future if nothing is done about it. We need now young expert psychologists who in their training have perceived the psychology of population as an acceptable and desirable research and teaching focus. We cannot just talk about the fact that we *should* be integrating population and psychology; we must simply take the plunge and do it if we sincerely believe it is a challenge we must meet. The nature of the course obviously depends on the instructor involved; again, however, no matter what the course design or content, we want to avoid simple discussions of population problems and aim instead to approach population from the theories and methodologies with which we are most familiar and by means of which we can make the most contribution.

Questions We Would Ask

There are a number of questions or issues that one needs to raise about the possibility and desirability of a focus on population in the psychology curriculum. Further, one must examine these issues carefully from several points of view, ranging from the unpopular but necessary question of administrative feasibility to consideration of the pedagogical value of such approaches. One of these questions is whether there should be a disciplinary (i.e., departmental) focus on problems such as population. A second issue is where the focus should be for population in a curriculum (i.e., should it be on the graduate or undergraduate level?). A third question concerns what kinds of more intensive (possibly professional) programs should be available. The fourth, and not independent, concern is the crucial issue of the advisability of a strictly population focus in psychology (i.e., to the exclusion of other social concerns). Before considering these issues, however, it might be helpful explicitly to distinguish between undergraduate, graduate, and professional education. It is the belief of the authors that these are three quite distinctive forms of education, each with its own goals and objectives (although we recognize a current trend toward the eradication of these distinctions). What may be a wise policy in graduate education may be highly inappropriate for undergraduate programs. Thus each of the previously mentioned issues must be considered in terms of the group of students involved.

First, should we have a disciplinary or subdisciplinary focus on psychology and population? It seems quite obvious that population is indeed not solely a psychological problem any more than it is strictly a demographic, sociological, or political problem. To approach it as strictly psychological, we think, would be to perpetuate disciplinary myths. For psychologists and nonpsychologists alike there would seem to be a need for an integrated focus on population—psychology should be there, but should be only part of a multidisciplinary focus. Thus in bringing population into the psychology curriculum we ourselves may distort and isolate the problem in our attempts to view it as a disciplinary or, worse, a subdisciplinary problem.

We could attempt to avert this disciplinary focus by bringing in the thinking and research of other disciplines, and we could do this from the very broad course down to the extremely specific one. Still, bringing in the thinking is not the same as bringing in the expertise. We in psychology flinch a bit when other disciplines embark on vast attitude and attitude-change studies with nary a psychologist on the research team, or when we read intricate population theories that we think have ignored psychological variables (or, even worse, have included them without realizing that they "belong" to us). There now seems to be a demand for and a trend toward interdisciplinary studies in population. We might wonder (from our own experiences) how well we can mesh different concepts and approaches if we confront them for the first time with (perhaps) rigidly set, completely disciplinary ideas of "appropriate" research techniques and focuses.

At the undergraduate level, at least, one may be tempted to suggest that the interdisciplinary problem be handled by teaching "our bit" in psychology courses and sending our students elsewhere to acquire other information (both content and methodology) from other departments also concerned with population issues. This approach, although appealingly simple, has many problems. First, there is no assurance that other departments are concerned with or, at any rate, teaching in the population area. Indeed, the rather sad performance of psychology departments in focusing on population should force us to consider this problem seriously.

A second, and even more major, problem centers around degree requirements that many, if not most, undergraduates must meet. At most colleges and universities students must take at least a certain prescribed number of courses in their major as well as required general courses. In addition the major department establishes requirements to assure that a minimal range of topics is covered by all majors in the discipline. Within psychology, for instance, a sequence of introductory courses, a statistics course, and several "advanced level" courses from several subareas are typically required of all majors. Thus an undergraduate might be limited in the number of population courses offered by his major department that he could take. Distributional requirements outside the major department may further limit the range and number of related population courses open to him, a particular problem if these courses are intended to produce an interdisciplinary understanding of the area. This last problem is augmented by the fact that most, but certainly not all, of the work in population studies of interest to psychologists (and psychology students) is being done in disciplines loosely grouped into the social sciences; relatively little (outside of botany and zoology) is currently being taught by departments in the natural sciences and less by those in humanities and fine arts.

Another approach to the interdisciplinary problem is to bring in the other areas rather than to send our students out. What disciplines we should bring together obviously depend on the research or theoretical focus of the individual instructor, but let us make a couple of suggestions for the sake of elaboration. Suppose we would like to focus on human crowding and density problems or, on a broader plane, on environmental psychology. Immediately we can perceive a number of disciplines whose members might conceivably collaborate in conceptualizing theoretical and research problems: psychology, obviously; urban planning; system theory (from the standpoint of psychology or from another discipline such as business administration); botany, biology, zoology (disciplines concerned with population dynamics across species); and sociology. Members of other disciplines might be included as regular members of a seminar team or as consultants for various aspects of the course.

In planning the development of a testable conceptual framework (e.g., in considering the development of an integrated theory concerning contraceptive behavior), we would again need not just one discipline—psychology—or even its subdisciplines. Perhaps we would need a team of psychologists—those concerned with values, attitudes, norms, motivation, decision-making, and so on. This might incorporate social, clinical, developmental, and other areas of psychology. However, we should also include an able anthropologist and sociologist so that we could include and effectively deal with more sociological and cultural aspects of attitude-value development and maintenance or change.

As a final example, suppose we wished to develop a broad field study or experiment as a course focus. If we were interested in a field study on attitudes toward population policy, we might include a political scientist, a sociologist, a psychologist, and someone who is expert in the mechanics of accomplishing good-public opinion research; such a combination is at work on such a study here at Carolina (Allen, Beza, Prothro, and Thompson, in progress).[4] As a class venture, with training and research a goal, it would be to the students' and our advantage to incorporate the various experts in the education and training for such interdisciplinary and applied projects; only in this way can we more assuredly guarantee a student's functioning on such teams when he becomes a professional psychologist. Given that one wishes only a psychological focus, it might also be profitable to include psychologists of different interests. To develop theory and research, a good blend could be made of any variety of combinations of social, clinical, experimental, developmental, and quantitative psychologists with each contributing his own expertise in consideration of the issues at hand.

Our second issue was *where* in the curriculum the initial focus on population properly belongs—on the undergraduate level or on the graduate level. Our hunch would be that, given a choice, the undergraduate level

---

[4] James Allen, Angell Beza, James Prothro, and Vaida Thompson. Development of instruments to measure readiness for population policies, University of North Carolina, in progress.

would be more ideal. If the issues were properly integrated and an inter-disciplinary perspective achieved, we would try to generate a set toward research and theory development as the student moves toward the graduate level. If we delayed until the graduate student had completed his basic training in his specialized discipline before attempting to provide electives, we might merely perpetuate the problems we cited earlier (namely, the difficulties faced by persons trained in more traditional ways when attempting to move out and contribute to a relatively foreign discipline). Obviously if both undergraduate and graduate programs could be provided, we would favor having both: a broad undergraduate program (which we will explore later) to prepare the student and an *integrated* focus on the graduate level (not just broad electives after basic training).

Our third question concerns what kind of programs *should* be available for graduate and undergraduate students. We are aware that increasingly graduate students in psychology are concerned with the application of their discipline to real social problems. Such students express concern with the lack of opportunity to focus on such problems as part of their training; they are further concerned that they will not be able to deal with these problems when the time comes.

At this point we should take a cautious position on a specialized grad-uate degree program in population developed independently (i.e., having no specific disciplinary emphasis). In such a Ph.D. program we see the kinds of problems discussed in relation to the general survey course. It seems preferable to continue to train professionals in a substantive area so that they will be able to approach and will be interested in approaching population problems, rather than to train generalists with broad interests who lack sufficient or adequate methodological or theoretical skills to make meaningful contributions to the understanding of the population field. While this result may not be the logically necessary outcome of such broadly based programs as a Ph.D. in population, we feel that at this time there is sufficient danger to caution against a program of this type.

Our aim of achieving an interdisciplinary focus on the undergraduate level and the related problem of distributive educational requirements lead us to favor an approach *other than* the psychology major with a pop-ulation emphasis. Although our suggested approach means additional ad-ministrative problems, at least in the short run, the experience of one of the authors (Appelbaum), in establishing such a program at the University of North Carolina at Chapel Hill, provides sufficient evidence of its possi-bility and practicability. This approach involves the establishment of a Bachelor of Arts in Interdisciplinary Studies. The results of such a degree program have implications far beyond the study of population problems, but we shall limit ourselves to this area.

The A.B. in Interdisciplinary Studies established at the University of North Carolina was designed to allow undergraduate students to pursue interdisciplinary or cross-disciplinary studies in accordance with their unique interests and abilities, while not abrogating the general liberal arts philosophy of the undergraduate division of the university. The program is seen as offering an alternative to the standard degree programs rather than replacing them. A student desiring to receive the Interdisciplinary A.B. must submit to the Associate Dean for Experimental and Special Studies (an associate dean of the College of Arts and Sciences) a sixty-hour (four-semester) course of study developed with the advice and approval of a full-time member of the faculty. The program is subject to a minimum number of restraints. These restraints assure that the program is truly interdisciplinary in nature; thus there is a limit on the maximum number of hours that may be taken in a single department and a requirement that in general courses should be taken from at least six departments. The usual distributional requirements and grouping of disciplines into divisions are not required, and the student stands reasonably free to pursue his inter-disciplinary subject as dictated by his interests and the nature of his study.

We feel that this program has certain features that make it highly desir-able for the incorporation of population studies into the undergraduate cur-riculum. First, the curriculum is planned by the individual student and his faculty sponsor. In addition to the obvious motivational benefits the indi-vidual faculty guidance should lead to greater depth and understanding of some aspect of the population problem than would usually be achieved by the student selecting courses on the basis of vague catalogue descriptions. A program with depth and breadth would more likely emerge if the faculty advisor was himself experienced both in his own field and in population. Second, the greater flexibility of the program should allow for the incor-poration of new courses as they become available. Finally, since the usual distributional requirements are eliminated, the concentration of population work in the social sciences departments should no longer prove problematic.

On the graduate level this same issue seems to be subject to rather differ-ent issues. First, graduate programs are usually highly specific programs for professional training in a particular discipline. Second, graduate programs are more nearly controlled at the departmental level than are undergrad-uate programs and are consequently more flexible about specific require-ments and general outlook. Nevertheless, while some departments may be able to see a population-psychology division, we would be inclined to think that at this point elective courses—to the extent of a minor, perhaps—would be better. If there were enough courses of an elective nature for a minor in population, the departmental personality would still determine the content and continue to achieve the general goal of professional training in the discipline of psychology. Some departments appear to require merely a number of courses outside the major (of, e.g., social psychology) but still within the department. Enough psychologists are interested in population that a first successful attempt by us and a little student demand might well lead to at least a small ground swell, so that a sufficient number of courses would soon emerge to fulfill part of this requirement. Arranging a series of courses in an organized format would require more department and instructor collaboration than is currently required, but this would seem to be only a slight obstacle. We believe that such a minor is not an impossible dream and that it may be realized in the not-too-distant future in some departments—if it does not already exist.

In departments that require an extradepartmental minor there should be no difficulty whatsoever in guiding the interested graduate student toward a good core of population courses. Our own graduate bulletin is replete with excellent courses that examine relevant issues in population from a wide interdisciplinary perspective.

We should also think about a minor in psychology for students who are currently majoring in population in other departments; this is a matter to which we have given virtually no attention. At this point it would seem that population students who seek a minor in psychology must merely pick out psychology courses, presumably with their advisors, that might be useful. While there rarely are psychology courses developed especially for students outside the department (particularly for a specific group of students), almost all of the courses we have envisioned throughout would surely be very useful for the student interested in the psychology of population. As a case in point, in our own department several years ago a visiting psychologist developed a course on motivational concepts as they related to population. This was developed with the population student in mind, and we understand that students from other disciplines who enrolled in the course developed a great deal of insight into motivation as it related to population in general and to their own disciplinary concepts. Given a behavioral science division of which psychology is a part, or a departmental orientation toward providing courses for nonmajors, a minor program at the graduate level should not be too difficult to accomplish.

Our final question pertains to the *advisability* of a specific population focus, in lieu of a more broad social problems focus. Despite all our own grandiose proposals, we might wonder aloud if, as responsible psychologists, we are *really* asking for psychologists to become interested *only* in population. We must face up to the recent concerns expressed by Albee (1970) in his APA address at Miami and focused upon in a recent issue of the APA *Monitor* and in a recent article by Sanford (1970): shouldn't our goal be to move toward a broad range of socially relevant issues? Do we really want only population psychologists—or are we seeking psychologists who have the capability and interest to deal with a vast array of social problems? If we seek a broader interest perhaps we would be doing a disservice to focus merely on population; instead, we would benefit the field and humanity more by incorporating diverse social problems into our real-life problem-oriented courses. What we might do is to make population an example and our approach a model for considering numerous real-life social problems. Several of our graduate students have suggested that this should be our intent—that a measurements course or a field research course might indeed focus on population, but that the overall goal should be to familiarize the student with such approaches to *any* real-life issues; otherwise, they suggest, we have merely offered another isolated focus. It is our conviction that a concentrated focus on the psychological approach to population *would* be highly generalizable and that students would not suffer from a concern with population, even if their subsequent concerns should be with some other (perhaps yet nonexistent) social problem. Many of the current social problems (e.g., pollution, urban and ghetto problems, racial issues, women's role issues, or poverty) are so interrelated with population that they often enter into considerations of population. Thus the population area might better serve as the predominant real-life focus than one of the other seemingly interrelated areas; a focus on another issue (such as roles of women or poverty) might more poorly accommodate considerations of other issues, particularly population. Still, we maintain that our concern should be with training that develops the capability for and interest in dealing with social problems rather than with training for isolated theoretical and research problems. Indeed, in the vein of concern expressed by others we might ask if psychology should continue to exist as a major discipline if it avoids training that deals with the problems of society.

Concluding Comments

Ours was more a conceptual than a reportorial charge. We were asked and asked ourselves how might population be introduced into a psychology curriculum? Of the psychologists now involved with population issues, only a handful have attempted courses on population, and these courses appear to be more isolated offerings than a move toward a minor or major focus on the psychology of population. Further, most of the course descriptions we have examined, while both provocative and undoubtedly productive, have been principally issue- or research-oriented. As we have noted, a focus on population issues (even those that seem patently psychological) may not derive from or apply extant psychological theories. A research focus, on the other hand, may adequately utilize psychological methodology but have no theoretical base. In suggesting courses or course content our constant theme was that either of the above approaches may not readily permit the psychologist to approach population as he would other more familiar issues; thus he is prevented from using his expertise most effectively. We have suggested throughout that psychologists attempt to perceive population issues principally through their own psychological eyes. We have urged that they attempt both to analyze population issues from the perspective of their own theories and to derive research from these same theories. We have further urged that familiar psychological research methodologies be utilized in exploring population questions, rather than methodologies of other disciplines with which psychologists are less familiar and less adept. In sum we have suggested that if psychologists are to contribute maximally to an understanding of population-related behaviors, they should not stray too far from their own theoretical and methodological expertise.

It is no doubt clear that our suggestions concerning course development are largely speculative, based on a few personal and a few reported experiences. We have not contended that any specific courses should be taught but have suggested that interested persons must develop the type of course and the content with which they are most familiar and most comfortable. Aside from commenting on the possibilities for a minor in population, we have offered no curriculum (i.e., course series) suggestions. We believe that a minor (or a major) focus on population within psychology cannot be instantaneously instituted; our hunch would be that such a minor will emerge where there is both a departmental interest and a corps of psychologists interested in providing courses, and that the initial content of a minor will vary with the interests and expertise of the faculty involved. We have not toyed with a major in population within psychology; we feel that such a goal is not an immediate possibility. We would contend that much more psychological theory is needed concerning the psychology of population-related behaviors before a population major could be considered.

We would like to conclude with our repeated comment that this chapter is indeed speculative. Our suggestions bear some resemblance to our own current and proposed attempts to incorporate population. However, we would hope that the reader would not attempt simply to follow (or reject out of hand) our skeletal models of courses but to generate courses or series of courses in which his own theoretical and technical skills would best serve him, his students, and the fields of both population and psychology.

REFERENCES

Abelson, R. P. 1959. Modes of resolution of belief dilemmas. *Journal of Conflict Resolution* 3:343–352.

Abelson, R. P. and Zimbardo, P. G. 1970. *Canvassing for peace: a manual for volunteers.* Ann Arbor: Society for the Psychological Study of Social Issues.

Albee, G. W. 1970. The uncertain future of clinical psychology. *American Psychologist* 25:1071–1080.

Allen, V. L. 1965. Situational factors in conformity. In L. Berkowitz, ed., *Advances in experimental social psychology.* New York: Academic Press 2:133–175.

Barker, R. G. 1968. *Ecological psychology.* Stanford: Stanford University Press.

Baughman, E. E. and Dahlstrom, W. G. 1968. *Negro and white children: a psychological study in the rural South.* New York: Academic Press.

Biddle, B. J. and Thomas, E. J., eds. 1966. *Role theory: concepts and research.* New York: Wiley.

Brehm, J. W. 1966. *A theory of psychological reactance.* New York: Academic Press.

Campbell, D. T. and Fiske, D. W. 1959. Convergent and discriminant validation by the multitrait-multimethod matrix. *Psychological Bulletin* 56:81–105.

Cannell, C. F. and Kahn, R. L. 1968. Interviewing. In G. Lindzey and E. Aronson, eds., *The handbook of social psychology.* Reading, Mass.: Addison-Wesley. 2:526–595.

Cohen, J. 1970a. Secondary motivation I. Personal motives. *Eyewitness series in psychology.* Chicago: Rand McNally.

———. 1970b. Secondary motivation II. Social motives. *Eyewitness series in psychology.* Chicago: Rand McNally.

Collins, B. E. and Guetzkow, H. 1964. *A social psychology of group processes for decision-making.* New York: Wiley.

Collins, B. E. and Raven, B. H. 1969. Group structure: Attraction, coalitions, communication, and power. In G. Lindzey and E. Aronson, eds., *The handbook of social psychology.* Reading, Mass.: Addison-Wesley. 4:102–204.

Craik, K. 1970. Environmental psychology. In *New directions in psychology.* New York: Holt, Rinehart & Winston. 4:1–121.

Crawford, T. J.; Heredia, R.; and Stocker, E. 1968. Family planning attitudes and behavior as a function of the perceived consequences of family planning. Unpublished manuscript, University of Chicago Community and Family Study Center.

Edwards, A. L. 1957. *Techniques of attitude scale construction.* New York: Appleton-Century-Crofts.

Evans, R. I. and Rozelle, R. M. 1970. *Social psychology in life.* Boston: Allyn and Bacon.

Fawcett, J. T. 1970. *Psychology and population.* New York: The Population Council.

Festinger, L. 1957. *A theory of cognitive dissonance.* Stanford: Stanford University Press.

Fishbein, M. 1963. An investigation of the relationships between beliefs about an object and the attitude toward that object. *Human Relations* 16:233–240.

———. 1965a. A consideration of beliefs, attitudes, and their relationships. In I. D. Steiner and M. Fishbein, eds., *Current studies in social psychology.* New York: Holt, Rinehart & Winston. Pp. 107–120.

———. 1965b. The prediction of interpersonal preferences and group member satisfaction from estimated attitudes. *Journal of Personality and Social Psychology* 1: 633–667.

———. 1967. A behavioral theory approach to the relations between beliefs about an object and the attitude toward the object. In M. Fishbein, ed., *Readings in attitude theory and measurement.* New York: Wiley. Pp. 389–400.

Freedman, D. 1963. The relation of economic status to fertility. *The American Economic Review* 53:414–426.

Gergen, K. J. 1969. *The psychology of behavior exchange.* Reading, Mass. Addison-Wesley.

Greenwald, A. G.; Brock, T. C.; and Ostrom, T. M., eds. 1968. *Psychological foundations of attitudes.* New York: Academic Press.

Guilford, J. P. 1954. *Psychometric methods.* New York: McGraw-Hill.

Hardin, G. 1968. The tragedy of the commons. *Science* 162:1243–1248.

Hill, R.; Stycos, J. M.; and Back, K. 1959. *The family and population control: a Puerto Rican experiment in social change.* Chapel Hill: University of North Carolina Press.

Hovland, C. I.; Harvey, O. J.; and Sherif, M. 1957. Assimilation and contrast effects in reaction to communication and attitude change. *Journal of Abnormal Social Psychology* 55:244–252.

Insko, C. A.; Blake, R. R.; Cialdini, R. B.; and Mulaik, S. A. 1970. Attitude toward birth control and cognitive consistency: theoretical and practical implications of survey data. *Journal of Personality and Social Psychology* 16:228–237.

Insko, C. A. and Schopler, J. 1967. Triadic consistency: a statement of affective-cognitive-conative consistency. *Psychological Review* 74:361–376.

Janis, I. L. 1967. Effects of fear arousal on attitude change: recent developments in theory and experimental research. In L. Berkowitz, ed., *Advances in experimental social psychology.* New York: Academic Press. 3:166–224.

Janis, I. L.; Mahl, G. F.; Kagan, J.; and Holt, R. R. 1969. *Personality: dynamics, development, and assessment.* New York: Harcourt Brace Jovanovich.

Jones, E. E. and Davis, K. E. 1965. From acts to dispositions: the attribution process in person perception. In L. Berkowitz, ed., *Advances in experimental social psychology.* New York: Academic Press. 2:219–266.

Jones, E. E. and Gerard, H. B. 1967. *Foundations of social psychology.* New York: Wiley.

Kahan, J. P. 1970. Rationality, the prisoner's dilemma, and the commons. Unpublished manuscript, University of North Carolina, L. L. Thurstone Psychometric Laboratory.

Katz, D. 1960. The functional approach to the study of attitudes. *Public Opinion Quarterly* 24:163–204.

Kelley, H. H. 1952. The two functions of reference groups. In G. E. Swanson, T. M. Newcomb, and E. L. Hartley, eds., *Readings in social psychology.* New York: Holt, Rinehart & Winston. Pp. 410–414.

———. 1966. A classroom study of the dilemmas in interpersonal negotiations. In K. Archibald, ed., *Strategic interaction and conflict.* Berkeley: University of California, Institute of International Studies. Pp. 49–73.

———. 1967. Attribution theory in social psychology. In D. Levine, ed., *Nebraska symposium on motivation.* Lincoln: University of Nebraska Press. Pp. 192–238.

Kelman, H. C. 1958. Compliance, identification, and internalization: three processes of attitude change. *Journal of Conflict Resolution* 2:51–60.

Korten, F. F.; Cook, S. W.; and Lacey, J. I. 1970. *Psychology and the problems of society.* Washington, D.C.: American Psychological Association.

Kothandapani, V. 1971. A psychological approach to the prediction of contraceptive behavior. University of North Carolina, Carolina Population Center Monograph Series no. 15.

Lowman, J. C. 1970. Development and field-testing of a self-administered measure of family functioning. Unpublished manuscript, University of North Carolina.

McClelland, D. S. 1961. *The achieving society.* New York: The Free Press.

McGuire, W. J. 1967. Personality and susceptibility to social influence. In E. Borgatta and W. Lambert, eds., *Handbook of personality theory and research.* Chicago: Rand McNally. Pp. 1130–1187.

Maslow, A. H. 1970. *Motivation and personality.* New York: Harper & Row.

Milgram, S. 1970. The experience of living in cities. *Science* 167:1461–1468.

Osgood, C. E.; Suci, G. J.; and Tannenbaum, P. H. 1957. *The measurement of meaning.* Urbana: University of Illinois Press.

Osgood, C. E. and Tannenbaum, P. H. 1955. The principle of congruity in the prediction of attitude change. *Psychological Review* 62:42–55.

Pareek, Udai, 1968. Motivational patterns and planned social change. *International Social Sciences Journal* 20:464–473.

Pettigrew, T. F. 1967. Social evaluation theory: convergences and applications. In D. Levine, ed., *Nebraska symposium on motivation.* Lincoln: University of Nebraska Press. Pp. 241–311.

Rainwater, L. 1960. *And the poor get children.* Chicago: Quadrangle Books.

———. 1965. *Family design: marital sexuality, family size, and contraception.* Chicago: Aldine.

Rapoport, A. 1970. *N-person game theory.* Ann Arbor: University of Michigan Press.

Rokeach, M. 1968. A theory of organization and change within value-attitude systems. *Journal of Social Issues* 24:13–33.

Rosenberg, M. J. 1956. Cognitive structure and attitudinal affect. *Journal of Abnormal and Social Psychology* 53:367–372.

———. 1960. A structural theory of attitude dynamics. *Public Opinion Quarterly* 24: 319–340.

Sanford, N. 1970. The activist's corner. *Journal of Social Issues* 26:155–161.

Sarbin, T. R. and Allen, V. L. 1968. Role theory. In G. Lindzey and E. Aronson, eds., *The handbook of social psychology.* Reading, Mass.: Addison-Wesley. 1:488–567.

Sommer, R. 1969. *Personal space: the behavioral basis of design.* Englewood Cliffs, N.J.: Prentice-Hall.

Stokols, D. 1970. The relationship between behavioral science and urban design: human crowding—a case in point. Unpublished manuscript, University of North Carolina.

Strodtbeck, F. L. 1951. Husband-wife interaction over revealed differences. *American Sociological Review* 16:468–473.

Thibaut, J. W. and Kelley, H. H. 1959. *The social psychology of groups.* New York: Wiley.

Thompson, V. D. 1970. Does family size make a difference? Unpublished manuscript, University of North Carolina.

Thompson, W. R. 1960. Early environmental influences on behavioral development. *American Journal of Orthopsychiatry* 30:306–314.

Waldrop, M. F. and Bell, R. Q. 1964. Relation of preschool dependency behavior to family size and density. *Child Development* 35:1187–1195.

————. 1966. Effects of family size and density on newborn characteristics. *American Journal of Orthopsychiatry* 36:544–550.

Wohwill, J. F. 1966. The physical environment: a problem for a psychology of stimulation. *Journal of Social Issues* 22:29–38.

Wyatt, F. 1967. Clinical notes on the motives of reproduction. *Journal of Social Issues* 23:29–56.

Wynne-Edwards, V. C. 1962. *Animal dispersion in relation to social behavior.* London: Oliver and Boyd.

Zimbardo, P. and Ebbesen, E. B. 1969. *Influencing attitudes and changing behavior.* Reading, Mass.: Addison-Wesley.

ACKNOWLEDGMENTS

The author wishes to express his gratitude for permission to reprint the following.

BACK, K. W., and HESS, P. H. From Ellis, A. 1970. "Group marriage: A possible alternative?" in H. A. Otto (ed.): *The family in search of a future: Alternative models for moderns.* Pp. 91, 92. Copyright © 1970 by Meredith Corporation. By permission of Appleton-Century-Crofts.

BACK, K. W. and HESS, P. H. From Pohlman, E. W. 1969. *The psychology of birth planning.* Cambridge: Schenkman Publishing Co., Inc. Pp. 98, 349.

BACK, K. W. and HESS, P. H. From Rainwater, L. 1965. *Family design: Marital sexuality, family size and contraception.* Chicago: Aldine Publishing Company. P. 232.

CLAUSEN, J. A. and CLAUSEN, S. R. From pp. 3–6, *Inside, looking out* by Harding Lemay. Copyright © 1971 by Harding Lemay. Originally appeared in *The New Yorker.* Reprinted by permission of Harper & Row, Publishers, Inc.

DAVID, H. P. From Callahan, D. 1970. *Abortion: Law, choice and morality.* New York: The Macmillan Company. P. 48. Copyright © 1970 by David Callahan.

DAVID, H. P. From Pohlman, E. W. 1969. *The psychology of birth planning.* Cambridge: Schenkman Publishing Co., Inc. P. 282.

DAVID, H. P. From Simon, N. 1970. Psychological and emotional indications for therapeutic abortion. *Seminars in Psychiatry,* 2:283–301. Reprinted by permission of the author and the publisher. This article was subsequently published in a 1971 Grune & Stratton publication: *Abortion: Changing views and practice.* P. 89.

DAVID, H. P. From Simon, N. and Senturia, A. G. 1966. Psychiatric sequelae of abortion. *Archives of general psychiatry,* 15:378–389. Copyright 1966, American Medical Association.

DAVID, H. P. From Tietze, C. 1970. Abortion on request: The consequences for population trends and public health. *Seminars in psychiatry,* 2:375–381. Reprinted by permission of the author and the publisher. This article was subsequently published in a 1971 Grune & Stratton publication: *Abortion: Changing views and practice.* P. 170.

FAWCETT, J. and BORNSTEIN, M. From Kahl, J. A. 1968. *The measurement of modernism: A study of values in Brazil and Mexico.* Austin: The University of Texas Press. P. 133.

FAWCETT, J. and BORNSTEIN, M. From Smith, P. H. and Inkeles, A. 1966. The OM scale: A comparative socio-psychological measure of individual modernity. *Sociometry,* 21:353–377. Washington: The American Sociological Association. Reprinted by permission of the author and the publisher.

FAWCETT, J. and BORNSTEIN, M. From Useem, J. and Useem, R. H. 1968. American-educated Indians in America: A comparison of two modernizing roles. *Journal of social issues,* 24: No. 4, 143–158. Ann Arbor: Society for the Psychological Study of Social Issues. Reprinted by permission of the author and the publisher.

GOUGH, H. From Ziegler, Rogers, Kriegsman, and Martin. 1968. Ovulation supressors, psychological functioning and marital adjustment. *Journal of the American medical association,* **204**:849–853. Copyright 1968, American Medical Association.

HOFFMAN, L. W. and HOFFMAN, M. L. From Hess, E. H. 1970. "Ethology and developmental psychology" in Mussen (ed.): *Carmichael's manual of child psychology.* New York: John Wiley & Sons, Inc., Publishers. P. 20. Copyright © 1946, 1954, and 1970 E. H. Hess. By permission of John Wiley & Sons, Inc.

HOFFMAN, L. W. and HOFFMAN, M. L. From Rainwater, L. 1960. *And the poor get children.* Chicago: Quadrangle Books, Inc. P. 87.

ROSEN, B. C. and SIMMONS, A. B. 1971. Industrialization, family and fertility: A structural-psychological analysis of the Brazilian case. *Demography,* **8**: 49–68.

SMITH, M. B. From Hardin, G. 1968. The tragedy of the commons. *Science,* **162**:1243–1248, 13 December 1968. Copyright 1968 by the American Association for the Advancement of Science. Reprinted by permission of the author and the publisher.

ZIMBARDO, P. and EBBESON, E. B. From Zimbardo-Ebbeson. 1969. *Influencing attitudes and changing behavior.* Addison-Wesley, Reading, Mass. Pp. 20–23.

INDEX